Spinal Cord Injury: An Issue of the Neurological Clinics

Spinal Cord Injury: An Issue of the Neurological Clinics

Edited by Carson Diaz

hayle medical
New York

Hayle Medical,
750 Third Avenue, 9th Floor,
New York, NY 10017, USA

Visit us on the World Wide Web at:
www.haylemedical.com

ISBN: 978-1-63241-684-1

Cataloging-in-Publication Data

Spinal cord injury : an issue of the neurological clinics / edited by Carson Diaz.
p. cm.
Includes bibliographical references and index.
ISBN 978-1-63241-684-1
1. Spinal cord--Wounds and injuries. 2. Spinal cord--Wounds and injuries--Treatment.
3. Nervous system--Diseases--Hospitals. I. Diaz, Carson.

RD594.3 .S75 2019
617.482 044--dc23

Table of Contents

Preface

This book has been an outcome of determined endeavour from a group of educationists in the field. The primary objective was to involve a broad spectrum of professionals from diverse cultural background involved in the field for developing new researches. The book not only targets students but also scholars pursuing higher research for further enhancement of the theoretical and practical applications of the subject.

A spinal cord injury refers to a damage to the spinal cord, which inhibits its function in a temporary or permanent capacity. Some of the symptoms may be loss of muscle sensation, function or autonomic function. Depending on the degree of the loss of muscle function and sensation, spinal injuries can be complete or incomplete. There can be full recovery from the injury or permanent tetraplegia may happen. Complications such as pressure sores, muscle atrophy, breathing problems and infections may also occur. The treatment of such an injury starts by restricting further motion of the spinal cord and maintaining adequate blood pressure. In cases where it interferes with daily activities, spinal injuries require occupational therapy and long-term physical therapy. This book explores all the important aspects of spinal cord injury in the present day scenario. It provides significant information of this discipline to help develop a good understanding of the treatment and management of spinal cord injury. It will help the readers in keeping pace with the rapid changes in this field.

It was an honour to edit such a profound book and also a challenging task to compile and examine all the relevant data for accuracy and originality. I wish to acknowledge the efforts of the contributors for submitting such brilliant and diverse chapters in the field and for endlessly working for the completion of the book. Last, but not the least; I thank my family for being a constant source of support in all my research endeavours.

Editor

1

Human Mesenchymal Cells from Adipose Tissue Deposit Laminin and Promote Regeneration of Injured Spinal Cord in Rats

Karla Menezes[1], Marcos Assis Nascimento[2], Juliana Pena Gonçalves[2], Aline Silva Cruz[1], Daiana Vieira Lopes[1], Bianca Curzio[3], Martin Bonamino[3], João Ricardo Lacerda de Menezes[1], Radovan Borojevic[4], Maria Isabel Doria Rossi[1], Tatiana Coelho-Sampaio[1]*

1 Institute of Biomedical Sciences, Federal University of Rio de Janeiro, Rio de Janeiro, Rio de Janeiro, Brazil, **2** Institute of Biophysics Carlos Chagas Filho, Federal University of Rio de Janeiro, Rio de Janeiro, Rio de Janeiro, Brazil, **3** National Institute of Cancer, Rio de Janeiro, Rio de Janeiro, Brazil, **4** Excellion, Petrópolis, Rio de Janeiro, Brazil

Abstract

Cell therapy is a promising strategy to pursue the unmet need for treatment of spinal cord injury (SCI). Although several studies have shown that adult mesenchymal cells contribute to improve the outcomes of SCI, a descripton of the pro-regenerative events triggered by these cells is still lacking. Here we investigated the regenerative properties of human adipose tissue derived stromal cells (hADSCs) in a rat model of spinal cord compression. Cells were delivered directly into the spinal parenchyma immediately after injury. Human ADSCs promoted functional recovery, tissue preservation, and axonal regeneration. Analysis of the cord tissue showed an abundant deposition of laminin of human origin at the lesion site and spinal midline; the appearance of cell clusters composed of neural precursors in the areas of laminin deposition, and the appearance of blood vessels with separated basement membranes along the spinal axis. These effects were also observed after injection of hADSCs into non-injured spinal cord. Considering that laminin is a well-known inducer of axonal growth, as well a component of the extracellular matrix associated to neural progenitors, we propose that it can be the paracrine factor mediating the pro-regenerative effects of hADSCs in spinal cord injury.

Editor: Eva Mezey, National Institutes of Health, United States of America

Funding: This work was supported by grants from the Conselho Nacional de Desenvolvimento Científico e Tecnológico (CNPq) and Fundação Carlos Chagas Filho de Apoio à Pesquisa do Estado do Rio de Janeiro (FAPERJ). KM and JPG are recipients of fellowships from CNPq, and MAN and DVL received fellowships from Coordenação de Aperfeiçoamento de Pessoal de Ensino Superior (CAPES) and FAPERJ, respectively. ASC received an undergraduate fellowship from CNPq. The funders had no role in study design, data collection and analysis, decision to publish, or preparation of the manuscript.

Competing Interests: Radovan Borojevic is an employee of the company Excellion.

* E-mail: tcsampaio@histo.ufrj.br

Introduction

Traumatic brain and spinal cord injuries affect individuals of all ages, causing various degrees of disability [1,2]. Despite intensive research over the last decade aiming to develop new cell-based therapies to treat trauma in the Central Nervous System (CNS), there is no consensus about the most appropriate cell types to reach this goal [3,4]. Embryonic stem cells previously differentiated into neural precursors, motor neurons, or pre-oligodendrocytes have been used in animal studies [5–8] and more recently, in a clinical study [9]. Adult stem/progenitor cells have also been used in both animal research and clinical studies. The primary source of progenitor cells is the bone marrow, where at least the hematopoietic stem cell and a population of mesenchymal stromal/stem cells co-exist (MSC) [10]. Both cell types have been used to treat experimental spinal cord injury (SCI) in animals, as well as injured human patients [11]. Given the potential of MSC to differentiate into several adult cell types, including neurons [12], these cells have attracted great interest.

In the last years, a growing number of studies have reported the effects of MSCs in promoting functional improvement, tissue sparing, and axonal growth after spine cord injury [13–23]. More recently, a new type of MSC isolated from adipose tissue has been investigated. Adipose tissue constitutes a more readily available deposit of adult progenitors due to its greater abundance of MSC-like cells, if compared to bone marrow, and because liposuction is a minimally invasive procedure. Known as adipose-derived stromal cells (ADSCs), these cells are isolated by selective adhesion and correspond to the perivascular stromal fraction of the adipose tissue [10,24,25]. ADSCs have recently been used to treat SCI in rats and dogs [26–28]. In particular, a recent study compared the effectiveness of hADSCs with that of human bone marrow stromal cells in a model of section injury in immunossupressed rats and reported the superior regenerative effect of hADSCs [29].

In the present study we investigated the regenerative potential of hADSCs in a model of ballon-induced spinal compression using immunocompetent rats. We show that hADSCs promote complete recovery of motor function after 8 weeks, while improving tissue preservation, restricting inflammation and stimulating axonal growth. In addition we propose that the regenerative effects of hADSCs are related to the secretion of the extracellular matrix protein laminin that accumulates in the spinal cord in colocalization with neural precursors.

Results

hADSC Promotes Functional and Morphological Recovery after Compressive SCI

In order to evaluate if human subcutaneous ADSCs (hADSCs) would improve the functional outcome after compressive SCI, we compared the open field locomotion (BBB scores) of animals receiving cells or culture medium (DMEM). Rats were subjected to moderate balloon compression and treated with either hADSCs or DMEM, delivered by intraspinal injection 30 minutes after injury. The BBB score for the DMEM group was 7.2 one week post injury/injection (wpi) and it increased to 15.6 after eight weeks (Fig. 1A). On the other hand, animals treated with hADSCs exhibited superior scores from the first evaluation, whereas such superiority became statistically significant from the fifth week on. From the fourth week on the BBB scores for the treated group were indistinguishable from those found for the sham operated group (Fig. 1A), indicating that hADSCs promoted complete functional recovery after a moderate compressive injury.

Mesenchymal stromal/stem cells are known to have immunosuppressive properties [30,31], enabling the use of human cells in immunocompetent animals as done in this study. We evaluated the distribution of the rat macrophages/microglia marker, ED1 in the spinal cord one week after compression. In the control animals, macrophages/microglia were profusely distributed in both white and gray matter (Fig. 1B). In animals receiving hADSC, macrophages were concentrated in lesion borders (Fig. 1C), suggesting that the injection of hADSC restrained the spread of inflammatory cells in the spinal cord parenchyma.

The compression injury led to the formation of cystic cavities in the spinal cord. Eight weeks after injury, control animals showed a large cavity surrounded by activated astrocytes (Fig. 1D, G). Animals receiving hADSC displayed smaller cavities and a reduction of GFAP expression of approximately 50% (Fig. 1E, H, I). Quantitative analysis of the cavity area was performed in a region encompassing 400 μm of the spinal cord tissue along the dorsal–ventral axis (Fig. 1F). Treatment with hADSCs reduced the cavity area by more than 90% at the lesion epicenter, whereas tissue sparing was seen at all levels analyzed (Fig. 1F). These results demonstrate that hADSC injection results in improved preservation of the nervous tissue after SCI.

hADSC Promotes Regeneration of Axonal Fibers

The presence of descending serotonergic fibers was evaluated in animals one and eight weeks after injury. One week after injury, hADSC-treated rats presented a large number of serotonergic fibers crossing the spared tissue in the lateral funiculus region surrounding the injury site (Fig. 2B). These fibers, which were less abundant in control animals, were apparently thicker than individual axons (Fig. 2A). Their superficial location corresponds to the region of descending serotonergic raphe fibers, indicating that they result from axonal regrowth after injury. In addition, seven days after injury we found several fibers displaying bulging tips, which are indicative of the occurrence of axonal regeneration (Fig. 2B, insert). Rostral to the lesion site the total lengths of serotonergic axons were similar in treated and non-treated rats (Fig. 2C). However, at the level of the epicenter (lateral to it) and caudal to the lesion, the total lengths of serotonergic axons were consistently higher after treatment with hADSC. Eight weeks after injury the fiber lengths decreased in comparison to those found one week after injury (Fig. 2D, E). Nevertheless, the total length of serotonergic fibers in the spinal cord was 8 times higher in the group treated with hADSCs (Fig. 2F). These results indicate that the regeneration of serotonergic axons promoted by hADSCs remains for a considerable time.

Axonal regeneration was further evaluated by using either the Tuj1 antibody, which stains young neurons more intensely [32], or anti-GAP-43, which labels neurons in regeneration [33]. Data are presented in series of three pictures taken from the spare tissue lateral to the lesion area. As shown in Figure 2G–R, the treatment with hADSCs substantially increased axonal regeneration. At both 1 and 8 weeks Tuj1-positive fibers in hADSC-treated animals ran straight and were aligned parallel to each other (Fig. 2J and high magnification in K). On the other hand, in control animals these fibers were tangled and randomly aligned (Fig. 2G and high magnification in H). The thicker bundles and aligned fibers observed in hADSC-treated animals are indicative of axonal fasciculation, which did not occur in control animals (Fig. 2, high magnifications in H and K). Tuj1 labeling presented a very faint and even distribution in normal unlesioned animals as this monoclonal antibody identifies preferentially young neurons [32]. Quantification of Tuj1 labeled fibers after one or eight weeks showed that treatment with hADSC led to an increase in the total length of young fibers of 3 or 3.5 times, respectively. Panels M to Q in Figure 2 show the results obtained by using the anti-GAP-43 antibody. One week after injury the total length of regenerating fibers increased 3-fold in the hADSC group relative to the control (Fig. 2M, P, O). Eight weeks after SCI, a large number of GAP-43 positive fibers was observed in rats treated with hADSCs, while control animals showed little staining (Fig. 2N, Q, R). No labeling was detected when anti-GAP43 was used in sections of normal unlesioned rats.

hADSCs Induce Foci of Increased Cellularity in Spinal Cord

We next sought to investigate the mechanisms by which hADSCs exert regenerative effects in the spinal cord. GFP-transduced hADSCs were injected 30 minutes after compression and animals were euthanized at different times. One day after injection, cells were densely packed and accumulated mainly in the meningeal surface, the central canal, and at the lesion site (Fig. 3A). One week later, the injected cells were detected at the region of the canal and at the injury site (Fig. 3B–D). In the fourth week, only a few isolated clusters of cells were identified near the lesion (Fig. 3E), while cells were not detected at the eighth week after injection.

A remarkable feature of hADSC-treated animals was the increase in tissue cellularity detected in DAPI-stained sections one week after cell injection. One large cluster of cells was found at the lesion site and smaller clusters were distributed along the spinal midline (Fig. 3G). Such clusters were not observed in normal unlesioned rats (Fig. 3F). In transversal sections it was possible to localize the clusters at the midline in the vicinity of the central canal (Fig. 3I–K). GFP-hADSCs were found in the center of these areas of high cellularity (Fig. 3K, L). Analysis of the section containing the central canal revealed that the vimentin-positive ependymal cell layer was enlarged in animals treated with hADSCs (compare Fig. 3M and N). Reconstruction of the central canal in the z axis showed regions with more than 10 stacked cells, indicative of a partial reconfiguration of the canal's architecture (Fig. 3P). We additionally observed an increased number of DAPI-stained nuclei throughout the spinal parenchyma, in the region between the central canal and the individual clusters (Fig. 3N, asterisk) and blood vessels in the vicinity of the reconfigured canal (Fig. S1).

Cell clusters did not correspond to inflammatory infiltrates given that most of them were not positive for the macrophage/microglia marker, CD68 (Fig. 3Q), and neither for the T

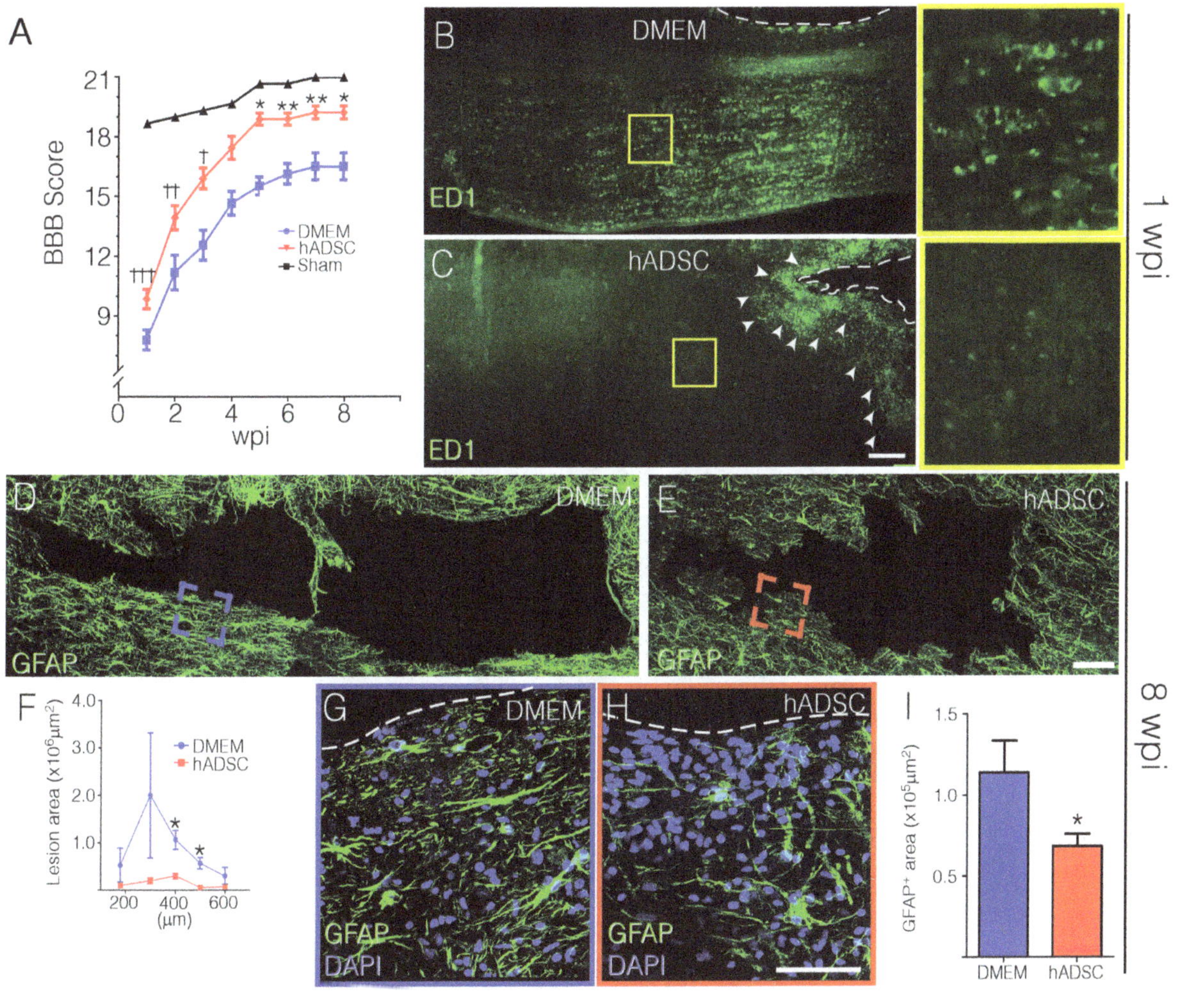

Figure 1. hADSCs induce functional recovery and reduce cavitation and cellular inflammatory response. The locomotor performance was assessed by the BBB score. Animals were evaluated weekly, during eight weeks after spinal compression (A). Asterisks indicate statistic differences between hADSC (n = 9) and DMEM groups (n = 9) and crosses indicate differences between hADSC and sham groups (n = 3). B,C) Low-magnification photomontages showing the marked difference in distribution of macrophages in the spinal cord of rats treated with hADSC (C) and DMEM (B). Note that ED1-positive cells concentrate in the immediate surroundings of the lesion cavity in hADSC-treated animals (arrowheads), in contrast to the dispersed distribution in DMEM-treated animals. D, E) GFAP immunoreactivity delineates the cavity and reveals astrocyte activation following injury, in vehicle (DMEM) (D) and hADSC (E) treated animals. F) Graph representing the area of the lesion cavity of 5 different dorso–ventral sections (represented in the x axis) in DMEM (blue) and hADSC (red) treated animals (n = 3 per condition). Note that cavitation in hADSC-treated animals is smaller. G,H) High magnification images of the boxed areas in *D* (blue) and *E* (red) are shown in *G* and H, respectively. Note the few GFAP-positive cells at the vicinity of the lesion and that very few cells are seen at the cavity border in hADSC-treated rat (H). I) Graph representing the total area of positive staining for GFAP (see *Materials and Methods*) in the immediate surroundings of the cavity in DMEM (blue) and hADSC (red) treated animals (n = 3 per condition). Dashed line delineates the cavity borders in G and H. *$P<0.05$, **$P<0.01$, ***: $p<0.001$. Bars: B and C = 500 µm, D and E = 100 µm and G and H = 50 µm.

lymphocyte marker, CD3 (Fig. 3R, S). Scattered macrophages were detected in the vicinity of the clusters, as well as T lymphocytes, which tended to form small aggregates surrounding the core of the DAPI-stained clusters. In contrast, DiI-labeled human fibroblasts injected into the intact rat spinal cord attracted large amounts of macrophage/microglial cells (Fig. 3T).

Since the increase in tissue cellularity was not related to injury-induced inflammation, we next investigated whether it would also occur upon injection of the cells into the undamaged spinal cord. We therefore included a third experimental group in which GFP-hADSCs were delivered directly into the spinal cord of normal rats and their distribution was analyzed one week after injection. Cells presented a clear tropism for the spinal midline, where they remained distributed along the central axis of the spinal cord (Fig. 3U'). It was noteworthy that more GFP positive cells were present in uninjured than in the injured spinal cord. Surprisingly we observed a large increase in tissue cellularity, which was more pronounced than that observed when hADSCs were injected after injury (Fig. 3U). Cells within the infiltrate in uninjured spinal cord did not stain for the CD68, which indicate that they were not inflammatory cells (Fig. S2).

hADSCs Led to the Appearance of Perivascular Spaces in between Endothelial and Astrocytic Basement Membranes

Another remarkable feature observed in animals treated with hADSCs was the presence, in the vicinity of the spinal axis, of blood vessels exhibiting two clearly definable separated basal

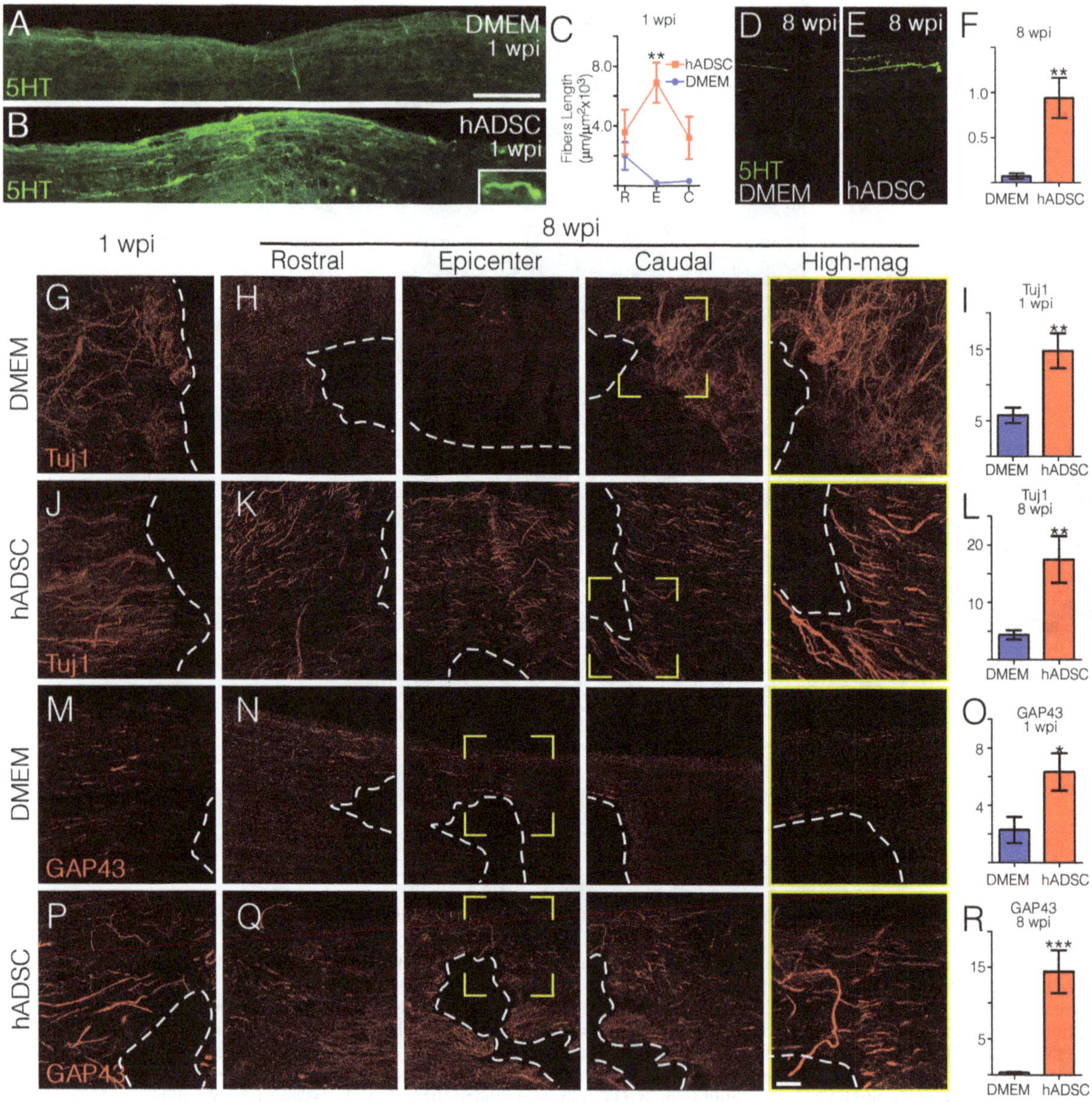

Figure 2. hADSCs promote axonal regeneration. A–D) Photomontages showing the expression pattern of 5HT-positive serotonergic fibers in horizontal sections spanning the pre- and post-lesion regions in DMEM (A) and hADSC (B) treated animals one week after compression. The inset shows an example of a hogback termination in the post-lesion area. Note that the hADSC-treated cord exhibits a larger number of serotoninergic fibers crossing the injury site. C) Graph representing the total length of 5-HT fibers in each experimental group (n = 3 in each group). D–E) 5HT expression was greatly reduced in the chronic phase (8 wks) in DMEM-treated rats (D), while it was slightly reduced in hADSC (E) treated group. F) Quantification of the total length of 5-HT positive axons, eight weeks after SCI (n = 3 in each group). G–R) Progression of axonal regeneration was followed by Tuj1 (G–L) or anti-GAP-43 (M–R) immunoreactivity. Panels on the left show Tuj1 (G, J) or GAP-43 (M, P) positive fibers one week after compression at the epicenter of the lesion. Panels H, K, N, Q and rows on the right show respective rostral (left), epicenter (center), and caudal (right) regions of the same section eight weeks after SCI. Far column on the right (yellow frame) shows boxed areas in higher magnification. The dashed line indicates the border of the lesion cavity. Graphics show the quantification of the total lengths of Tuj1 (I, L) or GAP-43 (O, R) positive fibers one week (I, O) and eight weeks (L, R) after SCI in the peri-cavity region (n = 3 in each group). Tuj1 and GAP-43 positive axons in DMEM (blue) and hADSC (red) treated groups were quantified in an area of approximately 900 μm in extension along the longitudinal axis. Both white and grey matter was analyzed. The y-axes in panels F, I, L, O and R were omitted for aesthetic purpose and they represent fiber length per area ($\mu m/\mu m^2 \times 10^3$). The values in C, F, I, L, O, R represent means ± standard errors. *$P<0.05$, **$P<0.01$, ***$P<0.001$. Bars: A, B = 500 μm, D–Q = 100 μm, high magnification = 50 μm.

lamina, which were identified by immunostaining with an anti-pan-laminin antibody (Fig. 4C, D, Movie S1). The internal lamina corresponds to the basement membrane contributed by the endothelial cells, here identified by immunostaining with the rat endothelial marker, RECA1 (Fig. 4E). The external lamina, which is part of the blood brain barrier in the CNS, is produced by the astrocytes and normally remains connected to the internal one. The separation of these two membranes suggests an increased traffic of cells in the perivascular compartment along blood vessels. A series of confocal images of a blood vessel suggests that cells accumulating in between the two laminas can be released at the spinal parenchyma upon disruption of the outer membrane (Fig. 4F). Separation of two basement membranes around blood

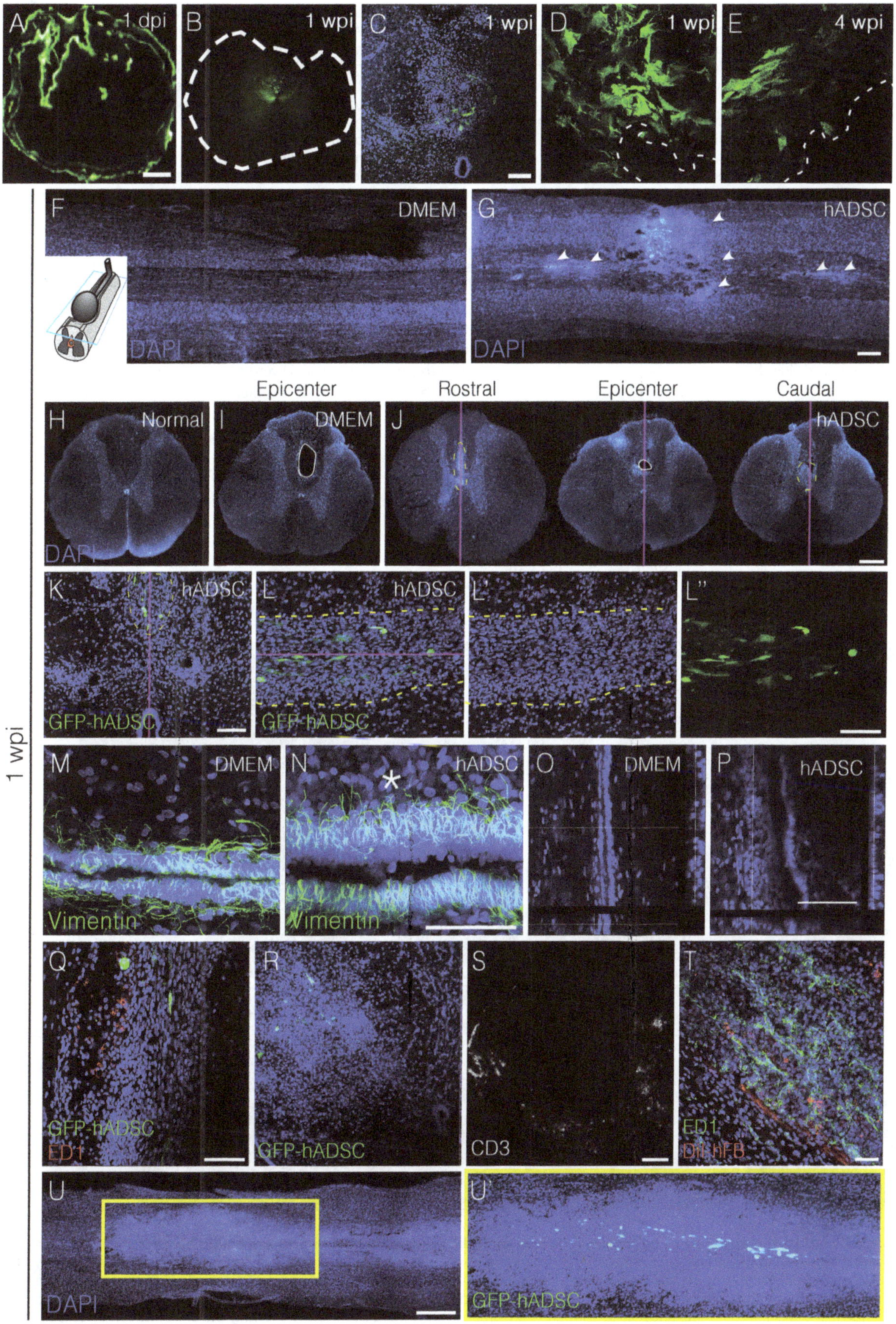
A
1 dpi
B
1 wpi
C
1 wpi
D
1 wpi
E
4 wpi
F
DMEM
DAPI
G
hADSC
DAPI
Epicenter
Rostral
Epicenter
Caudal
H
Normal
I
DMEM
J
hADSC
DAPI
K
hADSC
GFP-hADSC
L
hADSC
GFP-hADSC
L'
L''
M
DMEM
Vimentin
N
hADSC
Vimentin
O
DMEM
P
hADSC
Q
GFP-hADSC
ED1
R
GFP-hADSC
S
CD3
T
ED1
Dil hFB
U
DAPI
U'
GFP-hADSC
1 wpi

Figure 3. hADSCs increased cellularity in three distinct, but contiguous compartments (the central canal, midline parenchyma, and perivascular region). A–E) Time-course distribution and cell morphology after injection of hADSCs. A) Transverse section of the spinal cord one day after lesion and injection of GFP-transduced hADSCs, showing that these cells accumulate in the pial surface, central canal, and peri-lesional area. After one week (1 wpi), hADSCs were detected predominantly in the canal area and peri-lesionally (B, C). D, E) High magnification images of the GFP-positive cells clusters at one (D) and four wpi (E). F, G) DAPI-stained horizontal sections 200–250 μm above the central canal showing an increase in cellularity (G) mainly along the midline in hADSC-treated cord (arrowheads). H–J) DAPI-stained transversal sections of spinal cord from a normal rat (H), DMEM (I) and hADSCs–treated animals (J), 1 wpi. Sequential analysis of histological sections from treated animals (J) showed that initially there is an increased cellularity along the midline, crossing the region of the central canal of the spinal cord. In the following sections this cell cluster is observed at the margin of the lesion and persisted there until the end of the lesion. K–L'') Confocal images of transversal (K) and horizontal (L, L', L'') sections of spinal cord of hADSC-treated animal at 1 wpi. Note that the increased cellularity occurs in the region around the GFP-positive cells. M–P) Confocal images of horizontal sections of spinal cord immunostained with anti-vimentin in the central canal at 1 wpi. Note the increased thickness of the ependymal lining of the central canal, and the high cell density in hADSC-treated animal above the canal (asterisk). O, P) Orthogonal views of DAPI-stained section of the central canal. Q–S) Images showing infiltration of macrophages (ED1, panel Q) or T lymphocyte (CD3+ cells, panels R and S). T) Human fibroblasts (stained with CM-DiI, hFB) 1 week post injection into an intact spinal cord. Note the abundance of ED1-positive cells in hFB-treated rat. Confocal images of the cells cluster one week after injection of the hADSC-GFP positive cells into an uninjured spinal cord. The purple line represents the midline of the spinal cord. Bars: A, E, F, H–J = 500 μm; B–D, T = 50 μm; G = 25 μm, K. L, Q, R, S = 100 μm, U = 1 mm.

vessels was also observed when hADSCs were injected into the undamaged spinal cord (Fig. S2).

Cells within the Infiltrates Express Markers of Neural Precursors

In order to indentify the nature of the cells accumulating in the spinal cord of rats treated with hADSC after SCI we used antibodies against pericytes and/or neural cells. Cell within the infiltrates were positive for smooth muscle α-actin (αSMA), a marker for pericytes; Tuj1 and Olig2, markers for neural precursors; and for nestin, vimentin, and NG2, markers for both neural cells and pericytes (Fig. 5,A–F). Cells accumulating in between the two separated vascular basement membranes were negative for Olig2 or Tuj1 and positive for nestin, vimentin, NG2, and αSMA (Fig. 5G–M). Proliferative cells, positive for Ki67 were detected at lesion-associated cell clusters, which correlated with high nestin expression (Fig. 5N–Q). A similar profile of markers expression as well of proliferation was observed after injecting hADSCs into the undamaged spinal cord (Fig. S2), which indicates that the injection of these cells leads to an increased number of neural precursors and/or pericytes in the spinal cord.

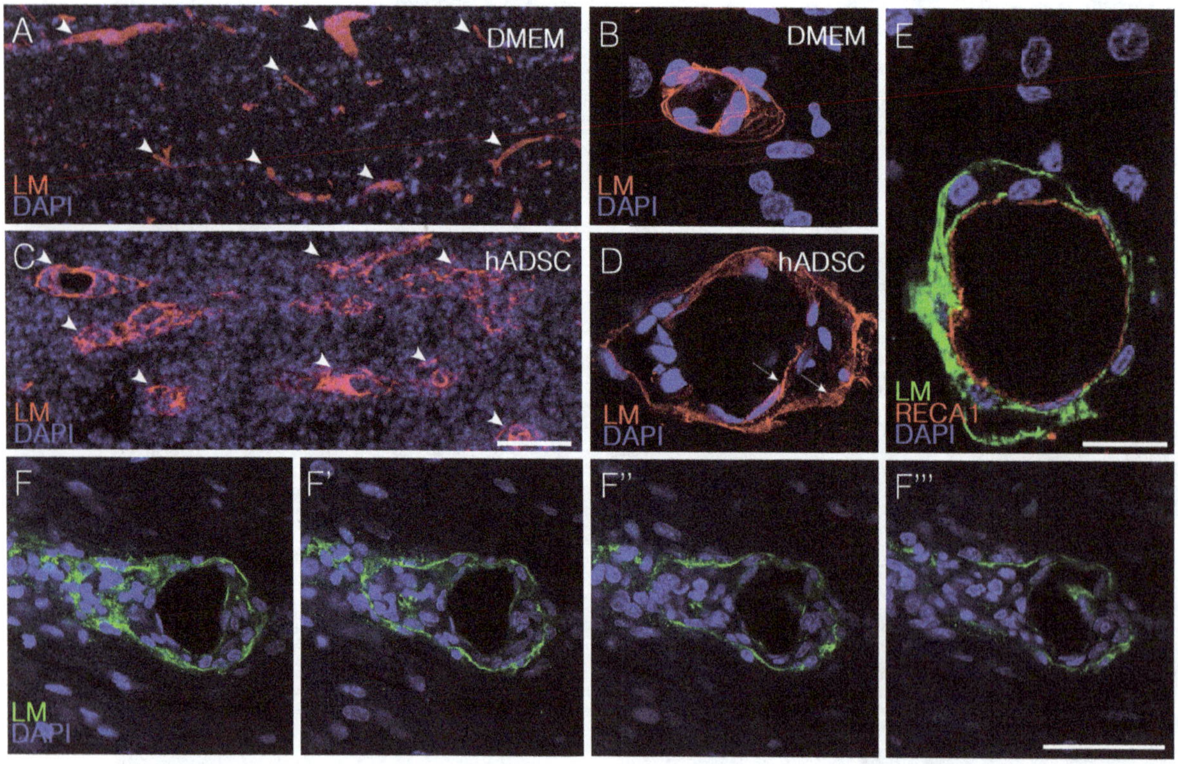

Figure 4. hADSCs led to the appearance of perivascular spaces in between endothelial and astrocytic basement membranes one week after injection. A–D) Confocal images of horizontal sections immunostained with anti-pan-laminin antibody (red) one week after injury. Note that in DMEM animals (A,B) there is no separation between the two membranes whereas in hADSCs-treated animals (C,D) these membranes are separated (arrows in D). E) Confocal images of a horizontal section immunostained with anti-pan-laminin (green) and RECA-1(red). F–F'') Confocal imagens of sequential optical sections immunostained with anti-pan-laminin (green) and DAPI (blue) showing the extravasation of cells from the blood vessels. Bars: C, F = 50 μm B, D, E = 25 μm.

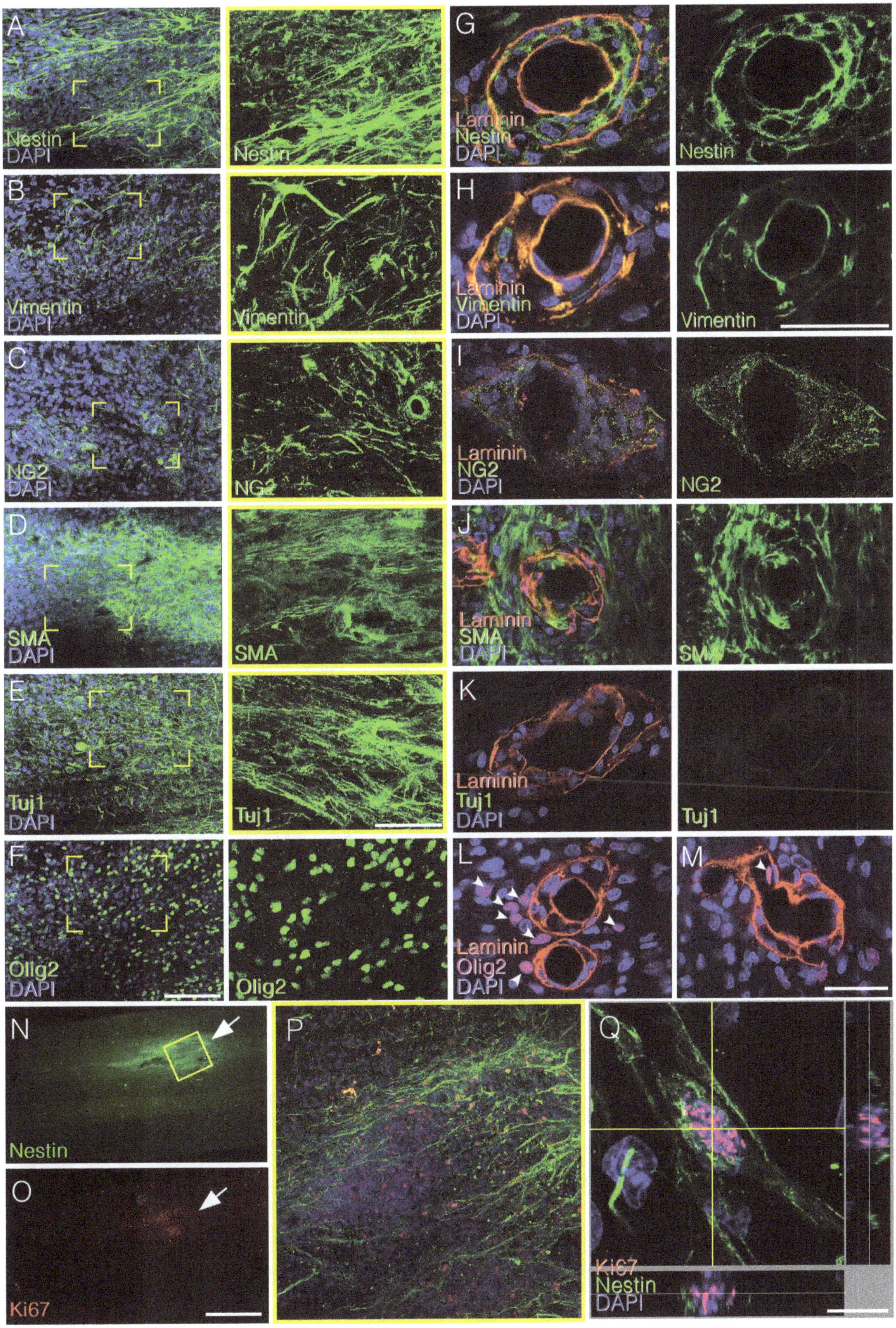
A
Nestin
DAPI
Nestin
G
Laminin
Nestin
DAPI
Nestin
B
Vimentin
DAPI
Vimentin
H
Laminin
Vimentin
DAPI
Vimentin
C
NG2
DAPI
NG2
I
Laminin
NG2
DAPI
NG2
D
SMA
DAPI
SMA
J
Laminin
SMA
DAPI
SMA
E
Tuj1
DAPI
Tuj1
K
Laminin
Tuj1
DAPI
Tuj1
F
Olig2
DAPI
Olig2
L
Laminin
Olig2
DAPI
M
N
Nestin
O
Ki67
P
Q
Ki67
Nestin
DAPI

Figure 5. Areas of increased cellularity induced by hADSC are mainly composed of neural precursors, but cell types differ in the vascular and parenchymal compartments. A–F) Confocal images of horizontal sections of the spinal cord showing immunostaining for nestin (A), vimentin (B), NG2 (C), smooth muscle α-actin (αSMA, D), Tuj1 (E), and Olig2 (F) in clusters of high cell density along the midline, one week after SCI. Note that cells in the clusters are positive for all of these markers, suggesting that clusters are mostly composed of neural progenitors and possibly of invading pericytes. Panels on the right correspond to high-magnification images of the boxed areas, showing the labeling for each phenotypic marker. G–M) Blood vessels immunostained with pan-laminin (red) and nestin (G), vimentin (H), NG2 (I), αSMA (J), Tuj1 (K) (green). Panels L and M show that most Olig2 positive cells (purple) are out of blood vessels (L). Panel M depicts one Olig2-labeled nucleus in close proximity with a region where the basal lamina seems to be disrupted (arrow). (N–Q) Correspondence between immunoreactivities for nestin (N) and Ki67 (O) in photomontages of horizontal sections of an injured spinal cord one week after injury/injection. Confocal images showing proliferative activity (anti-Ki67, red) in the spinal parenchyma (P) and a perivascular region (Q) of nestin positive cells. Bars: A–F = 100 μm; G–M = 50 μm; N, O = 1 mm, Q = 10 μm.

hADSCs Secrete Human Laminin in the Spinal Cord

A distinguished feature of niches of neural stem and neural precursors cells in the central nervous system is the presence of the protein laminin in their extracellular matrix [34–36]. We therefore investigated if hADSCs would produce laminin *in vivo*, which could be related to the accumulation of neural precursors in the tissue. Using monoclonal antibodies specific for laminin of human origin, we searched for a morphological correlation between areas of high cell density and the deposition of the protein. In a photomontage of a whole horizontal section it is possible to appreciate the high degree of co-localization between cell clusters and laminin deposits both in the injured (Fig. 6A–C) and in the uninjured spinal cord (Fig. 6D–E). Immunostainings for human fibronectin and human collagen IV showed that these two proteins were also present in the cell infiltrates but the deposits were less expressive than those of laminin (Fig. S3).

In order to support the interpretation that laminin associated to cell clusters was produced by hADSCs and not by the rat tissue it was important to confirm the specificity of the anti-human laminin antibodies. We used two different anti-human laminin antibodies to detect the protein. The first one was a mouse monoclonal raised against human laminin (clone LAM-89; Fig. 6E), which is commercially available and described as a reagent that does not cross-react with laminin of rat origin. This monoclonal recognizes the α5 chain and has been extensively used in the literature to label basement membranes in human tissue, particularly those associated to blood vessels [37,38]. We found no labeling of blood vessels in the rat spinal cord (Fig. 6, compare E' and E''). The second antibody was an anti-human α2 (clone 5H2; Fig. 6B–D). To assess the specificity of this antibody we performed immunostainings in rat skeletal muscle, a tissue in which laminin α2 is highly expressed. While a polyclonal anti-pan laminin stained the basement membranes around muscle fibers, monoclonal 5H2 did not recognize the rat muscle tissue (Fig. S4). These results indicate that the laminin matrix associated to the infiltrates of neural precursors was not produced by the rat host but, instead, by the injected human cells.

Results up to here indicate that hADSCs produce laminin α2 and α5 *in vivo*. We next used a panel of anti-human laminin antibodies to investigate which laminin chains appeared in the spinal parenchyma injected with hADSCs. Out of the six isoforms tested, we confirmed expression of α2 and α5 and also found positivity for β2 and γ1 laminin chains (Fig. 7A, C, E, F). The matrix associated to cell clusters was negative for α4 and β1 (Fig. 7B, D). In vitro, hADSCs we did not detect expression of α2, α4, α5 or β1 (Fig. 7G–I). We found positivity only for the β2 and the γ1 chains (Fig. 7K, L) and for anti-pan laminin (Fig. 7M).

Based on the recent observation that neurogenic niches in the adult CNS contain a novel type of laminin-rich basal lamina termed fractones [39], we next investigated whether the laminin secreted by hADSCs present the same morphology of fractones. Tissue sections of animals receiving hADSCs into the undamaged spinal cord were immunostained for pan-laminin one week after injection. The polyclonal pan-specific anti-laminin antibody stained all laminin-containing structures present in the tissue. Blood vessels were identified by their overall morphology and diameter above 5 μm (Fig. 8A and E, blue box). Fractones were identified by their organization in puncta with diameter between 1–4 μm and thin lines with 0.1–05 μm width and 5–50 μm length [40] (Fig. 8A and C, red box). In addition, we observed a reticular laminin matrix (Fig. 8A and D, yellow box) similar to the one of human origin secreted by hADSCs (Fig. 6C, E). While a clear increase in cellularity was observed along the whole spinal axis, the location of the most packed cells coincided with the reticular deposit (Fig. 8B, arrowheads). Panels C and D were reconstructed in the z axis to provide views of their 3D organization (Fig. 8F, G). Puncta present in fractones were spherical dense deposits, and the thin lines did not correspond to the side view of sheet-like matrices but instead, resembled essential lines (Fig, 8F). On the other hand, the reticular deposit presented a 3D structure in which each strut was connected to the neighboring one (Fig. 8G). Such reticular mesh is similar to the z-stack obtained using the anti-human α2 laminin antibody (Fig. 8H). DAPI counterstaining showed that cells appearing in the spinal parenchyma seemed trapped into the human laminin mesh secreted by hADSCs (Fig. 8H).

Discussion

In this study, we showed that treatment with cells isolated from human adipose tissue (hADSCs) improve open field locomotion after a compression injury in rats. We also found that hADSCs secreted human laminin, which accumulates in the spinal cord and increases the presence of neural precursors in the tissue.

The lesion area and the expression of the glial scar marker GFAP were both reduced after treatment with hADSCs, characteristics compatible with a resolutive inflammatory reaction. The treatment also resulted in increased numbers of regenerating fibers. A noteworthy finding was the many 5HT-positive descending axons, particularly at the injury epicenter, observed in hADSC rats as early as one week after lesion. Although the number of fibers decreased at the eighth week after lesion, it still remained much higher than that of non-treated animals. To our knowledge, no studies using cell therapy obtained such a marked improvement in axonal growth as the one promoted by hADSCs in our study.

In the present study, we delivered cells immediately after spinal cord injury. The advantage of this experimental design is that the therapy can contribute to reduce the secondary damage, which initiates within hours after trauma. On the other hand, the disadvantage of the early treatment is that the hemorrhagic and ischemic environment of SCI reduces the survival of the injected cells in the host tissue. Accordingly, the number of GFP-labeled cells progressively decreased between 1 and 7 days after injury and virtually disappeared 8 weeks later. In a previous study, Arboleda

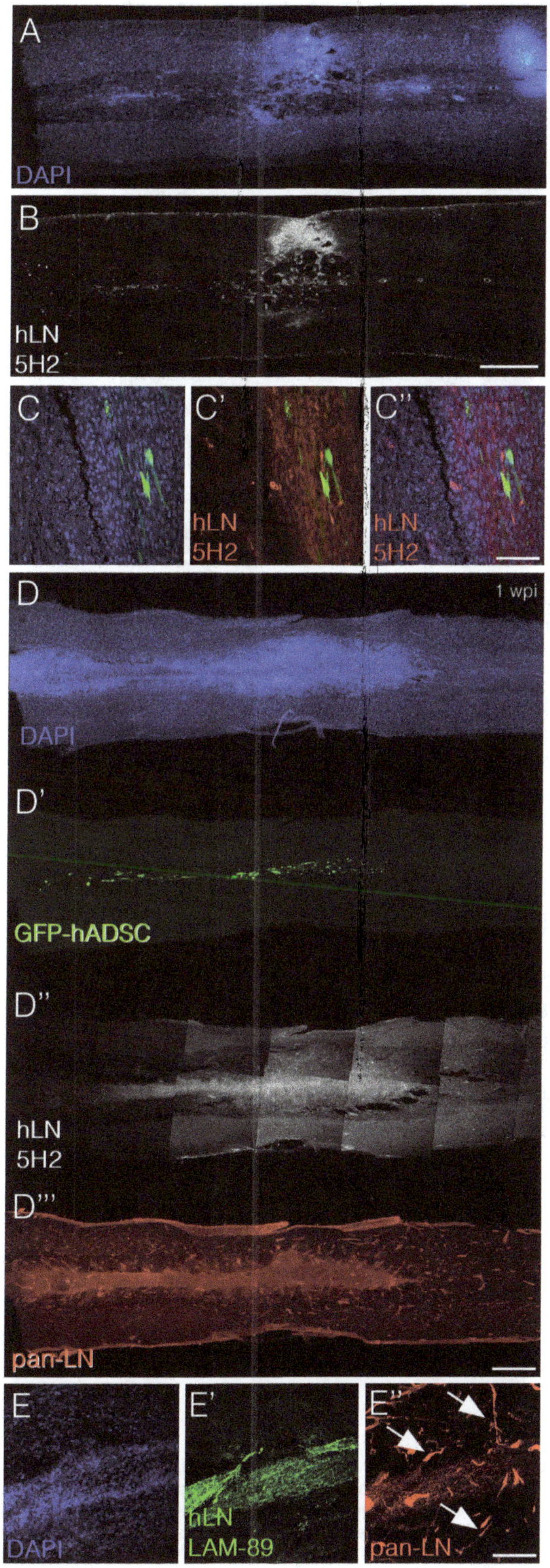

Figure 6. hADSCs secrete laminin in the spinal cord independently of SCI. A–C) Horizontal section of an animal subjected to spinal compression and injected with GFP-hADSCs one week after injury/injection. Panels A and B show photomontages depicting DAPI staining (A) and immunoreactivity for anti-human laminin (B). Note that cell infiltrates and laminin are located in corresponding regions. Panel C shows confocal images demonstrating the coincident localization of GFP-positive hADSCs (green), cell infiltrates (blue) and human laminin (red). D–E) Horizontal section of an uninjured animal one week after transplantation with GFP-hADSCs. Panels D to D''' show photomontages depicting DAPI staining (blue, D), GFP-positive hADSCs (D', green), immunoreactivity for anti-human laminin (D'', white) and immunoreactivity for anti-pan laminin (D''', red). Panel E shows confocal images to demonstrate that while the anti-pan laminin antibody labels rat blood vessels (E'', red), the anti-human laminin does not (E'). Bars: A, B, D = 1 mm, C = 100 μm, E = 200 μm.

and co-workers [26] injected rat ADSCs in immunosuppressed rats one week after injury and reported that living cells remained in the spinal cord during the eight weeks of the experiment. However, these cells did not integrate into the host tissue and their survival did not correlate with the extent of the functional improvements. More recently, Zhou and co-workers [29] reported results compatible with ours, showing that more than 30% of human ADSCs transplanted in immnosuppressed rats survived one week after injection, but that less than 1% remained in the spinal tissue three weeks later. These observations suggest that the regenerative effects of ADSCs were due to the induced secretion of paracrine factors that would stimulate endogenous precursors to regenerate the tissue. It has already been shown that co-culture with BMSCs can prime embryonic stem cells to produce pyramidal neurons able to integrate into the cerebral cortex and to project to the appropriate targets [41,42]. In addition, a recent study has demonstrated that factors produced by BMSCs can indeed prime neural precursors toward an oligodendrocyte fate [43]. Our results in combination with those of the literature suggest that it is not necessary that injected cells remain in the spinal cord during the regeneration process and that their beneficial priming effects are exerted within the first days after injury.

One important effect of hADSCs was the reduction of the spatial diffusion of macrophage/microglia, restraining these cells to the site of injury. To our knowledge, this is the first time that such an effect has been described as a corollary of cell therapy. It is possible that hADSCs accumulating in the lesion secrete cytokines that attract macrophages to the injury site. Indeed, in agreement with a previous study showing that ADSCs secrete 20 times more IL-6 than BMSCs *in vitro* [44], we observed that hADSCs secrete large amounts of IL-6 in the lesion area (MAN, KM, RB, TC-S, unpublished). Secretion of other cytokines such as IL-10, which is largely produced by hADSCs [45], may also play a role in regeneration, due to its ability to favor the differentiation of M2 macrophages. It has already been shown that BMSCs can shift macrophage differentiation towards the M2 pro-regenerative phenotype [46–48].

The present study describes three major novel observations that shed light on the mechanisms of neural tissue regeneration promoted by adult MSC cells. First, hADSCs induced an increase in cellularity at the lesion site and in clusters distributed along the spinal midline above the central canal. Cells in the clusters expressed markers of neural precursors. Likewise, in the non-injured spinal cord progenitor cells accumulated in a single large spindle-like cluster, indicating that the observed increase in cellularity does not depend on the occurrence of a lesion.

In animals receiving hADSCs, the vimentin-positive ependymal cell layer that lines the central canal [49] expanded, indicating that molecules secreted by hADSCs can increase the proliferation of neural precursors in the normal neurogenic area of the spinal cord.

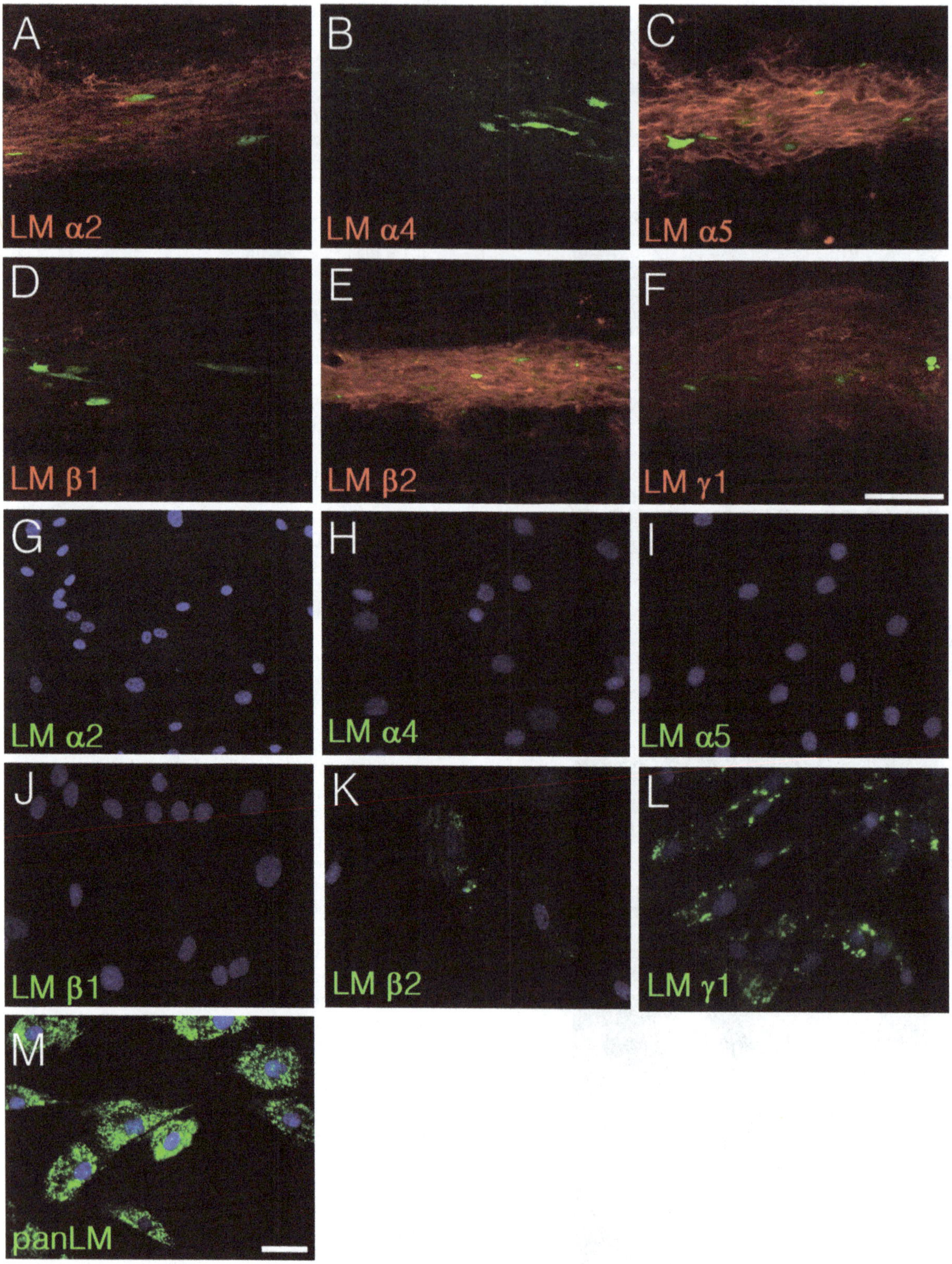

Figure 7. Identification of laminin chains produced by hADSCs *in vivo* and *in vitro*. A–F) Uninjured rats were injected with GFP-hADSCs and the human laminin chains produced in the spinal cord were analyzed one week after transplantation. Confocal images of horizontal sections taken at the spinal midline show that hADSCs are localized in areas rich in human laminin α2 (A), α5 (C), β2 (E) and γ1 (F). Immunoreactivity for human laminin α4 (B) and β1 (D) was not detected in the spinal cord (D). G–M) Analysis of the laminin chains produced by hADSCs cultivated *in vitro*. *In vitro*, the only laminin chains detected were β2 (K) and γ1 (L). Note that hADSCs did not produce α2 (G) nor α5 (I), which suggests that secretion of these two chains is triggered by the contact with the environment of the spinal cord. Panel M shows immunostaining for laminin using an anti-pan laminin antibody. Bars: A–F = 100 μm, G–M = 50 μm.

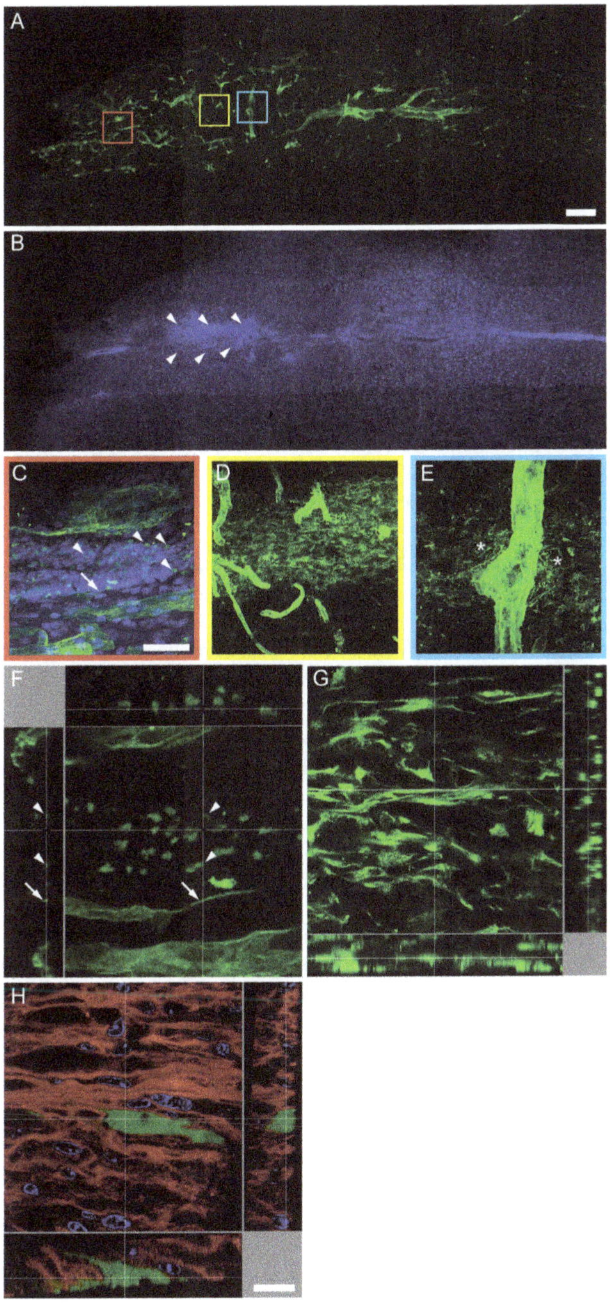

Figure 8. Laminin produced by hADSC forms reticular-like deposits independent of fractones. Photomontage of a horizontal section of the undamaged spinal cord one week after injection of hADSCs (A) immunostained with a pan-specific anti-laminin antibody (green) and (B) counterstained with DAPI (blue). The arrowheads in B delimit the region of the highest increase in cellularity, corresponding to reticular laminin in A. Boxed areas in A were amplified to show the detailed morphology of the types of laminin deposits in the spinal cord. C) The red box shows fractones characterized by the presence of thin lines (arrow) and puncta (arrowhead). D) The yellow box shows an independent reticular-like deposit. E) The blue box shows laminin around a blood vessel. Note that laminin seems to detach from the perivascular basal lamina and to spread in the spinal parenchyma (asterisks). Panels C and D were reconstructed in the z axis to provide a 3D view of the fractones (F) and of the reticular deposits (G). In F, lines (arrow) and puncta (arrowheads) presented similar shapes in 2D or 3D. Panel H shows a 3D view of laminin deposits stained with an antibody specific for the α2 chain of human laminin (red) and counterstained with DAPI (blue). The 3D structure of laminin secreted by hADSCs is similar to the one depicted in G and different from the one depicted in F. Note that DAPI-stained nuclei are nested within reticular laminin (red) and that the protein produced by GFP-transduced hADSCs (green) largely surpasses the borders of the secreting cells.

Cells from the ependymal layer have already been shown to proliferate after spinal cord injury [50]. This phenomenon could account for the scattered cell clusters seen in the white matter above the canal in animals submitted to injury. In these animals, a second focus of increased cellularity was the lesion epicenter. Progenitor cells could migrate from the neurogenic area of the canal toward the lesion using two alternative routes; directly through the parenchyma or along the perivascular space. Although we cannot presently discriminate between these possibilities, the presence of blood vessels near the expanded lining of the central canal reinforces the latter hypothesis. Similar to our results, it has been previously shown that the injection of bone marrow MSCs stimulated subventricular zone neurogenesis in the mouse brain [51].

The second remarkable feature observed in this study was the appearance of perivascular spaces limited by two clearly definable basement membranes in the spinal cord tissue. Separation of the two basal laminas, which are close together in physiological conditions, creates a perivascular compartment suitable for cell trafficking, associated to inflammation [52,53]. Recently, it has been proposed that mesenchymal precursors that differentiate into vascular mural cells use conduits in the extracellular matrix called "vascular guiding tunnels" to approach the newly formed endothelial tubes to which they will associate [54].

Cells located between the two membranes expressed nestin, vimentin, and NG2, which are markers for neural precursors and for perivascular cells. They were also positive for αSMA, which is expressed by pericytes of the nervous system [55], but not considered as a marker for neural precursors. This antigenic profile does not allow us to identify these perivascular cells as neural precursors derived from remote neurogenic areas into the lesion site or to perivascular cells with the potential to divide and differentiate into neural lineages. Corroborating the latter, pericytes have recently been proposed to correspond to a heterogeneous population [56] containing multipotent mesenchymal cells with the potential to differentiate into neural precursors [57]. Nevertheless, at this point we cannot determine if neural progenitors originate from the central canal or from the perivascular compartment. Tuj1 and Olig2 expression were not detected in the perivascular compartment, but were detected in the cellular infiltrate at the lesion site and also in the spindle-like cluster in non-damaged spinal cord. Thus, if progenitor cells do in fact migrate through the perivascular compartment they must differentiate into neuroblasts or glial precursors only upon contact with the neural parenchyma.

The third finding providing new information on the mechanisms involved in hADSC-induced regeneration is the accumulation of human laminin in the same areas of the spinal cord where precursor cells have also accumulated. Grafted cells produced a cloud-like pattern of laminin deposition, which corresponded to the location of neural precursors in both injured and non-injured spinal cord. Given that laminins, particularly those containing the α2 and α5 chains [36], are present in CNS regions where neural stem and progenitor cells reside, both during development and in the adult [34,35,58,59], we hypothesize that laminin can be the molecule produced by hADSCs that mediated the accumulation of neural precursors along the midline and at the injury site. In line with this hypothesis is our previous demonstration that acute injection of the protein laminin alone, as long as it is delivered in its polymeric form, promotes regeneration after spinal cord injury [60]. Although in that study we did not search for the presence of neural precursors in the tissue, we did find that laminin treatment led to regeneration of descending axons, to decreases in astrogliosis and cystic cavity size and to an expressive reduction of macrophage spreading in the spinal parenchyma, all events similar to those described here as elicited by hADSC.

This is the first time that a link between laminin and the pro-regenerative effects of mesenchymal cells in the central nervous system is proposed. Previous studies had proposed a connection between laminin and MSCs in other tissues such as the peripheral nerve and skeletal muscle [61,62]. However, those studies were conducted in laminin deficient animals in which MSCs were injected exactly as an attempt to restore tissue integrity. Furthermore, none of these two studies demonstrated a strong correlation between the localization of endogenous progenitors and laminin deposited by MSC, as shown here.

Bone marrow stromal cells have been shown to express laminin α4, α5, β1, β2 and γ1 [63]. Here we tested whether hADSCs *in vitro* produced these laminin chains, but we found reactivity only for β2 and γ1. In addition, we found no positivity for the α2 chain, which, together with α5, β2 and γ1, was detected *in vivo*. Considering that laminin α2 and α5 of human origin appeared in spinal cord of rats injected with hADSCs (injured or uninjured), we propose that the exposure of the cells to the spinal cord environment was capable of switching the production of laminin chains α2 and α5. These laminin chains secreted only after transplantation of hADSC may stimulate the proliferation and migration of neural precursors from the ependymal layer around the central canal or from other neurogenic niches around blood vessels. The attracted precursor cells accumulate mainly in the lesion site, contributing to regeneration of the nervous tissue and ultimately to functional recovery. In line with this hypothesis, it has previously been shown that laminin isoforms containing the α chains 2, 4 and 5 are essential components of the subependymal neurogenic niche of adult mice [36].

Our results show that hADSCs are efficient in promoting regeneration after SCI and suggest laminin as a mediator of the beneficial effects of these cells. A better understanding of the mechanisms underlying the regenerative effects of stem/progenitor cells in the nervous system is essential for development of future cell-based therapies to treat spinal cord injury in humans.

Experimental Procedures

Ethics Statement

All experimental procedures adhered to the guidelines of the American National Institute of Health and the Brazilian COBEA and were approved by the animal welfare committee of the Federal University of Rio de Janeiro/Center of Health Sciences [DAHEICB 041]. All the procedures involving human samples were approved by the Investigational Review Board at HUCFF (protocol numbers 043/09 and 088/04). Bone marrow samples were collected from discharged bone marrow collection kits after aspirates were transferred to infusion bags. Informed consent exemption was approved by the Investigational Review Board at HUCFF since data were analyzed anonymously and derived from discarded samples. Adipose tissue and lipoaspirates were collected after the patients signed a written informed consent.

Animals

We used adult female Sprague-Dawley rats (200–250 g), bred at the animal facility of the Federal University of Rio de Janeiro. Rats were kept in 12-hour light/dark cycles with free access to food and water in an isolated animal room. Sixty seven rats were used in this study. Forty-eight animals were included in the injured group submitted to spinal cord compression and were further subdivided in cell treated group (n = 27; 3 euthanized at 1 dpi, 12 at 1 wpi, 3 at 4 wpi and 9 at 8 wpi) and vehicle control (n = 21; 3 euthanized at 1 dpi, 6 at 1 wpi, 3 at 4 wpi and 9 at 8 wpi). Non-injured animals that received cells (n = 12; euthanized at 1 wpi) and sham operated animals (n = 6; 3 euthanized at 1 wpi and 3 at 8 wpi) were included. One uninjured animal was injected with human fibroblasts and euthanized one week later.

Samples and Cells

Fragments of subcutaneous adipose tissue and lipoaspirates were obtained from the abdominal region of patients undergoing plastic surgery at the Clementino Fraga Filho University Hospital (HUCFF), Federal University of Rio de Janeiro, Brazil. Human skin fibroblast cell line was obtained from the Cell Bank of Rio de Janeiro (BCRJ, Rio de Janeiro, RJ, Brazil).

Plasmid Construct and Lentivirus Production

The pLL3.7 plasmid, originally described by Dr. van Parijs's group [64], was provided by Dr. Guido Lenz (UFRGS – Porto Alegre, Brazil). Lentiviral vectors were produced as previously described [65,66].

Isolation and Transduction of hADSCs

Human adipose tissue-derived stromal cells were obtained as previously described [24,25,67]. Briefly, subcutaneous adipose tissue fragments and lipoaspirates were submitted to enzymatic digestion with 10 mg/mL collagenase IA (Sigma-Aldrich, St. Louis, MO) for 1 hour at 37°C under agitation. Cells were plated at $1–2\times10^4$ cells/cm^2 in Dulbecco's (DMEM Low-glucose, LGC, São Paulo, SP, Brazil) supplemented with 10% fetal bovine serum (FBS, Cultilab, Campinas, SP, Brazil) and antibiotics (100 U/ml of penicillin and 100 μg/ml of streptomycin, both from Sigma-Aldrich) and maintained overnight at 37°C with 5% CO_2. Non-adherent cells were removed and adherent cells were maintained as above and expanded by enzymatic digestion with 0.125% trypsin and 0.78 mM EDTA (Sigma-Aldrich). Lentivirus transduction was performed by addition of 1 mL of lentiviral vector stock with polybrene at the concentration of 8 μg/mL and 7 mL of DMEM. Cells were then incubated at 5% $C0_2$ and 37°C overnight. After incubation, the medium was replaced by fresh DMEM medium with 10% FCS. Cells were kept under these conditions until they were prepared for *in vivo* analysis. The typical multiplicity of infection (MOI) used for ADSC transduction ranged from 10 to 50. Transduced cells were trypsinized, fixed with 4% paraformaldehyde in PBS, and GFP expression was analyzed by flow cytometry (BD FACScalibur Flow Cytometer; Becton Dickinson) using CellQuest software.

Surgical Procedures

Animals were anesthetized with an i.m. injection (300 μl) of a cocktail containing xylazine (3.2 mg/kg; Syntec, Cotia, SP, Brazil), ketamin (62.5 mg/kg; Syntec), and acepromazin (0.625 mg/kg; Syntec) diluted in water, and were subjected to dorsal laminectomy. For the compression injury, T7 vertebra was removed and a 2-French Fogarty catheter (Baxter Healthcare Corporation, Irvine, CA) was inserted into the dorsal epidural space caudally to T8–T9 spinal level (1 cm distance from the incision). The balloon was inflated with 15 μl of water for 5 min. Rats were kept anesthetized for 30 min before application of acute experimental treatment or control buffers. Soft tissue and skin were sutured in anatomical layers and the animals were allowed to recover in warmed cages and kept in pairs during survival. As specific surgical and post-surgical care, all animals had their eyes lubricated during surgery, received subcutaneous 10 ml injections of Ringer solution for hydration immediately after being sutured, and were treated with gentamicin sulfate (40 mg/kg; Neoquímica, Anápolis, GO, Brazil) for 3 days to avoid urinary infection. The bladder was manually expressed until spontaneous function was reestablished 3 days after injury.

Spinal Cord Injections

Cell suspensions or vehicle (10 μl) were stereotaxically injected using a 10 μl Hamilton syringe, immediately after injury or after laminectomy in non-injured animals. The total volume was injected once, 1 cm rostrally to the lesion epicenter. In animals, which were not subjected to SCI, injections were made at T8–9 level.

Histology and Immunofluorescence

Rats were anesthetized and perfused transcardially with 4% paraformaldehyde in 0.1 M phosphate buffer (pH 7.4). Spinal cords were removed and a 1 cm segment between T7–T10 levels was removed. For immunofluorescence analysis, segments were cut in the transversal or horizontal planes in a vibratome (model 3000, Vibratome Co; 40 μm thick), and collected serially onto gelatin-coated glass slides. Tissue samples of gastrocnemius muscle of rats were cut in a cryostat for the anti-human laminin immunolabeling.

Prior to immunolabeling, slides were extensively washed with PBS, permeabilized with 0.3% Triton-X-100 (Sigma), blocked with 10% bovine serum albumin (Sigma) or normal goat serum (Sigma), and finally incubated overnight at 4°C with primary antibodies. The following mouse antibodies were used: anti-GAP-43 (1:4.000; Sigma); anti-GFAP (1:500; Sigma); anti-CD68 (ED1; 1:30; AbD Serotec, Oxford, UK); anti-RECA-1 (1:100; AbD Serotec), anti-CD3 (clone 1F4; 1:100; BioLegend, San Diego, CA); anti-αSMA (1:400; Sigma), anti-class III β-tubulin (Tuj1; 1:500; Covance, Princeton, NJ), anti-vimentin (1:100; Sigma), anti-human fibronectin (1:400; Sigma), anti-human collagen IV (1:500; Sigma), anti-human laminin α5 chain (clone LAM-89; 1:1000; Sigma), anti-human laminin α2 chain (clone 5H2; 1:1000; Millipore), anti-human laminin α2, α4, α5, β1, β2 and γ1, corresponding to clones 5A4, 3D12, 6A11, IIID9, 9F8 and IIID10, were kindly provided by Dr. Lydia Sorokin (University of Muenster, Germany). The following rabbit antibodies were used: anti-serotonin (5HT; 1:1000; Sigma); anti-Ki67 (1:100; Abcam); anti-nestin (1:500; Millipore); anti-Olig2 (1:500; Millipore); anti-NG2 (1:150; Millipore); and pan-laminin (polyclonal antibody raised against EHS laminin; 1:50; Sigma). After rinsing with PBS, sections were incubated for 2 h at room temperature with fluorescent dye-conjugated goat anti-mouse or anti-rabbit IgGs (1:500; Cy3-conjugated from Sigma and Alexa 488-conjugated from Molecular Probes/Invitrogen). After an additional wash with PBS and one with distilled water, slides were mounted with n-propyl galate (Sigma). In negative controls the primary antibodies were omitted (Fig. S5).

Image Analysis

Tissue and cells were analyzed in a TE200 fluorescence inverted microscope (Nikon), with standard DAPI/FITC/TRITC filters coupled to a color CCD camera (Evolution vf, Media Cybernetics) and using the software Image Pro Plus 6.0 for image processing (Media Cybernetics Inc.). Images were alternatively acquired with a TCS-SP5 confocal microscope (Leica).

Lesion epicenters and the largest diameter of cavity size were determined by digitalizing the cavity contours of GFAP-stained horizontal sections of the dorsal–ventral plane of the injured cord. The analyses were confined to the middle 640 μm, ranging from 120 to 760 μm below the first section from the top of the spine. For quantification, the section with the largest cavity size was chosen as the epicenter and 5 sections in 5 successive slides on each side of this putative epicenter had their areas calculated using the software Image Pro Plus 6.0 (Media Cybernetics Inc.) and plotted against a spatial axis. We evaluated three animals of each experimental group.

GAP-43 and 5-HT fibers were evaluated in conventional fluorescence images and plotted as the sum of the total length of positive fibers, at 3 different regions (injury epicenter; 500 μm rostral and caudal to epicenter), in 3 animals (1 section per animal).

Behavioral Assessment

Locomotor activity was evaluated using the open-field walking test, BBB [68]. One animal at a time was allowed to move freely inside a circular plastic tray for 5 min, and two independent examiners who were blinded to the experiment attributed scores. The final score of each animal was the mean value of both examiners.

Statistics

Comparisons between different experimental groups were performed using GraphPad Prism version 5.00 for Windows (GraphPad Software, San Diego, USA) to analyze the variance (ANOVA) with post-hoc Kruskal-Wallis test for multiple comparisons (BBB assays). For comparison between 2 groups we used the Student's t test (cavity size, ED1, GAP-43, and 5-HT labeling). Differences were considered significant when $p<0.05$.

Supporting Information

Figure S1 Neighboring blood vessels interact with the expanded wall of the central canal. (A–F) Consecutive confocal images in the z axis of a horizontal section at the level of the central canal processed for DAPI staining (blue) 1 week after injury. It is possible to see the transition between a single cell (A) and a multiple cell (B) lining of the canal wall (dashed line); the progressive thickening of the canal wall (D–E); a blood vessel approaching the canal area (arrows in B–F); and cells from the canal wall contacting the lumen of this blood vessel (F). (G–I) Higher magnification images of boxed areas in D–F, showing the area of interaction between the blood vessel and the central canal with high cell density. GFAP immunoreactivity (red) reveals the areas of tissue as opposed to hollow structures such as the blood vessel and the canal. Dashed lines delineate the border between the wall of the central canal and the spinal grey matter. Bars: A–F = 50 μm and G–I = 25 μm.

Figure S2 Areas of increased cellularity in the uninjured spinal cord injected with hADSC contain neural precursors and/or pericytes. A–C) Confocal images of a transverse section of the spinal cord immunostained with anti-CD68 (ED1, red), one week after the injection of GFP-hADSC into the undamaged spinal cord. Note that only a few scattered cells correspond to macrophages/microglial cells appearing in cell infiltrates (DAPI, blue). D–S) Confocal images of horizontal sections of the undamaged spinal cord one week after injection of hADSCs, showing the presence of neural precursors and/or pericytes, identified by immunostaining with anti-nestin (D–G, R,

S, green), anti-vimentin (H, I, red; J, K, green), Tuj1 (L,M, red), anti-SMA (N,O, red) and anti-Olig2 (P, Q, green). Note that the phenomenon of separation of the two laminas around blood vessels also occurs in the absence of lesion (F, G, J, K). Nestin-positive cells (green) present Ki67-positive nuclei (red), indicating that neural precursors proliferate in the cell infiltrates (R, S). Bars: A, H, I, P, Q = 100 μm; B, C, F–I, K, S = 25 μm; D, E, L–O, R: = 50 μm.

Figure S3 Extracellular matrix proteins secreted by the hADSCs in the undamaged spinal cord. Confocal images of horizontal sections of the spinal cord, one week after injection of GFP-hADSCs (green). Images show immunoreactivity for anti-human fibronectin (B, C, red), anti-human collagen IV (E, F, red) and anti-human laminin (clone 5H2, H, I, red) counterstained with DAPI (blue) to reveal cell infiltrates (A, D, G). Note that human laminin is more abundant than the other proteins. Bars: A–I = 100 μm.

Figure S4 The anti-human α2 laminin antibody does not cross-react with rat α2 laminin. The specificity of the anti-human laminin α2 antibody (clone 5H2) was investigated by testing its ability to recognize the rat muscle, where α2 is the major component of the basal lamina. Rat gastrocnemius muscle was cut transversally and stained with an anti-pan laminin antibody (A) or with 5H2 (B). Note that basement membranes around muscle fibers were labeled by anti-pan but not by anti-human α2 laminin. A negative control obtained by omitting the primary antibodies is shown in panel C. DAPI counterstaining appears in panels D–F. Scale bar = 100 μm.

Figure S5 Negative controls for immunolabeling analyses. A–F) Confocal images of horizontal sections of the spinal cord incubated with fluorescent dye-conjugated goat Cy3-anti-rabbit (A, red), Alexa 488-anti-mouse (B, green), Cy3-anti-mouse (D, red), Alexa 488-anti-rabbit (E, green). Red and green channels are shown superimposed (C, F) together with DAPI counterstaining (blue). Bars: A–F = 200 μm.

Movie S1 Cells accumulate in between the two laminin-rich basement membranes around blood vessels in the spinal cord of hADSC-treated animals. The animation was generated from a series of confocal optical slices of a horizontal section (50 μm thick) of the rat spinal cord 1 week after injury and injection of hADSC. The slice was immunostained for PAN-laminin (red) and nestin (green) and counterstained with DAPI (blue). Cells tend to accumulate in nestin-rich areas both between the two basement membranes and in the spinal parenchyma. Note that in the inferior part of the image cells seem to escape from the vessel in a region where the laminin membrane appears disrupted. Confocal micrographs were analyzed using a free trial version of Imaris software (version 7.2, Bitplane Scientific Software).

Acknowledgments

We would like to thank Laina Martins Cunha and Rosana Maria Assis Silva for excellent technical assistance. The authors are indebted to Dr. César Cláudio da Silva and Dr. Marcelo C. Acineto Souza, both from the Faculty of Medicine (UFRJ), who provided the adipose tissue fragments and lipoaspirates for isolation of hADSCs and to Dr. Lydia Sorokin from the University of Muenster for the kind gift of anti-laminin antibodies.

This manuscript was reviewed by a professional science editor and by a native English-speaking copy editor to improve readability.

Author Contributions

Conceived and designed the experiments: KM MB JRLM RB MIDR TCS. Performed the experiments: KM MAN JPG ASC DVL BC JRLM. Analyzed the data: KM MAN JRLM RB MIDR TCS. Contributed reagents/materials/analysis tools: MB JRLM RB MIDR TCS. Wrote the paper: KM JRLM MIDR TCS.

References

1. Burns AS, O'Connell C (2012) The challenge of spinal cord injury care in the developing world. J Spinal Cord Med 35: 3–8.
2. Devivo MJ (2012) Epidemiology of traumatic spinal cord injury: trends and future implications. Spinal Cord 50: 365–372.
3. Bradbury EJ (2002) Re-wiring the spinal cord: introduction to the special issue on plasticity after spinal cord injury. Exp Neurol 235: 1–4.
4. Ruff CA, Wilcox JT, Fehlings MG (2012) Cell-based transplantation strategies to promote plasticity following spinal cord injury. Exp Neurol 235: 78–90.
5. Hatami M, Mehrjardi NZ, Kiani S, Hemmesi K, Azizi H, et al. (2009) Human embryonic stem cell-derived neural precursor transplants in collagen scaffolds promote recovery in injured rat spinal cord. Cytotherapy 11: 618–630.
6. Keirstead HS, Nistor G, Bernal G, Totoiu M, Cloutier F, et al. (2005) Human embryonic stem cell-derived oligodendrocyte progenitor cell transplants remyelinate and restore locomotion after spinal cord injury. J Neurosci 25: 4694–4705.
7. McDonald JW, Howard MJ (2002) Repairing the damaged spinal cord: a summary of our early success with embryonic stem cell transplantation and remyelination. Prog Brain Res 137: 299–309.
8. Wyatt TJ, Rossi SL, Siegenthaler MM, Frame J, Robles R, et al. (2011) Human motor neuron progenitor transplantation leads to endogenous neuronal sparing in 3 models of motor neuron loss. Stem Cells Int 2011: 207230.
9. Lebkowski J (2011) GRNOPC1: the world's first embryonic stem cell-derived therapy. Interview with Jane Lebkowski. Regen Med 6: 11–13.
10. da Silva Meirelles L, Caplan AI, Nardi NB (2008) In search of the in vivo identity of mesenchymal stem cells. Stem Cells 26: 2287–2299.
11. Wright KT, El Masri W, Osman A, Chowdhury J, Johnson WEB (2011) Concise review: Bone marrow for the treatment of spinal cord injury: mechanisms and clinical applications. Stem Cells 29: 169–178.
12. Scuteri A, Miloso M, Foudah D, Orciani M, Cavaletti G, et al. (2011) Mesenchymal stem cells neuronal differentiation ability: a real perspective for nervous system repair? Curr Stem Cell Res Ther 6: 82–92.
13. Ankeny DP, McTigue DM, Jakeman LB (2004) Bone marrow transplants provide tissue protection and directional guidance for axons after contusive spinal cord injury in rats. Exp Neurol 190: 17–31.
14. Chopp M, Zhang XH, Li Y, Wang L, Chen J, et al. (2000) Spinal cord injury in rat: treatment with bone marrow stromal cell transplantation. Neuroreport 11: 3001–3005.
15. Cízková D, Rosocha J, Vanický I, Jergová S, Cízek M (2006) Transplants of human mesenchymal stem cells improve functional recovery after spinal cord injury in the rat. Cell Mol Neurobiol 26: 1167–1180.
16. Führmann T, Montzka K, Hillen LM, Hodde D, Dreier A, et al. (2010) Axon growth-promoting properties of human bone marrow mesenchymal stromal cells. Neurosci Lett 474: 37–41.
17. Hofstetter CP, Schwarz EJ, Hess D, Widenfalk J, El Manira A, et al. (2002) Marrow stromal cells form guiding strands in the injured spinal cord and promote recovery. Proc Natl Acad Sci USA 99: 2199–2204.
18. Osaka M, Honmou O, Murakami T, Nonaka T, Houkin K, et al. (2010) Intravenous administration of mesenchymal stem cells derived from bone marrow after contusive spinal cord injury improves functional outcome. Brain Res 1343: 226–235.
19. Pal R, Gopinath C, Rao NM, Banerjee P, Krishnamoorthy V, et al. (2010) Functional recovery after transplantation of bone marrow-derived human mesenchymal stromal cells in a rat model of spinal cord injury. Cytotherapy 12: 792–806.
20. Park H-W, Lim M-J, Jung H, Lee S-P, Paik K-S, et al. (2010) Human mesenchymal stem cell-derived Schwann cell-like cells exhibit neurotrophic effects, via distinct growth factor production, in a model of spinal cord injury. Glia 58: 1118–1132.
21. Pedram MS, Dehghan MM, Soleimani M, Sharifi D, Marjanmehr SH, et al. (2010) Transplantation of a combination of autologous neural differentiated and undifferentiated mesenchymal stem cells into injured spinal cord of rats. Spinal Cord 48: 457–463.
22. Zhang W, Yan Q, Zeng Y-S, Zhang X-B, Xiong Y, et al. (2010) Implantation of adult bone marrow-derived mesenchymal stem cells transfected with the

neurotrophin-3 gene and pretreated with retinoic acid in completely transected spinal cord. Brain Res 1359: 256–271.
23. Zurita M, Vaquero J, Bonilla C, Santos M, De Haro J, et al. (2008) Functional recovery of chronic paraplegic pigs after autologous transplantation of bone marrow stromal cells. Transplantation 86: 845–853.
24. Baptista LS, da Silva KR, da Pedrosa CSG, Claudio-da-Silva C, Carneiro JRI, et al. (2009) Adipose tissue of control and ex-obese patients exhibit differences in blood vessel content and resident mesenchymal stem cell population. Obes Surg 19: 1304–1312.
25. Zuk PA, Zhu M, Mizuno H, Huang J, Futrell JW, et al. (2001) Multilineage cells from human adipose tissue: implications for cell-based therapies. Tissue Eng 7: 211–228.
26. Arboleda D, Forostyak S, Jendelova P, Marekova D, Amemori T, et al. (2011) Transplantation of predifferentiated adipose-derived stromal cells for the treatment of spinal cord injury. Cell Mol Neurobiol 31: 1113–1122.
27. Oh JS, Kim KN, An SS, Pennant WA, Kim HJ, et al. (2011) Cotransplantation of mouse neural stem cells (mNSCs) with adipose tissue-derived mesenchymal stem cells improves mNSC survival in a rat spinal cord injury model. Cell Transplant 20: 837–849.
28. Park S-S, Lee YJ, Lee SH, Lee D, Choi K, et al. (2012) Functional recovery after spinal cord injury in dogs treated with a combination of Matrigel and neural-induced adipose-derived mesenchymal Stem cells. Cytotherapy 14: 584–597.
29. Zhou Z, Chen Y, Zhang H, Min S, Yu B, et al. (2013) Comparison of mesenchymal stem cells from human bone marrow and adipose tissue for the treatment of spinal cord injury. Cytotherapy, 15: 434–448.
30. Aggarwal S, Pittenger MF (2005) Human mesenchymal stem cells modulate allogeneic immune cell responses. Blood 105: 1815–1822.
31. Le Blanc K, Mougiakakos D (2012) Multipotent mesenchymal stromal cells and the innate immune system. Nat Rev Immunol 12: 383–396.
32. Menezes JR, Luskin MB (1994) Expression of neuron-specific tubulin defines a novel population in the proliferative layers of the developing telencephalon. J Neurosci 14: 5399–5416.
33. Benowitz LI, Routtenberg A (1997) GAP-43: an intrinsic determinant of neuronal development and plasticity. Trends Neurosci 20: 84–91.
34. Lathia JD, Patton B, Eckley DM, Magnus T, Mughal MR, et al. (2007) Patterns of laminins and integrins in the embryonic ventricular zone of the CNS. J Comp Neurol 505: 630–643.
35. Shen Q, Wang Y, Kokovay E, Lin G, Chuang S-M, et al. (2008) Adult SVZ stem cells lie in a vascular niche: a quantitative analysis of niche cell-cell interactions. Cell Stem Cell 3: 289–300.
36. Kazanis I, Lathia JD, Vadakkan TJ, Raborn E, Wan R, et al. (2010) Quiescence and activation of stem and precursor cell populations in the subependymal zone of the mammalian brain are associated with distinct cellular and extracellular matrix signals. J Neurosci 30: 9771–9781.
37. Hamann GF, Okada Y, Fitridge R, del Zoppo GJ (1995) Microvascular basal lamina antigens disappear during cerebral ischemia and reperfusion. Stroke 26: 2120–2126.
38. Chen X, Ai Z, Rasmussen M, Bajcsy P, Auvil L, et al. (2003) Three-dimensional reconstruction of extravascular matrix patterns and blood vessels in human uveal melanoma tissue: techniques and preliminary findings. Invest Ophthalmol Vis Sci 44: 2834–2840.
39. Mercier F, Kitasako JT, Hatton GI (2002) Anatomy of the brain neurogenic zones revisited: fractones and the fibroblast/macrophage network. J Comp Neurol 451: 170–188.
40. Mercier F, Schnack J, Chaumet MSG (2011) Fractones: Home and conductors of the neural stem cell niche. In Neurogenesis in the adult brain I: Neurobiology, eds Seki T et al. (Springer, Heidelberg), 109–133.
41. Barberi T, Klivenyi P, Calingasan NY, Lee H, Kawamata H, et al. (2003) Neural subtype specification of fertilization and nuclear transfer embryonic stem cells and application in parkinsonian mice. Nat Biotechnol 21: 1200–1207.
42. Ideguchi M, Palmer TD, Recht LD, Weimann JM (2010) Murine embryonic stem cell-derived pyramidal neurons integrate into the cerebral cortex and appropriately project axons to subcortical targets. J Neurosci 30: 894–904.
43. Steffenhagen C, Dechant F-X, Oberbauer E, Furtner T, Weidner N, et al. (2012) Mesenchymal stem cells prime proliferating adult neural progenitors toward an oligodendrocyte fate. Stem Cells Dev 21: 1838–1851.
44. Nakanishi C, Nagaya N, Ohnishi S, Yamahara K, Takabatake S, et al. (2011) Gene and protein expression analysis of mesenchymal stem cells derived from rat adipose tissue and bone marrow. Circ J 75: 2260–2268.
45. Castelo-Branco MTL, Soares IDP, Lopes DV, Buongusto F, Martinusso CA, et al. (2012) Intraperitoneal but not intravenous cryopreserved mesenchymal stromal cells home to the inflamed colon and ameliorate experimental colitis. PloS One 7: e33360.
46. Busch SA, Hamilton JA, Horn KP, Cuascut FX, Cutrone R, et al. (2011) Multipotent adult progenitor cells prevent macrophage-mediated axonal dieback and promote regrowth after spinal cord injury. J Neurosci 31: 944–953.
47. Kim J, Hematti P (2009) Mesenchymal stem cell-educated macrophages: a novel type of alternatively activated macrophages. Exp Hematol 37: 1445–1453.
48. Nakajima H, Uchida K, Guerrero AR, Watanabe S, Sugita D, et al. (2012) Transplantation of mesenchymal stem cells promotes an alternative pathway of macrophage activation and functional recovery after spinal cord injury. J Neurotrauma 29: 1614–1625.
49. Alfaro-Cervello C, Soriano-Navarro M, Mirzadeh Z, Alvarez-Buylla A, Garcia-Verdugo JM (2012) Biciliated ependymal cell proliferation contributes to spinal cord growth. J Comp Neurol 520: 3528–3552.
50. Meletis K, Barnabe?-Heider F, Carlén M, Evergren E, Tomilin N, et al. (2008) Spinal cord injury reveals multilineage differentiation of ependymal cells. PLoS Biol 6: e182.
51. Kan I, Barhum Y, Melamed E, Offen D (2011) Mesenchymal stem cells stimulate endogenous neurogenesis in the subventricular zone of adult mice. Stem Cell Rev 7: 404–412.
52. Sixt M, Engelhardt B, Pausch F, Hallmann R, Wendler O, et al. (2001) Endothelial cell laminin isoforms, laminins 8 and 10, play decisive roles in T cell recruitment across the blood-brain barrier in experimental autoimmune encephalomyelitis. J Cell Biol 153: 933–946.
53. Takigawa T, Yonezawa T, Yoshitaka T, Minaguchi J, Kurosaki M, et al. (2010) Separation of the perivascular basement membrane provides a conduit for inflammatory cells in a mouse spinal cord injury model. J Neurotrauma 27: 739–751.
54. Stratman AN, Davis GE (2012) Endothelial cell-pericyte interactions stimulate basement membrane matrix assembly: influence on vascular tube remodeling, maturation, and stabilization. Microscopy Microanal 18: 68–80.
55. Krueger M, Bechmann I (2010) CNS pericytes: concepts, misconceptions, and a way out. Glia 58: 1–10.
56. Göritz C, Dias DO, Tomilin N, Barbacid M, Shupliakov O, et al. (2011) A pericyte origin of spinal cord scar tissue. Science 333: 238–242.
57. Paul G, Özen I, Christophersen NS, Reinbothe T, Bengzon J, et al. (2012) The adult human brain harbors multipotent perivascular mesenchymal stem cells. PloS One 7: e35577.
58. Belvindrah R, Hankel S, Walker J, Patton BL, Müller U (2007) Beta1 integrins control the formation of cell chains in the adult rostral migratory stream. J Neurosci 27: 2704–2717.
59. Loulier K, Lathia JD, Marthiens V, Relucio J, Mughal MR, et al. (2009) Beta1 integrin maintains integrity of the embryonic neocortical stem cell niche. PLoS Biol 7: e1000176.
60. Menezes K, de Menezes JR, Nascimento MA, Santos RS, Coelho-Sampaio T (2010) Polylaminin, a polymeric form of laminin, promotes regeneration after spinal cord injury. FASEB J 24: 4513–4522.
61. Carlson KB, Singh P, Feaster MM, Ramnarain A, Pavlides C, et al. (2011) Mesenchymal stem cells facilitate axon sorting, myelination, and functional recovery in paralyzed mice deficient in Schwann cell-derived laminin. Glia 59: 267–277.
62. Fukada S-I, Yamamoto Y, Segada M, Sakamoto K, Nakajima M, et al. (2008) CD90-positive cells, an additional cell population, produce laminin α2 upon transplantation to dy^{3k}/dy^{3k} mice. Exp Cell Res 314: 193–203.
63. Siler U, Seiffert M, Puch S, Richards A, Torok-Storb B, et al. (2000) Characterization and functional analysis of laminin isoforms in human bone marrow. Blood 96: 4194–4203.
64. Rubinson DA, Dillon CP, Kwiatkowski AV, Sievers C, Yang L, et al. (2003) A lentivirus-based system to functionally silence genes in primary mammalian cells, stem cells and transgenic mice by RNA interference. Nat Genet 33: 401–406.
65. Lima LG, Oliveira AS, Campos LC, Bonamino M, Chammas R, et al. (2011) Malignant transformation in melanocytes is associated with increased production of procoagulant microvesicles. Thromb Haemost 106: 712–723.
66. Bonamino M, Serafini M, D'Amico G, Gaipa G, Todisco E, et al. (2004) Functional transfer of CD40L gene in human B-cell precursor ALL blasts by second-generation SIN lentivectors Gene therapy 11: 85–93.
67. Baptista LS, Pedrosa CSG, Silva KR, Otazú IB, Takiya CM, et al. (2007) Bone marrow and adipose tissue-derived mesenchymal stem cells: How close are they? J Stem Cells, 2: 73–90.
68. Basso DM, Beattie MS, Bresnahan JC (1995) A sensitive and reliable locomotor rating scale for open field testing in rats. J Neurotrauma 12: 1–21.

2

Persistent At-Level Thermal Hyperalgesia and Tactile Allodynia Accompany Chronic Neuronal and Astrocyte Activation in Superficial Dorsal Horn following Mouse Cervical Contusion Spinal Cord Injury

Jaime L. Watson, Tamara J. Hala, Rajarshi Putatunda, Daniel Sannie, Angelo C. Lepore*

Department of Neuroscience, Farber Institute for Neurosciences, Sidney Kimmel Medical College at Thomas Jefferson University, Philadelphia, Pennsylvania, United States of America

Abstract

In humans, sensory abnormalities, including neuropathic pain, often result from traumatic spinal cord injury (SCI). SCI can induce cellular changes in the CNS, termed central sensitization, that alter excitability of spinal cord neurons, including those in the dorsal horn involved in pain transmission. Persistently elevated levels of neuronal activity, glial activation, and glutamatergic transmission are thought to contribute to the hyperexcitability of these dorsal horn neurons, which can lead to maladaptive circuitry, aberrant pain processing and, ultimately, chronic neuropathic pain. Here we present a mouse model of SCI-induced neuropathic pain that exhibits a persistent pain phenotype accompanied by chronic neuronal hyperexcitability and glial activation in the spinal cord dorsal horn. We generated a unilateral cervical contusion injury at the C5 or C6 level of the adult mouse spinal cord. Following injury, an increase in the number of neurons expressing ΔFosB (a marker of chronic neuronal activation), persistent astrocyte activation and proliferation (as measured by GFAP and Ki67 expression), and a decrease in the expression of the astrocyte glutamate transporter GLT1 are observed in the ipsilateral superficial dorsal horn of cervical spinal cord. These changes have previously been associated with neuronal hyperexcitability and may contribute to altered pain transmission and chronic neuropathic pain. In our model, they are accompanied by robust at-level hyperaglesia in the ipsilateral forepaw and allodynia in both forepaws that are evident within two weeks following injury and persist for at least six weeks. Furthermore, the pain phenotype occurs in the absence of alterations in forelimb grip strength, suggesting that it represents sensory and not motor abnormalities. Given the importance of transgenic mouse technology, this clinically-relevant model provides a resource that can be used to study the molecular mechanisms contributing to neuropathic pain following SCI and to identify potential therapeutic targets for the treatment of chronic pathological pain.

Editor: Guglielmo Foffani, Hospital Nacional de Parapléjicos, Spain

Funding: This work was funded by the NIH (1R01NS079702 to A.C.L.) and the Craig H. Neilsen Foundation (#190140 to A.C.L.). The funders had no role in study design, data collection and analysis, decision to publish, or preparation of the manuscript.

Competing Interests: The authors have declared that no competing interests exist.

* Email: Angelo.Lepore@jefferson.edu

Introduction

Spinal cord injury (SCI) is a debilitating condition with widespread symptoms that affect patient quality of life. As many as 327,000 SCI patients are currently living in the United States, and approximately 12,000 new cases are reported each year [1]. Clinical studies propose that 64–82% of SCI patients experience some form of pathological pain following injury, and this pain has been associated with mood changes as well as difficulty with work and social activities [2]. Neuropathic pain constitutes a significant percentage of pain resulting from SCI; 41% of patients encounter at-level and 34% experience below-level neuropathic pain [3] following injury. Although SCI most often involves an acute injury to the spinal cord, the resulting pathological pain is often chronic and can increase in severity over time [4]. Thus, SCI-related neuropathic pain and its treatment is an important focus of spinal cord research.

In this study, we wanted to identify the molecular changes accompanying the alterations of at-level pain sensitivity in a mouse model of cervical contusion SCI. We induced SCI in the mouse and measured changes in pain behavior, specifically thermal hyperalgesia and tactile allodynia. Additionally, we studied the expression of various proteins in the dorsal horn of the spinal cord that may contribute to neuropathic pain and the cell types expressing these proteins. Importantly, we chose to utilize a mouse model of SCI that is clinically relevant but has not previously been used to study neuropathic pain.

Currently, mouse models of SCI-induced neuropathic pain are available, but do not address cervical contusion injury. According to the National Spinal Cord Injury Statistical Center, the majority of SCI patients in the United States experience injury to the cervical regions of the spinal cord [1], but most rodent SCI models involve injury to thoracic regions. Therefore, we chose to target our SCI to the cervical region of the spinal cord.

Additionally, contusion-type injury is most common in human patients [5] and is a popular model of SCI in rodents [6]. The respiratory and other dysfunctions that commonly accompany cervical contusion injuries make this model difficult to study [7]. To date, our group [8], [9], [10] and others [11] have used models of cervical contusion SCI in the mouse and rat to study motor deficits following injury. In the study of neuropathic pain, however, contusive injury to the cervical regions of the spinal cord has not been utilized in mice. Instead, transection, compression, contusion and other procedures are used primarily at thoracic levels to induce SCI in mice for studying neuropathic pain [6]. Here, we designed a model of moderate hemicontusive injury to the cervical spinal cord in the mouse that does not develop significant respiratory or other life-threatening complications for the study of neuropathic pain.

The development of neuropathic pain following SCI involves the disruption of neurons involved in nociception in the dorsal horn of the spinal cord. Under normal circumstances, neurons in the superficial laminae of the dorsal horn are responsible for pain transmission from peripheral nociceptors to the thalamus and, ultimately, the sensory cortex. Upon injury to the spinal cord, however, local changes can occur that alter how nociceptive neurons respond to peripheral stimuli [12]. These changes, termed central sensitization, can underlie pathological pain behaviors such as allodynia and hyperalgesia [12], [13].

One mechanism involved in central sensitization is the hyperexcitability of pain transmission neurons. Neuronal hyperexcitability results in an increase in the response of neurons to electrical input or even the firing of neurons in the absence of input. Hyperexcitability is characterized by spontaneous neuronal activity, aberrant responses to subthreshold stimuli, and increased transmission of suprathreshold input [12], [13]. In SCI, pain projection neurons in the dorsal horn can become more easily excited by noxious as well as non-noxious stimuli, resulting in pathological pain transmission. Changes to the neuron itself, as well as to its extracellular environment, can alter the neuron's electrophysiological profile, increasing its resting membrane potential and/or decreasing its action potential threshold. As one example of a mechanism underlying central sensitization, increased activity of transcription factors can trigger changes in gene expression that lead to long-term alterations in neuronal function and excitability. For instance, ΔfosB, a commonly used marker of persistent neuronal activation, has been associated with plasticity of pain transmission circuits in inflammatory pain, possibly through downstream targets such as CDK5 [14], [15].

Underlying hyperexcitability and central sensitization in SCI are changes in glial activation and glutamate transporter function. Astrocytes play an essential role in the central nervous system, providing support to neurons, regulating the uptake of glutamate and other factors from the extracellular space, and modulating synapse formation and function [13], [16]. Soon after insult, astrocytes can become activated (marked by glial fibrillary acidic protein (GFAP)) and possibly even proliferative and act to minimize the effects of the injury by reestablishing the blood brain barrier, releasing antioxidants, and protecting the lesion site from detrimental molecules. Activation of astrocytes, however, can also be harmful to neighboring neurons; when persistently active, astrocytes can contribute to neuronal hyperexcitability through the release of factors such as proinflammatory molecules, nitric oxide, and ATP [13], [17], [18].

The loss of glutamate transporters by activated astrocytes and the resulting imbalance in glutamate homeostasis may also contribute to the development of post-SCI neuropathic pain. Under normal conditions, glutamate is cleared from the synapse via glutamate transporters, such as GLT1 and GLAST, located in the plasma membrane of neurons and, more often, astrocytes. However, elevated release of glutamate from presynaptic neurons and/or injured neurons and glia or from damage to the glutamate transporter system can cause an excess of glutamate to linger in synaptic and extra-synaptic locations [13]. This disruption in glutamate homeostasis leads to overactivation of glutamate receptors, which can in some instances result in increased Ca^{2+} concentrations in the postsynaptic neuron. These changes can have negative impacts on cell health and function and alter the activation state of the neuron [19], [20], [21]. In SCI, glutamate excitotoxic damage to inhibitory interneurons can also indirectly boost the excitability of nociceptive neurons in the dorsal horn [18]. In this way, the loss of GLT1 in astrocytes observed following injury by our group [22], [23], [24] and others [25], [26] may contribute to central sensitization and neuropathic pain.

Recently published data from our group showed changes in neuronal and astrocyte activation as well as GLT1 expression in the superficial dorsal horn following cervical contusion SCI-induced hyperalgesia in the rat [24]. The study characterized a moderate hemicontusion injury to cervical regions of the rat spinal cord, which resulted in ipsilateral hyperalgesic behavior. Accompanying hyperalgesia were chronic increases in ΔfosB expression in neurons, astrocyte activation and proliferation in addition to a loss of GLT1 both at the site of the injury and in intact spinal cord caudal to the contusion site [24].

In the current study we characterize increases in pain sensitivity in a mouse model of cervical contusion SCI and the accompanying molecular alterations in the dorsal horn of the spinal cord. Our model exhibits at-level thermal hyperalgesia and tactile allodynia in addition to increases in neuronal and astrocyte activation and a decrease in astrocyte glutamate transporter expression in the superficial dorsal horn. Alterations in pain behavior, as well as neuronal and glial activation and glutamate transport expression in the dorsal horn, have not previously been characterized in mice receiving cervical contusion SCI. Thus, this study provides an observation of the molecular and behavioral changes that occur following cervical SCI in the mouse that can be used to further study the mechanisms underlying neuropathic pain in SCI.

Methods

Animal Studies

Ethics Statement. All animal care and treatment were conducted in strict accordance with the *European Communities Council Directive* (2010/63/EU, 86/609/EEC and 87-848/EEC) and the *NIH Guide for the Care and Use of Laboratory Animals*. Experimental protocols were approved by the Thomas Jefferson University Institutional Animal Care and Use Committee.

Animals. Fifty-six male C57BL/6 mice (25–30 g; The Jackson Laboratory, USA) and 26 transgenic BAC-GLT1-eGFP reporter mice [27] were used. The BAC-GLT1-eGFP reporter mice were created by Regan et al. [27]. The transgene in these mice involves cDNA for eGFP inserted into the start codon of a mouse BAC encompassing the entire GLT-1 gene. Thus, in these mice, eGFP expression is driven by the GLT1 promoter. Mice were housed 5 per cage in a controlled light-dark environment in the Thomas Jefferson University Animal Facility and were given food and water *ad libitum*. To prevent suffering, a combination of ketamine/xylazine and isofluorane was used to anesthetize animals during surgical procedures.

SCI Models. We chose to utilize two models in the C57BL/6 mice in this study; one with injury at the C5 level and another with injury at the C6 level. We did this to show that contusion injury to various levels of the cervical spinal cord has the potential to produce at-level neuropathic pain. Mice were anesthetized initially with ketamine (100 mg/kg) and xylazine (5 mg/kg) injected intraperitoneally, and the anesthetic plane was maintained with 1% isofluorane for the duration of the surgery. The body was immobilized by taping the forelegs to a fixation plate, and the head was immobilized by the isofluorane nose cone. The skin and muscle overlying the spinal column were retracted from levels C3 to T1, and spinal cord was exposed by unilateral laminectomy from the midline blood vessel to the lateral edge of the vertebral lamina at the level of C5 or C6. The spinal column was stabilized at the C3 and T1 spinous processes by microforceps attached to the fixation plate and the far right and left corners. C57BL/6 mice received unilateral contusion injuries at the exposed portion of the spinal cord using the Infinite Horizon Impactor (Precision Systems and Instrumentation; Lexington, KY) with an impactor tip of 0.7 mm in diameter, a force of 40 kilodynes, two seconds of dwell time, and an approximately perpendicular impact angle, parameters similar to our previously published cervical contusion SCI paradigms [8], [9], [10]. Injury parameters for BAC-GLT1-eGFP mice included a 1.0 mm diameter tip, 50 kilodyne force, and no dwell time at the C5 level. Control animals received unilateral laminectomy but not contusion injury to the spinal cord. Following injury, the forceps were removed and the muscle layers were secured with a sterile 4-0 silk suture. Sterile wound clips were used to close the skin, and 1 ml of lactated Ringers solution and 0.1 mg/kg of buprenorphine-HCl were administered subcutaneously.

Unilateral Hargreaves Thermal Test. A modified version of the Hargreaves test for thermal hyperaglesia, based on previously established methods [28], was conducted for the forepaws of each animal. This test detects sensitivity to thermal nociceptive stimuli by determining the latency to withdrawal of the paw from an infrared stimulus of a particular intensity. Prior to surgery, baseline measures were collected once weekly for two weeks. Following contusion SCI or laminectomy, each animal was tested weekly for six weeks. Before the first baseline test, the animals were acclimated to the testing room for an hour each day for five days. Prior to each session, mice were also acclimated to the testing room for an hour. Individually, the mice were restrained manually by the scruff only and placed on a thin glass pane, with one of the forepaws directly above the source of the infrared stimulus (UgoBasile; Comerio, VA). The animals continued to be restrained, but movement of the forepaw was unimpeded. The stimulus was initiated, and a fiber optic sensor on the movable infrared heat source measured the time to forepaw withdrawal. Forepaw withdrawal was defined as a quick movement of the paw away from the infrared stimulus often accompanied by licking of the forepaw. Spontaneous movements of the forepaw were not considered forepaw withdrawal and resulted in discarding the data and repeating the trial. Three trials were conducted for each forepaw of each animal, alternating the left and right forepaws, with an inter-trial interval of 120 seconds.

von Frey Filament Test. Semmes-Weinstein monofilaments (Stoetling Company; Dale, IL) ranging from 1.65 grams to 4.56 grams of force were utilized to measure tactile allodynia using the up-down method. Testing occurred twice prior to surgery to obtain baseline data and once weekly for six weeks after injury. Acclimation procedures were the same as those used for the Hargreaves test. Each mouse experienced ten trials per testing day with an inter-trial interval of 120 seconds. The first trial of each testing day utilized a filament of 3.84 grams. A single trial involved directing a monofilament at the center of the plantar surface of the forepaw of interest and application until the filament buckled. Mice were not restrained for this testing. The response of the mouse was then recorded as a positive or negative withdrawal response. The filament application was considered to produce a positive response if the mouse rapidly withdrew its forepaw, which was mostly accompanied by vocalization and/or licking of the forepaw. If the response was positive, the filament used in the next trial would be the next smaller filament. If instead the response was negative, the next larger filament would be used in the next trial. Withdraw threshold was determined as the lowest filament/force that evoked a positive withdrawal response in greater than 50% of the trials with that particular filament.

Grip Strength Testing. Grip strength was measured by the DFIS-2 Series Digital Force Gauge (Columbus Instruments, OH) [26], used previously by our group [8]. Attached to the force gauge is a triangular metal pull bar that allows for the transduction of force from the mouse to the gauge. The Digital Force Gauge measures the strength with which the mouse is able to grasp and hold onto a thin metal bar. Three baseline measures spread across two weeks were obtained prior to surgery, and mice were tested once weekly for six weeks following injury. In each trial, the mouse was allowed to grab the bar with one forepaw and was then quickly pulled away from the gauge so its grip was released, providing a measurement of the force with which the mouse gripped the bar. During each testing session, three trials for each forepaw were performed with an inter-trial interval of at least 60 seconds.

Histological Analyses

Tissue Processing. Mice were sacrificed at two days or two or six weeks following injury or laminectomy by anesthetic overdose and transcardial perfusion with 0.9% saline followed by 4% paraformaldehyde. The spinal cord was harvested following perfusion, fixed in 4% paraformaldehyde at room temperature for 24 hours, washed in 0.1M phosphate buffer at 4°C for 24 hours and then cryoprotected in 30% sucrose in 0.1M phosphate buffer at 4°C for three days. The cervical/rostral thoracic spinal cord was dissected from the rest of the cord, embedded in freezing medium, and flash-frozen with dry ice. Embedded tissue was cut transversely by cryostat at a thickness of 30 μm and mounted directly onto slides. Slides were stored at −20°C.

Motor Neuron Counts. A representative sample (i.e. every fifth section) of spinal cord tissue was used to locate the injury epicenter. Slides were thawed at room temperature for an hour and stained with 0.5% Cresyl violet acetate/Eriochrome cyanine. For each section, large motor neurons ventral to the central canal in the grey matter were counted for the ipsilateral and contralateral sides [9]. The motor neuron cell bodies were identified by their size and characteristic morphology. The injury epicenter was defined as the section with the fewest large motor neurons in the ipsilateral ventral grey matter.

Immunohistochemistry. Immunohistochemical analysis was performed both ipsilaterally and contralaterally to the unilateral injury at the injury epicenter as well as 1.05 mm caudal to the epicenter (Figure 1A–B). Sectioned tissue was thawed and dried at room temperature for an hour and then washed in TBS. Sections were blocked in 10% normal goat serum/0.2% Triton/TBS at room temperature for one hour followed by primary antibody incubation in 2% goat serum/0.5% Triton/TBS at 4°C overnight. Secondary antibody was incubated in 2% goat serum/0.5% Triton/TBS at room temperature for two hours. Primary and secondary antibodies used were rabbit polyclonal ΔfosB (IHC 1:100; Santa Cruz, USA) [30], rabbit polyclonal Ki67 (IHC 1:200; Abcam, USA) [31], mouse monoclonal GFAP (IHC 1:400, Sigma Aldrich, USA) [32], rabbit polyclonal GLT1 (IHC 1:800, kindly

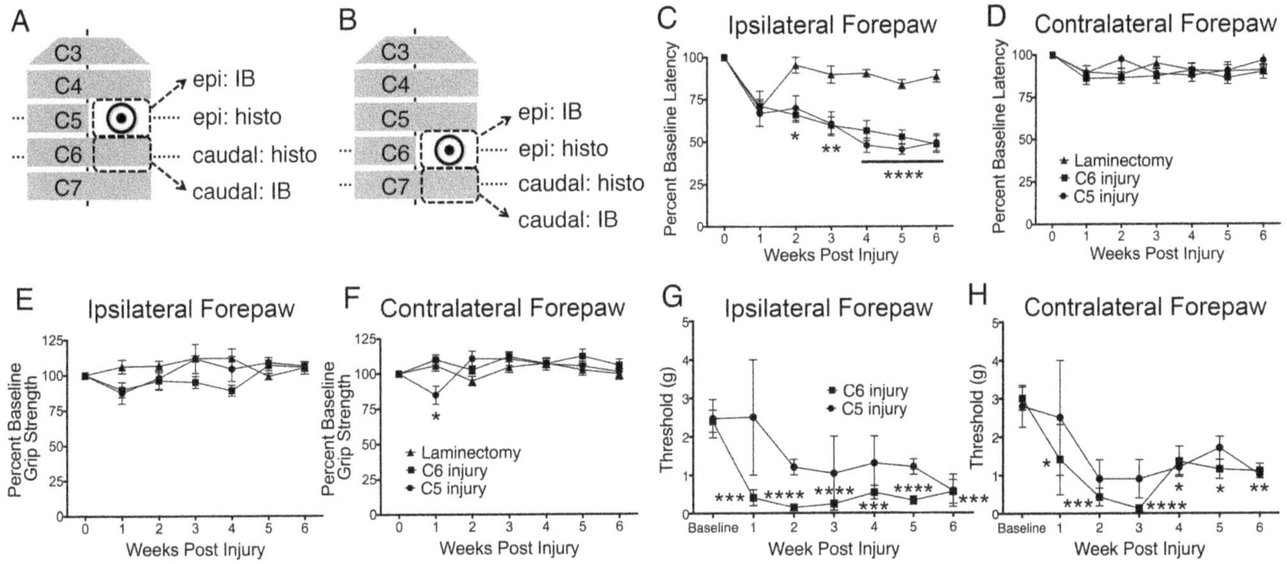

Figure 1. Animals receiving unilateral cervical contusion SCI exhibited persistent thermal hyperalgesia and tactile allodynia in the forepaw. Cervical contusion SCI was administered at the C5 or C6 level of the spinal cord while uninjured control animals received only laminectomy at the C6 level. Tissue from the level of laminectomy or epicenter of the injury and from the region immediately caudal was harvested for either immunoblotting or histology (A–B). Thermal hyperalgesia was measured using a modified version of the Hargreaves test. Animals receiving contusion injury showed a decrease in latency to withdrawal in the ipsilateral forepaw, measured as a percentage of baseline latency, compared to control animals (C). This difference was first observed at two weeks after injury and persisted until the animals were sacrificed at six weeks after injury. No change in withdrawal latency was seen in injured vs. uninjured animals in the contralateral forepaw (D). Animals receiving SCI were also tested for tactile allodynia using von Frey filament testing. In animals receiving C6 injury, but not C5 injury, a significant decrease compared to pre-injury baseline in the force threshold required to elicit a withdrawal response was evident both ipsilaterally (E) and contralaterally (F) for each of the six weeks following injury. The decrease in ipsilateral forepaw withdrawal latency and bilateral force threshold in injured animals occurred in the absence of changes in grip strength in either forepaw (G–H). Epi = epicenter; IB = immunoblotting; histo = histology; * = $p<0.05$; ** = $p<0.01$; **** = $p<0.0001$.

provided by Jeffrey Rothstein's lab at Johns Hopkins University) [29],, mouse monoclonal CD11b (IHC 1:4,000, AbD Serotec, USA), rhodamine-conjugated goat-anti-rabbit IgG (1:100; Jackson Immuno, USA) and FITC-conjugated goat-anti-mouse IgG (1:100; Jackson Immuno, USA).

Fluorescence Imaging and Quantification. Imaging and quantification of fluorescence immunostaining and BAC-GLT1-eGFP tissue were performed using a Zeiss Imager M2 upright fluorescence microscope [23]. Images were taken and analyses performed on saved PNG images for analyses. All immunostaining was quantified in the most superficial laminae (I–II) or lamina III of the spinal cord dorsal horn (Figure 2F–G). Laminae I–III were delineated by beginning at the most lateral portion of the dorsal horn, drawing a horizontal line across the gray matter, and following the outline of the gray matter back to the lateral extension of the dorsal horn. The border between laminae I–II and lamina III was identified by the change in tissue morphology represented by darker tissue in laminae I–II and lighter tissue in lamina III. Quantification analyses were performed using Metamorph software (Molecule Devices; Sunnyvale, CA). ΔfosB- and Ki67-positive cells were quantified by counting the stained nuclei in the superficial laminae. GFAP and GLT1 staining was more diffusely distributed and was therefore quantified in laminae I–II as an integrated intensity, or the sum of the intensity of pixels over a region, at constant exposure, brightness, and contrast. In BAC-GLT1-eGFP tissue, quantification was performed for laminae I–II and lamina III. eGFP-positive cells were counted separately for these regions [23].

Biochemical Analyses

Tissue Harvesting. Sacrifice occurred at two or six weeks after injury or laminectomy. Following anesthetic overdose, animals were perfused with 0.9% saline and the cervical spinal cord removed, dissected, and flash-frozen in dimethylbutane. The spinal cord was sub-dissected to collect the ipsilateral cord at the level of the injury and the segment directly caudal to the injury (Fig. 1A–B). To identify the regions of interest, the muscles were first removed to expose the spinal column. The laminectomy area was located, and the contralateral vertebral lamina was removed. Microdissection scissors were used to cut the spinal cord along the midline, and a 1.0 mm piece of tissue between the remaining laminae was collected. Flash-frozen tissue was stored at −80°C.

Western Blotting. Tissue samples were homogenized on ice in 50 µl of RIPA buffer containing 50 mM TRIS-HCl pH 7.6, 150 mM NaCl, 2 mM EDTA, 0.1% SDS, 0.01% NP-40, and Protease Inhibitor Cocktail (Roche Diagnostics, Indianapolis, IN). Protein concentration was determined by the Bradford assay, and equal amounts of protein were run on 4–12% Bis-Tris gels and transferred to nitrocellulose membranes. Odyssey blocking buffer (Li-Cor; Lincoln, NE) was used to block the membranes at room temperature for one hour. Primary antibodies for GLT1 (1:2,000) and actin (1:2,000; Abcam) were diluted in Odyssey blocking buffer and membranes were incubated at 4°C overnight. The membranes were then probed with IRDye-conjugated goat anti-rabbit or goat anti-mouse IgG (1:20,000; Li-Cor) at room temperature for one hour. Imaging was performed by the Li-Cor Odyssey infrared imaging system, and GLT1 band intensity was measured and normalized to actin band intensity using ImageJ software [22].

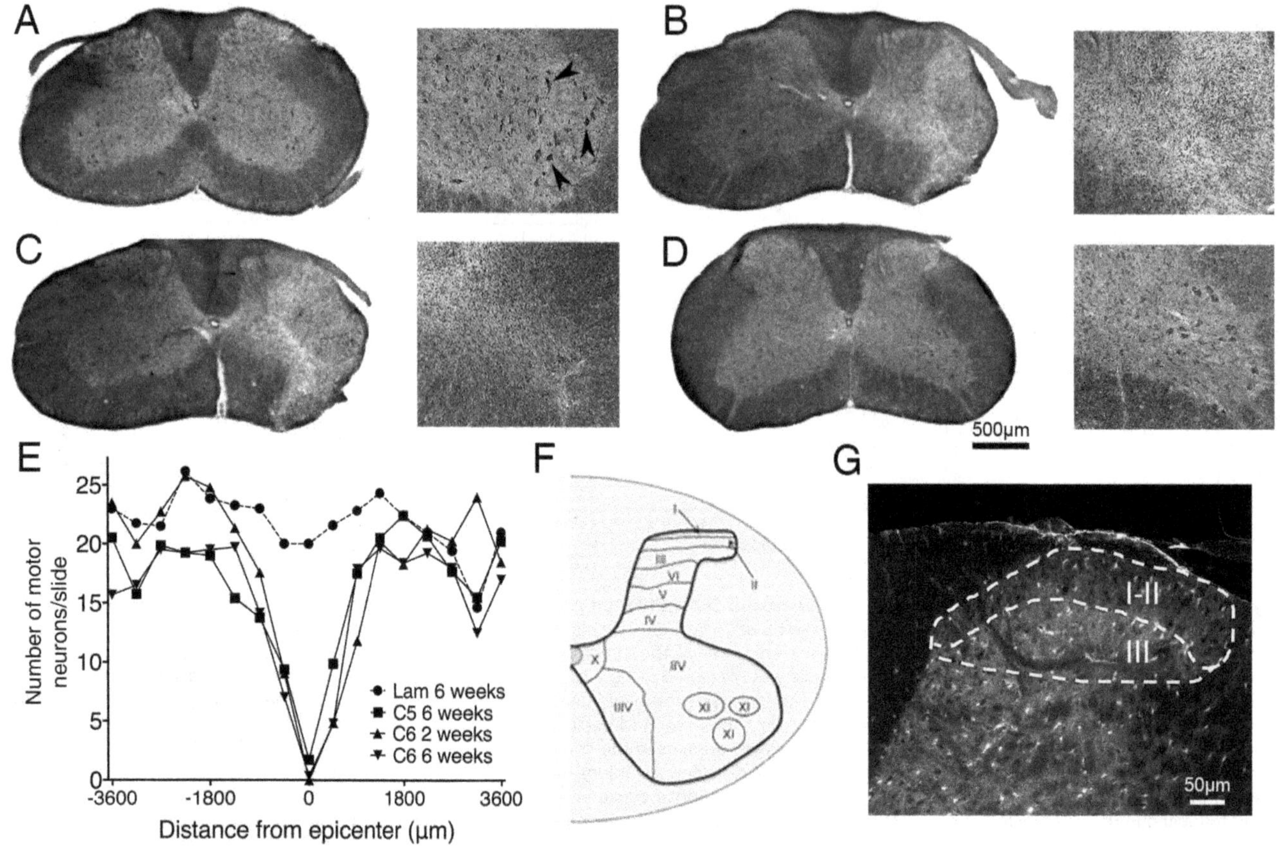

Figure 2. Unilateral contusion SCI induced a loss of ventral horn motor neurons at the injury epicenter. Harvested tissue was stained with Cresyl violet and Eriochrome cyanine. At the level of the laminectomy, uninjured control animals (A) exhibited large motor neurons in the ventral horn (arrowheads). At six weeks post-injury, animals receiving unilateral C5 (B) or C6 (C) contusion SCI showed a loss of these motor neurons at the injury epicenter but not 1.0 mm caudal to the injury (D). The spread of ventral horn motor neuron loss was approximately 1.0 mm rostrally and 1.0 mm caudally (2.0 mm total) from the epicenter (E). Immunohistochemical analyses of the injury models were performed in laminae I–II and lamina III of the cervical spinal cord dorsal horn (F–G). Lam = laminectomy.

Statistical Analyses

All data are presented as mean ± SEM. Statistical analyses were performed using GraphPad Prism (GraphPad Software, Inc.; La Jolla, CA). Bar graphs are presented as averages with error bars representing standard error. The Hargreaves test and von Frey threshold data were analyzed using a two-way ANOVA with repeated measured to compare the means within each group (laminectomy, C5 injury, or C6 injury) at each time point. The immunohistochemical and biochemical data were assessed with one-way ANOVA, comparing each group (laminectomy, C6 2 weeks, or C6 6 weeks) to one another. Statistical significance is defined as $p<0.05$ for all analyses.

Results

Robust and persistent forepaw thermal hyperalgesia and tactile allodynia were observed following unilateral cervical contusion SCI

Here we present a model of unilateral cervical contusion SCI in the mouse that exhibits persistent changes in pain behavior in the absence of motor deficits. Following baseline behavior testing, animals received unilateral laminectomy and contusion injury of 40 kilodyne of force with two seconds of dwell time at either the C5 (Fig. 1A) or C6 (Fig. 1B) level of the spinal cord. Control animals underwent laminectomy without injury. In both injury models, no grossly observable deficits in respiratory or other vital functions were present.

Beginning one week after injury, thermal hyperalgesia, tactile allodynia and grip strength were measured in laminectomy (n = 8) and injured animals (C5: n = 8; C6: n = 10) for six weeks. A modified version of the Hargreaves test was utilized to measure sensitivity to noxious thermal stimuli in the ipsilateral and contralateral forepaws. In both injured and uninjured animals, forepaw withdrawal upon noxious thermal stimulation was deliberate and was often accompanied by licking or scratching of the paw. Two-way ANOVA was used to compare withdrawal latency between animals with C5 injury, C6 injury, and laminectomy only at each time point. Post-injury measurements of latency to forepaw withdrawal are reported as a percentage of the baseline average for each animal. In laminectomy-only animals, withdrawal latency non-significantly decreased in the ipsilateral forepaw at one week post-injury but returned to and persisted at baseline levels until six weeks after injury (Fig. 1C). Beginning two weeks after injury and persisting for the length of testing, ipsilateral forepaw withdrawal latencies for animals receiving unilateral contusion SCI at the C5 or C6 level were significantly reduced compared to uninjured laminectomy animals (Fig. 1C). In the contralateral forepaw, no significant changes amongst the three experimental groups were seen (Fig. 1D).

In addition, tactile allodynia was assessed in C5 injured and C6 injured animals. The threshold force required to elicit a withdrawal response in each of the forepaws was measured by the von Frey test. In the C6 injury group, but not as robustly in the C5 injury group, tactile allodynia was evident (Fig. 1E–F). Animals were tested prior to injury to obtain baseline data and were then assessed for six weeks following injury. When values for each testing week were compared to pre-injury baseline data, animals receiving C6 injury exhibited a significant decrease in threshold force both ipsilaterally (Fig. 1E) and contralaterally (Fig. 1F). Although the data were not significant for animals receiving C5 injury, there was a similar trend in decreased response threshold.

While thermal and mechanical sensitivity increased in injured animals, this was not associated with changes in grip strength. Grip strength results were analyzed by two-way ANOVA to identify significance between each group at each time point. For the ipsilateral forepaw, no changes were observed between injured and uninjured animals for the six weeks following surgery (Fig. 1G). A significant decrease in contralateral grip strength for animals receiving injury at the C5 level was seen one week after injury compared to laminectomy or C6 injury (Fig. 1H). However, because the change occurred so soon after surgery and grip strength recovered to baseline levels by the next testing session, a spinal shock mechanism may be responsible for this unexpected change.

Together, the Hargreaves, von Frey, and grip strength data suggest hypersensitivity to noxious thermal and tactile stimuli in the absence of altered grip strength, indicating that the observed changes in forepaw withdrawal resulted from aberrant pain processing rather than motor deficits.

Unilateral cervical contusion SCI produced an injury characterized by a focal loss of ventral horn motor neurons

The animals that received unilateral contusion SCI exhibited loss of large motor neurons in the ventral grey matter as well as a disruption of lateral grey matter, dorsolateral funiculus, and ventrolateral funiculus of the ipsilateral hemicord (Fig. 2B–C). In laminectomy-only animals (n = 8), large motor neurons of distinct morphology were present throughout the ipsilateral ventral horn (Fig. 2A). These motor neurons were absent or their numbers were greatly reduced, however, at the injury site in animals receiving C5 (Fig. 2B; n = 8) or C6 (Fig. 2C; 2 weeks: n = 8; 6 weeks: n = 10) injury. This effect was limited to the injury site, as motor neuron populations and white matter were intact in regions rostral and caudal to the injury (Fig. 2D). Additionally, no loss of motor neurons was observed on the contralateral side of the spinal cord at any point along the rostral-caudal axis (data not shown). Thus, the anatomical disruption sustained by injured animals was restricted to the injury site ipsilaterally.

In order to quantify the contusion injury sustained by the animals and identify the injury epicenter along the rostral-caudal axis, sections were stained with Cresyl violet acetate/Eriochrome cyanine and motor neurons in the ventral horn were counted. The epicenter of the injury was determined by the extent of motor neuron loss, and the motor neuron counts were plotted by distance from this site (Fig. 2E). Significance was determined using one-way ANOVA to compare motor neuron counts between each group. Compared to laminectomy animals, a significant decrease in ventral horn motor neurons was observed for animals receiving injury at either cervical level and at both time points. The spread of both C5 and C6 injuries was approximately 2.0 mm (1.0 mm rostrally and 1.0 mm caudally from the epicenter) with a gradual decrease in motor neurons immediately rostral and caudal to the epicenter. The epicenter identified by this method was used for further immunohistochemical analyses of the neuronal and glial populations of the spinal cord dorsal horn, which were performed in laminae I–II and laminae III (Fig. 2F–G).

Chronic neuronal activation in the superficial laminae of the dorsal horn resulted from contusion SCI

Because injury at either the C5 or C6 level produced thermal hyperalgesia and tissue damage to a similar extent, we chose to move forward with a single model, the C6 injury, for further analyses. ΔfosB, a truncated splice version of the immediate early gene c-fos, is a transcription factor and marker of persistent neuronal activation. Chronic upregulation of this gene has been implicated in plasticity and inflammatory pain [14], [15] and has the potential to contribute to neuropathic pain. To study the extent of ΔfosB expression in our SCI model, we sacrificed animals at two weeks and six weeks after injury (n = 7–10) or six weeks after laminectomy (n = 8). Immunohistochemistry for ΔfosB was performed at the injury epicenter and 1.0 mm caudal to the injury in laminae I–II.

We found that ΔfosB-positive cells exhibited a defined pattern of nuclear staining in the superficial laminae. In our SCI model, we observed a persistent increase in the number of Δfos-expressing cells, suggesting chronic neuronal activation following cervical contusion injury. One-way ANOVA was used to compare the number of ΔfosB-positive cells between each group. Following laminectomy, limited-to-no ΔfosB expression was seen in the dorsal horn (Fig. 3A). Two weeks after injury (Fig. 3B), there was an increase in ΔfosB-positive cells on the ipsilateral side at and caudal to the injury epicenter. At six weeks (Fig. 3C), ΔfosB was upregulated bilaterally in the superficial laminae at the injury epicenter and 1.0 mm caudal. These changes are quantified in Figure 3D. The greatest increase in ΔfosB expression was observed at six weeks, suggesting that its expression was persistent and cumulative over time. Additionally, the expression of ΔfosB in the injured animals was specific to the dorsal horn of the spinal cord. There were few to no ΔfosB-positive cells in other regions of the spinal cord, including the ventral horn. This suggests that the effects of our injury paradigm on chronic neuronal activation were focal to the dorsal horn, an important region of the spinal cord for pain transmission and modulation.

Astrocytes were activated and proliferated in the dorsal horn of the spinal cord following cervical contusion SCI

Astrocytes play important protective and homeostatic roles in both the immediate and delayed response to CNS injury. Chronic activation in the spinal cord, however, can contribute to neuronal hyperexcitability of pain transmission neurons that underlies neuropathic pain [12], [13]. When astrocytes become activated, they express distinct proteins and in some cases proliferate [21]. In order to measure the spatial and temporal change in astrocyte activation in our model of SCI, we used immunohistochemistry to stain for GFAP, expressed by activated astrocytes, and Ki67, a marker of cellular proliferation. As in the previous immunohistochemical analyses, animals were studied two or six weeks after injury (n = 7–10) or six weeks after laminectomy (n = 8). For each analysis, one-way ANOVA was utilized to identify significance between the three groups.

Figure 4B shows the distinct morphology of activated astrocytes observed following injury compared to uninjured control (Fig. 4A). We found that injury induced diffuse GFAP expression throughout the gray matter of the spinal cord; therefore, we quantified astrocyte expression in laminae I–II by measuring GFAP intensity.

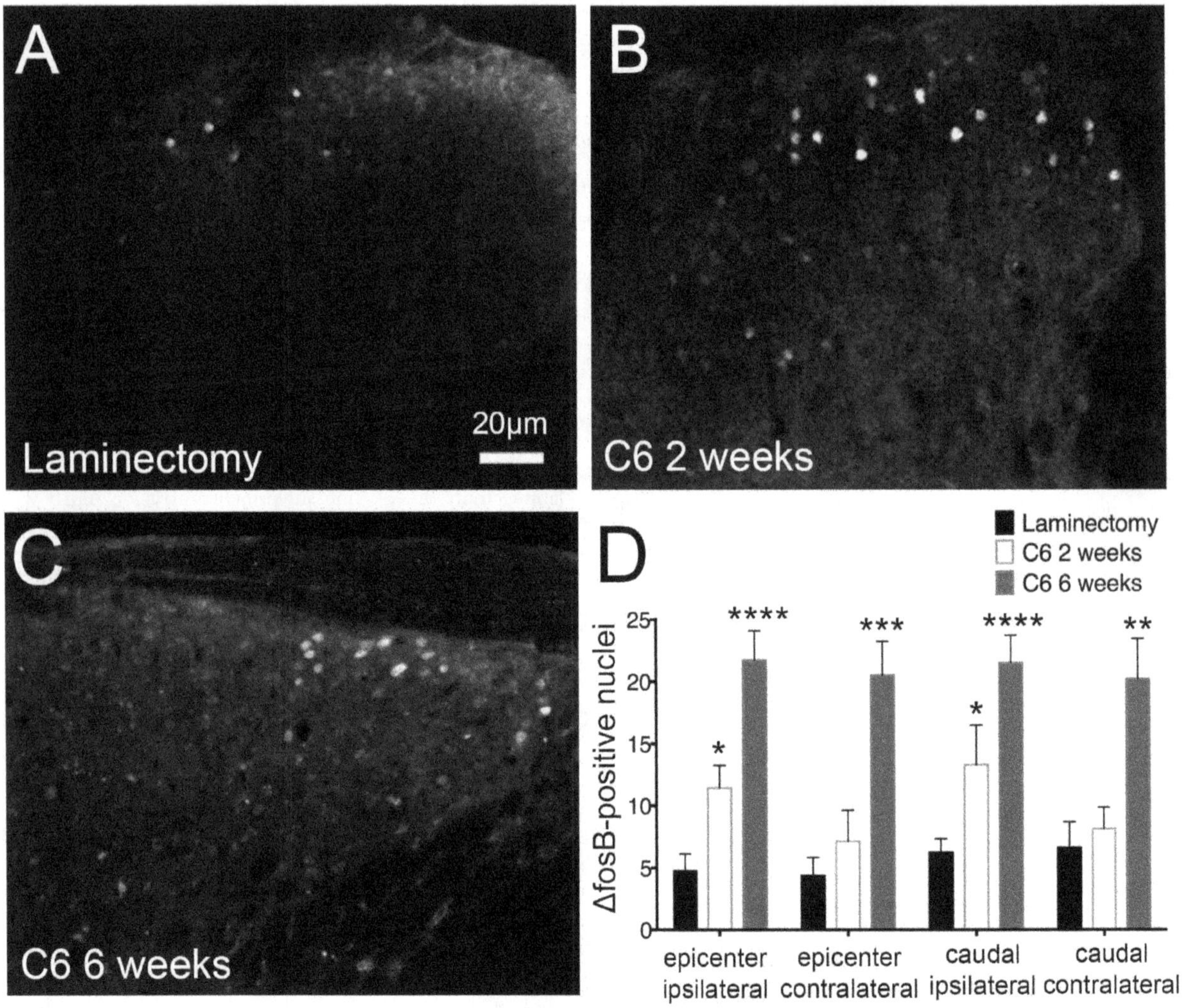

Figure 3. Chronic neuronal activation in the dorsal horn resulted from cervical contusion SCI. ΔfosB staining was used to measure the extent of persistent neuronal activation in the spinal cord. Following injury, ΔfosB-positive nuclei (arrowheads) were evident in laminae I–II (A–C). At all regions, laminectomy control animals (A) showed little-to-no ΔfosB expression (D). Two weeks after C6 injury (B), a significant increase in numbers of ΔfosB expressing cells in the superficial laminae of the ipsilateral dorsal horn was observed at the injury epicenter and caudal to the injury (D). ΔfosB levels were further increased at all regions in animals sacrificed six weeks post-injury (C, D). * = $p<0.05$; ** = $p<0.01$; *** = p 0.001; **** = $p<0.0001$.

Compared to laminectomy (Fig. 4C), GFAP intensity was significantly greater at both time points in animals receiving contusion SCI (Fig. 4D–E). These changes were observed ipsilaterally at the injury epicenter, with no alterations in GFAP expression at the other regions analyzed (Fig. 4F). GFAP expression was highest two weeks after injury, which suggests that, while post-injury astrocyte activation is chronic, it may lessen over time.

We next sought to study the extent of astrocyte proliferation in the dorsal horn to further support our assertion that astrocytes respond to the spinal cord insult we induced. We confirmed using confocal microscopy that, after injury, the majority of Ki67-expresing cells in the superficial were GFAP-positive astrocytes (Fig. 5A). Basally, proliferating cell numbers, and thus Ki67 expression, in the spinal cord were low (Fig. 5B). Two weeks following injury (Fig. 5C), the superficial laminae expressed a robust increase in bilateral Ki67 that was also seen in the ipsilateral dorsal horn caudal to the injury (Fig. 5E). At six weeks (Fig. 5D), an increase in Ki67 was also observed but did not reach the levels seen at two weeks.

We identified the phenotypes of these Ki67-positive proliferative cells. First, we quantified microglial activation in the superficial dorsal horn by immunostaining for CD11b (Fig. 5G–I). Like astrocytes, microglia play a role in both immediate and delayed responses to injury to the spinal cord and may contribute to the development of pathological pain (13). Compared to laminectomy (Fig. 5G), the intensity of CD11b expression was greater in animals with C6 SCI at both two (Fig. 5H–I) and six (Fig. 5I) weeks after injury. This increase was significant at the injury site both ipsilaterally and contralaterally, as well as caudal to the injury on the ipsilateral side (Fig. 5I).

We also quantified the percentage of Ki67-positive cells that were either GFAP-positive or CD11b-positive. This allowed us to determine if the proliferative cells are, in fact, astrocytes (GFAP-positive) or microglia (CD11b-positive). One-way ANOVA was used to identify significance in Ki67 and GFAP or CD11b colocalization. In laminectomy animals, the percentage of cells

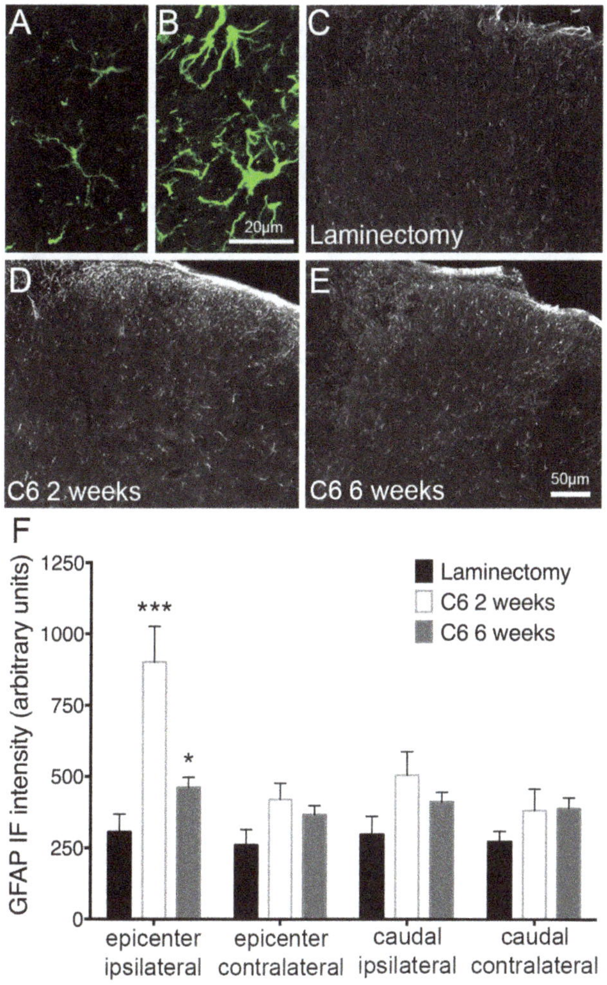

Figure 4. Astrocytes were activated and proliferated in the dorsal horn following cervical contusion SCI. Astrocyte activation in the superficial dorsal horn was characterized by quantification of GFAP expression in laminae I–II. (A) and (B) show representative images of dorsal horn GFAP expression at high magnification in laminectomy and injured animals, respectively. At the injury epicenter, compared to uninjured control animals (C), an increase in GFAP expression in the ipsilateral dorsal horn was evident at two (D) and six weeks (E) following injury. No significant changes in GFAP expression were observed at the other regions studied (F). IF = immunofluorescence; * = $p<0.05$; *** = $p<0.001$.

that are positive for both Ki67 and GFAP or CD11b is zero because there are no Ki67-positive cells present (Fig. 5F). At both two weeks and six weeks after C6 injury, there is a significant increase in the percentage of Ki67-positive cells that are also GFAP-positive or CD11b-positive (Fig. 5F). No significant difference exists between the percentage of Ki67-positive cells that are GFAP-positive or those that are CD11b-positive (Fig. 5F). Thus, both astrocytes and microglia are proliferative following cervical contusion SCI. These data further support the notion that activated astrocytes are present in the spinal cord following injury but retreat over time and/or that proliferation is mostly an early process of astrocyte activation post-SCI. The effects of astrocyte activation can be lasting, however, through the release of factors, for example, that can contribute to hyperexcitability.

Cervical contusion SCI led to reduced expression of GLT1 in the superficial dorsal horn of the spinal cord

The most abundant glutamate transporter in the CNS is GLT1, and its greatest expression is in astrocytes [33]. Through GLT1 and other glutamate transporters, astrocytes clear excitatory amino acids from the synapse after they are released, regulating glutamate's duration of action, controlling normal synaptic communication, and protecting cells from excitotoxic effects [33]. After SCI, we and others [23], [24], [25], [26] have reported a loss in astrocyte GLT1 expression. In this study, we utilized two animal models to study localized decreases in GLT1 in the context of neuropathic pain in the superficial dorsal horn.

In BAC-GLT1-eGFP reporter mice, the GLT1 promoter drives expression of eGFP [27]. Following injury, we sacrificed animals at two days (n = 7), two weeks (n = 9), and six weeks (n = 8) and quantified eGFP-positive cells separately in laminae I–II and lamina III. We used one-way ANOVA to compare the number of eGFP-positive cells at each time point. In uninjured animals (Fig. 6D; n = 6), eGFP expression was robust and widespread throughout the grey and white matter. Furthermore, almost all of the GFAP-expressing astrocytes in these regions co-localized with eGFP-positive cells (Fig. 6A–B). eGFP-positive cells were decreased, however, at two days, two weeks, and six weeks (Fig. 6E) at various regions in the spinal cord. Despite the increase in GFAP expression after injury, there were few cells co-expressing eGFP and GFAP, suggesting a loss of GLT1 expression in activated astrocytes (Fig. 6C). At the injury epicenter, eGFP expression was downregulated at two days ipsilaterally (Fig. 6F) and at all time points contralaterally in laminae I–II (Fig. 6G). In lamina III, a decrease in eGFP-positive cells was observed bilaterally at the injury epicenter (Fig. 6F–G). Caudal to the injury, we report a decrease in eGFP at all time points in laminae I–II and at two days and six weeks in lamina III (Fig. 6H). No changes in the contralateral dorsal horn caudal to the injury were observed (Fig. 6I).

In wild-type C57BL/6 animals, we employed immunohistochemical staining for GLT1 after C6 injury (n = 7–10) or laminectomy (n = 8). One-way ANOVA was used to identify significant differences in GLT1 staining between laminectomy, injured animals at 2 weeks, and injured animals at six weeks. Compared to laminectomy-only animals (Fig. 7A), animals receiving injury two weeks (Fig. 7B) or six weeks (Fig. 7C) prior to analysis showed a decrease in diffuse GLT1 protein expression in laminae I–II. These changes were seen at all regions analyzed (Fig. 7D). We further quantified the extent of GLT1 protein expression in injured (n = 7–8) and uninjured animals (n = 7) using immunoblotting techniques. At the injury epicenter, we observed a decrease in GLT1 protein in the ipsilateral hemicord at both time points after injury (Fig. 7E). Caudal to the injury, however, this glutamate transporter loss was not observed (Fig. 7F).

These data seem to contradict the immunohistochemical results we reported above. Thus, we performed immunohistochemical quantifications in regions outside of the superficial dorsal horn to try to identify the source of these contradictory results. At six weeks after injury, there is a significant loss of GLT1 expression in the ventral horn ipsilaterally at the epicenter compared to laminectomy animals (Fig. 7G). No significant change is seen in the ventral horn or white matter ipsilaterally caudal to the injury (Fig. 7G). These data suggest that, focally at the injury site, GLT1 loss occurs in multiple anatomical regions. However, caudal to the injury, the decrease in GLT1 expression may be more specific to the superficial dorsal horn (Fig. 7G). The changes in GLT1 from the immunoblotting data may not be evident due to the lack of anatomical specificity.

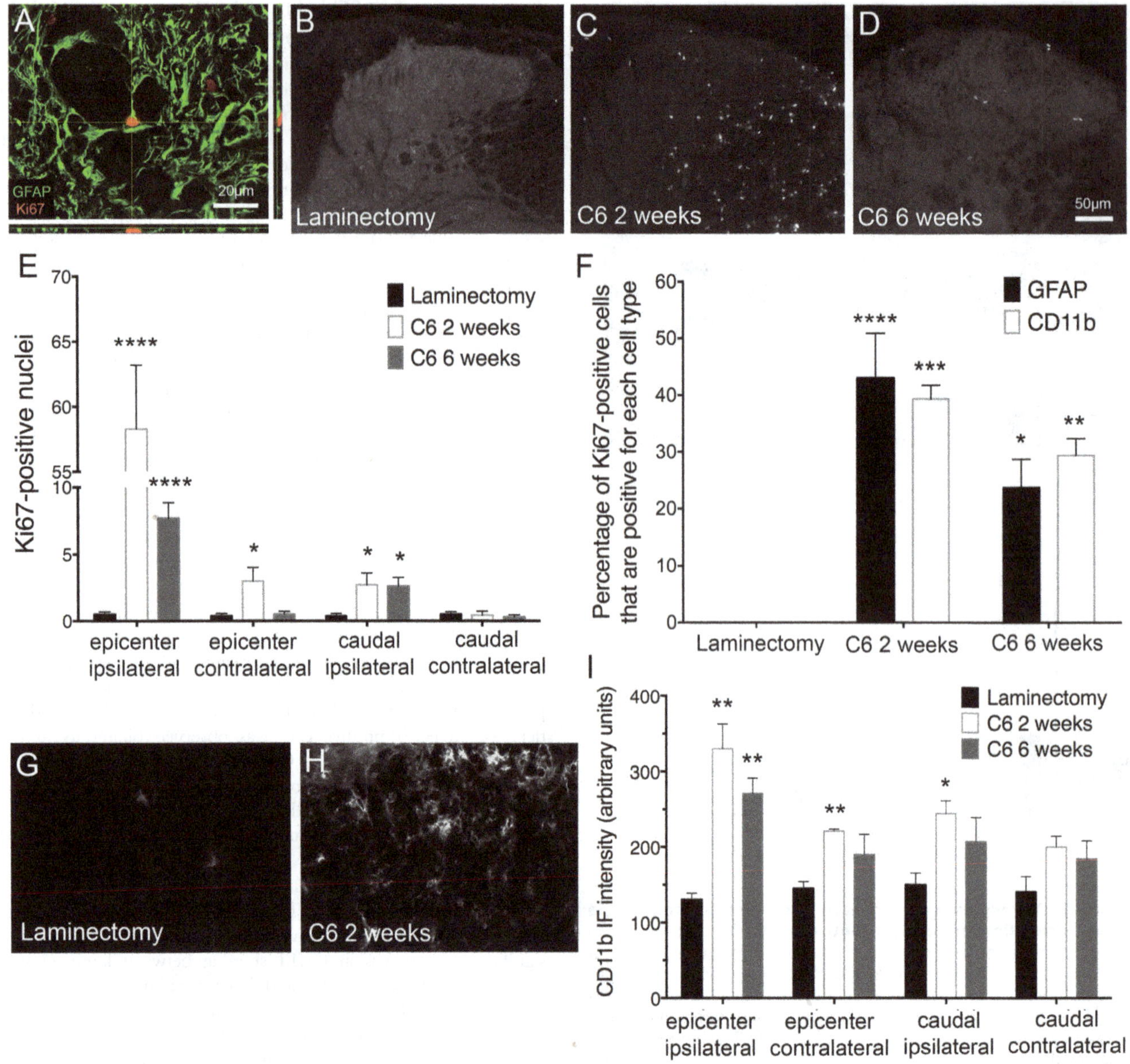

Figure 5. Enhanced cell proliferation, including proliferation of astrocytes, was evident after cervical contusion SCI. In the superficial laminae of the injured ipsilateral dorsal horn, we observed cells co-expressing GFAP and Ki67 (A), representing activated and proliferating astrocytes. In laminectomy control animals, little to no cell proliferation was evident (B). However, the number of Ki67-positive cells was significantly increased at two weeks (C) and six weeks (D) after injury on the ipsilateral side both at the level of and caudal to the injury (E). Additionally, at two weeks, there was a significant increase in proliferating cells contralaterally at the injury site (E). At both two and six weeks, a significant percentage of Ki67-positive cells were also either GFAP-positive or CD11b-positive (F). Compared to laminectomy (G), the intensity of CD11b expression in the superficial dorsal horn was greater in animals with C6 SCI at both two (H–I) and six (I) weeks after injury. This increase was significant at the injury site both ipsilaterally and contralaterally, as well as caudal to the injury on the contralateral side (I). * = $p<0.05$; ** = $p<0.01$; **** = $p<0.0001$.

Discussion

Here we describe changes in neuronal, astrocyte and microglial activation and GLT1 expression accompanying at-level thermal hyperalgesia in a cervical contusion SCI mouse model. In our model, robust and persistent thermal hyperalgesia and tactile allodynia are evident beginning one-two weeks after injury. Additionally, cervical contusion SCI induces an upregulation of ΔfosB, a marker of neuronal activity, in the superficial laminae of the dorsal horn. Astrocyte and microglial activation and proliferation, as measured by increases in GFAP, CD11b and Ki67 immunostaining, are also increased in these regions. We also observe a decrease in GLT1 expression and the number of GLT1-expressing cells in this model. These molecular changes that accompany hyperalgesia and allodynia in this study may contribute to the development of this aberrant pain response and represent important targets for better understanding the development of and treating neuropathic pain in SCI.

Hyperalgesia, defined as an increase in sensitivity to noxious stimuli, whether due to a decrease in pain threshold or an increase in response to stimuli above the pain threshold [36], is common in humans and is associated with sensory changes resulting from

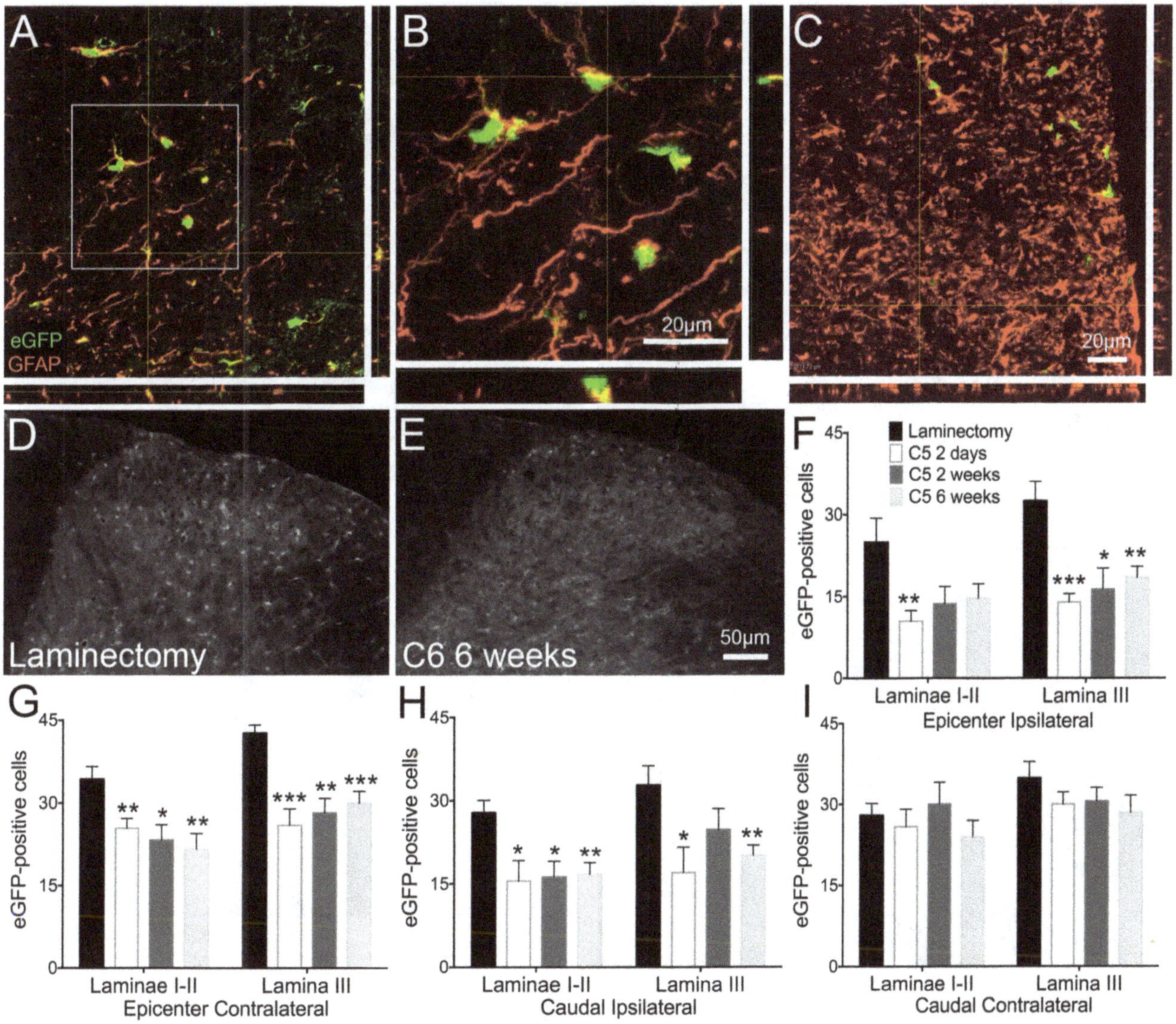

Figure 6. Astrocyte GLT1 promoter activity was reduced in injured BAC-GLT1-eGFP transgenic reporter mice. Following cervical contusion SCI, GLT1 expression/promoter activity, represented by eGFP-positive cells, was decreased in the superficial dorsal horn. In laminectomy animals, there were low levels of GFAP, although many of the cells that were GFAP-positive also expressed GLT1 (A–B). Following injury, however, an increase in GFAP was observed, but fewer of these activated astrocytes co-expressed GLT1 (C). Laminectomy control animals (D) had greater numbers of eGFP-positive cells compared to animals that received contusion injury two days, two weeks, or six weeks (E) prior to analysis. This decrease in GLT1 expression was observed at the injury epicenter in both the ipsilateral (F) and contralateral (G) superficial laminae as well as caudal to the injury on the ipsilateral side (H). No change in the number of eGFP-positive cells was found caudal to the injury on the contralateral side (I). * = $p<0.05$; ** = $p<0.01$; *** = p 0.001.

neuronal hyperexcitability [34], [35]. In mice, hyperalgesia in response to thermal stimuli can be measured using the Hargreaves test, in which a noxious infrared heat stimulus is placed under the paw and the paw withdrawal is recorded. In the models presented here, we observe thermal hyperalgesia in the ipsilateral forepaw beginning two weeks following cervical contusion SCI and persisting for the duration of the experiment. This is consistent with data from other groups, which report the development of hyperalgesia between two and three weeks after contusion SCI at various spinal levels in the mouse [37], [38] [39]. In the rat, our group and others observed thermal hyperalgesia as early as one week after cervical contusion injury [24], [40].

Like injured animals, laminectomy control animals show a decrease in withdrawal latency one week after surgery in the ipsilateral forepaw. This finding was unexpected, but not previously unreported. The development of post-laminectomy pain has been studied in the context of the extent of laminectomy, spinal deformation, and the loss of spinal stability following surgery [41], [42]. Researchers also showed that minimal laminectomy can induce transient hyperalgesic behavior at about one week after surgery [41]. While the cause of this pain behavior is unknown, it could reflect peripheral changes or spinal deformity rather than central sensitization or only transient central sensitization.

The ipsilateral development of thermal hyperalgesia in the mouse after SCI is consistent with the injury we see histologically. At the site of the injury, we observe a loss of ventral horn motor neurons and a disruption of normal tissue anatomy on the ipsilateral but not contralateral side. This suggests a disruption of

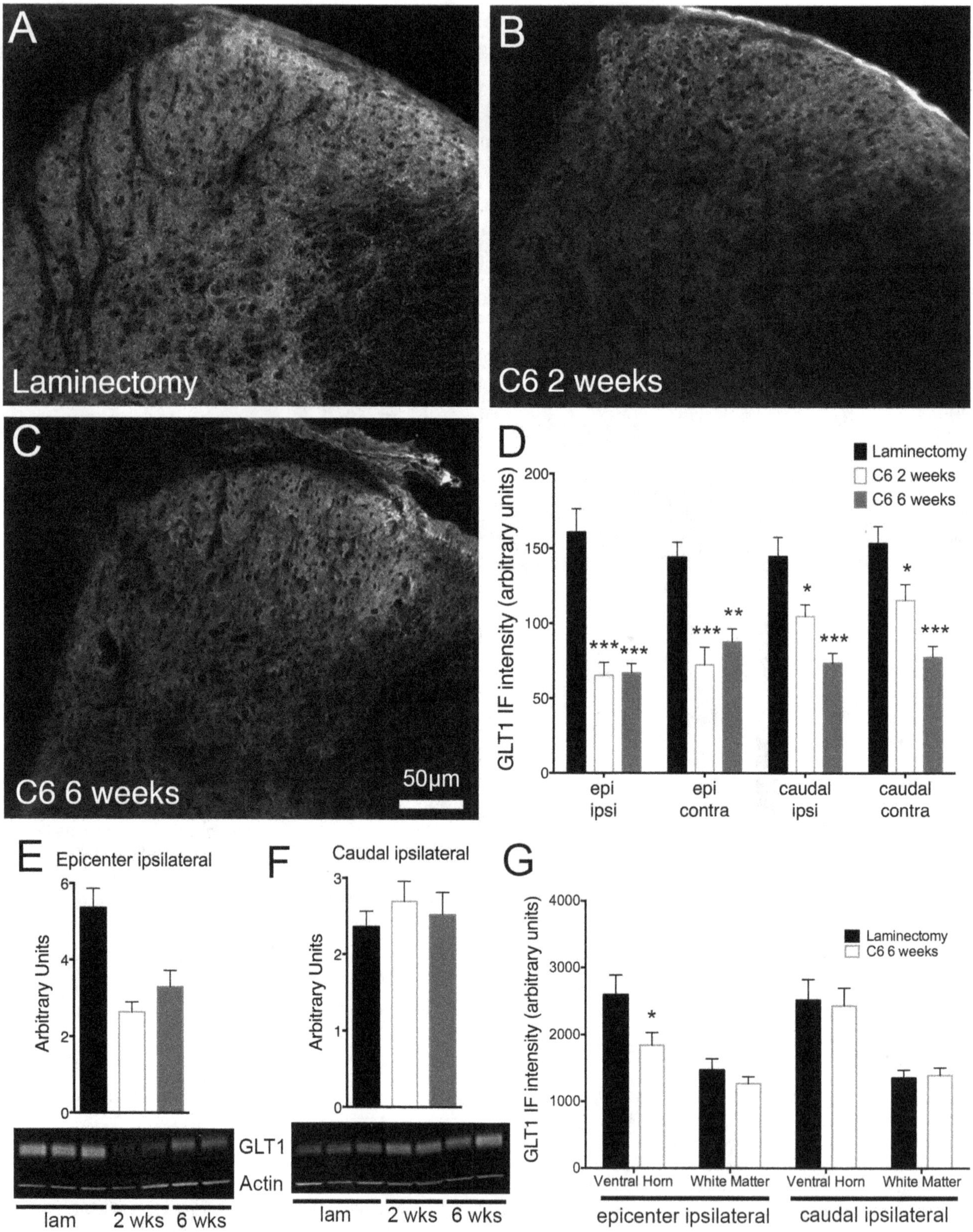

Figure 7. Cervical contusion SCI resulted in decreased astrocyte GLT1 expression in the dorsal horn. Immunohistochemical analysis revealed a decrease in GLT1 protein expression two (B) and six weeks (C) after cervical contusion SCI compared to laminectomy (A). This downregulation of the glutamate transporter was seen in the superficial dorsal horn on both sides of the spinal cord both at the injury site and caudal to the injury (D). Immunoblots of spinal cord tissue also showed a significant loss of GLT1 expression on the ipsilateral side at both time points following injury. However, this difference was seen only at the epicenter (E) and not caudal to the injury (F). Representative immunoblots are shown for each region (E–F). Analysis of GLT1 levels in regions of the spinal cord other than the superficial laminae at six weeks after injury reveal a loss of GLT1 expression in the ventral horn at the epicenter with no changes caudal to the injury (G). IF = immunofluorescence; epi = epicenter; ipsi = ipsilateral; contra = contralateral; lam = laminectomy; * = $p<0.05$; ** = $p<0.01$; *** = p 0.001.

pain transmission circuitry on the side of the injury, which may contribute to the hyperalgesia in the ipsilateral forepaw displayed by injured animals. The unilateral extent of the injury is also consistent with previous findings from our group; we previously reported damage to the ipsilateral dorsolateral and ventrolateral funiculi that did not extend bilaterally following moderate unilateral cervical SCI [10].

Unlike other studies [40], [44], we observe thermal hyperalgesia ipsilaterally but not contralaterally to the site of the injury. This discrepancy may reflect the modified version of the Hargreaves test that we utilized compared to these other groups. The Hargreaves test is most often used to measure thermal hyperalgesia in the hindpaw rather than the forepaw. Despite attempts to perform the Hargreaves test without restraint, including changes to the environment and longer acclimation times, we were unable to obtain reliable results. To overcome these difficulties, we restrained the mice in a way that did not impede forepaw movement but ensured that the mice remained still long enough to respond to the thermal stimulus. This method was introduced previously by Menendez, Lastra, Hidalgo, and Baamonde [28] for the study of hyperalgesia in the mouse forepaw. While the restraint improved the reliability of our thermal hyperalgesia measures, however, it may have affected the sensitivity of the mice to pain, which could have influenced the results we observed contralaterally.

Interestingly, while the hyperalgesia behavior changes we see are limited to the injured side of the spinal cord, we observe some molecular changes both ipsilaterally and contralaterally. ΔfosB and Ki67 expression is increased and GLT1 levels are decreased contralaterally after injury. The one alteration that is present ipsilaterally but not contralaterally is the activation of astrocytes. One possible explanation for the lack of hyperalgesic behavior in the contralateral forepaw is that the molecular changes we see are all required to elicit changes in pain behavior. There may be some interaction between activated neurons and glia that can disrupt pain transmission in the superficial laminae of the spinal cord following injury. Without activation of glia, pain transmission may continue normally.

Using von Frey filament testing, we assessed tactile allodynia following SCI. Allodynia, defined as a pain response to a previously non-noxious stimulus, is a common form of neuropathic pain [34]. In our model, we were able to identify allodynia following injury compared to baseline in the C6 injury group, but a similar significant effect was not observed in animals receiving C5 injury. We observed persistent tactile allodynia in both forepaws, which unlike the thermal testing results coincides with the anatomy of the histological findings.

Both hyperalgesia and allodynia are evoked pain behaviors in that they require a stimulus, whether noxious or non-noxious. We did not, however, study spontaneous pain, meaning pain that occurs in the absence of an external stimulus [43]. Spontaneous pain could potentially result, for example, from spontaneous activity in dorsal horn nociceptive neurons. Furthermore, while we measured at-level pain in the forepaw, we did not investigate below-level pain, which describes pain in dermatomes caudal to the level of injury and has been observed in the hindpaws of rats receiving cervical contusion SCI [40].

In this study, changes in pain behavior are exhibited in the absence of changes in motor behavior, as measured by grip strength. Because measures of evoked pain, such as the Hargreaves test and von Frey test, rely on motor activity (i.e. forepaw withdrawal) as a response, any dysfunction in motor behavior could affect test outcomes. The decrease in grip strength seen in the contralateral forepaw of C5 injury animals at one-week post injury was unexpected and could reflect transient local changes to the cervical spinal cord rather than a global alteration of pain transmission circuitry. Importantly, grip strength returns to baseline levels after this first week, at which point hyperalgesia and allodynia have developed.

Despite the maintenance of forepaw grip strength, we observed a significant loss of ventral horn motor neurons at the injury epicenter on the ipsilateral side following injury. One likely explanation for this disconnect is that our current injury model is milder and results in less motor neuron loss compared to our previous unilateral cervical contusion model in the mouse [9], which did produce persistent forelimb motor dysfunction. There is presumably some level of motor neuron loss necessary to result in quantifiable motor deficits.

At the molecular level, changes in ΔfosB and GLT1 were observed in the superficial dorsal horn of the injured spinal cord of our SCI model. Alterations in the expression of these proteins may contribute to central sensitization of pain transmission neurons in the cervical spinal cord. Central sensitization, including post-translational and transcriptional changes to dorsal horn neurons, affects the output of nociceptive neurons and the way in which peripheral stimuli are perceived. Thus, the observed changes may contribute to the hyperalgesic and allodynic phenotypes seen in our cervical contusion SCI.

C-fos is a member of the Fos family of transcription factors, which are induced quickly and transiently by a variety of stimuli. Because its expression is stimulated by an influx of calcium into neurons, c-fos acts as a marker of neuronal activity [45]. Previously, researchers have shown an induction of c-fos expression in the dorsal horn of the spinal cord following exposure to noxious stimuli in various forms [46],[47], [48], [49], [50]. ΔfosB is a truncated splice variant of the Fos family member, FosB. Unlike c-fos, which is expressed quickly but returns to basal levels within hours after stimulation, ΔfosB is induced gradually and is stable, so it accumulates over time and persists on the order of weeks or months [50]. ΔfosB has been implicated in a number of processes in the nervous system, including addiction, plasticity, and stress [45], [50] but may also play a role in neuronal changes associated with pain [14], [15].

In our SCI model, we see long-term elevation in the levels of ΔfosB in the superficial dorsal horn of the spinal cord, suggesting persistently increased activation of these neurons. These results are in accordance with another study that reported an increase in ΔfosB expression following pain induction, specifically carrageenan-induced inflammation [14]. Additionally, we previously reported an increase in ΔfosB expression in the rat following cervical contusion SCI [24]. While ΔfosB expression is significantly increased ipsilaterally at two weeks after injury, there is an even greater increase that spreads bilaterally at the six-week time point. This is consistent with the protein's stability and tendency to accumulate over time [46]. Furthermore, this persistent expression of the protein in the dorsal horn suggests an increase in the activity of these nociceptive neurons, possibly due to an increase in spontaneous firing and/or synaptic input, which may contribute to central sensitization. Thus the expression of ΔfosB that we see in our injury model is likely in accordance with its role in pain and plasticity.

In the nucleus accumbens and cortex, identified targets of ΔfosB include GluA2 and GluN1. In these regions, ΔfosB has been shown to upregulate these two proteins [50]. These targets are subunits of the glutamate receptors AMPAR and NMDAR, and their upregulation may contribute to increased glutamatergic transmission. Excessive stimulation of glutamate receptors can lead to hyperexcitability directly by increased activation of dorsal horn neurons and indirectly via glutamate excitotoxic loss of inhibitory interneurons [18]. It is unknown whether ΔfosB also targets these AMPAR and NMDAR subunits in the spinal cord following SCI. However, researchers have reported changes in GluA1 trafficking and expression in spinal neurons following central and peripheral injury and pain [51], [52], [53] as well as an upregulation of GluN1 and GluN2A in the ventral horn as a result of contusion SCI [54]. Despite this potential connection between ΔfosB and glutamate receptor subunits, ΔfosB does not definitively measure hyperexcitability. Instead, a continuation of this experiment to provide more conclusive evidence of the hyperexcitability could include electrophysiological measures of dorsal horn neurons.

Also following injury, we observe an increase in GFAP, a protein upregulated in activated astrocytes, in the dorsal horn of the spinal cord. We see this change at both time points, but it is more pronounced two weeks after injury. These data are in accordance with our group and others who have shown localized increases in markers of astrocyte activation following SCI [23], [24], [55], [56]. The observed increase in GFAP is seen only at the injury epicenter on the ipsilateral side, suggesting that this change is region-specific and may not play a role in potential above- or below-level changes, at least in our model.

The increase in activated astrocytes in our model of SCI could potentially have negative effects on the injured spinal cord and pain transmission circuitry. Often, activated astrocytes in the context of SCI and other injuries are considered detrimental because of their role in the formation of the glial scar, which can inhibit axon regeneration and plasticity, and the release of pro-inflammatory and other harmful molecules that can alter the excitability of neurons. Astrocytes, however, play many beneficial roles in the CNS, such as maintaining extracellular ion and neurotransmitter homeostasis, providing neurotrophic factor support, aiding in metabolic functions, and regulating the formation and maintenance of synapses [57].

Interestingly, while at-level thermal hyperalgesia is maintained through six weeks after injury, GFAP levels decrease slightly by this time point. Activated astrocytes play a significant role in the structural and molecular maintenance of the injury site [13], [17], [18], [57], [58]. The repair process following spinal cord injury, however, occurs in various phases, including acute, sub-acute, and chronic. While the effects of the glial scar and other repair processes can last months or years, not all of the molecules contributing to post-injury repair may be present at all stages. Thus, some astrocytes may return to the basal state in the days or weeks following injury, explaining the decrease in GFAP we see at six weeks compared to two weeks. Another explanation for the persistence of thermal hyperalgesia and tactile allodynia despite GFAP levels decreasing is that the loss of GLT1 also persists and contributes more strongly to the development of neuropathic pain after SCI. Alternatively, there may be irreversible damage to the spinal cord at this point that the inactivation of astrocytes may have no effect on.

Considering the various roles that astrocytes play following injury, it is important not only to study the reactive state of astrocytes in our model but also the effects of our injury on important homeostatic and protective functions of astrocytes. In light of this, we decided to investigate how our injury paradigm alters a centrally important function of astrocytes in the CNS, the uptake of glutamate through GLT1. Several groups have reported decreases in GLT1 levels following SCI [22], [23], [24], [25], [26], but the role of such changes has not been studied extensively in the context of neuropathic pain. To study GLT1 expression, we utilized both C57BL/6 wild-type and BAC-GLT1-eGFP reporter mice as well as both immunohistochemistry and western blotting. In our mouse cervical contusion SCI model, GLT1 levels are diminished in the dorsal horn at both time points at the epicenter and caudally on the ipsilateral side, suggesting a significant compromise in glutamate clearance in the injured spinal cord. Unlike with wild-type mice, in BAC-GLT1-eGFP mice, we see no change in the caudal contralateral region of the dorsal horn. This is likely due to a slightly different injury used in these two mouse paradigms.

Western blotting reveals that GLT1 protein levels are decreased ipsilaterally at the epicenter. However, no change in GLT1 levels is observed at the caudal ipsilateral region, which is contrary to the results we report using immunohistochemistry. This discrepancy likely reflects the difference in spatial resolution between these two techniques. Using immunohistochemistry, analyses of very specific regions, such as the superficial dorsal horn, are possible. For western blotting, however, we use a piece of tissue that encompasses an entire spinal cord level, including both the dorsal and ventral horn and surrounding white matter tracts. For our immunohistochemical analyses of the injured spinal cord, we examined the most superficial laminae of the dorsal horn, laminae I–II, as well as laminae III.

Importantly, co-localization analyses of GFAP and GLT1-eGFP at high-magnification reveal that, in control animals, most of the GLT1-positive cells are also GFAP-positive astrocytes. However, after injury, while the number of GFAP-positive cells is increased, the number and percentage of these astrocytes also expressing GLT1 is greatly reduced. This suggests that the loss of GLT1 that is observed in our animals occurs mostly in astrocytes, supporting our proposal that astrocytes activated after injury are deficient in glutamate clearance.

Like astrocytes, microglia play a major role in both immediate and delayed responses to injury to the spinal cord and may contribute to the development of pathological pain [13]. We also noted significant microglial activation in the superficial dorsal horn following cervical contusion SCI. Unlike astrocyte reactivity, we observed microglial activation not just at the ipsilateral epicenter region, but also at contralateral epicenter and caudal ipsilateral locations. Though we focused mostly on astrocyte changes, including down-regulation of GLT1 expression, it is likely that microglial activation also played a significant role in the persistent neuropathic pain phenotype observed in this study.

Here we present a model of unilateral cervical contusion SCI in the mouse that is representative of typical injury seen clinically in humans [1], [5]. The model exhibits at-level neuropathic pain accompanied by relevant molecular changes in the superficial dorsal horn. The protein expression changes suggest the presence of activated and proliferating astrocytes and a loss of GLT1 function, which may contribute to central sensitization, and underlie the development of neuropathic pain. We have identified a number of proteins that are altered by SCI and accompany thermal hyperalgesia and tactile allodynia, but their roles in the development of neuropathic pain have yet to be fully elucidated. Further research with the model may include identifying the factors and processes underlying the formation and maintenance of neuropathic pain in the spinal cord as well as recognizing targets for the treatment of chronic pathological pain resulting from SCI and similar injuries. Importantly, the availability of this model in the mouse allow for the use of valuable transgenic tools.

Acknowledgments

We would like to thank Drs. Luis Menéndez and Ana Baamonde for their assistance in the thermal testing procedures. We would also like to thank Dr. Jeannie Chin, Dr. Anupam Hazra and Brain Corbett for their advice and technical help with ΔFosB immunohistochemistry. Additionally, J.W.

would like to thank the members of her thesis committee, Dr. Piera Pasinelli and Dr. Lorraine Iacovitti, for their guidance and support.

Author Contributions

Conceived and designed the experiments: JLW ACL. Performed the experiments: JLW TJH RP DS ACL. Analyzed the data: JLW TJH RP DS ACL. Wrote the paper: JLW ACL.

References

1. National Spinal Cord Injury Statistical Center, University of Birmingham, Alabama (2013) Spinal cord injury facts and figures at a glance. Available: https://www.nscisc.uab.edu/PublicDocuments/fact_figures_docs/Facts%202013.pdf.
2. de Miguel M, Kraychete DC (2009) Pain in patients with spinal cord injury: A review. Rev Bras Anestheiol 59: 350–357.
3. Siddall PJ, McClelland JM, Rutkowski SB, Cousins MJ (2003) A longitudinal study of the prevalence and characteristics of pain in the first 5 years following spinal cord injury. Pain 103: 249–257.
4. Ravenscroft A, Ahmed YS, Burnside IG (2000) Chronic pain after SCI: A patient survey. Spinal Cord 38: 611–614.
5. McDonald JW, Becker D (2003) Spinal cord injury: Promising interventions and realistic goals. Am J Phys Med Rehabil 82: S38–S49.
6. Nakae A, Nakai K, Yano K, Hosokawa K, Shibata M, et al. (2011) The animal model of spinal cord injury as an experimental pain model. J Biomed Biotechnol 2011: 939023.
7. Kundi S, Bicknell R, Ahmed Z (2013) Spinal cord injury: Current mammalian models. Am J Neurosci 4: 1–12.
8. Nicaise C, Hala TJ, Frank DM, Parker JL, Authelet M, et al. (2012) Phrenic motor neuron degeneration compromises phrenic axonal circuitry and diaphragm activity in a unilateral cervical contusion model of spinal cord injury. Exp Neurol 235: 539–552.
9. Nicaise C, Putatunda R, Hala TJ, Regan KA, Frank DM, et al. (2012) Degeneration of phrenic motor neurons induces long-term diaphragm deficits following mid-cervical spinal contusion in mice. J Neurotrauma 29: 2748–2760.
10. Nicaise C, Frank DM, Hala TJ, Authelet M, Pochet R, et al. (2013) Early phrenic motor neuron loss and transient respiratory abnormalities after unilateral cervical spinal cord contusion. J Neurotrauma 30: 1092–1099.
11. Streijger F, Beernink TM, Lee JH, Bhatnagar T, Park S, et al. (2013) Characterization of a cervical spinal cord hemicontusion injury in mice using the infinite horizon impactor. J Neurotrauma 30: 869–883.
12. Latremoliere A, Woolf CJ (2009) Central sensitization: A generator of pain hypersensitivity by central neural plasticity. J Pain 10: 895–926.
13. Hulsebosch CE, Hains BC, Crown ED, Carlton SM (2009) Mechanisms of chronic central neuropathic pain after spinal cord injury. Brain Res Rev 60: 202–213.
14. Luis-Delgado OE, Barrot M, Rodeau JL, Ulery PG, Freund-Mercier MJ, et al. (2006) The transcription factor deltafosB is recruited by inflammatory pain. J Neurochem 98: 1423–1431.
15. Pareek TK, Kulkarni AB (2006) Cdk5: A new player in pain signaling. Cell Cycle 5: 585–588.
16. Clarke LE, Barres BA (2013) Emerging roles of astrocytes in neural circuit development. Nat Rev Neurosci 14: 311–321.
17. Karimi-Abdolrezaee S, Billakanti R (2012) Reactive astrogliosis after spinal cord injury: Beneficial and detrimental effects. Mol Neurobiol 46: 251–264.
18. Nakagawa T, Kaneko S (2010) Spinal astrocytes as therapeutic targets for pathological pain. J Pharmacol Sci
19. Chen CJ, Liao SL, Kuo JS (2000) Gliotoxic action of glutamate on cultured astrocytes. J Neurochem 74: 1557–1565.
20. Mark LP, Prost RW, Ulmer JL, Smith MM, Daniels DL, et al. (2001) Pictorial review of glutamate excitotoxicity: Fundamental concepts for neuroimaging. AJNR Am J Neuroradiol 22: 1813–1824.
21. Doble A (1999) The role of excitotoxicity in neurodegenerative disease: Implications for therapy. Pharmacol Ther 81: 163–221.
22. Lepore AC, O'Donnell J, Kim AS, Yang EJ, Tuteja A, et al. (2011) Reduction in expression of the astrocyte glutamate transporter, GLT1, worsens functional and histological outcomes following traumatic spinal cord injury. Glia 59: 1996–2005.
23. Lepore AC, O'Donnell J, Bonner JF, Paul C, Miller ME, et al. (2011) Spatial and temporal changes in promoter activity of the astrocyte glutamate transporter GLT1 following traumatic spinal cord injury. J Neurosci Res 89: 1001–1017.
24. Putatunda R, Hala TJ, Chin J, Lepore AC (2014) Chronic at-level thermal hyperalgesia following rat cervical contusion spinal cord injury is accompanied by neuronal and astrocyte activation and loss of the astrocyte glutamate transporter, GLT1, in superficial dorsal horn. Brain Res: in press.
25. Vera-Portocarrero LP, Mills CD, Ye Z, Fullwood SD, McAdoo DJ, et al. (2002) Rapid changes in expression of glutamate transporters after spinal cord injury. Brain Res 927: 104–110.
26. Olsen ML, Campbell SC, McFerrin MB, Floyd CL, Sontheimer H (2010) Spinal cord injury causes a wide-spread, persistent loss of Kir4.1 and glutamate transporter 1: Benefit of 17 beta-oestradiol treatment. Brain 133: 1013–1025.
27. Regan MR, Huang YH, Kim YS, Dykes-Hoberg ML, Jin L, et al. (2007) Variations in promoter activity reveal a differential expression and physiology of glutamate transporters by glia in the developing and mature CNS. J Neurosci 27: 6607–6619.
28. Menendez L, Lastra A, Hidalgo A, Baamonde (2002) Unilateral hot plate test: a simple and sensitive method for detecting central and peripheral hyperalgesia in mice. J Neurosci Methods 113: 91–97.
29. Lepore AC, Rauck B, Dejea C, Pardo AC, Rao MS, et al. (2008) Focal transplantation-based astrocyte replacement is neuroprotective in a model of motor neuron disease. Nat Neurosci 11: 1294–1301.
30. Perrotti LI, Weaver RR, Robison B, Renthal W, Maze I, et al. (2008) Distinct patterns of DeltaFosB induction in brain by drugs of abuse. Synapse 62: 358–369.
31. Lepore AC, Dejea C, Carmen J, Rauck B, Kerr DA, et al. (2008). Selective ablation of proliferating astrocytes does not affect disease outcome in either acute or chronic models of motor neuron degeneration. Exp Neurol 211: 423–432.
32. Lepore AC, Fischer I. (2005) Lineage-restricted neural precursors survive, migrate, and differentiate following transplantation into the injured adult spinal cord. Exp Neurol 194: 230–242.
33. Maragakis NJ, Rothstein JD (2001) Glutamate transporters in neurologic disease. Arch Neurol 58: 365–370.
34. Jorum E, Warncke T, Stubhaug A (2003) Cold allodynia and hyperalgesia in neuropathic pain: The effect of N-methyl-D-aspartate (NMDA) receptor antagonist ketamine–double-blind, cross-over comparison with alfentanil and placebo. Pain 101: 229–235.
35. Gwak YS, Hulsebosch CE (2011) Neuronal hyperexcitability: A substrate for central neuropathic pain after spinal cord injury. Curr Pain Headache Rep 15: 215–222.
36. Sandkuhler J (2009) Models and mechanisms of hyperalgesia and allodynia. Physiol Rev 89: 707–758.
37. Hoschouer EL, Basso DM, Jakeman LB (2010) Aberrant sensory responses are dependent on lesion severity after spinal cord contusion injury in mice. Pain 148: 328–342.
38. Mesiner JG, Marsh AD, Marsh DR (2010) Loss of GABAergic interneurons in laminae I–III of the spinal cord dorsal horn contributes to reduced GABAergic tone and neuropathic pain after spinal cord injury. J Neurotrauma 27: 729–737.
39. Hoschouer EL, Yin FQ, Jakeman LB (2009) L1 cell adhesion molecule is essential for the maintenance of hyperalgesia after spinal cord injury. Exp Neurol 216: 22–34.
40. Detloff MR, Wade ER Jr, Houle JD (2013) Chronic at- and below-level pain after moderate unilateral cervical spinal cord contusion in rats. J Neurotrauma 30: 884–890.
41. Kosta V, Kojundzic SL, Sapunar LC, Sapunar D (2012) The extent of laminectomy affects pain-related behavior in a rat model of neuropathic pain. Eur J Pain 13: 243–248.
42. Busic Z, Kostic S, Kosta V, Carija R, Puljak L, et al. (2012) Postlaminectomy stabilization of the spine in a rat model of neuropathic pain reduces pain-related behavior. Spine 15: 1874–1882.
43. Djouhri L, Koutsikou S, Fang X, McMullan S, Lawson SN (2006) Spontaneous pain, both neuropathic and inflammatory, is related to frequency of spontaneous firing in intact C-fiber nociceptors. J Neurosci 26:1281–1292.
44. Christensen MD, Everhart AQ, Pickelman JT, Hulsebosch CE (1996) Mechanical and thermal allodynia in chronic central pain following spinal cord injury. Pain 68: 97–107.
45. Bullitt E (1990) Expression of c-fos-like protein as a marker for neuronal activity following noxious stimulation in the rat. J Comp Neurol 296: 517–530.
46. Abbadie C, Honore P, Besson JM (1994) Intense cold noxious stimulation of the rat hindpaw induces c-fos expression in lumbar spinal cord neurons. Neuroscience 59: 457–468.
47. Jinks SL, Simons CT, Dessirier JM, Carstens MI, Antognini JF, et al. (2002) C-fos induction in rat superficial dorsal horn following cutaneous application of noxious chemical or mechanical stimuli. Exp Brain Res 145: 261–269.
48. Yi DK, Barr GA (1995) The induction of Fos-like immunoreactivity by noxious thermal, mechanical and chemical stimuli in the lumbar spinal cord of infant rats. Pain 60: 257–265.
49. Bester H, Beggs S, Woolf CJ (2000) Changes in tactile stimuli-induced behavior and c-Fos expression in the superficial dorsal horn and in parabrachial nuclei after sciatic nerve crush. J Comp Neurol 428: 45–61.
50. McClung CA, Ulery PG, Perrotti L, Zachariou V, Berton O, et al. (2004) DeltaFosB: A molecular switch for long-term adaptation in the brain. Brain Res Mol Brain Res 132: 146–154.
51. Galan A, Laird JM, Cervero F (2004) In vivo recruitment by painful stimuli of AMPA receptor subunits to the plasma membrane of spinal cord neurons. Pain 112: 315–323.
52. Katano T, Furue H, Okuda-Ashitaka E, Tagaya M, Watanabe M, et al. (2008) N-ethylmaleimide-sensitive fusion protein (NSF) is involved in central sensitization in the spinal cord through GluR2 subunit composition switch after inflammation. Eur J Neurosci 27: 3161–3170.

53. Larsson M, Broman J (2008) Translocation of GluR1-containing AMPA receptors to a spinal nociceptive synapse during acute noxious stimulation. J Neurosci 28: 7084–7090.
54. Grossman SD, Wolfe BB, Yasuda RP, Wrathall JR (2000) Changes in NMDA receptor subunit expression in response to contusive spinal cord injury. J Neurochem 75: 174–184.
55. Iwasaki R, Matsuura Y, Ohtori S, Suzuki T, Kuniyoshi K, et al. (2013) Activation of astrocytes and microglia in the C3-T4 dorsal horn by lower trunk avulsion in a rat model of neuropathic pain. J Hand Surg Am 38: 841–846.
56. Cho DC, Cheong JH, Yang MS, Hwang SJ, Kim JM, et al. (2011) The effect of minocycline on motor neuron recovery and neuropathic pain in a rat model of spinal cord injury. J Korean Neurosurg Soc 49: 83–91.
57. Pekny M, Nilsson M (2005) Astrocyte activation and reactive gliosis. Glia 50: 427–434.
58. Rolls A, Schechter R, Schwartz M (2009) The bright side of the glial scar in CNS repair. Nat Rev Neurosci 10: 235–241.

3

β1-Integrin and Integrin Linked Kinase Regulate Astrocytic Differentiation of Neural Stem Cells

Liuliu Pan[1]*, Hilary A. North[1], Vibhu Sahni[1], Su Ji Jeong[1], Tammy L. Mcguire[1], Eric J. Berns[2], Samuel I. Stupp[3,4,5], John A. Kessler[1]

1 Department of Neurology, Northwestern University, Chicago, Illinois, United States of America, **2** Department of Biomedical Engineering, Northwestern University, Evanston, Illinois, United States of America, **3** Department of Materials Science and Engineering, Northwestern University, Evanston, Illinois, United States of America, **4** Department of Chemistry, Northwestern University, Evanston, Illinois, United States of America, **5** Department of Medicine and Institute for BioNanotechnology in Medicine, Northwestern University, Chicago, Illinois, United States of America

Abstract

Astrogliosis with glial scar formation after damage to the nervous system is a major impediment to axonal regeneration and functional recovery. The present study examined the role of β1-integrin signaling in regulating astrocytic differentiation of neural stem cells. In the adult spinal cord β1-integrin is expressed predominantly in the ependymal region where ependymal stem cells (ESCs) reside. β1-integrin signaling suppressed astrocytic differentiation of both cultured ESCs and subventricular zone (SVZ) progenitor cells. Conditional knockout of β1-integrin enhanced astrogliogenesis both by cultured ESCs and by SVZ progenitor cells. Previous studies have shown that injection into the injured spinal cord of a self-assembling peptide amphiphile that displays an IKVAV epitope (IKVAV-PA) limits glial scar formation and enhances functional recovery. Here we find that injection of IKVAV-PA induced high levels of β1-integrin in ESCs in vivo, and that conditional knockout of β1-integrin abolished the astroglial suppressive effects of IKVAV-PA in vitro. Injection into an injured spinal cord of PAs expressing two other epitopes known to interact with β1-integrin, a Tenascin C epitope and the fibronectin epitope RGD, improved functional recovery comparable to the effects of IKVAV-PA. Finally we found that the effects of β1-integrin signaling on astrogliosis are mediated by integrin linked kinase (ILK). These observations demonstrate an important role for β1-integrin/ILK signaling in regulating astrogliosis from ESCs and suggest ILK as a potential target for limiting glial scar formation after nervous system injury.

Editor: Michael Fehlings, University of Toronto, Canada

Funding: This project was supported by National Institutes of Health Grants R01 NS 20013 and R01 NS 20778. The funders had no role in study design, data collection and analysis, decision to publish, or preparation of the manuscript.

Competing Interests: The authors have declared that no competing interests exist.

* Email: liuliupan2012@u.northwestern.edu

Introduction

After injury to the nervous system, astrocytes undergo a series of morphologic and molecular changes that facilitate sealing of the blood brain barrier and functional recovery [10,11,42]. However, there is also an increase in the number of astrocytes and formation of a glial scar that significantly impedes axonal regeneration [10,48,50,54]. New astrocytes are generated after spinal cord injury (SCI) both by ependymal stem cells (ESCs) as well as by preexisting astrocytes [2]. Several signaling pathways are known to be involved in the generation of astrocytes after SCI [18,37], but the precise molecular mechanisms regulating astrogliosis are not known.

Injection into an injured spinal cord of a self-assembling peptide amphiphile (PA) that contains an IKVAV epitope (IKVAV-PA) markedly reduced glial scar formation after SCI [54]. IKVAV-PA also profoundly suppressed astrocytic differentiation of cultured neural stem/progenitor cells (NSCs) [47]. The IKVAV sequence is an important neuroactive site on the laminin A chain that can mimic the effects of laminin-1 on neurite outgrowth [36,46,53]. Some of the effects of the IKVAV epitope are mediated via the β1-integrin receptor subunit [14] which is the most ubiquitously expressed integrin subunit. This suggested the possibility that β1-integrin signaling might be involved in astrogliosis after SCI.

The integrin family of cell surface receptors is an important link between cells and the extracellular matrix (ECM) and acts both to anchor the cell surface to the ECM and to initiate a variety of intracellular signaling events. Integrin signaling is complex. Integrin heterodimer formation can be induced both by extracellular ligand binding and by cytoplasmic signaling [45], resulting in a conformational change into an activated form. Integrin activation eventually induces intracellular signaling through assembly of a signaling complex at its cytoplasmic tail [7]. Integrins play multiple roles during the development of the nervous system [34]. β1-integrin is highly expressed by neural stem/progenitor cells (NSCs) and in fact has been used as a cell surface marker for NSC enrichment [15,40]. β1-integrin signaling is an important pathway by which NSCs respond to cues from the ECM to regulate both survival and proliferation [25]. Higher levels of β1-integrin expression by cultured NSCs correlate with a higher capability for self-renewal mediated via the MAPK cascade [8].

Although β1-integrin signaling influences astrocytic morphology and gene expression, it does not alter astrocyte proliferation [43]. We therefore asked whether the effects of IKVAV-PA in limiting the glial scar might be mediated by interactions with β1-integrin expressed by ESCs, and what downstream signaling pathways might be involved. We report a series of observations that demonstrate an important role for β1-integrin/ILK signaling in regulating astrocytic differentiation of ESCs and suggest ILK as a potential target for limiting glial scar formation after nervous system injury.

Materials and Methods

Animals

Timed pregnant CD1 mice, 129 SvJ mice and Long Evans rats were supplied by Charles River Laboratories (Wilmington, MA). β1 integrin floxed mice were supplied by Jackson Laboratory (strain name: B6;129-Itgb1tm1Efu/J).

Cell Culture reagents

Neurosphere growth media were made from supplementing DMEM/F12 (Gibco/Invitrogen) with N2 Supplement (Gibco/Invitrogen) and B27 Supplement (Gibco/Invitrogen), along with Pen/Strap/Glut 100x Mix (Gibco/Invitrogen). ILK inhibitor Cpd 22 was purchased from Millipore and dissolved in DMSO. IKVAV-PA and VVIAK-PA were made by the laboratory of Dr. Samuel Stupp (Northwestern University, IL, US).

Generation of progenitor cell neurospheres and differentiation cultures

To isolate NSCs from spinal cord, the spinal cord of postnatal day 1 mice were mechanically dissociated using razor blades along with pipetting and grown in serum-free neurosphere growth medium with EGF (20 ng/ml, human recombinant, BD) plus bFGF (20 ng/ml, human recombinant, Millipore) supplemented with Heparin (Sigma) for 7 days, to generate neurospheres. Primary spheres were grown for 7 days *in vitro* (DIV), and then passaged by dissociating with 0.05% trypsin (Invitrogen) for 2 minutes followed by incubation with a soybean trypsin inhibitor (Sigma), a 5- minute spin, and repeated trituration. Secondary spheres were grown for an additional 5–7 DIV and used for subsequent studies.

To isolate NSCs from SVZ, the lateral ganglionic eminences of postnatal day 1 mice were dissociated and grown in serum-free neurosphere growth medium with EGF (20 ng/ml, human recombinant, BD) for 5 days, as previously described, to generate neurospheres [30,56]. Primary spheres were grown for 3–4 days *in vitro* (DIV), and then passaged by dissociating with 0.05% trypsin (Invitrogen) for 2 minutes followed by incubation with a soybean trypsin inhibitor (Sigma), a 5 minute spin, and repeated trituration. Secondary spheres were grown for an additional 3–4 DIV and used for subsequent studies.

For differentiation studies, neurospheres were dissociated and plated at a density of 1×10^4 cells/cm^2 onto poly-D-lysine-coated (PDL, Sigma) coverslips additionally coated with Laminin (Roche) within 24-well culture plates, and then grown for 7 DIV in neurosphere growth medium with low concentration EGF(1 ng/ml or 0.2 ng/ml).

Immunochemistry of cultures

Prior to PFA fixation, O4 antibody (mouse IgM, Chemicon) was added to cells for 30 minutes at 4°C. 10 μM thymidine analog 5-Ethyl-2′-deoxyuridine (EdU, invitrogen) was added to the cells for 12 hours. Fixed coverslips were incubated with primary antibodies at 4°C overnight in blocking media (0.2% Triton with 1% BSA in PBS). Antibodies were as follows: GFAP (Rabbit, Dako); βIII-tubulin (mouse IgG2b, Sigma); β1 integrin (Rat, Millipore); β1 integrin, activated, HUTS-4 (Mouse IgG2b, Millipore); phosphore-ILK, Ser246 (Rabbit, Millipore); ILK (Rabbit, Millipore); Sox2 (Goat, Santa Cruz). Primary antibodies were visualized with Alexa 647- (infrared) Alexa 555/594- (red), Alexa 488- (green) and Alexa 350- (blue) conjugated secondary antibodies (Invitrogen). Cells were counted in 26 alternate fields of each coverslip and verified in a minimum of three independent experiments.

Western Blot analysis

Cells were lysed in T-PER Tissue Protein Extraction Reagent (Pierce, Thermo Scientific), supplemented with complete protease and phosphatase inhibitor cocktail (Roche). After removal of cellular debris by centrifugation at 13200 g for 5 min at 4°C, the protein concentration of the lysate was determined using the Bio-Rad Protein Assay standardized to bovine serum albumin. The indicated amounts of cell lysate were resolved by sodium dodecyl sulfate–polyacrylamide gel electrophoresis (SDS–PAGE) and electro-transferred onto nitrocellulose membranes (Bio-Rad). The following primary antibodies were used at 1:1000 dilution unless otherwise noted: pFAK (Rabbit, Cell Signaling); FAK (Rabbit, Cell Signaling); GFAP (Rabbit, Dako); ILK (Rabbit, Millipore); GAPDH (Mouse IgG, Millipore); pAkt (Rabbit, Cell Signling); Akt (Rabbit, Cell Signaling). Horseradish peroxidases (HRP)-conjugated secondary antibodies (Santa Cruz) were used at 1:2000 dilutions. Detection was carried out using SuperSignal West Femto Maximum Sensitivity Substrate detection system (Pierce). Immunoblots were stripped and re-probed using Restore Western Blot Stripping Buffer (Pierce).

RT-qPCR (reverse transcriptase-quantitative polymerase chain reaction)

RNA was harvested from plated cells using Trizol (Invitrogen) and RNAqueous-Micro kit (Ambion). 500 ng of RNA was used to generate cDNA using oligo-dT primers (Thermoscript RT-PCR kit, Invitrogen). Real-time PCR was performed using SybrGreen Master Mix (Applied Biosystems). Three replicates were run for each cDNA sample with the test and control primers. An amplification plot showing cycle number versus the change in fluorescent intensity was generated by the Sequence Detector program (Applied Biosystems).

Retrovirus production and infection

The β1 integrin constructs were cloned into the pCLE-IRES-EGFP retroviral vector and the retrovirus production is as previously described [4]. 293 FT cells were transfected with pCLE retroviral and pCMV-VSVG helper plasmids using Lipofectamine 2000 transfection reagent (Invitrogen). The supernatant from the cells was collected on day 2, 4 and 7 post transfection, concentrated, tittered and then $\sim 10^7$ viral particles were used to infect 2.5 million cells for 48 hours in sphere forming media (containing 20 ng/ml EGF). Cells were then FACS sorted for GFP and then either used immediately for RNA isolation or plated on PDL-laminin as described above.

Thymidine analog labeling

For 5-ethynyl-2′-deoxyuridine (EdU) (Invitrogen) labeling of neurospheres in culture, cells were incubated in neurospheres media containing 10 μM EdU for 12 h and then processed for

EdU detection according to the protocol of the manufacturer (Click-IT Flow Cytometry Assay kit; Invitrogen).

Generation of mutated ILK, b1integrin constructs

Constitutive active ILK expressing construct ILK_S343D were generated by point mutation using QuikChange II XL Site-Directed Mutagenesis Kit (Agilent Technologies). Mutation backbone template was mouse ilk expressing vector ordered from OriGene (ilk (NM_010562) Mouse cDNA ORF Clone). Mutation primers were designed as follows: 5′-GGCTGATGTTAAGTTT-GATTTCCAGTGCCCTGGG-3′ and 5′-CCCAGGGCACTG-GAAATCAAACTTAACATCAGCC-3′. Kinase dead ILK expressing construct ILK_S343A were generated using mutation primers designed as follows:

5′-GCTGATGTTAAGTTTGCTTTCCAGTGCCCTG-3′.

5′-CAGGGCACTGGAAAGCAAACTTAACATCAGC-3′.

Mouse spinal cord injury and PA injection

All animal procedures were performed in accordance with the Public Health Service Policy on Humane Care and Use of Laboratory Animals and all procedures were approved by the Northwestern University Institutional Animal Care and Use Committee. Female 129 SvJ mice (10 weeks of age) or female Longs Evans Rats (8 weeks of age) were anesthetized by inhalation of 2.5% isoflurane anesthetic in 100% oxygen administered by a VetEquip Rodent anesthesia machine. A T11 vertebral laminectomy was performed to expose the spinal cord. The spinal cord was injured using an IH-0400 Spinal Cord impactor (Precision Systems) with a 1.25 mm tip with 70 Kdynes of force and 60 s of dwell time for mice and with a 2.50 mm tip with 185 Kdynes of force and 60 s of dwell time for rats. Skin was sutured using AUTOCLIPs (9 mm; BD Biosciences). For postoperative care, animals were kept on a heating pad for 24 h to maintain body temperature. Both mice and rats were given Buprenex (2.5 mg/kg, s.c.) and Baytril (5 mg/kg, s.c.) to minimize discomfort and infection. Bladders were manually expressed twice daily. A 5d Baytril treatment course (5 mg/kg daily, s.c.) was started in the event of hematuria.

PA (1% aqueous solution) or vehicle was injected 48 h after SCI using borosilicate glass capillary micropipettes (Sutter Instruments, Novato, CA) (outer diameter, 100 μm). The capillaries were loaded onto a Hamilton syringe using a female luer adaptor (World Precision Instruments, Sarasota, FL) controlled by a Micro4 microsyringe pump controller (World Precision Instruments). The amphiphile was diluted 1:1 with a 580 μM solution of glucose just before injection and loaded into the capillary. Under Avertin anesthesia, the autoclips were removed and the injury site was exposed. The micropipette was inserted to a depth of 750 μm measured from the dorsal surface of the cord for mice and a depth of 1250 μm measured for rats, and 2.5 μl for mice or 5.0 μl for rats of the diluted amphiphile solution or vehicle was injected at 1 μl/min. The micropipette was withdrawn at intervals of 250 μm to leave a trail (ventral to dorsal) of the PA in the cord. At the end of the injection, the capillary tip was left in the cord for an additional 1 min, after which the pipette was withdrawn and the wound closed. For all experiments, the experimenters were kept blinded to the identity of the animals.

Animal perfusions, tissue processing and immunohistochemistry

Animals were killed using an overdose of halothane anesthesia and transcardially perfused with 4% paraformaldehyde in PBS. The spinal cords were dissected and fixed for 2 h with 4% paraformaldehyde and subsequently overnight in 30% sucrose in PBS. The spinal cords were then frozen in Tissue-Tek embedding compound and sectioned on a Leica (Deerfield, IL) CM3050S cryostat.

20 μm thick frozen sections were cut on a leica (CM3050S) Cryostat and collected on Superfrost Bond Rite slides (Richard Allen Scientific). Every fifth section was placed on the same slide such that each adjacent section was 80 μm away from its neighbor. Four sections were placed on each slide and hence the width of the frozen cord spanned on each slide was 240 μm. We roughly averaged about 20 slides per cord. Sections were processed for immunohistochemistry in the same manner as described for the cells. Primary antibodies used were: GFAP (Sigma, mouse IgG1 1:500), β1integrin (Millipore, rat IgG, 1:500), HUTS-4 (Millipore, mouse IgG1 1:500).

Statistical analyses

Student's unpaired t test was used for all two group comparisons. Analysis of variance (ANOVA) with the Bonferroni post hoc test was used for all multiple group experiments. P values<0.05 were deemed significant. Values in graphs are shown are Mean ±S.E.M.

Results

Knockout of β1-integrin from cultured ESCs increases astrocytic differentiation

Immunocytochemical examination of adult spinal cord revealed that β1-integrin is expressed predominantly in the ependymal zone (Figure 1A) where ESCs reside [32]. ESCs are able to form neurospheres and can generate all three neural lineages, neurons, astrocytes and oligodendrocytes (Figure 1B and Meletis et al, 2008 [32]). To assess the role of β1-integrin signaling in this process, we isolated and cultured ependymal cells from β1-integrin$^{flx/flx}$ mice and ablated out β1-integrin by infecting cells with Adeno-Cre-GFP virus or a control Adeno-GFP virus. Two days after virus infection, neurospheres were dissociated, sorted by fluorescence activated cell sorting (FACS) to select virus infected cells, and grown again as neurospheres. Western blot analysis confirmed the depletion of β1-integrin in the Adeno-Cre-GFP treated cells (Figure 1C). One week later the cells were dissociated, plated in differentiating conditions for 7 days, and analyzed immunocytochemically (Figure 1B, 1D, 1E). The total number of cells did not differ between control and β1 integrin null cultures (Figure 1D). Control ESCs generated a large number of GFAP-expressing astrocytes (35.3±3.3%of the cells) and smaller numbers of βIIItubulin-immunoreactive neurons (3.3±0.1%) and CNPase-expressing oligodendrocytes (~3.0±1.3%) (Figure 1B, 1E). The remainder of the cells remained undifferentiated. Knockout of β1 integrin significantly increased the number of GFAP$^+$ cells by 67% (to a total amount of 59.1±3.7% of the cells; $p \leq 0.004$) without altering the numbers of neurons or oligodendroglia (Figure 1B, 1E). This suggests that β1-integrin signaling suppresses astrocytic differentiation by ESCs.

To determine whether this regulatory process is unique to the ependymal population of NSCs, we repeated the experiment using SVZ-derived NSCs with strikingly similar results. The total number of cells did not differ between control and β1 integrin null cultures (Figure 2C). Control SVZ-derived NPCs generated 37.3±3.1% astrocytes, 3.4±0.1% neurons, and 3.1±0.5% oligodendrocytes (Figure 2A, 2D). Knockout of β1-integrin (Figure 2B) did not alter neuronal or oligodendroglial lineage differentiation but significantly increased the number of GFAP$^+$ astrocytes generated to more than 55% (55.65±7.8%) of the cells (p≤

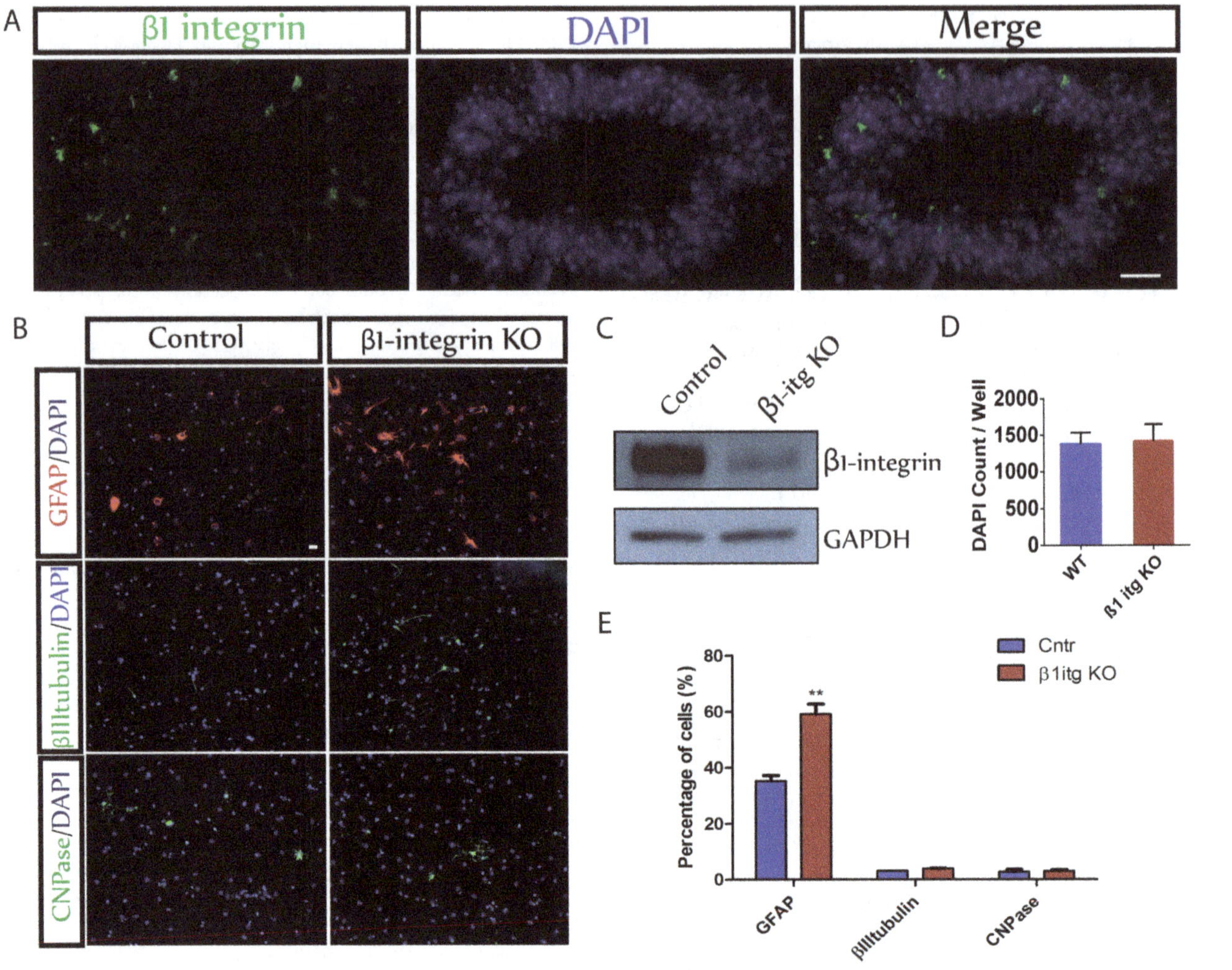

Figure 1. β1-integrin suppresses generation of astrocytes by NSCs derived from the spinal cord. A. Ependymal NSCs in adult mouse spinal cord express β1-integrin. B. NSCs derived from spinal cord are able to differentiate into astrocytes (GFAP -red), neurons (βIIItubulin-green) and oligodendrocytes (CNPase-green). β1-integrin Knock-Out (KO) increases astrocyte differentiation without altering neuronal or oligodendroglial differentiation. *Scale bar = 20 μm.* C. Western blot analysis shows depletion of β1 integrin protein levels in β1-itg KO NSCs derived from the spinal cord. D. Quantification of total cell numbers (DAPI) in the cultures of control and β1-integrin null cells analyzed for lineage commitment (E). There was no difference in overall cell numbers ($n = 12$, $p = 0.89$). Values are means ± SEM. E. Quantification of cell numbers of different lineages shows a significant increase (**$p \leq 0.004$) in astrocytes (67% of increase) in cultures of β1 integrin null cells at 7DIV without any change in neuronal or oligodendroglial differentiation.

0.046). Knockout of β1-integrin had an even greater effect on levels of GFAP mRNA which increased more than 2-fold compared to control, but levels of βIIItubulin and CNPase mRNAs were unchanged (Figure 2E). Thus the astrocyte-suppressive effects of β1-integrin are comparable in ESCs and in SVZ NSCs (Figure1E, 2D).

Inhibition of β1 integrin signaling by a dominant negative construct increases astrocytic differentiation

After binding to ligands, integrin receptors trigger an intracellular signaling cascade mediated predominantly via a small cytoplasmic domain of the β subunit [12]. This domain can cross talk with multiple intracellular signal transduction systems [28], thereby altering progenitor cell responses to extrinsic factors [13]. Specifically the cytoplasmic domain of β1 integrin mediates the majority of its intracellular signaling [12], and mutant forms of β1 integrin that lack this domain act as a dominant negative form of the receptor [20,22,41]. We misexpressed this form of β1 integrin, hereafter referred to as β1ΔC, in NSCs using retroviral mediated gene transfer. Cultured NSCs were transduced with either control pCLE-IRES-GFP or β1ΔC-IRES-GFP retroviruses, FAC-sorted 48 hours later for the positively transfected cells, and plated in differentiating conditions. Seven days after plating, the percentages of neurons (βIII tubulin), astrocytes (GFAP) and oligodendrocytes (O4) were assayed. Expression of β1ΔC increased the number of GFAP^{+} astrocytes more than 2.5-fold ($p \leq 0.005$) compared to control pCLE cultures (Figure 3A, 3B), without altering numbers of neurons or oligodendrocytes (Figure 3B). This further supports the conclusion that β1-integrin signaling suppresses astrocytic differentiation.

IKVAV-PA increases β1-integrin expression in cultured NSCs and suppresses astrocytic differentiation

We next tried to overexpress β1-integrin in cultured NSCs using techniques identical to those used to overexpress β1ΔC. Since the overexpressed cDNA lacked the 3′UTR, we could design PCR

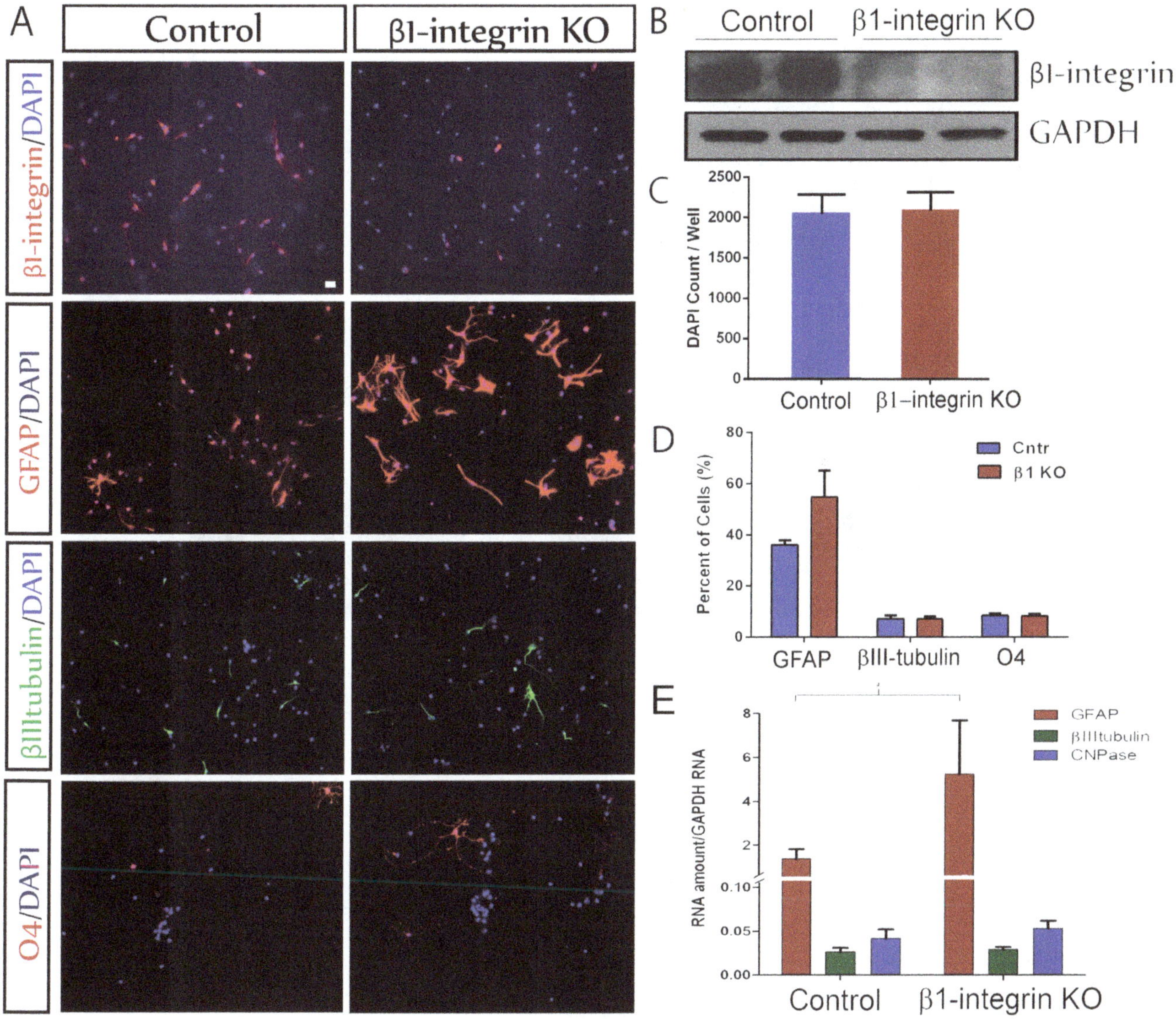

Figure 2. β1-integrin suppresses generation of astrocytes by NSCs derived from the SVZ. A. NSCs derived from the SVZ show a similar profile of differentiation as those derived from spinal cord. β1-integrin Knock-Out (KO) increases astrocytic differentiation (GFAP - red) without altering neuronal (βIIItubulin - green) or oligodendroglial (O4 -red) differentiation. *Scale bar = 20 μm*. B. Western blot analysis shows depletion of β1-integrin protein in the β1KO derived NSCs compared with control. C. Quantification of total cell numbers (DAPI) in the cultures of control and β1-integrin null cells analyzed for lineage commitment (D). There was no difference in overall cell numbers ($n = 20$, $p = 0.91$). Values are means ± SEM. D. Quantification of cell numbers of different lineages shows a significant increase (*$p \leq 0.046$) in astrocytes (56% increase) in the β1-integrin KO group compared with control at 7DIV without any change in neuronal or oligodendroglial differentiation. E. Quantification of mRNA levels by qPCR after 7DIV reveals a significant increase in GFAP mRNA in the β1-integrin KO group compared with control. βIIItubulin and CNPase mRNAs were unchanged.

primers that detect the endogenous transcript alone as well ones that detect total β1 integrin. At 2 days post infection, there was a significant (~3 fold) increase in the levels of total β1-integrin. However, even at this time levels of endogenous transcript had already decreased by 60%. At 7 days, we could detect no difference in the levels of β1-integrin between the two groups (not shown). Multiple attempts to overexpress β1-integrin failed, presumably due to a strong feedback loop that maintained β1-integrin expression at a stable level. By contrast, culture of NSCs in the presence of IKVAV-PA markedly increased levels of β1-integrin expression compared to control cells grown in the presence of laminin (Figure 3C, 3D, 3E, 3F). There were significant increases in expression of both β1-integrin protein (Figure 3C, 3D) and mRNA (Figure 3E, 3F).

We also evaluated the expression of different integrin subunits in cultured NSCs and found significant levels of α5, α6, and αV but no significant levels of β3 or β4 integrins. We then examined the levels of these integrin transcripts in NSCs cultured in IKVAV PA for 7 days using real time RT-PCR. There was a significant (~3 fold) increase in the β1 integrin transcript levels in cells cultured in IKVAV PA as compared to the control (Figure 3E, 3F). However, there were no changes in levels of the α5, α6 or αV subunits and no detectable levels of the β3 or β4 subunits. This suggests that IKVAV-PA is a uniquely effective tool for increasing β1-integrin expression by NSCs.

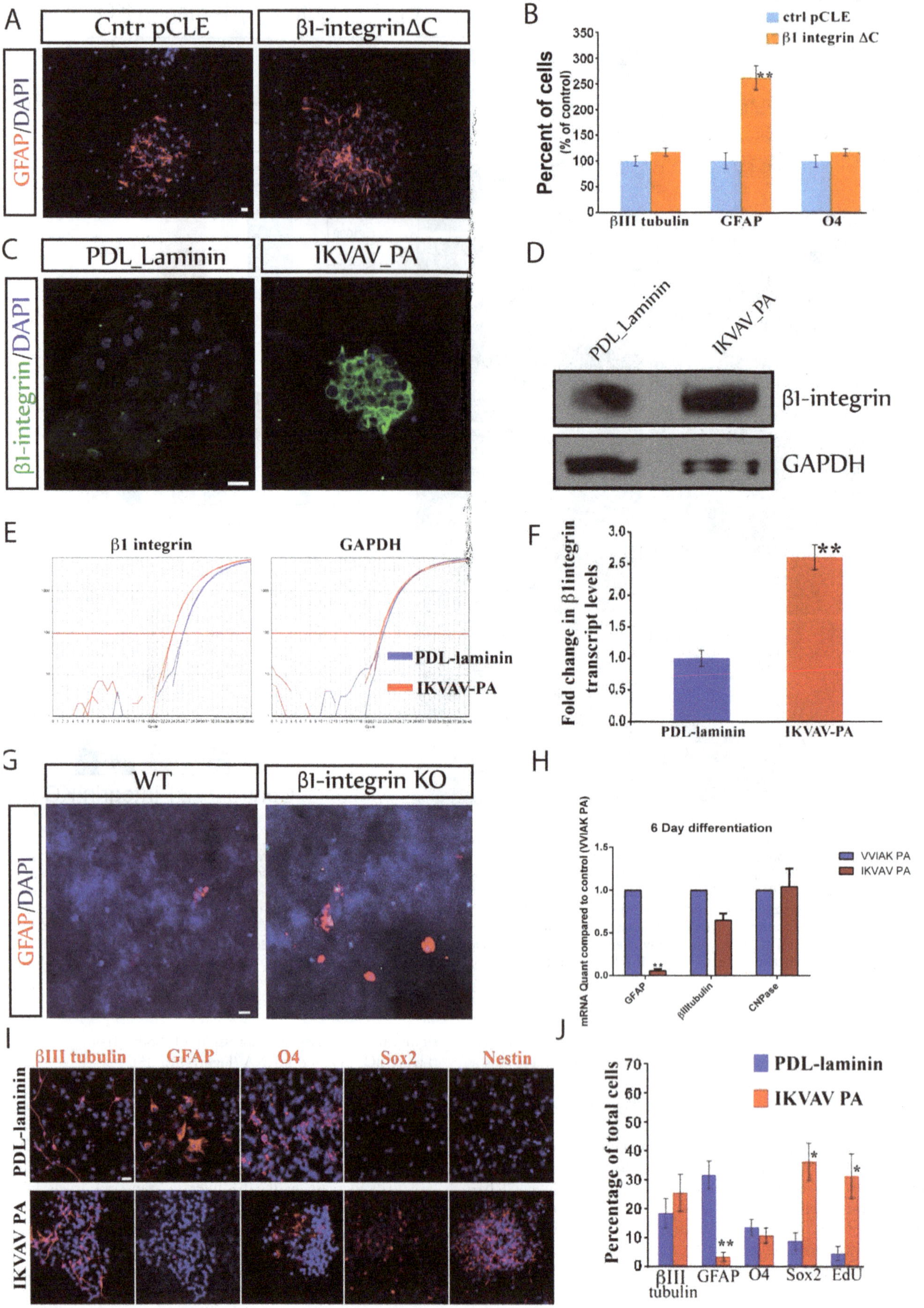

A
Cntr pCLE
β1-integrinΔC
GFAP/DAPI
B
ctrl pCLE
β1 integrin ΔC
Percent of cells
(% of control)
350
300
250
200
150
100
50
0
βIII tubulin
GFAP
O4
**
C
PDL_Laminin
IKVAV_PA
β1-integrin/DAPI
D
PDL_Laminin
IKVAV_PA
β1-integrin
GAPDH
E
β1 integrin
GAPDH
PDL-laminin
IKVAV-PA
F
Fold change in β1integrin transcript levels
3.0
2.5
2.0
1.5
1.0
0.5
0.0
PDL-laminin
IKVAV-PA
**
G
WT
β1-integrin KO
GFAP/DAPI
H
6 Day differentiation
mRNA Quant compared to control (VVIAK PA)
1.5
1.0
0.5
0.0
GFAP
βIIItubulin
CNPase
VVIAK PA
IKVAV PA
**
I
βIII tubulin
GFAP
O4
Sox2
Nestin
PDL-laminin
IKVAV PA
J
PDL-laminin
IKVAV PA
Percentage of total cells
70
60
50
40
30
20
10
0
βIII tubulin
GFAP
O4
Sox2
EdU
**
*
*

Figure 3. β1-integrin regulates astrocytic differentiation. A. NSCs were infected with retrovirus expressing GFP alone (ctrl pCLE) orβ1-integrinlacking the cytoplasmic domain (β1-integrin ΔC), cultured for 7 days on PDL-laminin and immunostained for GFAP (red) and DAPI (blue). *Scale bar = 20 μm.* B. Astrocytic differentiation (GFAP expression) increased more than 2.5 fold (**p≤0.005) in the β1- integrin ΔC group compared to control while neuronal (βIIItubulin) and oligodendroglial (O4) differentiation were unchanged. C. NSCs were cultured either on PDL-laminin or IKVAV-PA for one day and immunostained with β1- integrin (green) and DAPI (blue). Culture in IKVAV-PA dramatically increased expression of β1- integrin. *Scale bar = 20 μm.* D. Western Blot analysis shows that NSCs express higher levels of β1integrin protein when cultured for one day in IKVAV-PA compared to control (PDL-laminin). E. Real time PCR amplification plots showing that the β1integrin transcripts increase in cells cultured in IKVAV-PA compared to control (PDL-laminin). F. Quantitation of the increase in transcript levels of β1integrin in the IKVAV PA versus PDL-laminin group. (**p≤ 0.0007). G. KO of β1-integrin increases the number of astrocytes (GFAP – red) generated by NSCs cultured in IKVAV PA for 7 DIV. Blue = DAPI. H. NSCs were cultured in either control PA (VVIAK PA) or IKVAV PA for 7DIV, and RNA was extracted for qPCR quantification. The graph represents each lineage marker mRNA level in IKVAV PA normalized to levels in the control PA. Levels of GFAP mRNA were profoundly decreased (**p≤0.0005 in the IKVAV-PA group) without any significant change in levels of βIIItubulin of CNPase mRNAs. I. NPCs were cultured either on PDL-laminin or in IKVAV PA for 7DIV and immunostained with DAPI (blue) and several lineage markers (red). Note the absence of GFAP staining in the IKVAV PA group and the increase in the progenitor markers Sox2 and nestin. *Scale bar = 20 μm.* J. Quantification of the percentages of cells in the conditions described in (i) (*p≤0.017, **p≤0.005).

Culture of NSCs in the presence of IKVAV-PA increased levels of β1-integrin expression and suppressed astrocytic differentiation suggesting a causal relationship [47]. However, to directly test whether the suppressive effects on astrocyte development were due to the expression of β1-integrin, we examined the effects of IKVAV-PA on NSCs in which β1-integrin was knocked out using Adeno-Cre retrovirus as described above (Figure 3G). Culture of control NSCs in IKVAV-PA markedly suppressed astrocytic differentiation (12.5±1.4% of cells) as previously described [48]. However, more than 37% of cells (37.3±5.1%) in which β1-integrin was ablated differentiated into GFAP$^+$ astrocytes even in the presence of IKVAV-PA. Thus the suppressive effects of IKVAV-PA on astrogliosis depended upon the presence of β1-integrin in the cells. We next wanted to ascertain that the effects of IKVAV-PA depended upon the integrity of the IKVAV epitope and were not related to other physicochemical properties of the PA. We therefore compared the effects of IKVAV-PA on mRNA expression with those of a PA in which the amino acid sequence of the epitope was scrambled (VVIAK-PA) (Figure 3H). The profound inhibitory effects of IKVAV-PA on expression of GFAP mRNA were lost when the IKVAV epitope was scrambled. However, there were no significant differences in levels of either βIIItubulin or CNPase mRNAs in IKVAV-PA and VVIAK-PA treated cells, indicating the specificity of the effects of the IKVAV epitope on expression of GFAP mRNA.

IKVAV-PA consistently suppressed astrocyte differentiation by cultured NSCs without changing either neuronal or oligodendroglial differentiation. This suggested that the PA maintained cells in an undifferentiated stem/progenitor cell state. To directly test this hypothesis we examined the effects of the PA on expression of the NSC marker, SOX2, as well as incorporation of the thymidine analog EdU. We used the most optimal substratum for control cells, PDL-laminin, for comparison even though it presented to cells a small amount of the IKVAV epitope (Figure 3I, 3J). Again the IKVAV-PA almost completely suppressed astrocytic differentiation (3.2±0.8% of the cells expressed GFAP versus 32.4±4.7% in controls; p≤0.005) without altering neuronal (βIIItubulin) or oligodendroglial (O4) lineage differentiation. However, the decrease in the percentage of GFAP-expressing cells was almost exactly matched by an increase in the percentage of cells that expressed Sox2 and that were proliferative as measured by EdU incorporation. These observations indicate that IKVAV suppressed astrocytic differentiation by maintaining cells in the NSC state.

The ILK pathway mediates suppressive effects of β1-integrin on astrocytic differentiation

We next sought to determine whether IKVAV-PA actually activates β1-integrin and to define the signaling pathways mediating the effects of β1-integrin on astrocytic development by NSCs. Integrins are heterodimeric receptors, and the relationship between the α and β subunits changes after ligand binding resulting in an "activated" protein conformation [29]. This conformational change initiates intracellular signaling and also increases the affinity of ligand binding [9,52]. We used a conformation sensitive β1-integrin antibody, HUTS-4 [29], to detect the activated form of β1-integrin in NSCs one day after plating in either IKVAV-PA or VVIAK-PA (Figure 4A). Almost all cells cultured in IKVAV-PA immunostained for the activated conformation of β1-integrin whereas little immunostaining was detectable in cells culture in VVIAK-PA. This provides evidence that IKVAV-PA rapidly activated β1-integrin.

β1-integrin signals through a variety of different mechanisms including but not limited to associating with other membrane proteins, serving as a binding dock for intracellular signaling molecules to bind and aggregate, and activating a specific set of intracellular domain bound kinases such as focal adhesion kinase (FAK) and integrin-linked kinase (ILK) [1,5]. Integrin-linked kinase (ILK) is a 59kDa serine/threonine protein kinase that associates with the cytoplasmic domain of β-integrins and transduces signaling after activation of the integrin [17]. Western blot analysis showed no difference in levels of FAK in NSCs grown in IKVAV PA compared to cells grown in VVIAK PA (Figure 4B). By contrast, culture of the cells in IKVAV PA resulted in a very large increase in levels of ILK (Figure 4B). Similarly, immunostaining for ILK indicated that most NSCs cultured in IKVAV PA expressed ILK whereas little staining was apparent in cells cultured in VVIAK PA (Figure 4A).

This suggested that ILK might mediate suppressive effects of β1-integrin on astrocytic development. To explore this hypothesis, we designed a rescue experiment to determine whether expression of a constitutively active form of ILK was sufficient to block the effects of knockout of β1-integrin (Figure 4C). We created two functionally mutated ILK expression constructs based on the findings of Hannigan, Troussard et al [16]. We substituted serine 343 of the potential autophosphorylation site with aspartate (S343D), to get a constitutive active form of ILK (ILK_CA), and we substituted serine 343 with Alanine (S343A) to make a kinase-dead ILK (ILK_KD). NSCs were isolated from β1-integrin$^{flx/flx}$ mice and β1-integrin was knocked out as described above by infecting cells with Adeno-Cre or control virus. The cells were electroporated with either the ILK_CA or the ILK_KD construct, FAC- sorted two days later, and plated on PDL-Laminin for 7

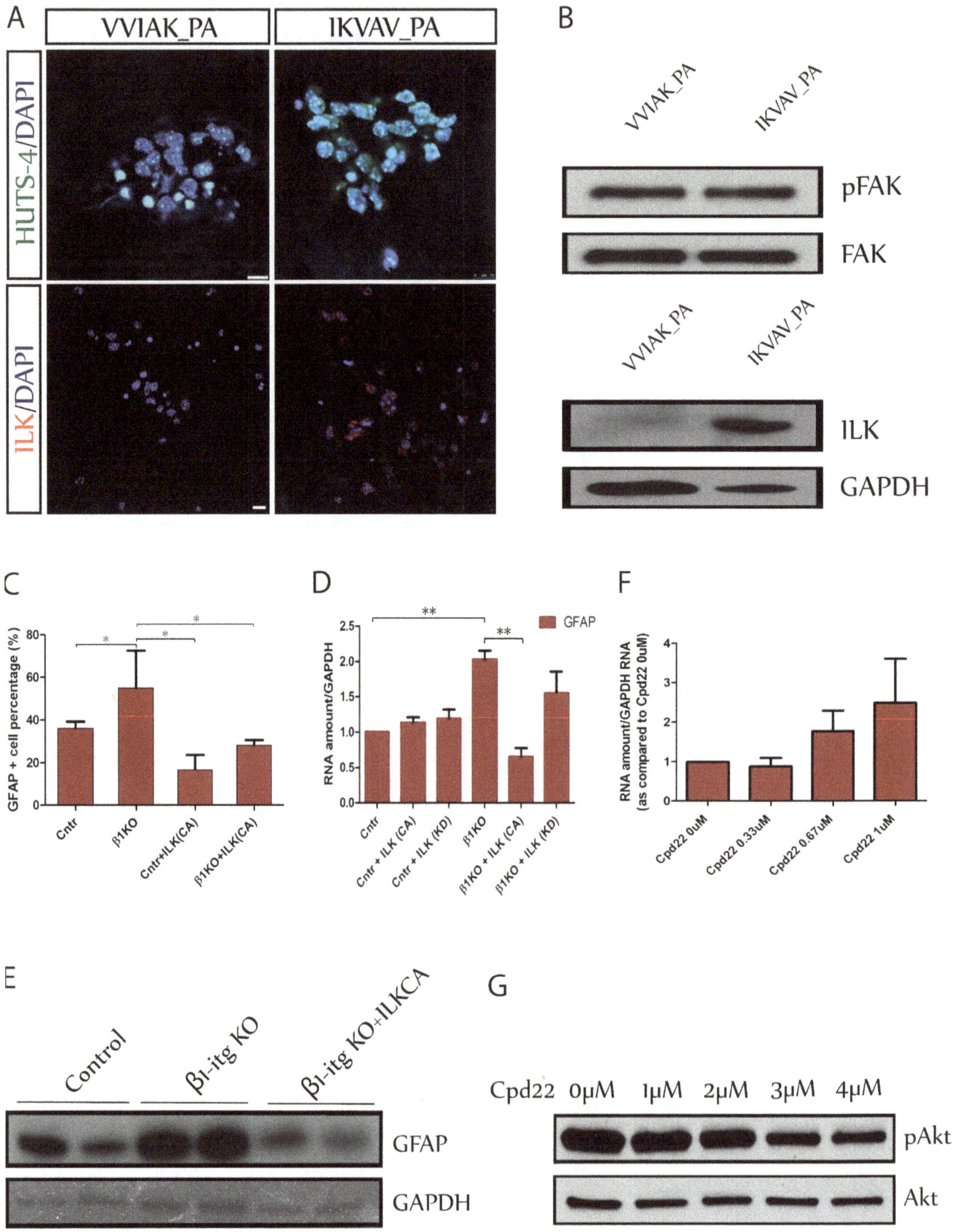

Figure 4. Integrin Linked Kinase (ILK) regulates astrocytic differentiation by NSCs. A. NSCs cultured in either control (scrambled) PA (VVIAK PA) or IKVAV PA for one day, and immunostained with activated β1integrin antibody HUTS-4 (green) or ILK (red). *Scale bar in HUTS-4 staining image = 10 μm, and in the ILK staining image = 20 μm.* B. Western blot analysis of NSCs cultured in either control PA (VVIAK PA) or IKVAV PA for one day. Note that levels of ILK are markedly elevated in the IKVAV-PA group without any change in FAK. C. β1-integrin KO and control NSCs were

transfected with either a control construct or a construct expressing a constitutively active form of ILK (ILK-CA). At 7DIV the cells were immunostained for GFAP and numbers of GFAP$^+$ cells were counted. (*$p \leq 0.05$) D. β1-integrin KO and control NSCs were transfected with a control construct, a construct expressing constitutively active ILK (ILK-CA), or a construct expressing kinase-dead ILK (ILK-KD) and cultured for 7DIV. RNA was extracted for qPCR measurement of GFAP mRNA graphed as a ratio compared to the control (**$p \leq 0.004$). Note that β1-integrin KO increased levels of GFAP mRNA, but this increase was blocked by expression of ILK-CA. E. Western blot analysis of GFAP expression in control NSCs and in β1-integrin KO NSCs transfected with either with a control construct or ILK-CA. Note that transfection with ILK-CA prevented the increase in GFAP expression in β1-integrin KO NSCs. F. NSCs were treated with different doses of the ILK inhibitor, Cpd22. After 6DIV RNA was extracted for qPCR quantification of GFAP. Note that GFAP expression increased in a dose dependent manner after treatment with Cpd22. H. NSCs were treated with different doses of the ILK inhibitor, Cpd22 for 3h, and protein was extracted for western blot analysis. Note that treatment with the drug reduced levels of phospho-Akt without any change in levels of AKT.

days in differentiating conditions. On day 7 cells were examined immunocytochemically (Figure 4C) and also were examined for levels of mRNAs for βIIItubulin, CNPase, and GFAP (Figure 4D). There were no detectable differences in the number of either βIIItubulin or CNPase immunoreactive cells across the different conditions (not shown). 37.3±3.1% of control cells expressed GFAP, but knockout of β1-integrin increased the percentage of GFAP-immunoreactive cells to 55.65±7.8% ($p \leq 0.05$) (Figure 4C). Overexpression of ILK-CA reduced the percentage of GFAP$^+$ cells to 16.7±4.0%, and overexpression of ILK-CA in β1-integrin knockout cells prevented the increase associated with knockout of β1-integrin (GFAP$^+$ cells number dropped to 28.1±1.4%). There were no detectable differences in levels of mRNA encoding either βIIItubulin or CNPase across the different conditions (not shown). Moreover neither construct exerted any effect on GFAP mRNA in control cells. However, knockout of β1-integrin increased levels of GFAP mRNA more than twofold, but expression of the ILK-CA construct prevented this increase and levels of mRNA in these cells actually trended lower than in control cells (Figure 4D). We then examined levels of GFAP protein in these cells by western blot analysis. Knockout of β1-integrin resulted in a very large increase in levels of GFAP protein (Figure 4E). Expression of the ILK-CA construct in β1-integrin knockout cells not only prevented the increase in GFAP but actually reduced it below control levels. There were no differences in proliferation (EdU$^+$ incorporation) among the groups. These observations indicate that ILK signaling suppresses astrogliogenesis, analogous to the effects of β1-integrin, and suggest that ILK mediates at least some of the effects of β1-integrin on astrocytic differentiation. To further test this hypothesis, we examined the effects of a chemical inhibitor of ILK, Cpd22 [23], on differentiation of NSCs. ILK has been shown act directly on Ser473 kinase in Akt [19]. To first verify that the inhibitor actually acted as expected in NSCs, the cells were treated with different concentrations of Cpd22 one day after plating (Figure 4G). 3 hours after drug application, we harvested protein for western blot analysis and found a dose-dependent inhibition of levels of phospho-Akt without any change in the overall levels of Akt. This suggested that the drug was able to penetrate NSCs and exert effects on a known ILK target. We therefore next assessed the effects of Cpd22 treatment on astrocytic differentiation. We chose a dose range that was tolerated well by the cells for a 6 day period of treatment without any evidence of cell death and examined the cells for levels of GFAP mRNA. Treatment of NSCs with the inhibitor resulted in a dose-dependent increase in levels of GFAP mRNA (Figure. 4F). These data are supportive of the hypothesis that ILK signaling inhibits astrocytic differentiation.

IKVAV PA activates β1-integrin and suppresses glial scar formation after SCI

Previously we reported that injection of IKVAV-PA into an injured spinal cord suppresses glial scar formation and enhances behavioral outcome [54]. Since our findings *in vitro* suggested that IKVAV-PA suppresses astrocytic development by activating β1-integrin, we sought to determine whether the PA actually activates β1-integrin signaling in the injured spinal cord. IKVAV-PA and a PA with a bioinert epitope (KKIAV-PA) were injected into the damaged spinal cord 24 hours after a contusion injury. The spinal cords were removed 3 weeks later for immunocytochemical analyses. As previously reported, injection of IKVAV-PA significantly reduced glial scarring as indicated by GFAP immunocytochemistry (Figure 5A, 5B). By contrast, the PA with an inert epitope had no demonstrable effect.

We then examined the spinal cords immunocytochemically using the HUTS-4 antibody to probe for the activated conformation of β1-integrin. IKVAV-PA and control vehicle were injected into the damaged spinal cord 48 hours after a contusion injury. The spinal cords were removed 1 week later for immunocytochemical analyses. Very little HUTS-4 staining was detectable in a vehicle-injected spinal cord (Figure 5C). By contrast, there was abundant HUTS-4 staining in the spinal cord injected with IKVAV-PA, demonstrating that the PA activated β1-integrin signaling *in vivo*.

Injection of IKVAV-PA into the injured spinal cord also consistently improved behavioral outcome [54] as measured by open field testing [3,21], but it was unclear whether the behavioral enhancement was also due to β1-integrin signaling. To help determine this we examined the effects of PAs displaying two different epitopes that are known to interact with β1-integrin, a Tenascin C epitope and the fibronectin epitope RGD [39,55]. The Tenascin C epitope, ADEGVFDNFVLK, is just a small portion of Tenascin C that interacts specifically with β1-integrin [31,33]. We injected these PAs into injured spinal cords of 8 weeks old adult rats two days after a standard impaction injury and followed behavioral outcome for 12 weeks. Similar to prior findings with IKVAV-PA, we found improvements with both Tenascin C-PA and RGD-PA (Figure 5D). Vehicle-injected animals reached an average score of 5.58±0.59 by 12 weeks after the injury. The Tenascin C-PA group reached an average score of 10.20±0.84 ($p \leq 0.002$) and the RGD-PA group achieved an average score of 8.5±2.1 ($p \leq 0.024$).

Discussion

β1-integrin is a transmembrane receptor protein expressed by stem cells in many organ systems [15,25]. β1-integrin signaling mediates a variety of stem cell functions including pluripotency maintenance, self-renewal, proliferation and regulation of migration [25]. In the present study, we report that β1-integrin signaling inhibits astrocytic differentiation by both spinal cord ependymal stem cells and subventricular zone stem cells and helps to maintain stemness. We further found that these effects are mediated, at least in part, by ILK. In previous studies we found that injection of IKVAV-PA into an injured spinal cord limited glial scar formation and enhanced behavioral outcome. In this present study, we report an underlying mechanism to be a ligand (IKVAV) mediated

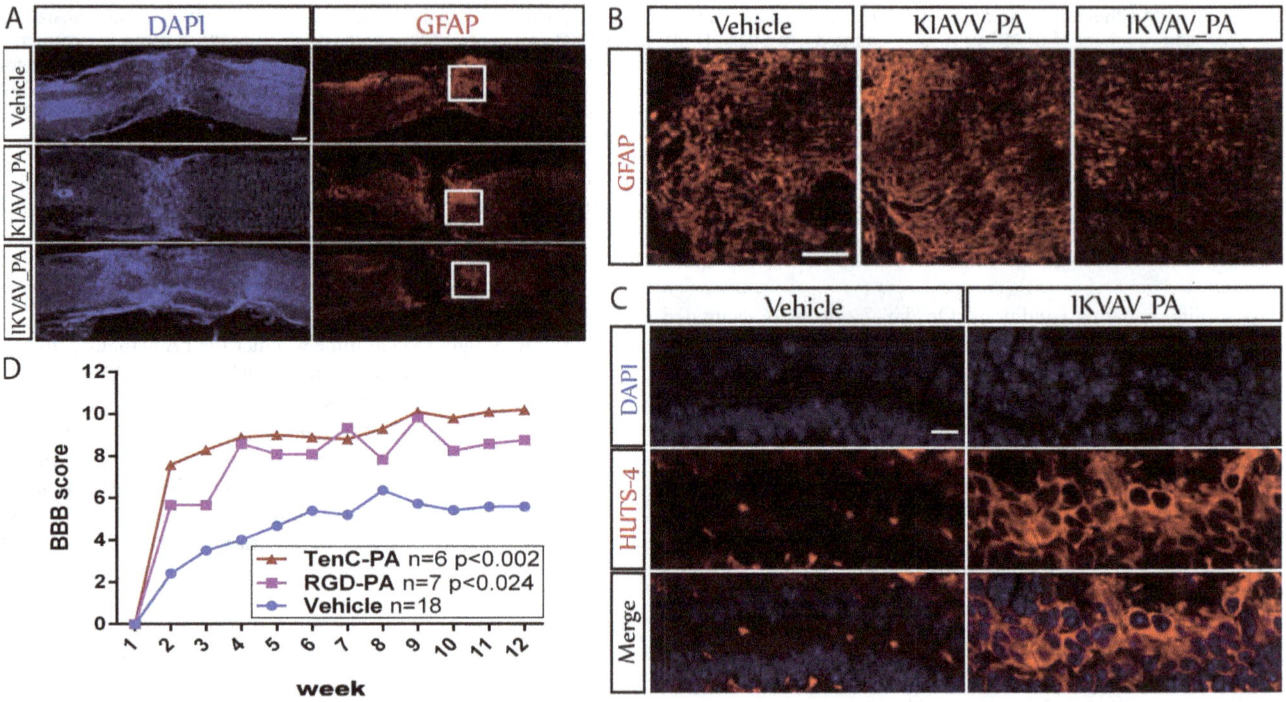

Figure 5. β1-integrin signaling in vivo regulates astrogliogenesis after spinal cord injury (SCI). A. Low magnification (10X) images of representative longitudinal sections of injured mouse spinal cords at 3 weeks post SCI, that were injected with either the IKVAV PA, scrambled KIAVV PA or vehicle injected at 24 hours post injury. Sections are stained with DAPI (blue) and GFAP (red). *Scale bar = 200 μm.* B. Representative confocal Z-stacks taken at higher magnification (20X) of the areas boxed in (a) showing reduced gliosis in the IKVAV PA injected animals at 3 weeks post SCI. *Scale bar = 100 μm.* C. High magnification (63x) confocal images of the ependymal regions stained with activated β1integrin antibody HUTS-4 (red) and DAPI (blue). Injured mouse spinal cords were injected either with IKVAV PA or vehicle 2 days post injury. *Scale bar = 20 μm.* D. Spinal cord injured rats were injected with either Tenascin-C epitope presenting PA, RGD epitope presenting PA or vehicle 2 days post injury, and monitored with BBB scoring for 12 weeks. Both PA groups showed significant improvement compared to the vehicle group.

increase of β1 integrin signaling in ependymal cells which suppresses astrogliosis.

Astrogliosis after SCI has both beneficial and detrimental effects on recovery. Astrocytic hypertrophy is necessary for repairing the damaged blood-brain barrier, and it is a beneficial process that limits inflammatory damage and restores homeostasis [10,27,38]. However, astrocytic hyperplasia leads to formation of a dense glial scar that inhibits axonal regeneration [48]. Therapeutic approaches to limiting glial scar formation after SCI must therefore seek to limit the detrimental effects of astrocytic hyperplasia while maintaining the beneficial effects of the initial reactive astrocytes. In previous studies we found that injection into an injured spinal cord of IKVAV-PA limited astrocytic hyperplasia without altering the early hypertrophic response to the injury [54]. However, the reason for these divergent effects was unclear. In the present study we found that ESCs expressed high levels of β1-integrin after SCI whereas levels of the protein were not demonstrably increased in resident astrocytes after the injury. Further, our findings suggested that the effects of the PA reflected limitation of ESC differentiation into astrocytes. By contrast, β1-integrin signaling does not alter astrocyte proliferation although it exerts effects on reactive gliosis [43]. Thus injection of IKVAV-PA into a damaged spinal cord was able to limit astrogliosis by limiting ESC differentiation into astrocytes without altering the beneficial responses of resident astrocytes to the injury. Our findings indicate a causal relationship between IKVAV PA application and β1-intregrin signaling activation in vivo. This conclusion is supported by our observation that ablation of β1-intregrin in ESCs significantly worsens behavioral outcome after SCI (unpublished observation).

Identification of the molecular mechanisms underlying the beneficial effects of the PA should enable design of new targeted molecules that are even more effective in promoting recovery after SCI. For example, we found that PAs displaying two other epitopes known to interact with β1-integrin, a Tenascin C epitope and the RGD epitope of fibronectin, facilitated behavioral recovery after SCI. Ultimately it should be possible to design molecules that are even more effective therapeutically. For example, PAs can be created that incorporate more than one β1-integrin-interacting epitope and that also include epitopes targeting other signaling molecules such BMP receptors [44] or cytokines that activate JAK-STAT signaling [37] that have been implicated in astrocytic responses after SCI.

The increase in GFAP expression after ablation of β1-integrin in NSCs was accompanied by an increase in the number of $GFAP^+$ astrocytes detected by immunocytochemistry suggesting an increase in astrocyte lineage commitment. Because this comparison was done under differentiation conditions with very low levels of EGF, proliferation was limited. However it is possible that the increase in GFAP expression simply allowed detection of preexisting astrocytes with previously undetectable levels of GFAP. In either case, our findings support our hypothesis that β1-integrin signaling suppresses astrocytic differentiation, and is consistent with our finding *in vivo* that increased β1-integrin signaling leads to reduced glial scar formation. It should also be noted that the increase in $GFAP^+$ cells *in vitro* in the presence of IKVAV-PA was matched by a decrease in the number of $Sox2^+$ stem cells suggesting an effect on lineage commitment.

Our observations indicate that at least some of the effects of β1-integrin signaling on astrocytic differentiation are mediated by ILK, but the precise mechanisms mediating the effects of ILK remain unclear. ILK is a serine/threonine protein kinase that directly affects numerous other signaling pathways [17,24]. For example, in dendritic formation ILK directly phosphorylates GSK-3beta thus inhibiting its signaling [35]. However, in addition to its kinase activity, ILK can initiate signal transduction through its function as a scaffolding protein. For example, in mouse kidney development, the auto-phosphorylation site of ILK is dispensable, whereas the alpha-parvin binding ability of ILK is critical for normal development [49]. In both cases the effects of ILK reflect modulation of other important signaling pathways in the cell. Possible candidates include the PI3K/Akt and PI3K/RhoA pathways, that are known downstream targets of ILK and that have been implicated in reducing the potential for astrocytic differentiation [6]. However in other systems ILK signaling has also been linked to BMP and JAK-STAT signaling which are the major pathways involved in astrocytic differentiation [26,51]. Delineation of the set of pathways that mediate the effects of ILK on astrogliosis will ultimately be required to design effective interventions for limiting gliosis after injury to the nervous system.

It is noteworthy that the effects of β1-integrin signaling on astrocytic development were almost identical in ESCs isolated from the adult spinal cord and NSCs isolated from the adult SVZ. In turn this suggests that this signaling system may be an important target for regulating astrogliosis after brain injury as well as after SCI. Although this study did not examine the responses of subgranular zone stem cells to β1-integrin signaling, we find that the molecule is expressed abundantly in the SGZ. Thus it is likely that β1-integrin signaling an important regulator of stem cell proliferation and differentiation throughout the adult nervous system.

Acknowledgments

We thank Mark Benton for his critical reading of this manuscript.

Author Contributions

Conceived and designed the experiments: LP HAN VS JAK. Performed the experiments: LP HAN VS SJ TLM EJB. Analyzed the data: LP VS JAK. Contributed reagents/materials/analysis tools: EJB SIS JAK. Contributed to the writing of the manuscript: LP VS JAK.

References

1. Anthis NJ, Campbell ID (2011) The tail of integrin activation. Trends Biochem Sci, 36(4): p. 191–8.
2. Barnabe-Heider F, Goritz C, Sabelstrom H, Takebayashi H, Pfrieger FW, et al. (2010) Origin of new glial cells in intact and injured adult spinal cord. Cell Stem Cell, 7(4): p. 470–82.
3. Basso DM, Beattie MS, Bresnahan JC, Anderson DK, Faden AI, et al. (1996) MASCIS evaluation of open field locomotor scores: effects of experience and teamwork on reliability. Multicenter Animal Spinal Cord Injury Study. J Neurotrauma, 13(7): p. 343–59.
4. Bonaguidi MA, McGuire T, Hu M, Kan L, Samanta J, et al. (2005) LIF and BMP signaling generate separate and discrete types of GFAP-expressing cells. Development, 132(24): p. 5503–14.
5. Brakebusch C, Fassler R (2005) beta 1 integrin function in vivo: adhesion, migration and more. Cancer Metastasis Rev, 24(3): p. 403–11.
6. Brozzi F, Arcuri C, Giambanco I, Donato R (2009) S100B Protein Regulates Astrocyte Shape and Migration via Interaction with Src Kinase: IMPLICATIONS FOR ASTROCYTE DEVELOPMENT, ACTIVATION, AND TUMOR GROWTH. J Biol Chem, 284(13): p. 8797–811.
7. Campbell ID, Humphries MJ (2011) Integrin structure, activation, and interactions. Cold Spring Harb Perspect Biol, 3(3)
8. Campos LS, Leone DP, Relvas JB, Brakebusch C, Fassler R, et al. (2004) Beta1 integrins activate a MAPK signalling pathway in neural stem cells that contributes to their maintenance. Development, 131(14): p. 3433–44.
9. Casar B, Rimann I, Kato H, Shattil SJ, Quigley JP, et al. (2012) In vivo cleaved CDCP1 promotes early tumor dissemination via complexing with activated beta1 integrin and induction of FAK/PI3K/Akt motility signaling. Oncogene.
10. Dusart I, Marty S, Peschanski M (1991) Glial changes following an excitotoxic lesion in the CNS–II. Astrocytes. Neuroscience, 45(3): p. 541–9.
11. Fawcett JW, Asher RA (1999) The glial scar and central nervous system repair. Brain Res Bull, 49(6): p. 377–91.
12. Giancotti FG (1997) Integrin signaling: specificity and control of cell survival and cell cycle progression. Curr Opin Cell Biol, 9(5): p. 691–700.
13. Giancotti FG, Ruoslahti E (1999) Integrin signaling. Science, 285(5430): p. 1028–32.
14. Hall DE, Reichardt LF, Crowley E, Holley B, Moezzi H, et al. (1990) The alpha 1/beta 1 and alpha 6/beta 1 integrin heterodimers mediate cell attachment to distinct sites on laminin. J Cell Biol, 110(6): p. 2175–84.
15. Hall PE, Lathia JD, Miller NG, Caldwell MA, ffrench-Constant C (2006) Integrins are markers of human neural stem cells. Stem Cells, 24(9): p. 2078–84.
16. Hannigan G, Troussard AA, Dedhar S(2005) Integrin-linked kinase: a cancer therapeutic target unique among its ILK. Nat Rev Cancer, 5(1): p. 51–63.
17. Hannigan GE, Leung-Hagesteijn C, Fitz-Gibbon L, Coppolino MG, Radeva G, et al. (1996) Regulation of cell adhesion and anchorage-dependent growth by a new beta 1-integrin-linked protein kinase. Nature, 379(6560): p. 91–6.
18. Herrmann JE, Imura T, Song B, Qi J, Ao Y, et al. (2008) STAT3 is a critical regulator of astrogliosis and scar formation after spinal cord injury. J Neurosci, 28(28): p. 7231–43.
19. Hill MM, Feng J, Hemmings BA (2002) Identification of a plasma membrane Raft-associated PKB Ser473 kinase activity that is distinct from ILK and PDK1. Curr Biol, 12(14): p. 1251–5.
20. Hynes RO (1992) Integrins: versatility, modulation, and signaling in cell adhesion. Cell, 69(1): p. 11–25.
21. Joshi M, Fehlings MG (2002) Development and characterization of a novel, graded model of clip compressive spinal cord injury in the mouse: Part 1. Clip design, behavioral outcomes, and histopathology. J Neurotrauma, 19(2): p. 175–90.
22. Lee KK, de Repentigny Y, Saulnier R, Rippstein P, Macklin WB, et al. (2006) Dominant-negative beta1 integrin mice have region-specific myelin defects accompanied by alterations in MAPK activity. Glia, 53(8): p. 836–44.
23. Lee SL, Hsu EC, Chou CC, Chuang HC, Bai LY, et al. (2011) Identification and characterization of a novel integrin-linked kinase inhibitor. J Med Chem, 54(18): p. 6364–74.
24. Legate KR, Montanez E, Kudlacek O, Fassler R (2006) ILK, PINCH and parvin: the tIPP of integrin signalling. Nat Rev Mol Cell Biol, 7(1): p. 20–31.
25. Leone DP, Relvas JB, Campos LS, Hemmi S, Brakebusch C, et al. (2005) Regulation of neural progenitor proliferation and survival by beta1 integrins. J Cell Sci, 118(Pt 12): p. 2589–99.
26. Leung-Hagesteijn C, Hu MC, Mahendra AS, Hartwig S, Klamut HJ, et al. (2005) Integrin-linked kinase mediates bone morphogenetic protein 7-dependent renal epithelial cell morphogenesis. Mol Cell Biol, 25(9): p. 3648–57.
27. Liberto CM, Albrecht PJ, Herx LM, Yong VW, Levison SW (2004) Pro-regenerative properties of cytokine-activated astrocytes. J Neurochem, 89(5): p. 1092–100.
28. Liu S, Calderwood DA, Ginsberg MH (2000) Integrin cytoplasmic domain-binding proteins. J Cell Sci, 113 (Pt 20): p. 3563–71.
29. Luque A, Gomez M, Puzon W, Takada Y, Sanchez-Madrid F, et al. (1996) Activated conformations of very late activation integrins detected by a group of antibodies (HUTS) specific for a novel regulatory region (355–425) of the common beta 1 chain. J Biol Chem, 271(19): p. 11067–75.
30. Mehler MF, Mabie PC, Zhu G, Gokhan S, Kessler JA (2000) Developmental changes in progenitor cell responsiveness to bone morphogenetic proteins differentially modulate progressive CNS lineage fate. Dev Neurosci, 22(1–2): p. 74–85.
31. Meiners S, Nur-e-Kamal MS, Mercado ML (2001) Identification of a neurite outgrowth-promoting motif within the alternatively spliced region of human tenascin-C. J Neurosci, 21(18): p. 7215–25.
32. Meletis K, Barnabe-Heider F, Carlen M, Evergren E, Tomilin N, et al. (2008) Spinal cord injury reveals multilineage differentiation of ependymal cells. PLoS Biol, 6(7): p. e182.
33. Mercado ML, Nur-e-Kamal A, Liu HY, Gross SR, Movahed R, et al. (2004) Neurite outgrowth by the alternatively spliced region of human tenascin-C is mediated by neuronal alpha7beta1 integrin. J Neurosci, 24(1): p. 238–47.
34. Milner R, Campbell IL (2002) The integrin family of cell adhesion molecules has multiple functions within the CNS. J Neurosci Res, 69(3): p. 286–91.
35. Naska S, Park KJ, Hannigan GE, Dedhar S, Miller FD, et al. (2006) An essential role for the integrin-linked kinase-glycogen synthase kinase-3 beta pathway during dendrite initiation and growth. J Neurosci, 26(51): p. 13344–56.
36. Nomizu M, Weeks BS, Weston CA, Kim WH, Kleinman HK, et al. (1995) Structure-activity study of a laminin alpha 1 chain active peptide segment Ile-Lys-Val-Ala-Val (IKVAV). FEBS Lett, 365(2–3): p. 227–31.
37. Okada S, Nakamura M, Katoh H, Miyao T, Shimazaki T, et al. (2006) Conditional ablation of Stat3 or Socs3 discloses a dual role for reactive astrocytes after spinal cord injury. Nat Med, 12(7): p. 829–34.

38. Pekny M, Nilsson M (2005) Astrocyte activation and reactive gliosis. Glia, 50(4): p. 427–34.
39. Pfaff M, Gohring W, Brown JC, Timpl R (1994) Binding of purified collagen receptors (alpha 1 beta 1, alpha 2 beta 1) and RGD-dependent integrins to laminins and laminin fragments. Eur J Biochem, 225(3): p. 975–84.
40. Pruszak J, Ludwig W, Blak A, Alavian K, Isacson O (2009) CD15, CD24, and CD29 define a surface biomarker code for neural lineage differentiation of stem cells. Stem Cells, 27(12): p. 2928–40.
41. Relvas JB, Setzu A, Baron W, Buttery PC, LaFlamme SE, et al. (2001) Expression of dominant-negative and chimeric subunits reveals an essential role for beta1 integrin during myelination. Curr Biol, 11(13): p. 1039–43.
42. Robel S, Berninger B, Gotz M(2011) The stem cell potential of glia: lessons from reactive gliosis. Nat Rev Neurosci, 12(2): p. 88–104.
43. Robel S, Mori T, Zoubaa S, Schlegel J, Sirko S, et al. (2009) Conditional deletion of beta1-integrin in astroglia causes partial reactive gliosis. Glia, 57(15): p. 1630–47.
44. Sahni V, Mukhopadhyay A, Tysseling V, Hebert A, Birch D, et al. (2010) BMPR1a and BMPR1b signaling exert opposing effects on gliosis after spinal cord injury. J Neurosci, 30(5): p. 1839–55.
45. Sanchez-Mateos P, Cabanas C, Sanchez-Madrid F (1996) Regulation of integrin function. Semin Cancer Biol, 7(3): p. 99–109.
46. Sephel GC, Tashiro KI, Sasaki M, Greatorex D, Martin GR, et al. (1989) Laminin A chain synthetic peptide which supports neurite outgrowth. Biochem Biophys Res Commun, 162(2): p. 821–9.
47. Silva GA, Czeisler C, Niece KL, Beniash E, Harrington DA, et al. (2004) Selective differentiation of neural progenitor cells by high-epitope density nanofibers. Science, 303(5662): p. 1352–5.
48. Silver J, Miller JH (2004) Regeneration beyond the glial scar. Nat Rev Neurosci, 5(2): p. 146–56.
49. Smeeton J, Zhang X, Bulus N, Mernaugh G, Lange A, et al. (2010) Integrin-linked kinase regulates p38 MAPK-dependent cell cycle arrest in ureteric bud development. Development, 137(19): p. 3233–43.
50. Stirling DP, Liu S, Kubes P, Yong VW (2009) Depletion of Ly6G/Gr-1 leukocytes after spinal cord injury in mice alters wound healing and worsens neurological outcome. J Neurosci, 29(3): p. 753–64.
51. Tabe Y, Jin L, Tsutsumi-Ishii Y, Xu Y, McQueen T, et al. (2007) Activation of integrin-linked kinase is a critical prosurvival pathway induced in leukemic cells by bone marrow-derived stromal cells. Cancer Res, 67(2): p. 684–94.
52. Tadokoro S, Shattil SJ, Eto K, Tai V, Liddington RC, et al. (2003) Talin binding to integrin beta tails: a final common step in integrin activation. Science, 302(5642): p. 103–6.
53. Tashiro K, Sephel GC, Weeks B, Sasaki M, Martin GR, et al. (1989) A synthetic peptide containing the IKVAV sequence from the A chain of laminin mediates cell attachment, migration, and neurite outgrowth. J Biol Chem, 264(27): p. 16174–82.
54. Tysseling-Mattiace VM, Sahni V, Niece KL, Birch D, Czeisler C, et al. (2008) Self-assembling nanofibers inhibit glial scar formation and promote axon elongation after spinal cord injury. J Neurosci, 28(14): p. 3814–23.
55. Yokosaki Y, Monis H, Chen J, Sheppard D (1996) Differential effects of the integrins alpha9beta1, alphavbeta3, and alphavbeta6 on cell proliferative responses to tenascin. Roles of the beta subunit extracellular and cytoplasmic domains. J Biol Chem, 271(39): p. 24144–50.
56. Zhu Y, Li H, Zhou L, Wu JY, Rao Y (1999) Cellular and molecular guidance of GABAergic neuronal migration from an extracortical origin to the neocortex. Neuron, 23(3): p. 473–85.

Influence of Delivery Method on Neuroprotection by Bone Marrow Mononuclear Cell Therapy following Ventral Root Reimplantation with Fibrin Sealant

Roberta Barbizan[1], Mateus V. Castro[1], Benedito Barraviera[2], Rui S. Ferreira Jr.[2], Alexandre L. R. Oliveira[1]*

1 Laboratory of Nerve Regeneration, Department of Structural and Functional Biology, University of Campinas - UNICAMP, Campinas, São Paulo, Brazil, **2** Center for the Study of Venoms and Venomous Animals (CEVAP), São Paulo State University (UNESP – Univ Estadual Paulista), Botucatu, São Paulo, Brazil

Abstract

The present work compared the local injection of mononuclear cells to the spinal cord lateral funiculus with the alternative approach of local delivery with fibrin sealant after ventral root avulsion (VRA) and reimplantation. For that, female adult Lewis rats were divided into the following groups: avulsion only, reimplantation with fibrin sealant; root repair with fibrin sealant associated with mononuclear cells; and repair with fibrin sealant and injected mononuclear cells. Cell therapy resulted in greater survival of spinal motoneurons up to four weeks post-surgery, especially when mononuclear cells were added to the fibrin glue. Injection of mononuclear cells to the lateral funiculus yield similar results to the reimplantation alone. Additionally, mononuclear cells added to the fibrin glue increased neurotrophic factor gene transcript levels in the spinal cord ventral horn. Regarding the motor recovery, evaluated by the functional peroneal index, as well as the paw print pressure, cell treated rats performed equally well as compared to reimplanted only animals, and significantly better than the avulsion only subjects. The results herein demonstrate that mononuclear cells therapy is neuroprotective by increasing levels of brain derived neurotrophic factor (BDNF) and glial derived neurotrophic factor (GDNF). Moreover, the use of fibrin sealant mononuclear cells delivery approach gave the best and more long lasting results.

Editor: Graca Almeida-Porada, Wake Forest Institute for Regenerative Medicine, United States of America

Funding: The present work was supported by a grant from Fundação de Amparo a Pesquisa do Estado de São Paulo – FAPESP, Brazil (2010/0986-5). Barbizan R. was supported by Fundação de Amparo a Pesquisa do Estado de Sao Paulo – FAPESP (process number: 2010/00729-2). This work was funded by grants from Coordenação de Aperfeiçoamento de Pessoal de Nível Superior (CAPES), Conselho Nacional de Desenvolvimento Cientifico e Tecnológico (CNPq) and Fundação de Amparo à Pesquisa do Estado de São Paulo (FAPESP). The funders had no role in study design, data collection and analysis, decision to publish, or preparation of the manuscript.

Competing Interests: The authors have declared that no competing interests exist.

* Email: alroliv@unicamp.br

Introduction

In order to enhance the success of adult stem cell (SC) translational medicine efforts, the source as well as the most effective delivery method has to be considered. The bone marrow contains endothelial progenitor cells and mononuclear cells (MC). The MC fraction corresponds to the totality of hematopoietic and mesenchymal stem cells. MC present clinical advantages over other stem cells, based on the minimally invasive harvesting procedures, which are fast and cost-effective. Also, the possibility of autografting avoids the use of immunosuppressants, present low oncogenic potential and does not raise ethical issues [1] as compared to other SC. Moreover, MCs have similar potential therapeutic outcome for nerve regeneration in comparison to mesenchymal cells [2]. The peripheral nerve regeneration after MC has been connected to the local production of neurotrophic factors [1,3,4]. Relevantly, stem cell therapy may also present an immunomodulatory effect, reducing pro-inflammatory events as well as glial reaction following lesion.

Ventral root avulsion in rats has been used as a model for brachial plexus lesion (BPL). BPL is frequently caused by motorbike accidents in young adults as well as following complicated child-birth delivery [5]. It causes paralysis in the corresponding muscle groups and loss of sensory functions [6]. The degenerative impact on motoneurons is well characterized and is potentiated by pulling out the ventral roots from the CNS/PNS interface at the spinal cord surface [6]. Similarly to BPL, VRA results in extensive loss of neurons in the first weeks after injury [7,8].

Reimplantation of avulsed roots can rescue motoneurons from degeneration, increasing the regenerative capacity of axonal regrowth [9,10]. As a result, anatomical and functional reinnervation of denervated muscles can be obtained [11–13]. As seen in a previous work [10], a snake venom derived fibrin sealant allowed successful and stable ventral root implantation. Nevertheless, additional therapeutic approaches need to be developed, since root reimplantation alone, although neuroprotective, results in insufficient functional sensory-motor recovery [12,14–16].

In order to improve the outcome following VRA, regarding neuronal survival, several attempts have been made to provide neurotrophic molecules at the site of injury. In this regard, the association of the root reimplantation with BDNF and CNTF resulted in rescue of injured motoneurons after avulsion in rabbits [17]. Therefore, the use of neurotrophic factors in combination with root reimplantation is a potential therapy to be used in patients.

The use of recombinant neurotrophic factors, however, present important drawbacks. One of them is the need of relatively large amounts of the purified substance, to reach the target lesioned area. Due to the short biological activity window of such substances, there is also need of constant perfusion, what may contribute to infection and further lesion of the affected spinal cord area. Additionally, it is improbable that a single neurothrophic molecule will be sufficient to provide the necessary conditions for optimal regeneration.

Based on such facts, the advent of stem cell technology brought new insights on cell therapy and local delivery of trophic substances. To date, however, there is not sufficient data on the delivery method to the nervous system, especially following VRA. So far, it is known that mesenchymal stem cells synthesize and possibly release BDNF and GDNF, when grafted to the VRA lesion area [18]. No data, however, indicates that MC exhibit the same properties.

Therefore, the present study investigated two delivery strategies of MC, comparing the local injection to the spinal cord with the possibility of mixing MC with fibrin sealant on the interface of the CNS/PNS. Local production of BDNF and GDNF were evaluated in both situations.

The results herein demonstrate that MC therapy is neroprotective and increases the transcript and protein levels of BDNF and GDNF in the lesioned spinal cord area. Moreover, the administration method significantly influenced treatment outcome, so that the use of fibrin sealant MC delivery approach gave the best and more long lasting results.

Material and Methods

2.1- Experimental animals

Adult female Lewis (LEW/HsdUnib) rats, 7 weeks old, were obtained from the Multidisciplinary Center for Biological Investigation (CEMIB/UNICAMP) and housed under a 12-hour light/dark cycle with free access to food and water. The study was approved by the Institutional Committee for Ethics in Animal Experimentation (Committee for Ethics in Animal Use – Institute of Biology - CEUA/IB/UNICAMP, proc. n° 2073-1). All experiments were performed in accordance with the guidelines of the Brazilian College for Animal Experimentation. The animals were subjected to unilateral avulsion of the L4-L6 lumbar ventral roots and divided into 4 groups: 1) VRA without reimplantation (AV 1 week, n = 5; AV 4 weeks, n = 15 and AV 8 weeks, n = 10); 2) VRA followed by lesioned roots reimplantation with fibrin sealant (AV+S 1 week n = 5, AV+S 4 weeks, n = 15 and AV+S 8 weeks, n = 10); 3) VRA followed by lesioned roots reimplantation with fibrin sealant and MC homogenized to the sealant (AV+S+HC 1 week, n = 5, AV+S+HC 4 weeks, n = 15 and AV+S+HC 8 weeks, n = 10) and 4) VRA followed by lesioned roots reimplantation with fibrin sealant and injection of MC (AV+S+IC 4 weeks, n = 15 and AV+S+IC 8 weeks, n = 10).

The peroneal functional index was calculated weekly up to 8 weeks after injury (n = 10 for each group). Animals were killed 1 week and 4 weeks after injury and their lumbar spinal cords were processed for PCR (n = 5 for each group). The animals were killed after 4 and 8 weeks after avulsion and the lumbar spinal cords were processed for immunohistochemistry (n = 5 for each group) and neuronal survival counting (n = 5 for each group). Each animal's unlesioned, contralateral spinal cord side, served as an internal control.

2.2- Bone Marrow Mononuclear Cells Extraction

MC were extracted from transgenic Lewis rats (LEW-Tg EGFP F455/Rrrc), with the EGFP (Enhanced green fluorescent protein) gene under Ubiquitin C promoter control. The animals were imported from Missouri University (EUA) and were provided by Dr. Alfredo Miranda Góes, Federal University of Minas Gerais – UFMG, Brazil.

The EGFP rats were killed with lethal dose of halothane (Tanohalo, Cristália Chemicals and Pharmaceuticals, Brazil), and the femur and tibia were dissected out from the muscular and connective tissue. The cells were isolated by density gradient centrifugation using Histopaque 1077 following the separation of mononuclear cells methods of Sigma-Aldrich n° 1119 protocol. The cell suspension consists of heterogeneous cell populations (13.2% CD11b, 1.52% CD3, 92.2% CD45, 20.8% CD34 of CD45). After 2 washing steps, cells were immediately transplanted.

2.3- Ventral root avulsion (VRA)

The rats were anesthetized with 50 mg/Kg of Ketamine (Fort Dodge) and 10 mg/Kg of xylasine (Köning) and subjected to unilateral avulsion of the lumbar ventral roots as previously described [19]. Right side avulsion was performed at the L4, L5 and L6 lumbar ventral root after laminectomy. A longitudinal incision was made to open the dural sac, the denticulate ligament was dissected and the ventral roots associated with the lumbar intumescence could be identified and avulsed with fine forceps (Nº 4). Finally, the musculature, fascia and skin were sutured in layers. Chlorhydrate of tramadol was administrated by gavage after the surgical procedures (20 mg/kg) and 2.5 mg/day soluble in water during 5 days.

2.4- Reimplantation of the motor roots

In AV+S, AV+S+MC and AV+S+IC groups, the roots were replaced at the exact point of detachment, on the ventral surface of the lumbar spinal cord at the avulsion site with the aid of a snake venom fibrin sealant [10]. The fibrin sealant was kindly provided by CEVAP/UNESP and is under the scope of the Brazilian Patents BR 10 2014 011432 7 and BR 10 2014 011436 0 [20–22]. The sealant used herein is composed of three separate solutions (1-fibrinogen, 2-calcium chloride and 3-thrombin-like fraction). During surgical repair of the avulsed roots, the first two components were applied and the avulsed roots were returned to their original sites. The third component was then added for polymerization. The reimplanted roots were then gently pulled from the spinal cord, and the stability of the fixation was observed to evaluate the success of the repair.

2.5- Mononuclear cells transplantation

In group 3 (AV+S+HC), 3×10^5 MCs were added to the fibrin sealant in avulsed roots reimplantation at the moment of implantation. In this case, the cells are grouped in the right ventrolateral surface of the spinal cord (Figure 1 A and B). In group 4, 3×10^5 MCs were placed directly into the lateral funiculus on the lesioned side (ipsilateral) in the segments L4–L6 of the spinal cord with the aid of a thick capillary Pasteur pipette coupled to a Hamilton syringe and then the avulsed roots were repaired with sealant. In this group, the cells are at the site of injection (Figure 1 C and D).

2.6- Specimen preparation

The animals were anaesthetized with an overdose of mixture of xylasine and Ketamine, and the vascular system was transcardially perfused with phosphate buffer 0.1 M (pH 7.4). For PCR, the rats

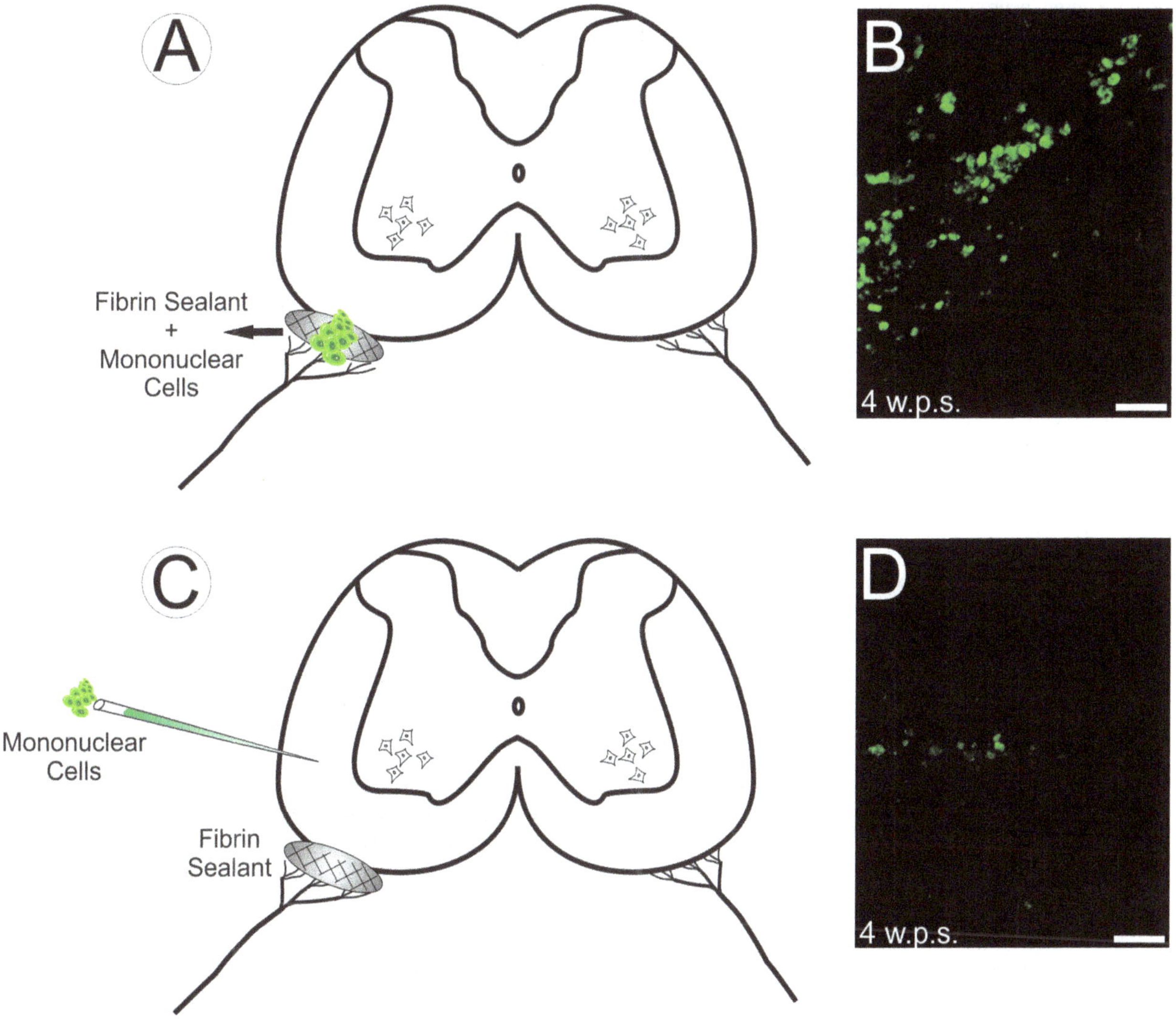

Figure 1. Scheme of the spinal cord subjected to motor root avulsion and reimplantation, with the two different cell delivery locations. A) Scheme of transverse spinal cord section subjected to motor avulsion followed by fibrin sealant reimplantation plus MC. B) MC are grouped in the right ventrolateral surface of the spinal cord (AV+S+HC), four weeks post surgery (4 w.p.s.). C) Scheme of the transverse spinal cord section subjected to motor root avulsion followed by fibrin sealant reimplantation and cell injection in the lateral funiculus. D) The cells are at the site of injection (AV+S+IC), 4 w.p.s. Such cells were E-GFP fluorescent donors. Scale bar = 50 µm.

were killed 1 and 4 weeks after VRA and their lumbar intumescences were frozen in liquid nitrogen. For neuron survival counting and immunohistochemistry the rats were killed 4 and 8 weeks after VRA and fixed by vascular perfusion of 10% formaldehyde in phosphate buffer (pH 7.4). The lumbar intumescence was dissected, post-fixed overnight and then washed in phosphate buffer and stored overnight in sucrose 20% before freezing. Transverse cryostat 12 µm thick sections of spinal cords were obtained and transferred to gelatin-coated slides and dried at room temperature for 30 min before being stored at −20°C.

2.7- Counting of motoneurons survival

Cell counts were performed on sections from the lumbar enlargement. Transverse cryostat sections of the spinal cords were stained for 3 min in aqueous 1% cresyl fast violet solution (Sigma-Aldrich, USA). The sections were then washed in distilled water, dehydrated and mounted with Entellan (Merck, USA). The motoneurons were identified (based on their morphology, size, and location in the dorsolateral lamina IX) and cells with a visible nucleus and nucleolus were counted. The absolute number of motoneurons on the lesioned and non-lesioned side of each section was used to calculate the percentage of surviving cells in each specimen. This percentage was calculated by dividing the number of motoneurons in the ipsilateral (lesioned) side by the number of neurons in the contralateral (non-lesioned) side and multiplying the result by 100. Abercrombie's formula was used to correct for the duplicate counting of neurons [23].

$$N = nt/(t+d)$$

where N is the corrected number of counted neurons, n is the counted number of cells, t is the thickness of the sections (12 µm) and d is the average diameter of the cells. Because differences in cell size can significantly affect cell counts, the value of d was calculated specifically for each experimental group and for both ipsilateral and contralateral neurons. The diameters of 15 randomly chosen neurons from each group were measured by using the ImageTool software (version 3.00, The University of Texas Health Science Center, San Antonio, USA).

2.8- Immunohistochemistry

Transverse sections of spinal cord were incubated with mouse anti-synaptophysin (Dako, 1:250), goat anti-GFAP (Dako, 1:900), and rabbit anti-Iba1 (Wako, 1:800) diluted in a solution containing 1% BSA in TBS-T (Tris-Buffered Saline and Tween) and 2% Triton X-100 in PB 0.1 M (phosphate buffer). All sections were incubated for 6 hours at room temperature in a moist chamber. After rinsing in TBS-T, the sections were incubated according to the primary host antibody (CY-3, Jackson Immunoresearch; 1:250) for 45 minutes in a moist chamber at room temperature. After 3 times washing in TBS-T, the slides were mounted in a mixture of glycerol/PBS (3:1) and observed with a Nikon eclipse TS100 inverted microscope (Nikon, Japan). For quantitative measurements, 3 representative images (with 2 MNs) of the spinal cord (L4–L6 at lamina IX, ventral horn) from each animal were captured at a final magnification of ×200. Double blind quantification was performed in IMAGEJ software (version 1.33 u, National Institute of Health, USA) using the enhanced contrast and density slicing two features [24]. The integrated density of pixels was systematically measured in six representative areas of the motor nucleus from each section, according to [19]. The integrated pixel density was calculated for each section of spinal cord, and then a mean value for each spinal cord was calculated. The data are represented as the mean ± standard error (SE).

2.9- Real time polymerase chain reaction (PCR)

Total RNA was extracted from the ipsilateral and contralateral sides of the frozen lumbar intumescences, 1 and 4 weeks after lesion, using the RNeasy Lipid Tissue Kit (cat n° 74804, Quiagen), according to the manufacturer's recommendations. The RNA was quantified using a NanoDrop Spectrophotometer (A260/280; model 2000, Thermo Scientific). The RNA (1 μg) obtained from five samples was reverse-transcribed using a commercial kit (AffinityScripts QPCR cDNA Synthesis Kit - Agilent Technologies, La Jolla, CA, USA) to achieve a final reaction volume of 20 μL. Real time quantitative PCR was performed on Mx3005P qPCR System (Agilent Technologies, La Jolla, CA, USA), after an initial denaturation for 10 minutes at 95°C, followed by 35 cycles of amplification (95°C for 30 seconds followed by 72°C for one minute). The reactions were carried out with 12.5 μL 2×SYBR Green PCR master mix (Agilent Technologies), 0.2 μM of each forward and reverse primer 100 ng cDNA template, in a final reaction volume of 20 μL. All quantifications were normalized to the house keeping gene β-actin. A non-template control with non-genetic material was included to eliminate contamination or nonspecific reactions. Each sample (n = 5) was tested in triplicate and then used for the analysis of the relative transcription data using the $2^{-\Delta\Delta CT}$ method [25]. The following forward (F) and reverse (R) primers were used: BDNF: (F) 5′-CCACAATGTTC-CACCAGGTG-3′, (R) 5′-TGGGCGCAGCCTTCAT-3′; GDNF: (F) 5′-CCACCATCAAAAGACTGAAAAG-3′, (R) 5′-CGGTTCCTCTCTCTTCGAGGA-3′; Iba-1 (F) 5′- CCC-CACCTAAGGCCACCAGC-3′, (R) 5′-TCCTGTTGGCTTT-CAGCAGTCC-3′; GFAP (F) 5′-TGCTGGAGGGCGAA-GAAAACCG-3′ 5′-CCAGGCTGGTTTCTCGGATCTGG-3′; β-actin (F) 5′-GGAGATTACTGCCCTGGCTCCTA-3′ (R) 5′-GACTCAICGTACTCCTGCTTGCTG-3′. The BDNF and GDNF were based on [18] and the β-actin was based on [26].

2.10- Functional Analysis

For the gait recovery analysis, the CatWalk system (Noldus Inc., The Netherlands; was used. In this set up, the animal crosses a walkway with an illuminated glass floor. A high-speed video camera Gevicam (GP-3360, USA) equipped with a wide-angle lens (8.5 mm, Fujicon Corp., China) is positioned underneath the walkway and the paw prints are automatically recorded and classified by the software. The paw prints from each animal were obtained before and after the VRA. Post-operative CatWalk data were collected twice a week for 12 weeks. The peroneal functional index (PFI) was calculated as the distance between the third toe and hind limb pads (print length) and the distance between the first and fifth toes (print width). Measurements of these parameters were obtained from the right (lesioned) and left (unlesioned) paw prints, and the values were calculated using the following formula [27].

$$PFI = 174.9\ x\ ((EPL - NPL)/NPL)$$
$$+ 80.3x\ ((ETS - NTS)/NTS)) - 13.4$$

Where N: normal, or non-operated side; E: experimental, or operated; PL: print length; TS: total toe spread, or distance between first to fifth toe.

The pressure exerted on the platform by individual paws was also evaluated. The Catwalk data from each day were expressed as an ipsi-/contralateral ratio.

2.11- Statistical analysis

Statistical analysis was performed with Graphpad Prisma 4.0 software. The neuronal survival, immunohistochemistry, and PCR were firstly evaluated with one-way ANOVA. Data from the functional analysis was evaluated with two-way ANOVA. Bonferroni post-test was used to identify intergroup differences. The data are presented as the mean ± SE and the differences between groups were considered significant when the P-value was <0.05 (*), <0.01 (**) and <0.001 (***).

Results

3.1- Neuroprotection after root reimplantation plus MC treatment after VRA

Neuronal survival was assessed as the ipsi-/contralateral ratio of motoneurons present in the lamina IX of the ventral horn. No significant differences between the numbers of motoneurons on the contralateral side in the different experimental conditions were observed. After four weeks, there was severe degeneration of affected motorneurons in the AV group (Fig. 2A). In implanted groups (Fig 2 C, E and G) a higher number of surviving neurons was observed. Such neuroprotection was even more evident in the AV+S+HC group (Fig. 2I) (AV 36.09%±3.67%; AV+S 65.19%±6.93%; AV+S+HC 89.44%±1.89%; AV+S+IC 64.60%±1.33% percentage of survival ipsi-/contralateral ± SEM; p<0.001).

Neuroprotection in the implanted groups remained superior to the avulsion only throughout the time course of the study, i.e. up to 8 weeks post lesion (Fig. 2 D, E and F). Nevertheless, the AV+S+HC group was similar to AV+S. Figure 2I shows the ipsi-/contralateral ratio for the groups where a statistically significant neuroprotective effect was observed (AV 34.58%±4.12%; AV+S 66.46%±3.88%; AV+S+HC 67.11%±4.83%; AV+S+IC 46.81%±5.87% percentage of survival ipsi-/contralateral ± SEM; p<0.001).

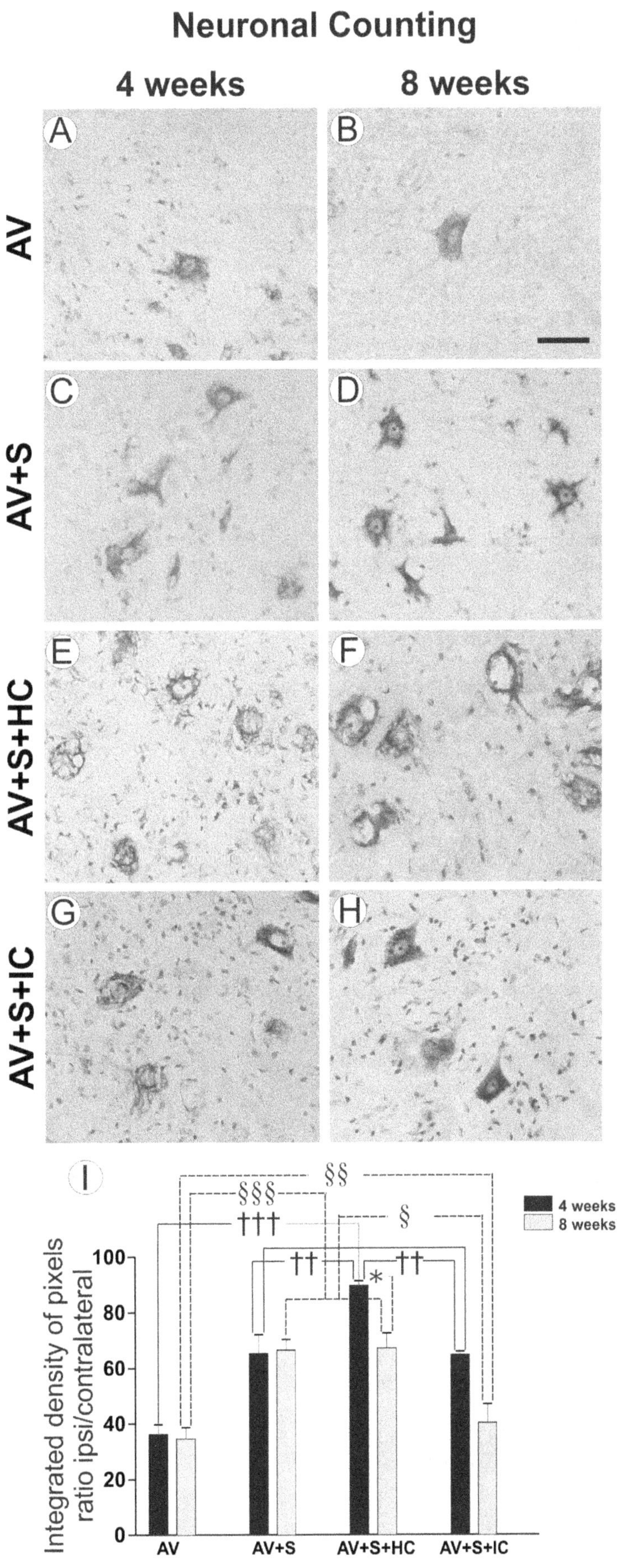
Neuronal Counting
4 weeks
8 weeks
A
B
C
D
E
F
G
H
AV
AV+S
AV+S+HC
AV+S+IC
I
4 weeks
8 weeks
Integrated density of pixels ratio ipsi/contralateral
100
80
60
40
20
0
AV
AV+S
AV+S+HC
AV+S+IC
§§
§§§
†††
§
††
††
*

Figure 2. Nissl-stained spinal cord transverse sections at lamina IX illustrating the neuroprotective effects of root reimplantation and MC treatment on motoneurons 4 and 8 weeks after VRA. Motoneuron cell bodies of the ipsilateral side of VRA after 4 weeks (A, C, E and G) and after 8 weeks (B, D, F and H). (A and B) AV, (C and D) AV+S, (E and F) AV+S+HC and (G and H) AV+S+IC. Scale bar = 50 μm. (I) Percentage of neuronal survival after ventral root avulsion, reimplantation and reimplantantion with MC. Note a significant rescue of lesioned neurons in the implanted groups with and without cells in two different survival times (4 and 8 weeks). This neuroprotection was even more intense in AV+S+HC 4 weeks after avulsion. (†† $p<0.01$ and ††† $p<0.001$ comparing all groups 4 weeks after avulsion, § $p<0.05$, §§ $p<0.01$ and §§§ $p<0.001$ comparing all groups 8 weeks after AV and *$p<0.05$ comparing AV+S+HC at two different times after avulsion, n = 5).

3.2- Decreased synaptic elimination after VRA followed by implantation and cell treatment

Synaptic network changes after root avulsion were evaluated in the ventral horn by immunohistochemistry with an antibody against synaptophysin. Quantitative measurements of synaptophysin immunoreactivity in the sciatic motor nuclei after avulsion (AV) and after avulsion followed by ventral root implantation (AV+S), implantation with cells homogenized on the sealant (AV+S+HC) and implantation with cell injection (AV+S+IC) were carried out. As shown in Fig. 3, AV only led to a significant decrease in synaptophysin expression four weeks after avulsion, which remained until 8 weeks. Such results indicate a significant decrease of complexity of intraspinal networks following lesion. In contrast, in implanted groups with or without cells, the repair resulted in preservation of synaptophysin immunoreactivity, in the immediate vicinity of the motoneurons. In AV+S+IC group the synaptic inputs decreased when comparing 4 and 8 weeks. Four weeks after avulsion: (AV 0.43±0.01; AV+S 0.66±0.09; AV+S+HC 0.65±0.07; AV+S+IC 0.60±0.01 mean ratio ipsi-/contralateral ± SE with $p<0.01$) and 8 weeks after avulsion: (AV 0.40±0.05; AV+S 0.72±0.05; AV+S+HC 0.84±0.07; AV+S+IC 0.855±0.03 mean ratio ipsi-/contralateral ± SE, $p<0.05$).

3.3- Astroglial reactivity is not further enhanced by mononuclear cells around motoneuron vicinity

Immunoreactivity against GFAP was used to analyze the degree of astroglial reactivity after lesion. This demonstrates the presence of GFAP-positive astrocytic processes in the vicinity of the avulsed motoneurons. Figure 4 shows that the astroglial reactivity was not significantly further increased after implantation and cell treatment in both experimental times: Four weeks after avulsion (AV 2.65±0.48; AV+S 2.49±0.60; AV+S+HC 2.62±0.43; AV+S+IC 2.17±0.12 mean ratio ipsi-/contralateral ± SE); eight weeks after avulsion (AV 3.45±0.61; AV+S 2.09±0.26; AV+S+HC 2.58±0.37; AV+S+IC 2.30±0.32 mean ratio ipsi-/contralateral ± SE).

The real-time PCR analysis was performed to measure GFAPmRNA in the RNA in all ventral horn after avulsion. Figure 4 demonstrated that the levels of GFAPmRNA were similar in all groups, 1 week (Fig 4 J) after lesion (AV 1.51±0.38; AV+S 1.20±0.24; AV+S+HC 1.65±0.26 mean ratio ipsi-/contralateral ± SE). However, 4 weeks (Fig 4 K) after avulsion, AV+S group presented a decreased number of transcripts to GFAP (AV 2.64±0.45; AV+S 1.35±0.14; AV+S+HC 2.11±0.12; AV+S+IC 2.00±0.12 mean ratio ipsi-/contralateral ± SE).

3.4- Microglial reactivity is enhanced by mononuclear cells one week after tranplantation

To detect possible changes in the microglial cells close to large motoneurons cell bodies after avulsion, the immunoreactivity against Iba-1 was evaluated in the ventral horn in the different experimental groups. Figure 5 shows that the microglial reactivity was not significantly further increased after implantation and cell treatment in both experimental times. However, the AV+S and AV+S+IC groups showed decreased microglia reaction in the course of experimental time. Four weeks after avulsion: (AV 4.71±0.41; AV+S 4.73±0.94; AV+S+HC 3.02±0.64; AV+S+IC 5.67±1.34; mean ratio ipsi-/contralateral ±SE with $p<0.01$) and 8 weeks after avulsion: (AV 2.70±0.51; AV+S 2.18±0.57; AV+S+HC 2.32±0.59; AV+S+IC 2.25±0.35 mean ratio ipsi-/contralateral ± SE, $p<0.05$).

The real-time PCR analysis was performed to measure Iba-1 mRNA in the in ventral horn RNA after avulsion. Figure 5 demonstrated that the levels of Iba-1 mRNA in AV+S+HC were significantly greater than in the AV and AV+S groups (AV 0.95±0.30; AV+S 1.63±0.60; AV+S+HC 4.15±0.48 mean ratio ipsi-/contralateral ± SE). Nevertheless, 4 weeks (Fig 5 K) after avulsion, Iba-1 mRNA were similar in all groups (AV 2.07±0.26; AV+S 1.07±0.18; AV+S+HC 1.64±0.26; AV+S+IC 1.73±0.03 mean ratio ipsi-/contralateral ± SE).

3.5- Mononuclear cells enhance BDNF and GDNF expression one week after avulsion

Real time PCR was used to detect BDNF and GDNF mRNAs in the lumbar spinal cord after avulsion (Figure 6). The results demonstrated the levels of both neurotrophic factors in the AV+S+HC group were significantly greater, when compared to the other groups, one week after surgery (A and C) (BDNF - AV 1.20±0.29; AV+S 1.33±0.18; AV+S+HC 2.48±0.10 mean ratio ipsi-/contralateral ± SE *$p<0.05$) and (GDNF - AV 1.71±0.56; AV+S 1.24±0.23; AV+S+HC 2.86±0.34; mean ratio ipsi-/contralateral ± SE *$p<0.05$). Four weeks after avulsion, BDNF and GDNF mRNA levels were similar in all groups (B and D) (BDNF - AV 2.04±0.18; AV+S 1.45±0.35; AV+S+HC 1.53±0.16; AV+S+IC 1.70±0.17 mean ratio ipsi-/contralateral ± SE) and (GDNF - AV 2.25±0.10; AV+S 1.92±0.43; AV+S+HC 1.72±0.30; AV+S+IC 1.77±0.01 mean ratio ipsi-/contralateral ± SE).

3.6- Functional motor recovery

The recovery of motor function was analysed by the CatWalk System. Post-operative assessments of peroneal function were performed for eight consecutive weeks. The preoperative peroneal functional index mean values (Figure 7A) did not significantly differ between groups. The peroneal functional index drastically declined after avulsion. The three implanted groups presented significantly better peroneal index performance as compared to AV group (AV −228.89±23.0; AV+S −139.75±12.5; AV+S+HC −155.50±17.2; AV+S+IC −205.14±18.6, mean ratio ipsi-/contralateral ± SE, *$p<0.05$, **$p<0.01$ and ***$p<0.001$. These results are consistent with the footprint paw pressure data (Figure 7B), indicating that all three implanted groups presented a better performance as compared to avulsion group (AV 0.20±0.07; AV+S 0.81±0.09726454; AV+S+HC 0.66±0.078; AV+S+IC 0.40±0.11 mean ratio ipsi-/contralateral ± SE with *$p<0.05$ and ***$p<0.001$).

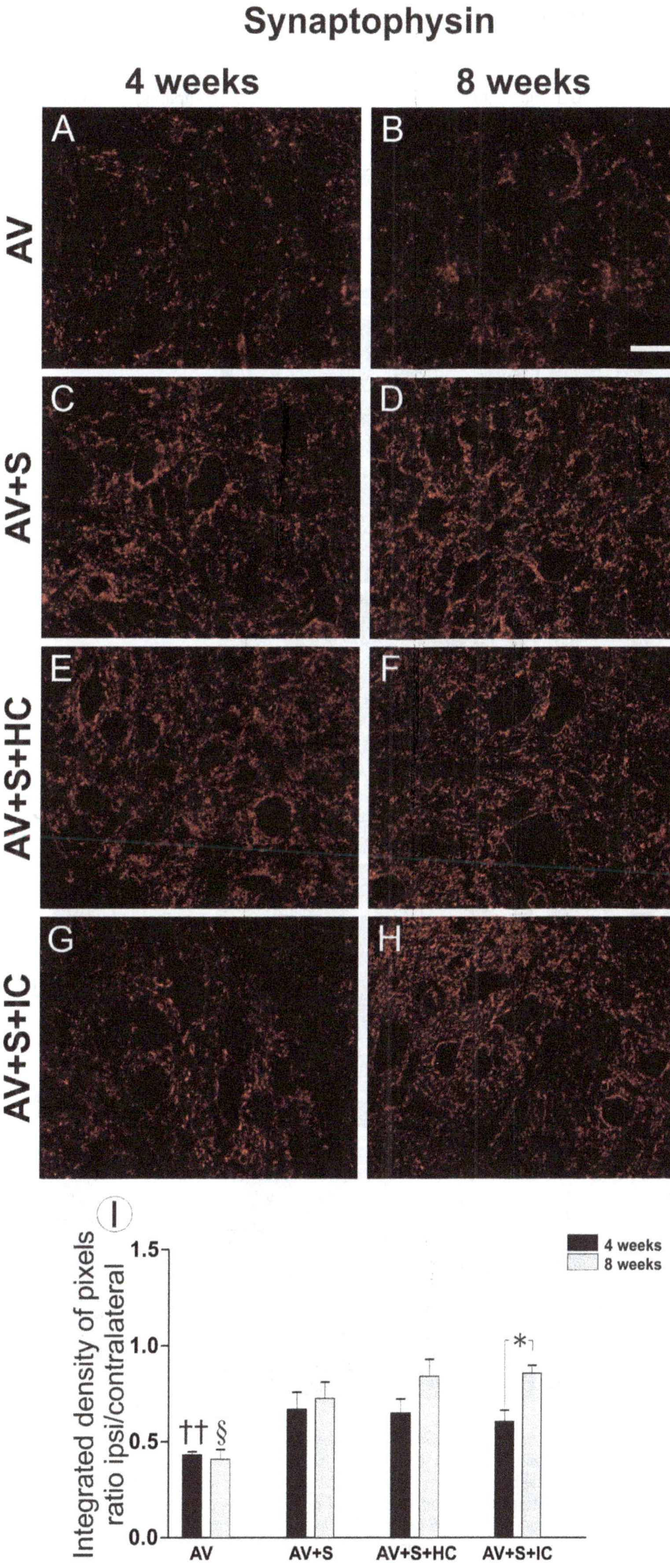
Synaptophysin
4 weeks
8 weeks
AV
AV+S
AV+S+HC
AV+S+IC
A
B
C
D
E
F
G
H
I
Integrated density of pixels ratio ipsi/contralateral
1.5
1.0
0.5
0.0
4 weeks
8 weeks
††
§
*
AV
AV+S
AV+S+HC
AV+S+IC

Figure 3. Immunohistochemical analysis of the spinal cord ventral horn stained with anti-synaptophysin 4 and 8 weeks after VRA. Observe the preservation of synaptophysin labeling, especially at the surface of the lesioned motoneurons in implanted group and both implanted with mononuclear cells treatment. After 4 weeks post lesion (A, C, E and G) and after 8 weeks (B, D, F and H). (A and B) AV, (C and D) AV+S, (E and F) AV+S+HC and (G and H) AV+S+IC. Scale bar = 50 μm. (I) Quantification of synaptic covering obtained by the ratio ipsi/contralateral sides of the integrated density of pixels at lamina IX four and eight weeks after injury. (†† $p<0.01$ comparing all groups 4 weeks after avulsion, § $p<0.05$ comparing all groups 8 weeks after AV and * $p<0.05$ comparing AV+S+IC at two different times after avulsion, n = 5).

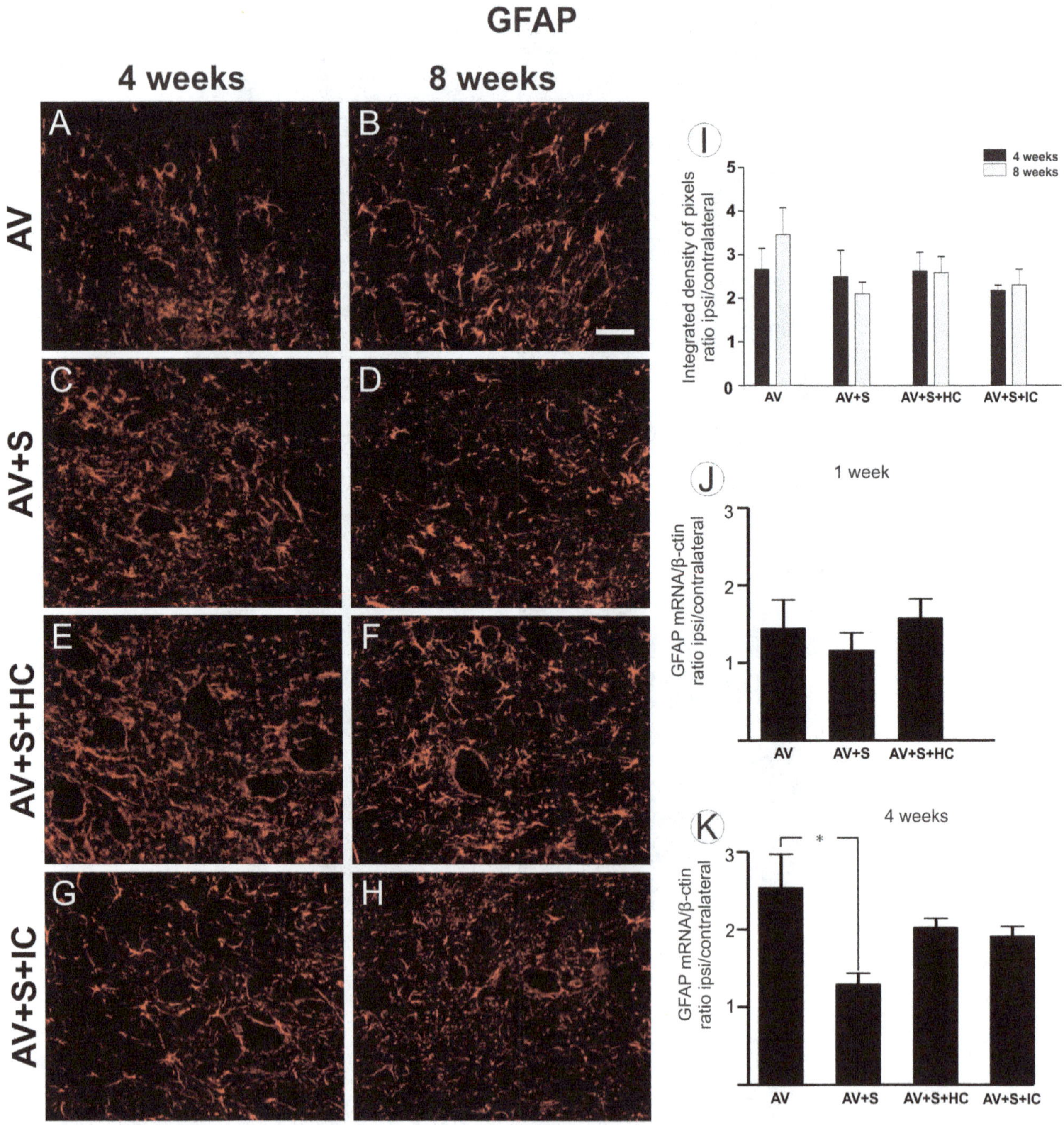

Figure 4. Glial fibrillary acidic protein (GFAP) in the spinal cord ventral horn. Immunohistochemical analysis of the anterior horn of the spinal cord was labeled with anti-GFAP, 4 and 8 weeks after injury to assess the degree of astroglial reactivity after root avulsion (A–H). Representative images of AV, AV+S, AV+S+HC and AV+S+IC. Scale bar = 50 μm. Observe that ventral root implantation and cell treatment did not increase astroglial reaction. (I) The mean ratio of the ipsi-/contralateral integrated intensity of pixels of the ipsilateral and contralateral sides in all groups. (* $p<0.05$, n = 5). (J) One week after avulsion, there were no differences between groups by GFAPmRNA analysis. (K) The RT-qPCR performed 4 weeks after avulsion demonstrated significant decrease in the synthesis of GFAP mRNA in AV+S group compared with AV (*$p<0.05$, n = 5).

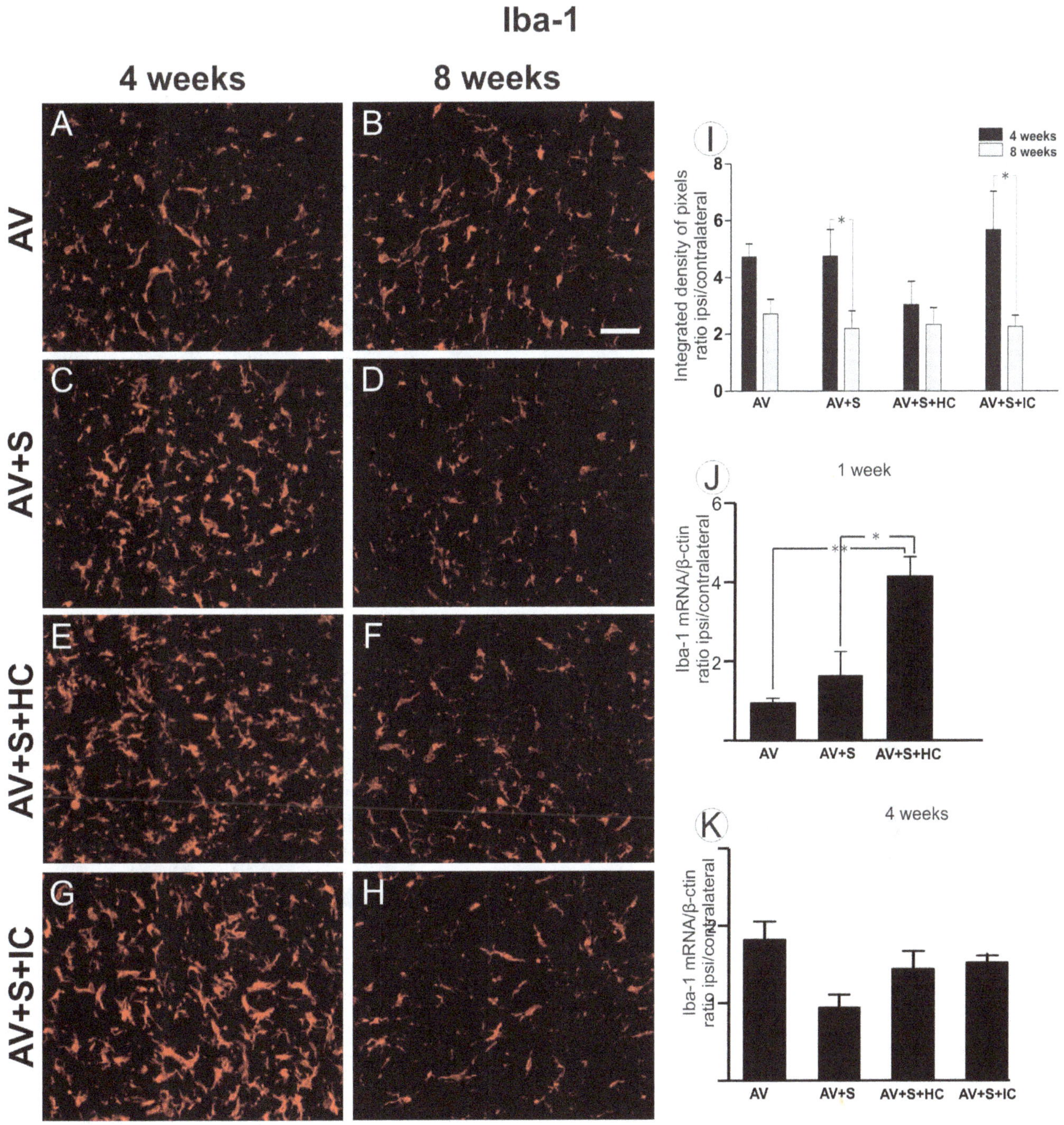

Figure 5. Microglial analysis of the spinal cord ventral horn 4 and 8 weeks after VRA. The quantification analysis on motoneuron cell bodies stained with anti- Iba1 of the ipsilateral side of VRA after 4 weeks (A, C, E and G) and after 8 weeks (B, D, F and H). (A and B) AV, (C and D) AV+S, (E and F) AV+S+HC and (G and H) AV+S+IC. Scale bar = 50 µm. (I) The mean ratio of the ipsil-/contralateral integrated intensity of pixels of the ipsilateral and contralateral sides in both groups. Note the decrease in microglial reactivity in AV+S and AV+S+IC as compared 4 and 8 weeks after injury. (J) There were significant increase in the synthesis of Iba-1 mRNA in the lumbar spinal cord one week after avulsion (*$p<0.05$ and **$p<0.01$, $n=5$). (K) The RT-qPCR, performed 4 weeks after avulsion, did not demonstrate significant differences between groups in Iba-1 mRNA.

Discussion

Brachial plexus lesions are particularly debilitating and usually affect young adults. To date, new technological refinements aiming at improving the repair of such traumatic injury are necessary. Although nerve reimplantation has been proposed [7,10] the relatively poor clinical outcome requires further attention. Treatment with neurotrophic factors, following root reimplantation, has proven to be efficient [17]. Importantly, it has been previously shown that mesenchymal stem cells naturally produce BDNF and GDNF when grafted to the VRA lesion area [18]. Considering it, the present study main objective was to compare the root reimplantation regenerative outcome by either injecting or engrafting the mononuclear cells at the wounded area,

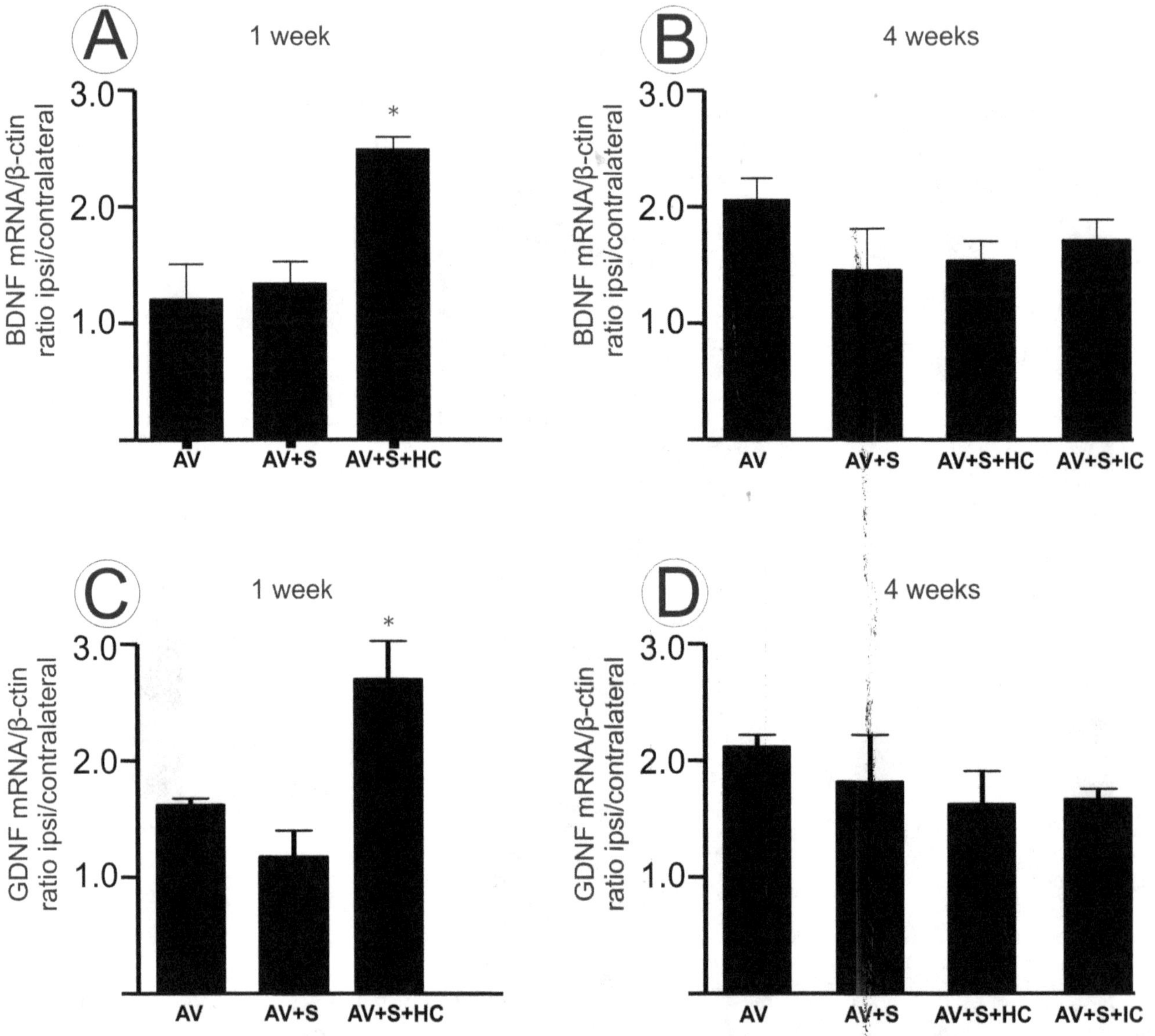

Figure 6. Neurotrophic factor expression (BDNF and GDNF) by RT-qPCR in the ventral horn spinal cord 1 and 4 weeks after avulsion. Expression of mean ratio of the ipsi-/contralateral mRNA for BDNF obtained by RT-qPCR in the lumbar spinal cord one (A) and four (B) weeks after avulsion. Note that one week after avulsion AV+S+HC enhanced the BDNF mRNA production compared to others groups (*$p<0.05$, $n=5$). Expression of mean ratio of the ipsi-/contralateral mRNA for GDNF obtained by RT-qPCR in the lumbar spinal cord one (C) and four (D) weeks after avulsion. Note that, one week after avulsion in the AV+S+HC group, there is enhanced GDNF mRNA production as compared to others groups (*$p<0.05$, $n=5$).

with aid of a fibrin sealant scaffold. However, evaluating the perspective of translational studies, the use of bone marrow MC has been preferred instead of mesenchymal stem cells.

The use of MC resulted in neuroprotection following peripheral nervous system lesion [1,3] and following spinal cord injury [28]. Furthermore, the mononuclear fraction is easy to obtain, implicating in lower costs and less processing time, as compared with other cell types [1,29].

An important point to be observed is the best moment for performing the cell therapy. Therefore, in some instances, it has been proposed a late cell transplantation, following the acute phase after injury [30]. However, immediate cell engrafting increases the survival of motoneurons after root avulsion [17].

Based on such observations, the present work was based on cells treatment immediately after avulsion, in order to obtain the best neuroprotective results possible. This is particularly important following CNS/PNS injuries that cause extensive degeneration of adult motoneurons [31–33]. Such neuronal loss reaches up to 80% of motoneuron degeneration in the first two weeks post injury [7]. Our results showed that both intraspinal administration and fibrin sealant implantation of MC preserved a significant number of motoneurons when compared to the untreated group (avulsion). The neuroprotective effect observed herein reinforces that the combination of root reimplantatio and cell therapy leads to enhancement of axotomized motoneurons. On the contrary, most of the motoneurons degenerated following AV, which reinforces the need of acute neuroprotective treatments following VRA.

Neuronal rescue was highest following root reimplantation and fibrin sealant cell engrafting, 4 weeks after injury. Such effect may be the result of stem cell neurotrophic factor release in the site of

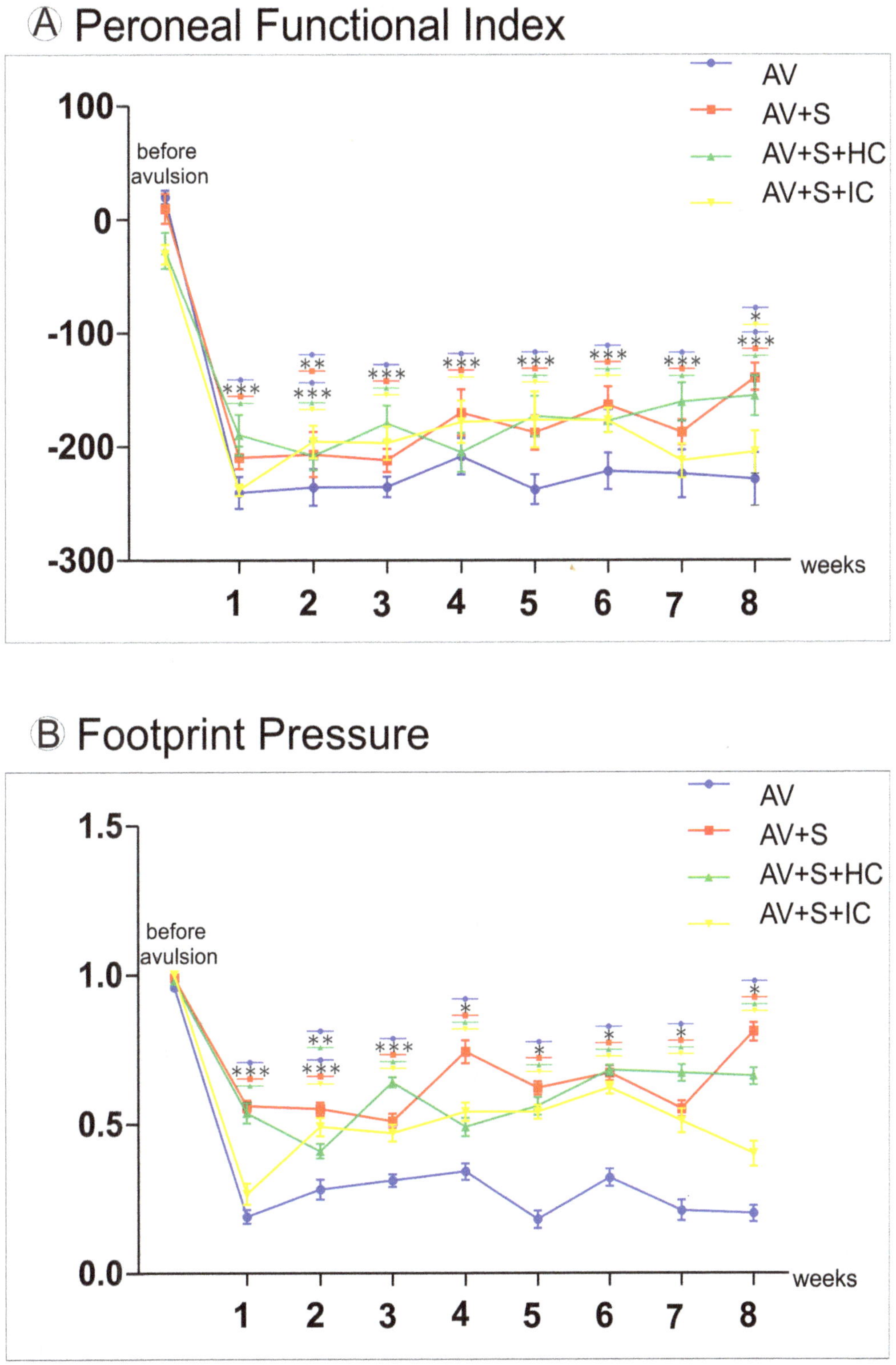

Figure 7. Motor function recovery after ventral root treatment. (A) Graph of the peroneal nerve functional index up to 8 weeks after avulsion. There is a significantly better performance of the three implanted groups compared to AV from the first week post lesion until the eighth week (***$p<0.001$, **$p<0.01$ and *$p<0.05$ $n=10$). (B) Restoration of weight-bearing capacity following avulsion. There is also a restoration of weight-bearing capacity following avulsion in implanted groups with or without cells from the first up to the eight week after injury. Values are expressed as the ratio of ipsi-/contralateral pressure exerted by the paw on the catwalk platform (***$p<0.001$ and *$p<0.05$, $n=10$).

injury [17,18]. Nevertheless, the production of extracellular matrix molecules has also been suggested as neuroprotective [34]. Neuronal survival decreased at 8 weeks post injury, indicating that the therapeutic window for MC is relatively short and further cell treatments may be necessary to maintain the axotomized neurons.

Cell injection to the spinal cord gave similar results to the reimplantation alone, 4 weeks post injury. However, neuronal degeneration increased up to 8 weeks, reaching the level of avulsion only. We believe that the injection into the CNS/PNS interface result in a late inflammatory response that cause delayed cell death. In this sense, using a similar reimplantation approach, followed by mesenchymal stem cell injection, neuron preservation has been shown without significant functional recovery [35]. Overall, the neuronal survival results indicate that fibrin sealant homogenized MC result in acutely better results as compared to intraspinal engrafting.

According to prior studies, MC express BDNF and GDNF [3] in the PNS following sciatic nerve injury. BDNF is also produced by MCs in the CNS, 3 and 7 days after MC therapy [4]. In line with this, several studies have demonstrated neuroprotective effects of such neurotrophic factors [7,32,36], especially after spinal cord injury [37]. Neuroprotection is also achieved in neonatal animals [38], where the effects of axotomy are more drastic than in adults. The results herein are in line with the literature and show BDNF and GDNF production by the MC, 1 week post injury.

Interestingly, BDNF, which is exacerbated in the implant group, promotes axonal sprouting and elongation after peripheral nerve injury and during development [39]. This is in line with the motor recovery observed in all root reimplanted groups, suggesting regeneration of axons after avulsion.

Functional analysis of the peroneal nerve, as well as the pressure exerted by the ipsilateral paw, provides reliable data on functional recovery of animals with motor problems [40,41]. The motor improvement observed herein is noteworthy because gait restoration is necessarily related to motor units recovery, together with cerebral cortex control [42]. Importantly, the preservation of pre-synaptic inputs to the injured motoneurons after implantation, observed by immunohistochemistry, indicates preservation of supraspinal contacts.

An important occurrence following VRA is the reduction of pre-synaptic terminals to motoneurons [42,43]. This synaptic decrease become irreversible if the regrowing axons within the root do not reach their target muscles [43]. Importantly, the groups subjected to root reimplantation showed a significant preservation of synapses as compared to the avulsion only group. In this case, cell treatment gave no further benefit, indicating that the restoration of CNS/PNS connection is sufficient to preserve spinal synaptic networks. Coupled with such synaptic changes, glial cells became reactive following VRA. Such reactive gliosis is characterized by hypertrophy of the cell body and processes of astrocytes and microglial hyperplasia [44–46].

Although the microglial reaction was morphologically decreased by MC treatment four weeks post lesion, at one week, an enhancement of Iba-1 gene transcripts was obtained. One possibility is that MCs increased or accelerated acute microglial response [47]. Regarding the astrogliosis, no differences were perceived between groups by immunohistochemical analysis. qPCR data, on the other hand, indicated a decreased number of GFAP gene transcripts following root reimplantation alone. This is in line with what has been observed 12 weeks after root reimplantation [10].

Conclusions

Taken together, the results of the present study indicate that MCs therapy further preserves injured motoneurons up to 4 weeks after implantation, in comparison to root reimplantation alone. Such fact is possibly related to the production of neurotrophic factors, such as BDNF and GDNF. Nonetheless, such difference was not seen at 4 weeks post injury. This may in turn indicate that restoration of the CNS/PNS connection must be carried out in a short period of time after avulsion. Importantly, the present data indicate that cell injection to the spinal cord does not result in long lasting neuroprotection. On the other hand, engrafting of MC at the site of injury with the aid of a fibrin scaffold is effective and may represent a more practical approach, with regard to translational medicine.

Acknowledgments

The authors are thankful to Prof. Dr. Alfredo M. Goes for providing the EGFP transgenic rats used in the present study. To Prof. Dr. Antonio C. Rodrigues for the fruitful discussions and to Prof. Dr. Dawidson A. Gomes and Prof. Dr. Ana Leda Longhini for expert flow cytometry analysis and comments.

Author Contributions

Conceived and designed the experiments: ALRO. Performed the experiments: ALRO MVC RB. Analyzed the data: ALRO MVC RB BB RSF. Contributed reagents/materials/analysis tools: ALRO BB RSF. Contributed to the writing of the manuscript: ALRO MVC RB BB RSF.

References

1. Goel RK, Suri V, Suri A, Sarkar C, Mohanty S, et al. (2009) Effect of bone marrow-derived mononuclear cells on nerve regeneration in the transection model of the rat sciatic nerve. J Clin Neurosci 16: 1211–1217.
2. de Freitas HT, da Silva VG, Giraldi-Guimaraes A (2012) Comparative study between bone marrow mononuclear fraction and mesenchymal stem cells treatment in sensorimotor recovery after focal cortical ablation in rats. Behav Brain Funct 8: 58.
3. Lopes-Filho JD, Caldas HC, Santos FC, Mazzer N, Simoes GF, et al. (2011) Microscopic evidences that bone marrow mononuclear cell treatment improves sciatic nerve regeneration after neurorrhaphy. Microsc Res Tech 74: 355–363.
4. Gubert F, Zaverucha-do-Valle C, Figueiredo FR, Bargas-Rega M, Paredes BD, et al. (2013) Bone-marrow cell therapy induces differentiation of radial glia-like cells and rescues the number of oligodendrocyte progenitors in the subventricular zone after global cerebral ischemia. Stem Cell Res 10: 241–256.
5. Thatte MR, Babhulkar S, Hiremath A (2013) Brachial plexus injury in adults: Diagnosis and surgical treatment strategies. Ann Indian Acad Neurol 16: 26–33.
6. Carlstedt T (2009) Nerve root replantation. Neurosurg Clin N Am 20: 39–50, vi.
7. Koliatsos VE, Price WL, Pardo CA, Price DL (1994) Ventral root avulsion: an experimental model of death of adult motor neurons. J Comp Neurol 342: 35–44.
8. Li L, Houenou LJ, Wu W, Lei M, Prevette DM, et al. (1998) Characterization of spinal motoneuron degeneration following different types of peripheral nerve injury in neonatal and adult mice. J Comp Neurol 396: 158–168.
9. Penas C, Casas C, Robert I, Fores J, Navarro X (2009) Cytoskeletal and activity-related changes in spinal motoneurons after root avulsion. J Neurotrauma 26: 763–779.
10. Barbizan R, Castro MV, Rodrigues AC, Barraviera B, Ferreira RS, et al. (2013) Motor recovery and synaptic preservation after ventral root avulsion and repair with a fibrin sealant derived from snake venom. PLoS One 8: e63260.
11. Cullheim S, Carlstedt T, Linda H, Risling M, Ulfhake B (1989) Motoneurons reinnervate skeletal muscle after ventral root implantation into the spinal cord of the cat. Neuroscience 29: 725–733.
12. Hoang TX, Nieto JH, Dobkin BH, Tillakaratne NJ, Havton LA (2006) Acute implantation of an avulsed lumbosacral ventral root into the rat conus medullaris promotes neuroprotection and graft reinnervation by autonomic and motor neurons. Neuroscience 138: 1149–1160.
13. Chang HY, Havton LA (2008) Surgical implantation of avulsed lumbosacral ventral roots promotes restoration of bladder morphology in rats. Exp Neurol 214: 117–124.

14. Carlstedt T (2008) Root repair review: basic science background and clinical outcome. Restor Neurol Neurosci 26: 225–241.
15. Eggers R, Tannemaat MR, Ehlert EM, Verhaagen J (2010) A spatio-temporal analysis of motoneuron survival, axonal regeneration and neurotrophic factor expression after lumbar ventral root avulsion and implantation. Exp Neurol 223: 207–220.
16. Giuffre JL, Kakar S, Bishop AT, Spinner RJ, Shin AY (2010) Current concepts of the treatment of adult brachial plexus injuries. J Hand Surg Am 35: 678–688; quiz 688.
17. Lang EM, Asan E, Plesnila N, Hofmann GO, Sendtner M (2005) Motoneuron survival after C7 nerve root avulsion and replantation in the adult rabbit: effects of local ciliary neurotrophic factor and brain-derived neurotrophic factor application. Plast Reconstr Surg 115: 2042–2050.
18. Rodrigues Hell RC, Silva Costa MM, Goes AM, Oliveira AL (2009) Local injection of BDNF producing mesenchymal stem cells increases neuronal survival and synaptic stability following ventral root avulsion. Neurobiol Dis 33: 290–300.
19. Oliveira AL, Thams S, Lidman O, Piehl F, Hokfelt T, et al. (2004) A role for MHC class I molecules in synaptic plasticity and regeneration of neurons after axotomy. Proc Natl Acad Sci U S A 101: 17843–17848.
20. Gasparotto VP, Landim-Alvarenga FC, Oliveira AL, Simoes GF, Lima-Neto JF, et al. (2014) A new fibrin sealant as a three-dimensional scaffold candidate for mesenchymal stem cells. Stem Cell Res Ther 5: 78.
21. Barros LC, Soares AM, Costa FL, Rodrigues VM, Fuly AL, et al. (2011) Biochemical and biological evaluation of gyroxin isolated from Crotalus durissus terrificus venom. The Journal of Venomous Animals and Toxins including Tropical Diseases 17: 23–33.
22. Barros LC, Ferreira RS, Jr., Barraviera SR, Stolf HO, Thomazini-Santos IA, et al. (2009) A new fibrin sealant from Crotalus durissus terrificus venom: applications in medicine. J Toxicol Environ Health B Crit Rev 12: 553–571.
23. Abercrombie M, Johnson ML (1946) Quantitative histology of Wallerian degeneration; nuclear population in rabbit sciatic nerve. J Anat 80: 37–50.
24. Freria CM, Velloso LA, Oliveira AL (2012) Opposing effects of Toll-like receptors 2 and 4 on synaptic stability in the spinal cord after peripheral nerve injury. J Neuroinflammation 9: 240.
25. Livak KJ, Schmittgen TD (2001) Analysis of relative gene expression data using real-time quantitative PCR and the 2(-Delta Delta C(T)) Method. Methods 25: 402–408.
26. Yao L, Chen X, Tian Y, Lu H, Zhang P, et al. (2012) Selection of housekeeping genes for normalization of RT-PCR in hypoxic neural stem cells of rat in vitro. Mol Biol Rep 39: 569–576.
27. Bain JR, Mackinnon SE, Hunter DA (1989) Functional evaluation of complete sciatic, peroneal, and posterior tibial nerve lesions in the rat. Plast Reconstr Surg 83: 129–138.
28. Yoshihara T, Ohta M, Itokazu Y, Matsumoto N, Dezawa M, et al. (2007) Neuroprotective effect of bone marrow-derived mononuclear cells promoting functional recovery from spinal cord injury. J Neurotrauma 24: 1026–1036.
29. Fernandes M, Valente SG, Fernandes MJ, Felix EP, Mazzacoratti Mda G, et al. (2008) Bone marrow cells are able to increase vessels number during repair of sciatic nerve lesion. J Neurosci Methods 170: 16–24.
30. Okada S, Ishii K, Yamane J, Iwanami A, Ikegami T, et al. (2005) In vivo imaging of engrafted neural stem cells: its application in evaluating the optimal timing of transplantation for spinal cord injury. FASEB J 19: 1839–1841.
31. Novikov L, Novikova L, Kellerth JO (1995) Brain-derived neurotrophic factor promotes survival and blocks nitric oxide synthase expression in adult rat spinal motoneurons after ventral root avulsion. Neurosci Lett 200: 45–48.
32. Kishino A, Ishige Y, Tatsuno T, Nakayama C, Noguchi H (1997) BDNF prevents and reverses adult rat motor neuron degeneration and induces axonal outgrowth. Exp Neurol 144: 273–286.
33. Oliveira AL, Langone F (2000) GM-1 ganglioside treatment reduces motoneuron death after ventral root avulsion in adult rats. Neurosci Lett 293: 131–134.
34. Ide C (1996) Peripheral nerve regeneration. Neurosci Res 25: 101–121.
35. Torres-Espin A, Corona-Quintanilla DL, Fores J, Allodi I, Gonzalez F, et al. (2013) Neuroprotection and axonal regeneration after lumbar ventral root avulsion by re-implantation and mesenchymal stem cells transplant combined therapy. Neurotherapeutics 10: 354–368.
36. Yan Q, Elliott J, Snider WD (1992) Brain-derived neurotrophic factor rescues spinal motor neurons from axotomy-induced cell death. Nature 360: 753–755.
37. Bregman BS, Coumans JV, Dai HN, Kuhn PL, Lynskey J, et al. (2002) Transplants and neurotrophic factors increase regeneration and recovery of function after spinal cord injury. Prog Brain Res 137: 257–273.
38. Sendtner M, Holtmann B, Kolbeck R, Thoenen H, Barde YA (1992) Brain-derived neurotrophic factor prevents the death of motoneurons in newborn rats after nerve section. Nature 360: 757–759.
39. Mendell LM, Munson JB, Arvanian VL (2001) Neurotrophins and synaptic plasticity in the mammalian spinal cord. J Physiol 533: 91–97.
40. Dijkstra JR, Meek MF, Robinson PH, Gramsbergen A (2000) Methods to evaluate functional nerve recovery in adult rats: walking track analysis, video analysis and the withdrawal reflex. J Neurosci Methods 96: 89–96.
41. Varejao AS, Meek MF, Ferreira AJ, Patricio JA, Cabrita AM (2001) Functional evaluation of peripheral nerve regeneration in the rat: walking track analysis. J Neurosci Methods 108: 1–9.
42. Purves D, Lichtman JW (1978) Formation and maintenance of synaptic connections in autonomic ganglia. Physiol Rev 58: 821–862.
43. Brannstrom T, Kellerth JO (1998) Changes in synaptology of adult cat spinal alpha-motoneurons after axotomy. Exp Brain Res 118: 1–13.
44. Privat A, Valat J, Fulcrand J (1981) Proliferation of neuroglial cell lines in the degenerating optic nerve of young rats. A radioautographic study. J Neuropathol Exp Neurol 40: 46–60.
45. Norton WT, Aquino DA, Hozumi I, Chiu FC, Brosnan CF (1992) Quantitative aspects of reactive gliosis: a review. Neurochem Res 17: 877–885.
46. Eng LF, Ghirnikar RS, Lee YL (2000) Glial fibrillary acidic protein: GFAP-thirty-one years (1969–2000). Neurochem Res 25: 1439–1451.
47. Grove JE, Bruscia E, Krause DS (2004) Plasticity of bone marrow-derived stem cells. Stem Cells 22: 487–500.

5

NK1 Receptor Blockade Is Ineffective in Improving Outcome following a Balloon Compression Model of Spinal Cord Injury

Anna Victoria Leonard[1]*, Emma Thornton[1], Robert Vink[2]

1 School of Medical Sciences, University of Adelaide, Adelaide, South Australia, Australia, **2** Division of Health Sciences, University of South Australia, Adelaide, South Australia, Australia

Abstract

The neuropeptide substance P (SP) is a well-known mediator of neurogenic inflammation following a variety of CNS disorders. Indeed, inhibition of SP through antagonism of its receptor, the tachykinin NK1 receptor, has been shown to be beneficial following both traumatic brain injury and stroke. Such studies demonstrated that administration of an NK1 receptor antagonist reduced blood-brain-barrier permeability, edema development and improved functional outcome. Furthermore, our recent studies have demonstrated a potential role for SP in mediating neurogenic inflammation following traumatic spinal cord injury (SCI). Accordingly, the present study investigates whether inhibition of SP may similarly play a neuroprotective role following traumatic SCI. A closed balloon compression injury was induced at T10 in New Zealand White rabbits. At 30 minutes post-injury an NK1 receptor antagonist was administered intravenously. Animals were thereafter assessed for blood spinal cord barrier (BSCB) permeability, spinal water content (edema), intrathecal pressure (ITP), and histological and functional outcome from 5 hours to 2 weeks post-SCI. Administration of an NK1 receptor antagonist was not effective in reducing BSCB permeability, edema, ITP, or functional deficits following SCI. We conclude that SP mediated neurogenic inflammation does not seem to play a major role in BSCB disruption, edema development and consequential tissue damage seen in acute traumatic SCI. Rather it is likely that the severe primary insult and subsequent hemorrhage may be the key contributing factors to ongoing SCI injury.

Editor: Pranela Rameshwar, Rutgers - New Jersey Medical School, United States of America

Funding: The study was funded by the Neil Sachse Foundation (http://www.nsf.org.au/) and the University of Adelaide. AVL is the Neil Sachse Foundation Fellow. The funders had no role in study design, data collection and analysis, decision to publish, or preparation of the manuscript.

Competing Interests: The authors have declared that no competing interests exist.

* E-mail: anna.leonard@adelaide.edu.au

Introduction

Spinal cord injury (SCI) remains a major cause of disability within society, frequently affecting individuals in the prime of their life. To date, therapies have very limited efficacy in attenuating any resultant functional deficits, and accordingly, novel therapeutic approaches are urgently required. SCI is characterized by both primary and secondary injury mechanisms. While the primary injury is clearly irreversible, secondary injury mechanisms are considered reversible and are thus targeted for potential therapeutic interventions. Edema is one of the major secondary injury mechanisms in CNS injury, being considered to significantly contribute to further potentiation of injury development and tissue damage. The development of edema following SCI has been well characterized both within the injury epicentre [1,2,3,4,5,6] and in the adjacent segments where a delayed rostrocaudal spread of edema has been demonstrated with time [7,8]. Such edema may be both vasogenic and cytotoxic in nature, however it has been hypothesized that the initial edema is predominantly vasogenic in nature given that blood-spinal cord-barrier (BSCB) disruption is also present [1,2,9,10,11]. Importantly, increased edema following injury may lead to raised intrathecal pressure (ITP) [12], which in turn can result in greater tissue damage, and ultimately profound functional deficits.

Neurogenic inflammation has recently been shown to play an important role in the development of edema following a range of CNS injuries [13,14,15,16,17,18,19,20]. Neurogenic inflammation is a response of perivascular, unmyelinated afferent nerve fibres to injury or infection and is typically characterized by vasodilation, protein extravasation and edema [13,14,21]. The vascular response is facilitated by the release of neuropeptides such as substance P (SP) and calcitonin gene related peptide (CGRP). SP is known to preferentially bind to the tachykinin NK1 receptor, activation of which results in increased barrier permeability and edema development [14]. Increased SP immunoreactivity has been associated with increased blood brain barrier (BBB) permeability and edema development following both TBI [13,17] and stroke [16], whilst antagonism of the NK1 receptor has been shown to reduce BBB permeability and edema, as well as improve functional outcome [13,17,22]. Furthermore, our recent investigation following SCI has demonstrated that SP stores are reduced following injury, indicative of SP release, whilst NK1 receptor immunoreactivity increased [20]. Such results implicate a role for SP as a mediator of neurogenic inflammation following

SCI. However, whether inhibition of SP may similarly produce a neuroprotective effect following SCI has not yet been investigated.

Accordingly, the current study investigates the effect of administration an NK1 receptor antagonist following a balloon compression model of SCI. Specifically, this paper will assess SP immunoreactivity, BSCB permeability, edema, ITP, histological outcome, and functional outcome from 5 hours to 2 weeks post-SCI. We have utilized the balloon compression model of SCI due to its closed nature, thus facilitating development of increased ITP, and its replication of key primary injury mechanisms in clinical SCI as previously reported [20,23,24,25].

Materials and Methods

All experimental protocols were conducted according to the guidelines established by the National Health and Medical Research Council and were approved by the animal ethics committees of the University of Adelaide (M-2010-140) and the Institute of Medical and Veterinary Sciences (98/10), Adelaide, South Australia.

2.1. Balloon compression model of SCI

New Zealand white rabbits (n = 88) were subject to a balloon compression spinal cord injury as previously described [26,27]. Briefly, during the 12-hour day cycle, animals were removed from their home cages and anesthetized via a subcutaneous injection of Ketamine (2.5 mg/kg) and Domitor (0.25 mg/kg) mixture. Once a surgical level of anesthesia was achieved, the animal was placed onto a thermostatically controlled heating pad in the prone position. Initially, the dorsal surface of the animal's back was shaved and a midline incision of approximately 10 cm in length was made along the spinous processors (approximately T11 – L2). Paraspinal muscles were retracted and a laminectomy performed. A balloon catheter (ApexTM MonorailTM 4 mm×8 mm, Boston Scientific) was then advanced approximately 4 cm to T10 and rapidly inflated using an inflation device (Boston Scientific) to 8 atm of pressure. The balloon remained inflated for a 5-minute period before being deflated and removed. The muscular wound was sutured closed followed by closure of the skin with surgical clips. An additional group of animals were subject to all surgical procedures except inflation of the balloon catheter (sham; surgery controls).

2.2. n-acetyl L-tryptophan (NAT)

Animals were randomly assigned to receive the NK1 receptor antagonist, n-acetyl tryptophan (NAT), or equal volume vehicle (0.9% saline). NAT was administered intravenously at 30 minutes post-SCI at 2.5 mg/kg, with this optimal dose of NAT having been previously determined in studies conducted in our laboratory [28]. For studies with survival times greater than 24 hours, 2 additional i.v. doses were administered daily on day 1 and 2 post-SCI.

2.3. BSCB permeability

The Evan's Blue (EB) dye extravasation method, as previously described [14], was used to assess BSCB permeability at 5 hours (vehicle, n = 5; NAT, n = 6) post-SCI (or sham, n = 5). Briefly, 30 minutes prior to perfusion, EB was injected intravenously. The animals were then saline perfused and the spinal cord dissected and 10 mm segments cut. Each segment was homogenized and the absorbance of the supernatant was measured at 610 nm using a spectrophotometer. The level of extravasated EB within each tissue sample was then determined using a previously obtained EB standard curve, and was expressed as ug/mg of spinal cord tissue.

2.4. Edema measurement

Animals were assessed for edema at 3 days post-SCI (NAT and vehicle; n = 4/group) or sham (n = 5) using the wet weight/dry weight method as previously described [14]. Briefly, animals were administered a lethal injection of pentobarbital and the spinal cord rapidly removed. The spinal cord was cut into 10 mm segments and the wet weight was obtained. Spinal cord segments were then oven dried at 100°C for 48 hours before the dry weight was measured. The percentage of tissue water content was then calculated using the equation: % Water Content = (Wet Weight – Dry Weight)/Wet weight) X 100

2.5. Intrathecal pressure measurement

Animals (vehicle, n = 6; NAT, n = 5; sham, n = 5) underwent a tracheotomy and the right and left femoral artery were dissected. The right femoral artery was cannulated and connected to a syringe pump containing saline, which was administered at 2 ml/h except when taking a blood sample for blood gas analysis. A Codman MICROSENSOR ICP probe was inserted into the left artery to monitor blood pressure. Following balloon compression, a Codman MICROSENSOR ICP probe was introduced into the intrathecal space and extended to the injury epicentre. The Codman probes were connected to an 8 channel Powerlab system (AD instruments) and the output was viewed live and recorded with Labchart (AD instruments). Intrathecal pressure was monitored for a 5 hour period. Blood pressure and blood gases were monitored to ensure physiological parameters were maintained.

2.6. Functional outcome

Animals were randomly assigned to sham, vehicle or NAT treated groups (n = 6 per group) and were assessed on days 3, 7, 10 and 14 post-SCI for both sensory and motor outcome. A modified Tarlov Score [23] was used to assess motor function of the hindlimbs. The criteria were as follows: 0 = No movement; 1 = minor movement of the hind limb joints; 2 = major movement of the hind limb joints; 3 = able to stand properly but unable to hop; 4 = able to hop, but not properly; 5 = normal movement. Animals were scored following a recorded 5-minute monitoring period. In addition, a forelimb to hindlimb ratio was calculated by recording the number of hindlimb movements per the first 20 forward moving forelimb steps. This ratio was then converted into a percentage.

The sensory outcome test involved applying the tip end of Dumont #4 fine forceps to the shaved plantar surface of animal's hind paw and assessing the withdrawal time. Animals were placed into an enclosed plastic box with a wire bottom with food provided as a distraction. The fine forceps were then applied to each hind paw 10 times with a 30 second interval between each application. The withdrawal response of the animals to the stimulus was graded as either; 0 = no response, 1 = weak response (slight movement of one joint of the hindlimb), 2 = moderate response (extensive movement of 2 or more joints of the hindlimb), or 3 = normal response. A sensory score out of 30 was given to each hind paw.

2.7. Histological outcome

Animals were randomly assigned to sham (n = 11), vehicle (n = 23) and NAT treated groups (n = 21) and were assessed for histological outcome using immunohistochemical techniques. Briefly animals were perfuse fixed with 10% formalin at 5 hours, 24 hours, 3 days, or 2 weeks post-SCI. Spinal cord tissue was then processed, embedded in paraffin and 5 μm cross sections were cut for assessment of morphological features (H&E stain), SP (Santa

Cruz Sc-9758; 1:2000, EDTA retrieval), NK1 receptor (Advanced Targeting Systems #AB-N33AP; 1:4000, Citrate retrieval), Albumin (Cappel #0113-0341; 1:20,000), microglia (Griffonia simplicifolia – Sigma L2140; 1:200), and AQP4 (Abcam Ab9512; 1:200, Citrate retrieval).

All sections underwent a similar immunohistochemical procedure, with all antibodies incubated at room temperature and PBS washes applied between each antibody. Briefly, sections were dewaxed, dehydrated and placed in methanol with 30% hydrogen peroxide. Specified microwave antigen retrieval was performed as required and sections incubated for 45 min in 3% normal horse serum. Primary antibody was added overnight before specific biotinylated secondary antibody (Vector,1:250) was added for 30 minutes. Tertiary streptavidin peroxidase conjugate (SPC; Pierce, 1:1000) was added for 1 hour and the immunocomplex visualised using 3,3′diaminobenzidine (DAB; Sigma) as a chromogen in the peroxidase reaction.

All sections were scanned at high resolution using the Hamamatsu Nanozoomer. Slides were viewed using the associated proprietary viewing software (NDP.view v1.1.27, Hamamatsu). Qualitative assessments were made by a blinded assessor using a ranking system (0 = no staining to 10 = extensive dark staining). Alternatively, whole sections were exported and assessed using our previously published color deconvolution method [29].

2.8. Statistical Analysis

All statistical tests were undertaken using GraphPad PRISM®. Evan's Blue extravasation, edema, ITP, Plantar prick test, and color deconvolution were analyzed using a two-way analysis of variance (ANOVA) followed by Bonferroni post-tests, with data expressed as mean ± standard error of the mean (SEM). Immunohistochemistry ranking and modified Tarlov score were analyzed using the Kruskal Wallis ANOVA followed by Dunn's multiple comparisons test. This data was expressed as the median and interquartile range (immunohistochemical ranking) or as the median and individual data points (Tarlov score).

Results

3.1. BSCB Permeability– Evan's Blue extravasation

Sham animals demonstrated minimal EB extravasation with an average of 6.93±1.25 µg EB/g tissue measured along all segments of the spinal cord (Figure 1A). After injury, a significant ($p<0.001$) increase in EB extravasation to 15.43±3.04 µg EB/g tissue was observed in vehicle treated animals within the injury epicentre at 5 hours post-SCI, with adjacent segments recording similar values to sham. NAT treated animals had similar EB extravasation to vehicles within the injury epicentre ($p<0.001$), however recorded significantly greater EB values ($0.01<p<0.05$) in the immediate adjacent segments when compared to shams. No significant differences were seen between vehicle and NAT treated groups.

3.2. Edema measurement

The spinal cord tissue water content of sham animals was 65.55±2.08% (Figure 1B). By 3 days post-SCI in vehicle treated animals, spinal cord water content had significantly increased ($p<0.001$) to 77.47±1.00% in the injury epicentre and to 68.82±1.39% and 70.4±1.56% within the immediate rostral ($p<0.05$) and caudal ($p<0.001$) segments, respectively. NAT treated animals had a similar edema profile to vehicle treated animals at this time, although a greater increase was apparent within the most distal caudal segment of the spinal cord, which was significant compared to sham ($p<0.05$).

3.3. Intrathecal pressure measurement

The intrathecal pressure of sham animals was 0.65±1.61 mmHg at the beginning of the recording period then stabilized and reached 3.75±1.26 mmHg by the end of monitoring (Figure 1C). An immediate significant increase in ITP was observed following injury with vehicle treated animals recording 5.31±3.98 mmHg ($p<0.001$) at 30 min post-SCI. ITP continued to gradually rise, reaching a maximal ITP of 7.36±0.79 mmHg by the end of 5 hour monitoring period ($p<0.001$). A similar significant increase in ITP was observed at the beginning of the monitoring period within the NAT treated group, with a recorded ITP measurement of 6.82±1.48 mmHg ($p<0.001$). Thereafter, a gradual increase in ITP was observed in the NAT treated group reaching a maximal recording of 9.42±1.34 mmHg at the end of the monitoring period ($p<0.001$). Whilst the NAT treated animals appear to trend slightly higher, no significant difference was observed between treatment groups over time.

3.4. Functional outcome

3.4.1. Motor function - Modified Tarlov Scale. Sham animals demonstrated normal motor function on all assessment days and ranked 5 (Figure 2A). Following injury, vehicle treated animals demonstrated a significant decrease in hindlimb motor function with severe paralysis observed on days 3 and 6 post-SCI. By day 10 and 14, vehicle treated animals ranked 1 and had regained some motor function. In contrast, NAT treated animals had recovered some minor hindlimb joint movement on day 6 post-SCI and accordingly had a significant improvement when compared to vehicle treated animals ($p<0.05$). However, from day 10 onwards, vehicle and NAT treated animals both had only minor motor function as assessed by the Tarlov score.

3.4.2. Motor function - hindlimb to forelimb ratio. The frequency of the hind limb movement was recorded as the number of hindlimb movements per 20 forelimb steps (Figure 2B). Sham animals demonstrated normal movement with every forelimb step followed by a hindlimb step, resulting in a 100% normal hindlimb movement. Vehicle treated injured animals showed no hind limb movement on day 3 and subsequently recorded 0% for the frequency of hind limb movement. Thereafter, a gradual increase in the frequency of hindlimb movement was observed, reaching 20±15.17% by day 14 post-SCI. As in the Tarlov score, NAT treated animals demonstrated earlier increases in the frequency of hindlimb movement with 10.83±12.81% recorded on day 6 post-SCI, and had a higher maximal frequency of movement of 25.83±18.82% observed on day 14 post-SCI. However, the improvement in hindlimb motor function produced by NAT treatment was only slight and was not significant.

3.4.3. Sensory function – prick test. Sham animals demonstrated normal sensory function over the 14 day assessment period, with only a slight deficit observed on day 3 in the left hindlimb. Such results suggest that the surgical procedure did not affect sensory function (Figure 2C and 2D). Vehicle treated animals demonstrated a significant decrease on day 3 post-SCI to 11.75±4.57 and 13.00±6.38 for the left and right hindlimbs, respectively ($p<0.001$). Some spontaneous improvement was observed over the assessment period and by day 14 the pain withdrawal score was 17.00±4.96 and 16.50±4.43 for the left and right hindlimbs, respectively ($p<0.001$). NAT animals similarly demonstrated a significant decrease in sensory function following injury, obtaining a pain withdrawal score of 13.00±2.98 and 10.00±4.99 for the left and right hindlimbs, respectively, on day 3 post-SCI ($P<0.001$). Similarly to vehicle treated animals, NAT treated animals recorded a slight spontaneous improvement in sensory function in both hindlimbs during the assessment period

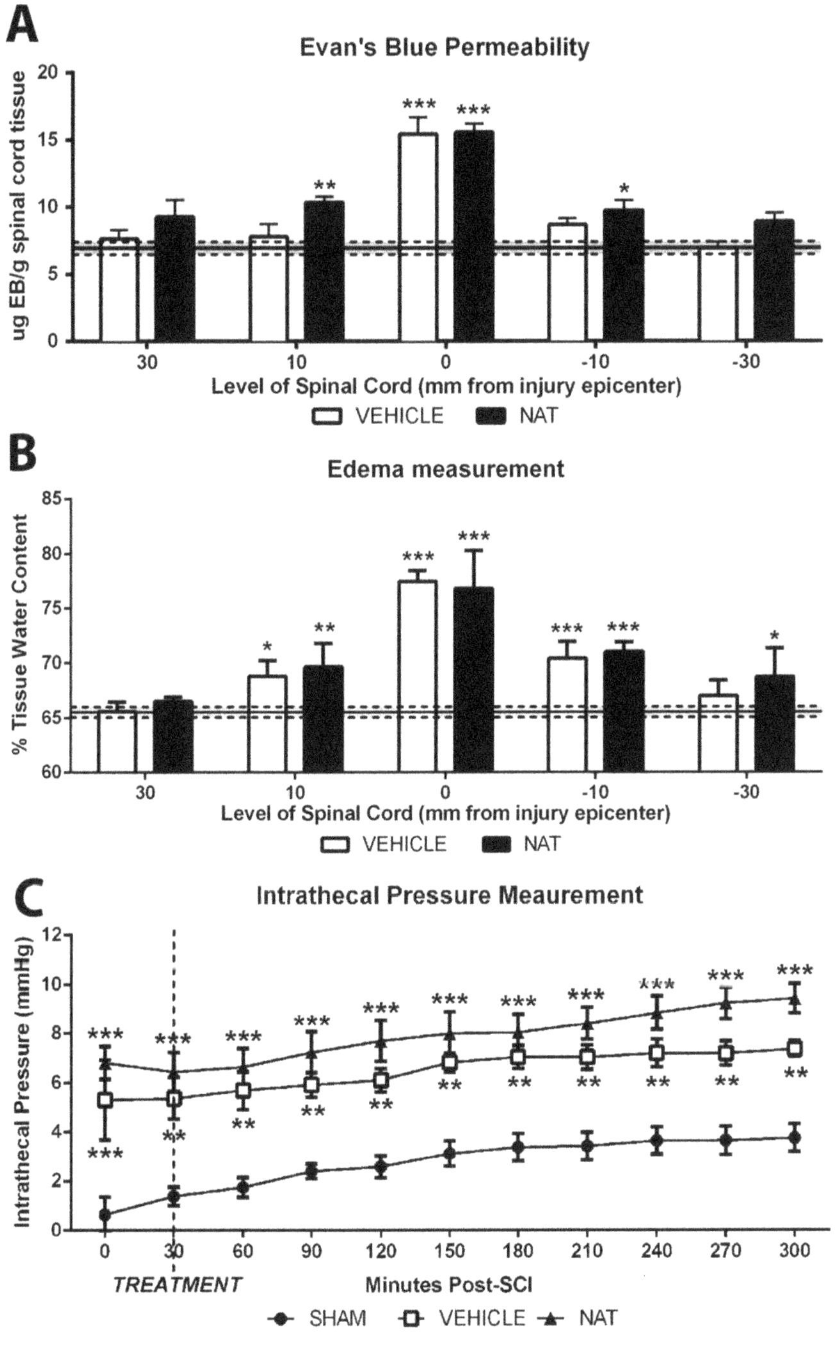

Figure 1. The effect of NAT administration on barrier permeability at 5 hours post-SCI was determined by the extent of EB extravasation (A). The percentage of spinal cord tissue water content was measured to determine the extent of edema development at 3 days post-SCI (B). The effect of NAT administration on ITP was measured for a 5 hour monitoring period (C). Sham levels indicated by the dashed line in (A) & (B). *denotes $p<0.05$, ** denotes $p<0.01$, *** denotes $p<0.001$ compared to sham.

recording a pain withdrawal score on day 14 post-SCI of 18±6.24 and 17.5±1.71 in the left and right hindlimbs respectively.

3.5. Histological outcome

3.5.1. Morphological features – H&E staining. Sham animals had normal tissue morphology and architecture (Figure 3). SCI resulted in focal areas of severe hemorrhage within the injury epicentre, predominantly within the grey matter, and substantial tissue disruption at 5 hours. The hemorrhage continued to spread and was diffusively located through the injury epicentre by 24 hours. Localized hemorrhage was also observed predominantly within the dorsal aspect of the white matter in the adjacent segments at this time. By 3 days post-SCI, moderate diffuse hemorrhage was observed within the injury epicentre, whilst minor hemorrhage was still apparent within the adjacent segments. Additionally by this time, loss of tissue morphology and architecture are clearly evident in the injury epicentre. By 2 weeks post-SCI extensive tissue loss was evident within the injury

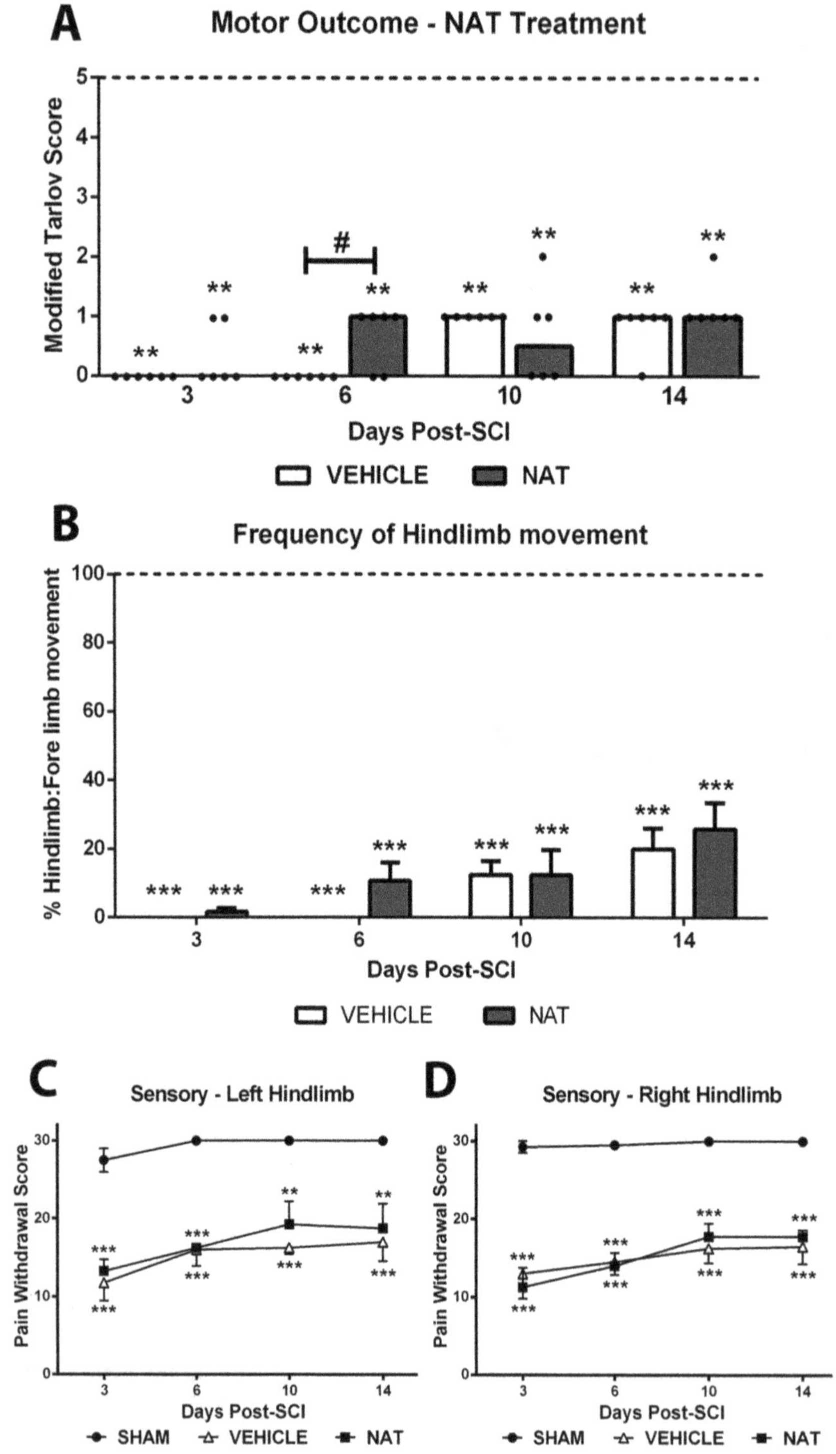

Figure 2. The effect of NAT administration on motor and sensory function following SCI. A modified Tarlov score was used to assess crude motor function (A), data is expressed as the median with individual data points plotted. Whilst a significant improvement was observed at 6 days post-SCI following NAT administration, this improvement was not significantly different to vehicle on days 10 and 14 post-injury. The frequency of hindlimb movement gradually increased in both treatment groups over time (B). Whilst NAT treated animals demonstrated earlier increases in movement frequency, no significant difference was observed between groups. A similar significant decrease in sensory function was observed in both the left (C) and right (D) hindlimbs of both treatment groups. ** denotes $p<0.01$, *** denotes $p<0.001$ when compared to sham. # denotes $p<0.05$ compared to vehicle.

epicentre with minimal white matter sparing and minor hemorrhage. The adjacent segments also demonstrated loss of tissue centred within the grey matter and radiating outwards. No differences in morphological features were observed between treatment groups at any time point post-SCI.

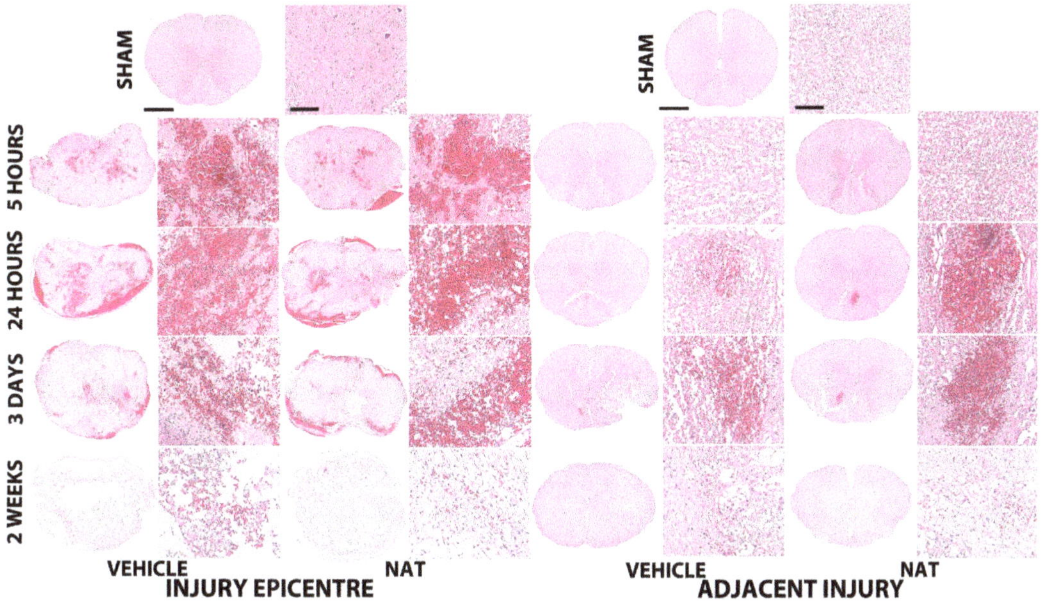

Figure 3. H&E staining demonstrates the morphological changes within the injury epicentre from 5 hours to 2 weeks post-SCI. Hemorrhage was predominant within 24 hours post-SCI, with marked tissue loss observed by 2 weeks post-SCI. No differences were observed between vehicle and NAT treatment groups. Cross section scale bar =1 mm, high magnification scale bar =100 μm.

3.5.2. Substance P immunoreactivity - Dorsal Horn region. Sham animals demonstrated a moderate level of SP immunoreactivity (median =6) within the grey matter with particular predominance in lamina I and II of the dorsal horn (Figure 4). Within the injury epicentre, there was a significant decrease in SP immunoreactivity in both treatment groups when compared to sham ($p<0.001$), with further decreases in both groups at 24 hours (vehicle =0 $p<0.001$; NAT=1 $p<0.01$) and 3 days post-SCI ($p<0.001$ for both groups). By 2 weeks, the injury epicentre in both groups was completely devoid of SP immunoreactivity ($p<0.001$). The loss in SP immunoreactivity within the adjacent sections was not as pronounced as in the injury epicentre until day 3 in the 10 mm caudal section (median =2; $p<0.001$) and 2 weeks in the 10 mm rostral section (median =2). Interestingly at day 3 within the 10 mm caudal section, NAT treated animals had greater SP expression, with a median ranking of 4. Similarly, in the rostral section at 2 weeks, NAT treated animals recorded a higher median ranking of 4 suggesting NAT treatment resulted in greater SP immunoreactivity.

3.5.3. Substance P immunoreactivity - Perivascular region. The perivascular region was assessed within the grey matter of the spinal cord (Figure 5). The injury epicentre could not be examined because of severe tissue disruption. Sham animals demonstrated moderate SP immunoreactivity surrounding the vasculature with a median of 6. At 5 hours post-SCI a slight decrease was observed within both adjacent segments in both treatment groups, with this trend remaining at 24 hours post-SCI. Interestingly in both adjacent segments, by 3 days post-SCI the NAT treated group had returned to sham levels, recording a median ranking of 6. By 2 weeks post-SCI, both treatment groups demonstrated comparable immunoreactivity to sham levels in the rostral segment, though remained below sham levels within the caudal segment. No significant differences were detected between treatment groups at any time post-SCI.

3.5.4. NK1 immunoreactivity - Grey Matter. Sham sections demonstrated diffuse immunoreactivity within the grey matter with greater intensity observed within the dorsal horn resulting in a median ranking of 7 (Figure 6). At 5 and 24 hours post-SCI within the injury epicentre, a significant increase in NK1 receptor immunoreactivity to a median ranking to 9 was observed within the injury epicentre in both treatment groups (vehicle = $p<0.01$, NAT = $p<0.05$–0.01). Such immunoreactivity remained elevated in both treatment groups on day 3 post-SCI. By 24 hours post-SCI, the adjacent segments also demonstrated a slight increase in NK1 expression centrally within the grey matter in both groups. However by day 3, a slight reduction in NK1 immunoreactivity within these segments was observed in both groups (median =5). By 2 weeks post-SCI, the loss of tissue made it difficult to assess NK1 immunoreactivity in the injury epicentre, whereas NK1 immunoreactivity had further decreased in the adjacent segments of both groups, recording a median ranking of 4 (rostral = $p<0.05$, caudal $p<0.001$).

3.5.5. NK1 immunoreactivity – Perivascular. Sham sections demonstrated faint NK1 receptor immunoreactivity surrounding the vasculature with a median ranking of 4 (Figure 7). Due to severe tissue disruption, NK1 immunoreactivity was not assessed within the injury epicentre. A slight increase in NK1 immunoreactivity was observed within the adjacent segments of both treatment groups at 5 hours post-SCI. Further increases were observed at 24 hours post-SCI within the caudal segment recording a median ranking of 7 for both treatment groups, whilst the rostral segment was only slightly increased to a median ranking of 6. By day 3, NAT treated caudal segments remained at a median of 7, whereas vehicle treated animals had slightly reduced further to 6, although this was still increased compared to shams. Similarly, within the rostral segment NAT treatment resulted in slightly greater immunoreactivity compared to both vehicle and sham, whereas vehicle treated animals had comparable NK1 immunoreactivity to shams. Vehicle treated animals remained at sham levels at 2 weeks post-SCI in both sections, whilst NAT treatment still recorded above sham levels (rostral median =5; caudal median 6).

3.5.6. Albumin immunoreactivity. Albumin immunoreactivity was assessed to quantify the effect of NAT administration on

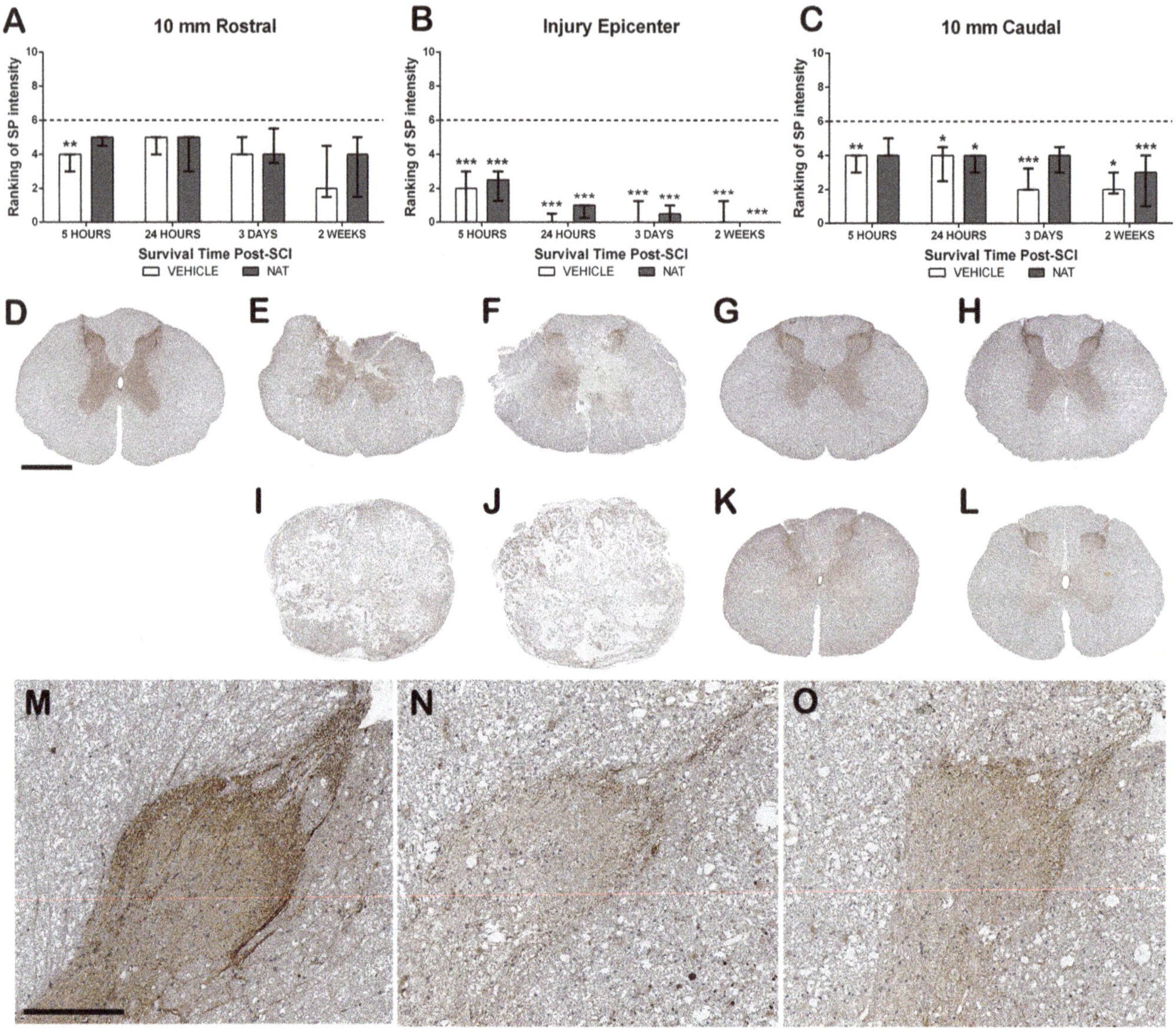

Figure 4. Assessment of the effect of NAT treatment on SP immunoreactivity within the dorsal horn region following SCI. Ranking of SP immunoreactivity within the injury epicentre (B) and at 10 mm rostral (A) and 10 mm caudal (C). Sham sections demonstrated moderate SP immunoreactivity (D). At 5 hours post-SCI reduced immunoreactivity was observed in both vehicle and NAT treatment groups within the injury epicentre (E = Vehicle, F = NAT), whilst a slight reduction was apparent within the adjacent segments (G = Vehicle, H = NAT). However, a significant loss was observed by 2 weeks post-SCI within the injury epicentre (I = Vehicle, J = NAT) and within the adjacent segments (K = Vehicle, L = NAT). Higher magnification images clearly demonstrate this difference (M = sham, N = 2 week Vehicle adjacent, O = 2 week NAT adjacent). Low magnification scale bar = 1 mm, High magnification scale bar = 200 μm. Dashed line (A–C) represents sham median.

the extent of BSCB permeability following SCI (Figure 8). Sham sections of spinal cord demonstrated minimal albumin immunoreactivity with a DABwt% of 4.7±0.42, indicating that sham surgery did not disrupt the BSCB. Following injury, a significant increase in albumin immunoreactivity was observed within the injury epicentre and became maximal at 24 hours post-SCI reaching 24.64±2.77 DABwt% ($p<0.001$). Albumin immunoreactivity then decreased over time, although was still significantly greater than shams at 2 weeks ($p<0.001$). The NAT treated animals had a similar expression of albumin to vehicle treated animals in the injury epicentre, although they recorded significantly greater albumin than vehicle treated animals at day 3 ($p<0.05$). However by 2 weeks, they had decreased below vehicle treated animals but were still had significantly greater albumin than sham ($p<0.05$). Similarly, the adjacent segments demonstrated maximal increases at 24 hours post-SCI for both treatment groups ($p<0.001$), with a decrease over time so that by 2 weeks both groups had returned to sham levels. Moreover, NAT treated animals were comparable to vehicles at all assessment times in the adjacent segments.

3.5.7. Microglial immunoreactivity (ISOB4) - White Matter. Sham sections demonstrated low numbers of resting microglia with long fine processes. After injury, small numbers of microglia were observed within the injury epicentre of both treatment groups (Figure 9A). At 24 hours post-SCI many cells with a small round phenotype suggestive of phagocytic activity can be seen. Furthermore, increased numbers of immunoreactive cells can also be seen within the adjacent segments at this time. At 3 days post-SCI, tissue loss is apparent and further increases in immunoreactive cells are seen within the injury epicentre in both

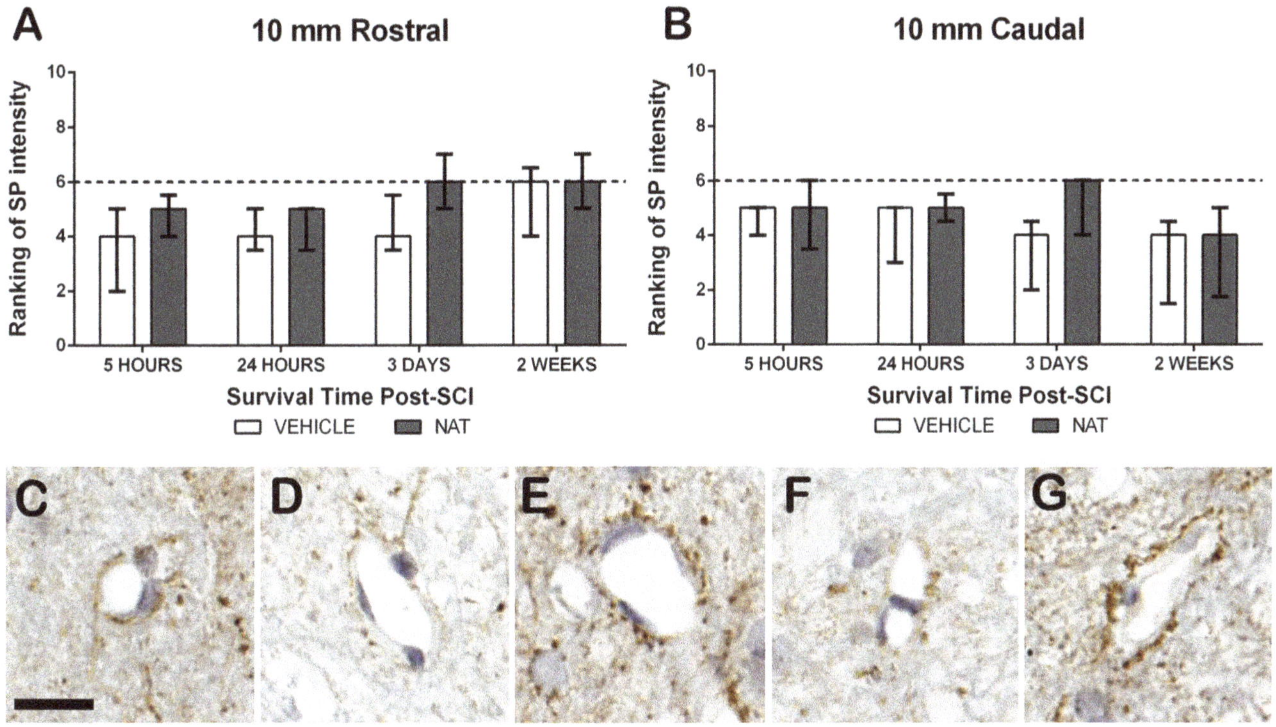

Figure 5. Assessment of the effect of NAT treatment on SP immunoreactivity within the perivascular region following SCI. Ranking of SP immunoreactivity at 10 mm rostral (A) and 10 mm caudal (B) to the injury epicentre. Sham sections demonstrated moderate SP immunoreactivity (C). At both 5 and 24 hours post-SCI a slight decrease was observed within both segments of vehicle and NAT treatment groups. However at 3 days post-SCI NAT treated sections at both 10 mm rostral (E) and caudal (G) demonstrated a return to sham levels whilst vehicle treated remained reduced (D = 10 mm rostral; F = 10 mm caudal). *denotes $p<0.05$, **denotes $p<0.01$, ***denotes $p<0.001$, sham median ranking indicated by the dashed line. Scale bar = 25 μm.

treatment groups. By 2 weeks post-SCI greater tissue loss is apparent and florid microglia are present within the white matter, becoming amoeboid in shape by 2 weeks post-SCI. At this time, the adjacent segments of spinal cord also demonstrate increased microglia immunoreacitivty, with many amoeboid cells apparent within the white matter of both treatment groups. No differences in microglia immunoreactivity were observed between vehicle and NAT treated animals.

3.5.8. Microglial immunoreactivity (ISOB4) - Grey Matter. Sham sections again demonstrate low numbers of resting microglia with fine long processes (Figure 9B). At 5 hours post-SCI, hemorrhage is visible in addition to small round immunoreactive cells, suggestive of phagocytic activity, present within the injury epicentre of both treatment groups. At 24 hours post-SCI florid microglia can be seen within the injury epicentre whilst the adjacent segments also demonstrate increased microglia particularly surrounding the blood vessels within both treatment groups. At 3 days post-SCI greater tissue loss was observed within the injury epicentre with many immunoreactive cells still present, and becoming larger in size. The adjacent segments demonstrated numerous activated microglia that appear ramified in nature. By 2 weeks post-SCI increased tissue loss was observed within the injury epicentre with larger phagocytic cells apparent within both vehicle and NAT treated sections. The adjacent segments similarly demonstrate florid microglial activity with many observed as fully ramified and amoeboid in appearance, representing phagocytic activity. No differences in microglial immunoreactivity between vehicle and NAT treated groups were observed.

3.5.9. AQP4 immunoreactivity - Perivascular region. Sham sections of spinal cord demonstrated faint AQP4 immunoreactivity surrounding the vasculature within the grey matter, assessed as a median ranking of 3 (Figure 10). Due to severe tissue disruption the injury epicentre was not assessed. Following injury increased AQP4 immunoreactivity was observed by 5 hours and reached a median ranking of 6 by 24 hours post-SCI. A slight decrease was observed at 3 days post-SCI in the caudal section, whereas the rostral section still ranked 6. A further decrease to below sham levels was apparent by 2 weeks (rostral = 2; caudal = 1). NAT treatment had a similar pattern of immunoreactivity to vehicle treated animals in the rostral section, apart from on day 3 when they ranked slightly less (median = 4). Within the caudal section, NAT treated animals recorded slightly higher than vehicles at 5 hours, but then decreased over time so that they were less than vehicles at 24 hours but similar at 3 days and 2 weeks.

3.5.10. AQP4 immunoreactivity - Central Canal region. Sham sections of spinal cord demonstrated faint AQP4 immunoreactivity in the ependymal cells of the central canal with a median ranking of 3 (Figure 10). The injury epicentre was too disrupted to accurately assess AQP4 immunoreactivity. Following injury an increase was observed in the rostral section by 5 hours (median = 4.5) with a slightly further rise to 5 at 24 hours and 3 days before returning to sham levels at 2 weeks. In contrast, NAT treated animals had maximal AQP4 immunoreactivity in this section by 5 hours (median = 5), which remained until day 3 when a reduced ranking of 4 was recorded. A further decrease was seen at 2 weeks, although they were still just above shams (median 3.5). Within the caudal section, AQP4 was not increased until 24 hours when a median ranking of 6 was recorded in the vehicle treated animals. AQP4 then declined over time to be near to sham

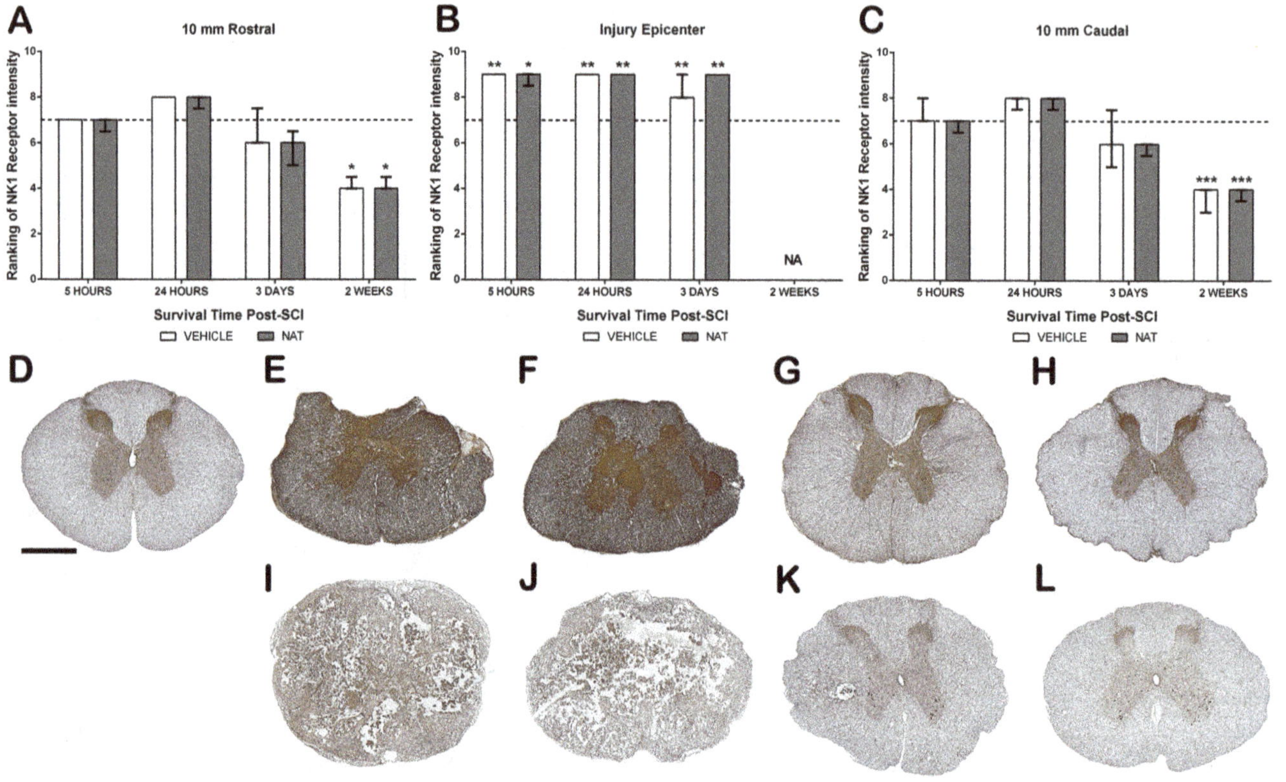

Figure 6. The effect of NAT administration on NK1 receptor immunoreactivity within the grey matter following SCI. Ranking of NK1 receptor immunoreactivity at 10 mm rostral (A), within the injury epicentre (B) and at 10 mm caudal (C). At 24 hours post-SCI a significant increase was observed within the injury epicentre (E= vehicle and F=NAT), whilst adjacent segments demonstrated a slight increase (G= vehicle and H=NAT). By 2 weeks post-SCI tissue loss was too great to assess NK1 immunoreactivity within the injury epicentre (I-vehicle, J-NAT) although adjacent segments had reduced immunoreactivity (K-vehicle, L-NAT). No differences were observed between treatment groups at any time point. *denotes $p<0.05$, **denotes $p<0.01$, ***denotes $p<0.001$, sham median ranking indicated by the dashed line (A,B & C). Scale bar =1 mm.

levels by 2 weeks. In contrast, NAT treatment resulted in a increase in AQP4 by 5 hours recording a median ranking of 5, however then declined to 4 at 24 hours and had returned to sham levels by day 3. No significant differences were observed between treatment groups at any assessment time.

Discussion

The present study has demonstrated that administration of the NK1 receptor antagonist, NAT, does not reduce BSCB permeability, edema, ITP or significantly improve neurological function following SCI. These results suggest that SP mediated neurogenic inflammation does not play a major role in the acute development of such injury processes following traumatic SCI. However, a release of SP was observed, demonstrated by reduced SP immunoreactivity, whilst perivascular NK1 receptor immunoreactivity initially increased before decreasing, which is suggestive of NK1 receptor activation and internalisation. This reflects manifestation of SP mediated neurogenic inflammation, albeit that neurogenic inflammation may not be the predominant driver of these injury processes in the acute phase of SCI.

Although only a bolus dose of NAT was administered on the day of surgery, and for two consecutive days for survival times of 3 days or more, such dosage regimes have previously been used in acute CNS injury with highly beneficial outcomes [13,17,22]. Indeed administration of an NK1 receptor antagonist at 30 minutes post-TBI reduced barrier permeability, edema and improved functional outcome, demonstrating that inhibition of SP effects was possible despite a 30 minute delay post-injury [13,17]. It is unlikely that a shorter timeframe for pharmacological intervention would be clinically relevant. Furthermore, whilst NAT is not barrier permeable, our results demonstrate that the BSCB was disrupted for at least 5 hours post-SCI. Given the severe extent of hemorrhage and destruction of vasculature observed at the site of impact, intravenous administration may have not provided sufficient delivery of NAT. Nonetheless, some differences between vehicle and NAT treated groups were observed in the current study beyond the injury site, indicating that NAT administration was likely successfully delivered centrally. A more direct route of administration, such as an injection into the intrathecal space may provide a more efficient method of administration for future investigations. Given the highly preserved nature of NK1 receptors across different vertebrate species [30], it is unlikely that any lack of effectiveness of NAT treatment was due to low affinity for the rabbit NK1 receptor.

Whilst two isoforms of the NK1 receptor exist, a long complete isoform and a truncated isoform, the binding site of the antagonist is identical in both, and thus the NK1 receptor antagonist used in the current study would be equally effective on both isoforms. However, the long NK1 isoform is known to predominate within the CNS whilst the truncated isoform is most represented within peripheral tissue [31]. Additionally, consideration must be given to related tachykinin receptors, the NK2 receptor and NK3 receptor. Our results do not exclude the possibility that the NK2 or NK3 receptors might play an important role and that inhibition of these receptors may be beneficial to outcome after SCI. However, SP

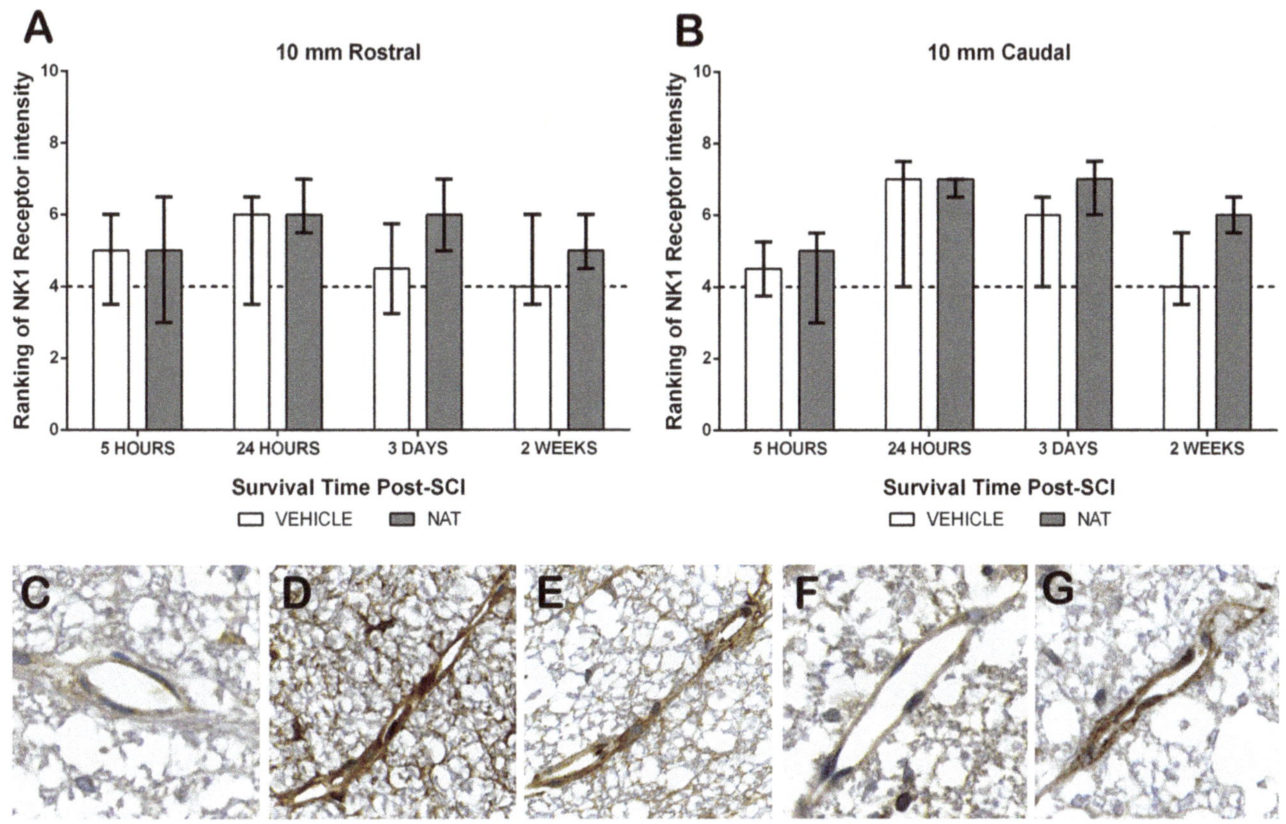

Figure 7. The effect of NAT administration on NK1 receptor immunoreactivity within the perivascular region following SCI. NK1 receptor immunoreactivity ranking at 10 mm rostral (A) and caudal (B). Sham sections demonstrated faint immunoreactivity surrounding the vasculature (C). Notably, at 24 hours post-SCI a marked increase was observed in both vehicle (D) and NAT (E) treatment groups. By 2 weeks post-SCI at 10 mm caudal vehicle treated (F) returned to sham levels, whilst NAT treated remained elevated (G). Median sham ranking indicated by the dashed line (A&B).

binds preferentially to the NK1 receptor [32], and it is only activation of this receptor that is thought to result in the initiation of neurogenic inflammation. Indeed, It has been demonstrated that the NK2 and NK3 receptors have no direct role in plasma protein extravasation within the CNS [33].

After receiving 3 consecutive daily doses of NAT or saline, NAT treated animals demonstrated a trend for greater perivascular and dorsal horn SP immunoreactivity than vehicle treated animals. Such increases in SP may be explained by the presence of an NK1 autoreceptor, which is thought to regulate SP release through a negative feedback loop [34,35]. In the current study, blockade of the NK1 autoreceptor due to NAT administration would prevent SP from exerting negative feedback on its own synthesis and release, resulting in greater expression of SP. However, the comparative increase in SP would not have been functional, as blockade of the NK1 receptor with NAT prevents SP from binding and mediating downstream effects.

Interestingly, at 3 days post-injury NAT treatment resulted in significantly higher BSCB permeability compared to vehicle as assessed by albumin. This finding paradoxically implies that inhibition of the NK1 receptor resulted in greater BSCB permeability. Such results are in contrast to previous studies where NAT treatment resulted in reduced BSCB permeability following TBI and stroke [13,22]. These findings imply that despite similar secondary injury processes arising following SCI, the role of SP may be vastly different in SCI than its role in other acute CNS injuries. One important difference may be the extent of primary mechanical damage, resulting in severe hemorrhage. Previous studies within our group have demonstrated that in severe subarachnoid hemorrhage, NAT administration worsened outcome [36]. These combined results suggest that in models of severe hemorrhage, the primary induced tissue and vasculature damage may dominate over SP mediated neurogenic inflammation in the development of BSCB permeability. Furthermore, as the current study provided evidence that NAT treatment worsened BSCB permeability, SP may actually play a protective role in such severe hemorrhage models. Indeed, a recent study demonstrated that SP treatment promoted a more anti-inflammatory environment following SCI by inducing interlukin-10 and M2 macrophages whilst suppressing nitric oxide synthase and tumour necrosis factor-α [37]. Our own results demonstrate an increase in microglial activity following SCI, though predominantly phagocytic in nature, with no differences between treatment groups. In addition, intrathecal administration of a SP antagonist has been shown to cause a marked decrease in spinal cord blood flow (SCBF) [38] and likely contributed to further damage and BSCB permeability by promoting an ischemic environment. These findings together with the current study suggest that SP may be beneficial following acute SCI.

Regardless of the role of SP following SCI, edema remains a serious complication leading to raised ITP [39,40], reduced SCBF [9,40] and myelin damage [1]. Indeed, numerous studies have shown that the extent of edema corresponds to the degree of functional deficits observed following injury [41,42,43,44,45]. The

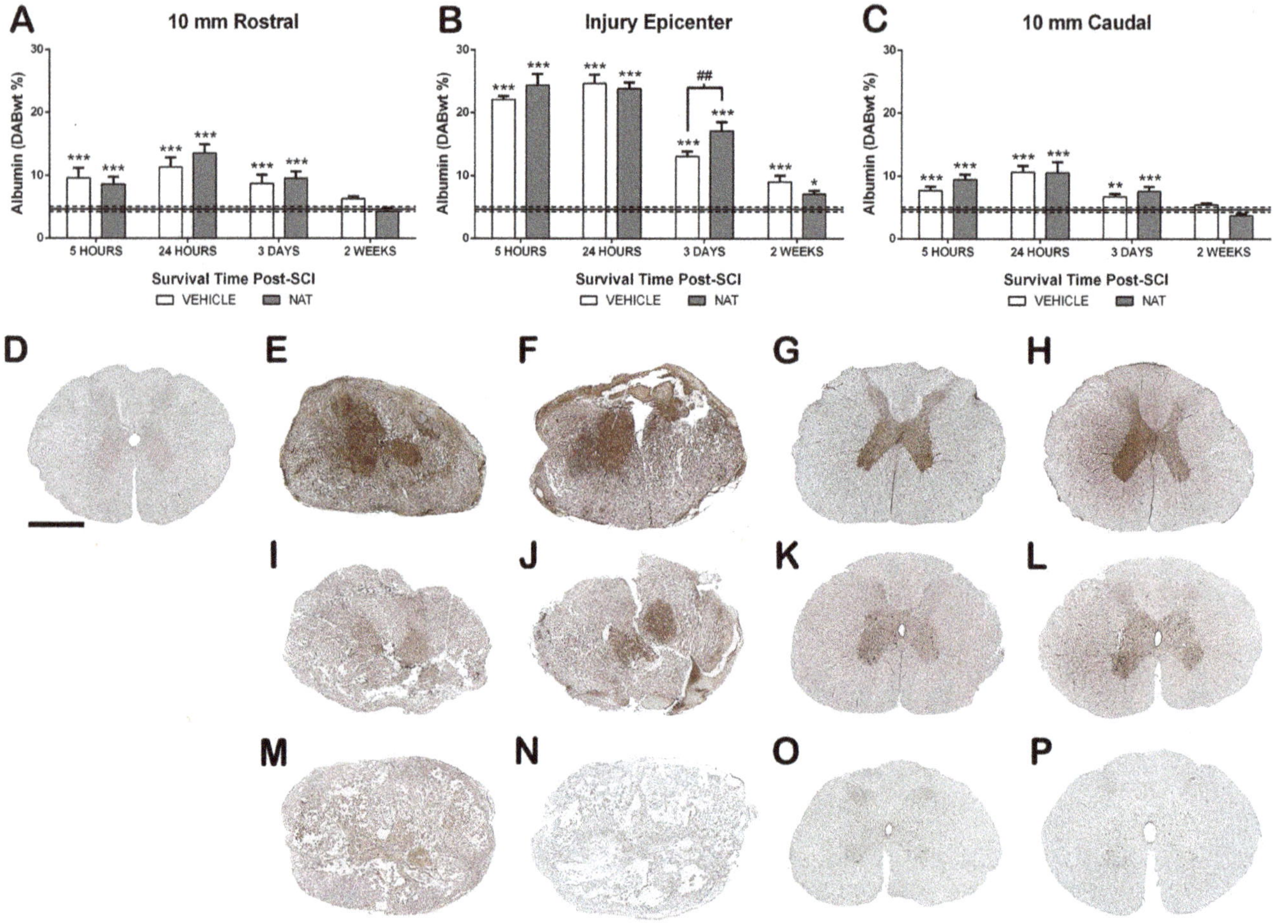

Figure 8. The effect of NAT treatment on albumin immunoreactivity following SCI. Albumin immunoreactivity at 10 mm rostral (A), within the injury epicentre (B) and at 10 mm caudal (C). Sham sections (D) demonstrated minimal immunoreactivity. Immunoreactivity was significantly increased at both 5 and 24 hours post-SCI. Representative images at 24 hours are shown within the injury epicentre (E-vehicle, F-NAT) and adjacent segment (G-vehicle, H-NAT). By 3 days post-SCI albumin immunoreactivity began to reduce within the injury epicentre (I-vehicle, J-NAT) and adjacent segment (K-vehicle, L-NAT), though NAT treatment resulted in significantly greater albumin immunoreactivity when compared to vehicle. Albumin immunoreactivity reduced further by 2 weeks post-SCI within the injury epicentre (M-vehicle, N-NAT), returning to sham levels within the adjacent segments (O-vehicle, P-NAT). *denotes $p<0.05$, **denotes $p<0.01$, ***denotes $p<0.001$ when compared to sham. Mean sham values indicated by the dashed line. Scale bar = 1 mm.

present study demonstrated increased edema associated with raised ITP following injury, which was maximal at 3 days post-SCI. Furthermore, at this time it was apparent that the adjacent segments, uninjured by the balloon compression, also demonstrated significant increases in edema. Therefore, substantial rostrocaudal spread of edema had occurred following the balloon compression model by 3 days post-SCI. However, albumin immunoreactivity, a marker of BSCB permeability, was maximal at 24 hours post-SCI with a reduction observed at 3 days post-SCI within the adjacent segments. Therefore, significant disparity exists between BSCB permeability and edema formation, indicating that the rostrocaudal spread of edema was not due to BSCB disruption and thus not vasogenic in nature. These results further suggest that neurogenic inflammation is not primarily responsible for the developed edema and may account for the ineffectiveness of NAT administration to reduce edema.

It is possible that the spread of edema may be a compensatory mechanism to reduce the edema present within the injury epicentre. Alternatively, the BSCB may in fact still remain permeable to smaller molecules than albumin. Previous studies have employed alternative smaller tracers of extravasation such as hydrazide [46], horseradish peroxidase [10,47,48], protein luciferase [49], and iodine [4,50] and found greater extension of BSCB permeability. Alternatively, such increases in edema may be due to an ultrafiltration mechanism rather than extravasation as previously described by Nemecek and colleagues [7]. Such ultrafiltration may be aided by reduced blood flow and severe hemorrhage. As NAT treatment has no ability to reduce hemorhage and SP antagonists can markedly reduce SCBF [38], the greater edema within the adjacent segments of NAT treated animals may be due to increased ultrafiltration. Alternatively, in the absence of BSCB disruption, the increased edema may be facilitated by AQP4 water channels.

Indeed, within the current study, AQP4 immunoreactivity was increased following injury at similar times to maximal edema. Although such an increase implies that AQP4 may facilitate edema development, NAT administration resulted in a slight increase in edema and a concurrent reduction in AQP4 immunoreactivity. Therefore, injury induced increases in AQP4 may actually be a compensatory mechanism to assist in fluid clearance. These changes in AQP4 and edema formation contrast to that in TBI, where injury reduced AQP4 expression and NAT

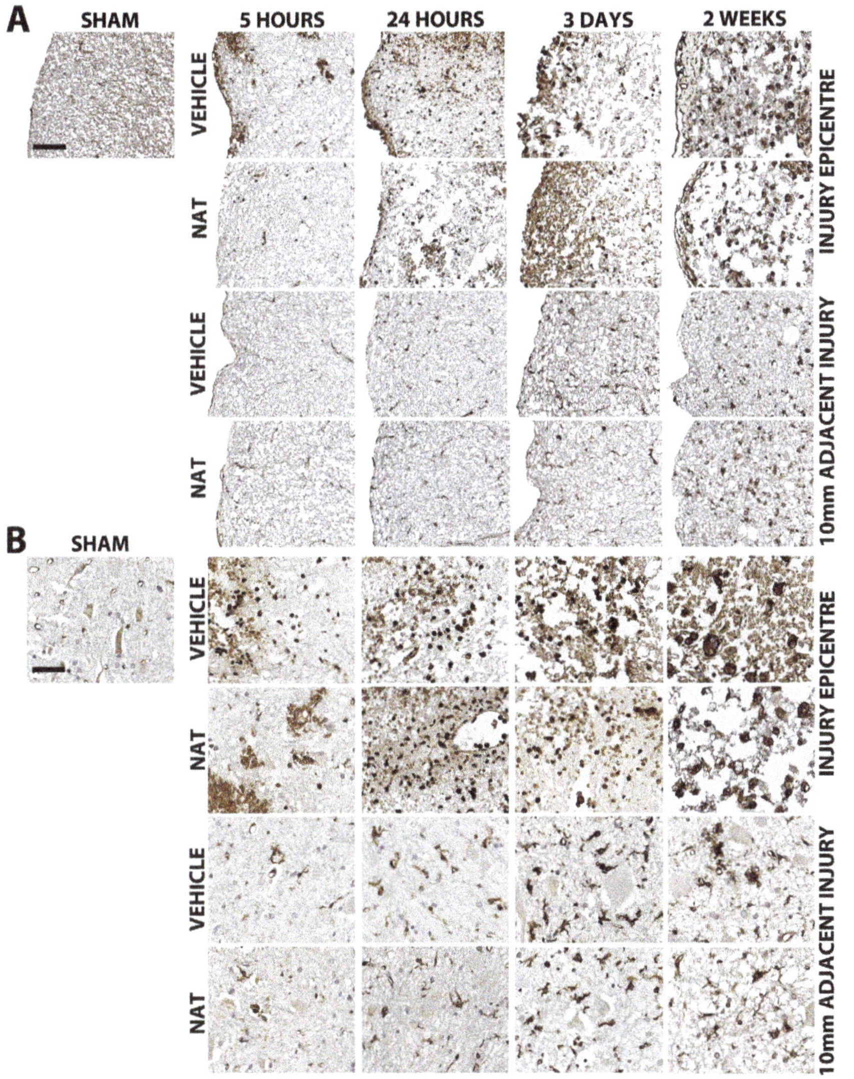

Figure 9. The effect of NAT administration on microglial immunoreactivity following SCI within the white matter (A) and grey matter (B). Sham sections demonstrate minimal microglial immunoreactivity in both the white and grey matter. Within the white matter microglia immunoreactivity is maximal by 2 weeks post-SCI within the injury epicentre and adjacent segment for both treatment groups. Within the grey matter, many small round microglia can be seen within the injury epicentre, increasing in size by 2 weeks post-SCI. Within the adjacent segment of the grey matter many ramified microglia can be seen by 3 days post-SCI and becoming amoeboid in shape by 2 week post-SCI. No differences between treatment groups were observed. Scale bar (A) = 200 μm, (B) = 50 μm.

treatment restored AQP4 levels, whilst reducing edema [28]. These opposing effects of NAT treatment in TBI and SCI further illustrate the differences in their injury mechanisms. Moreover, these results demonstrate that the relationship between SP and AQP4 warrants further investigation. Taken together, these results demonstrate that AQP4 may play an essential role in the elimination of excess fluid. Indeed, previous investigations have similarly demonstrated that AQP4 plays an integral role in facilitating water clearance following SCI [2,51,52]. However, to date, almost all studies of AQP4 following SCI have assessed its function through altered expression [2,51], or employed AQP4-null mice [12,52]. As such, further investigation to fully elucidate the role of AQP4 following SCI is required. Ideally, this could be through the pharmacological modulation of the AQP4 water channels, which may then be utilized as a novel therapeutic intervention.

Conclusions

The current study has demonstrated that despite a release of SP and therefore induction of SP mediated neurogenic inflammation, the severe primary damage that results in destruction of vasculature and hemorrhage may play a greater role in BSCB disruption, subsequent edema development and associated tissue damage and functional deficits following traumatic SCI. Thus, administration of the NK1 receptor antagonist, NAT, did not reduce BSCB permeability, edema, ITP, or improve neurological function following SCI. In contrast, SP may actually play a beneficial role in reducing this ongoing damage associated with traumatic SCI.

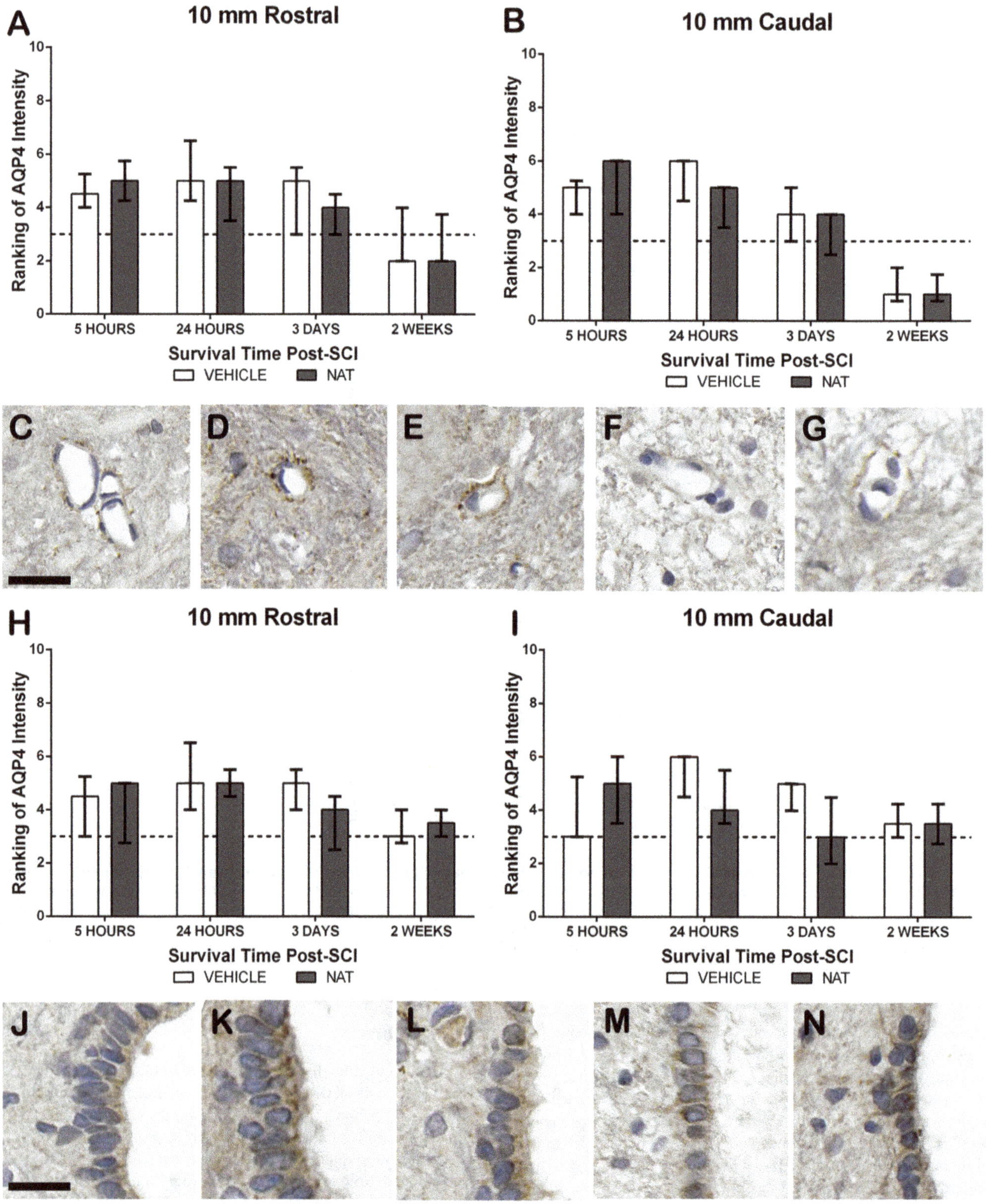

Figure 10. The effect of NAT administration on perivascular and ependymal AQP4 immunoreactivity following SCI. Ranking of perivascular AQP4 immunoreactivity at 10 mm rostral (A) and 10 mm caudal (B). Sham sections demonstrated faint immunoreactivity surrounding the vessels (C). Increased immunoreactivity can be seen at 24 hours following both vehicle (D) and NAT (E) treatment. Reduced immunoreacticity below sham levels was observed at 2 weeks (H-vehicle, I-NAT). Dashed line indicated mean sham values. Ranking of ependymal AQP4 immunoreactivity at 10 mm rostral (H) and 10 mm caudal (I). Sham sections demonstrated faint immunoreactivity within the ependymal cells of the central canal (J). At 24 hours post-SCI increases were apparent, with greater increases in the caudal segments of vehicle treated sections (K) than NAT treated (L). By 2 weeks post-SCI both treatment groups demonstrated comparable AQP4 immunoreactivity to sham levels (M-vehicle, N-NAT). Scale bars = 25 μm.

Author Contributions

Conceived and designed the experiments: AVL ET RV. Performed the experiments: AVL. Analyzed the data: AVL ET RV. Contributed to the writing of the manuscript: AVL ET RV.

References

1. Sharma HS (2005) Pathophysiology of blood-spinal cord barrier in traumatic injury and repair. Curr Pharm Des 11: 1353–1389.
2. Nesic O, Lee J, Ye Z, Unabia GC, Rafati D, et al. (2006) Acute and chronic changes in aquaporin 4 expression after spinal cord injury. Neuroscience 143: 779–792.
3. Sharma HS, Winkler T, Stalberg E, Olsson Y, Dey PK (1991) Evaluation of traumatic spinal cord edema using evoked potentials recorded from the spinal epidural space. An experimental study in the rat. J Neurol Sci 102: 150–162.
4. Sharma HS, Olsson Y, Nyberg F, Dey PK (1993) Prostaglandins modulate alterations of microvascular permeability, blood flow, edema and serotonin levels following spinal cord injury: an experimental study in the rat. Neuroscience 57: 443–449.
5. Winkler T, Sharma HS, Stalberg E, Olsson Y, Nyberg F (1994) Opioid receptors influence spinal cord electrical activity and edema formation following spinal cord injury: experimental observations using naloxone in the rat. Neurosci Res 21: 91–101.
6. Ates O, Cayli SR, Gurses I, Turkoz Y, Tarim O, et al. (2007) Comparative neuroprotective effect of sodium channel blockers after experimental spinal cord injury. J Clin Neurosci 14: 658–665.
7. Nemecek S, Petr R, Suba P, Rozsival V, Melka O (1977) Longitudinal extension of oedema in experimental spinal cord injury–evidence for two types of post-traumatic oedema. Acta Neurochir (Wien) 37: 7–16.
8. Demediuk P, Lemke M, Faden AI (1990) Spinal cord edema and changes in tissue content of Na+, K+, and Mg2+ after impact trauma in rats. Adv Neurol 52: 225–232.
9. Wang R, Ehara K, Tamaki N (1993) Spinal cord edema following freezing injury in the rat: relationship between tissue water content and spinal cord blood flow. Surg Neurol 39: 348–354.
10. Noble LJ, Wrathall JR (1989) Distribution and time course of protein extravasation in the rat spinal cord after contusive injury. Brain Res 482: 57–66.
11. Goodman JH, Bingham WG Jr, Hunt WE (1976) Ultrastructural blood-brain barrier alterations and edema formation in acute spinal cord trauma. J Neurosurg 44: 418–424.
12. Saadoun S, Bell BA, Verkman AS, Papadopoulos MC (2008) Greatly improved neurological outcome after spinal cord compression injury in AQP4-deficient mice. Brain 131: 1087–1098.
13. Donkin JJ, Nimmo AJ, Cernak I, Blumbergs PC, Vink R (2009) Substance P is associated with the development of brain edema and functional deficits after traumatic brain injury. J Cereb Blood Flow Metab.
14. Vink R, Young A, Bennett CJ, Hu X, Connor CO, et al. (2003) Neuropeptide release influences brain edema formation after diffuse traumatic brain injury. Acta Neurochir Suppl 86: 257–260.
15. Nimmo AJ, Cernak I, Heath DL, Hu X, Bennett CJ, et al. (2004) Neurogenic inflammation is associated with development of edema and functional deficits following traumatic brain injury in rats. Neuropeptides 38: 40–47.
16. Turner RJ, Blumbergs PC, Sims NR, Helps SC, Rodgers KM, et al. (2006) Increased substance P immunoreactivity and edema formation following reversible ischemic stroke. Acta Neurochir Suppl 96: 263–266.
17. Corrigan F, Leonard A, Ghabriel M, Van Den Heuvel C, Vink R (2012) A substance P antagonist improves outcome in female Sprague Dawley rats following diffuse traumatic brain injury. CNS Neurosci Ther 18: 513–515.
18. Harford-Wright E, Thornton E, Vink R (2010) Angiotensin-converting enzyme (ACE) inhibitors exacerbate histological damage and motor deficits after experimental traumatic brain injury. Neurosci Lett 481: 26–29.
19. Thornton E, Vink R (2012) Treatment with a substance P receptor antagonist is neuroprotective in the intrastriatal 6-hydroxydopamine model of early Parkinson's disease. PLoS One 7: e34138.
20. Leonard AV, Thornton E, Vink R (2013) Substance P as a mediator of neurogenic inflammation following balloon compression induced spinal cord injury. J Neurotrauma.
21. Thornton E, Ziebell JM, Leonard AV, Vink R (2010) Kinin receptor antagonists as potential neuroprotective agents in central nervous system injury. Molecules 15: 6598–6618.
22. Turner RJ, Helps SC, Thornton E, Vink R (2011) A substance P antagonist improves outcome when administered 4 h after onset of ischaemic stroke. Brain Res 1393: 84–90.
23. Tarlov IM, Klinger H (1954) Spinal cord compression studies. II. Time limits for recovery after acute compression in dogs. AMA Arch Neurol Psychiatry 71: 271–290.
24. Tarlov IM, Klinger H, Vitale S (1953) Spinal cord compression studies. I. Experimental techniques to produce acute and gradual compression. AMA Arch Neurol Psychiatry 70: 813–819.
25. Fukuda S, Nakamura T, Kishigami Y, Endo K, Azuma T, et al. (2005) New canine spinal cord injury model free from laminectomy. Brain Res Brain Res Protoc 14: 171–180.
26. Martin D, Schoenen J, Delree P, Gilson V, Rogister B, et al. (1992) Experimental acute traumatic injury of the adult rat spinal cord by a subdural inflatable balloon: methodology, behavioral analysis, and histopathology. J Neurosci Res 32: 539–550.
27. Vanicky I, Urdzikova L, Saganova K, Cizkova D, Galik J (2001) A simple and reproducible model of spinal cord injury induced by epidural balloon inflation in the rat. J Neurotrauma 18: 1399–1407.
28. Donkin J (2006) The effects of the neuropeptide Substance P on outcome following experimental brain injury in rats. Adelaide: University of Adelaide.
29. Helps SC, Thornton E, Kleinig TJ, Manavis J, Vink R (2012) Automatic nonsubjective estimation of antigen content visualized by immunohistochemistry using color deconvolution. Appl Immunohistochem Mol Morphol 20: 82–90.
30. Dietl MM, Palacios JM (1991) Phylogeny of tachykinin receptor localization in the vertebrate central nervous system: apparent absence of neurokinin-2 and neurokinin-3 binding sites in the human brain. Brain Res 539: 211–222.
31. Caberlotto L, Hurd YL, Murdock P, Wahlin JP, Melotto S, et al. (2003) Neurokinin 1 receptor and relative abundance of the short and long isoforms in the human brain. Eur J Neurosci 17: 1736–1746.
32. Harrison S, Geppetti P (2001) Substance p. Int J Biochem Cell Biol 33: 555–576.
33. O'Shaughnessy CT, Connor HE (1993) Neurokinin NK1 receptors mediate plasma protein extravasation in guinea-pig dura. Eur J Pharmacol 236: 319–321.
34. Malcangio M, Bowery NG (1994) Effect of the tachykinin NK1 receptor antagonists, RP 67580 and SR 140333, on electrically-evoked substance P release from rat spinal cord. Br J Pharmacol 113: 635–641.
35. Lever IJ, Grant AD, Pezet S, Gerard NP, Brain SD, et al. (2003) Basal and activity-induced release of substance P from primary afferent fibres in NK1 receptor knockout mice: evidence for negative feedback. Neuropharmacology 45: 1101–1110.
36. Barry CM, Helps SC, den Heuvel C, Vink R (2011) Characterizing the role of the neuropeptide substance P in experimental subarachnoid hemorrhage. Brain Res 1389: 143–151.
37. Jiang MH, Chung E, Chi GF, Ahn W, Lim JE, et al. (2012) Substance P induces M2-type macrophages after spinal cord injury. Neuroreport 23: 786–792.
38. Freedman J, Post C, Kahrstrom J, Ohlen A, Mollenholt P, et al. (1988) Vasoconstrictor effects in spinal cord of the substance P antagonist [D-Arg, D-Trp7,9 Leu11]-substance P (Spantide) and somatostatin and interaction with thyrotropin releasing hormone. Neuroscience 27: 267–278.
39. Yashon D, Bingham WG, Jr., Faddoul EM, Hunt WE (1973) Edema of the spinal cord following experimental impact trauma. J Neurosurg 38: 693–697.
40. Kwon BK, Curt A, Belanger LM, Bernardo A, Chan D, et al. (2009) Intrathecal pressure monitoring and cerebrospinal fluid drainage in acute spinal cord injury: a prospective randomized trial. J Neurosurg Spine 10: 181–193.
41. Flanders AE, Spettell CM, Friedman DP, Marino RJ, Herbison GJ (1999) The relationship between the functional abilities of patients with cervical spinal cord injury and the severity of damage revealed by MR imaging. AJNR Am J Neuroradiol 20: 926–934.
42. Leypold BG, Flanders AE, Burns AS (2008) The early evolution of spinal cord lesions on MR imaging following traumatic spinal cord injury. AJNR Am J Neuroradiol 29: 1012–1016.
43. Bozzo A, Marcoux J, Radhakrishna M, Pelletier J, Goulet B (2011) The role of magnetic resonance imaging in the management of acute spinal cord injury. J Neurotrauma 28: 1401–1411.
44. Koyanagi I, Iwasaki Y, Isu T, Akino M, Abe H (1989) Significance of spinal cord swelling in the prognosis of acute cervical spinal cord injury. Paraplegia 27: 190–197.
45. Shepard MJ, Bracken MB (1999) Magnetic resonance imaging and neurological recovery in acute spinal cord injury: observations from the National Acute Spinal Cord Injury Study 3. Spinal Cord 37: 833–837.
46. Maikos JT, Shreiber DI (2007) Immediate damage to the blood-spinal cord barrier due to mechanical trauma. J Neurotrauma 24: 492–507.
47. Noble LJ, Wrathall JR (1987) The blood-spinal cord barrier after injury: pattern of vascular events proximal and distal to a transection in the rat. Brain Res 424: 177–188.
48. Jaeger CB, Blight AR (1997) Spinal cord compression injury in guinea pigs: structural changes of endothelium and its perivascular cell associations after blood-brain barrier breakdown and repair. Exp Neurol 144: 381–399.
49. Whetstone WD, Hsu JY, Eisenberg M, Werb Z, Noble-Haeusslein LJ (2003) Blood-spinal cord barrier after spinal cord injury: relation to revascularization and wound healing. J Neurosci Res 74: 227–239.

50. Nyberg F, Sharma HS (2002) Repeated topical application of growth hormone attenuates blood-spinal cord barrier permeability and edema formation following spinal cord injury: an experimental study in the rat using Evans blue, ([125])I-sodium and lanthanum tracers. Amino Acids 23: 231–239.
51. Mao L, Wang HD, Pan H, Qiao L (2011) Sulphoraphane enhances aquaporin-4 expression and decreases spinal cord oedema following spinal cord injury. Brain Inj 25: 300–306.
52. Kimura A, Hsu M, Seldin M, Verkman AS, Scharfman HE, et al. (2010) Protective role of aquaporin-4 water channels after contusion spinal cord injury. Ann Neurol 67: 794–801.

6

CSF Proteomics of Secondary Phase Spinal Cord Injury in Human Subjects: Perturbed Molecular Pathways Post Injury

Mohor Biplab Sengupta[1], Mahashweta Basu[2], Sourav Iswarari[3], Kiran Kumar Mukhopadhyay[4], Krishna Pada Sardar[4], Biplab Acharyya[4], Pradeep K. Mohanty[2], Debashis Mukhopadhyay[1]*

1 Biophysics and Structural Genomics Division, Saha Institute of Nuclear Physics, Kolkata, West Bengal, India, **2** Condensed Matter Physics Division, Saha Institute of Nuclear Physics, Kolkata, West Bengal, India, **3** Department of Physical Medicine & Rehabilitation, Nil Ratan Sircar Medical College & Hospital, Kolkata, West Bengal, India, **4** Department of Orthopaedic Surgery, Nil Ratan Sircar Medical College & Hospital, Kolkata, West Bengal, India

Abstract

Recovery of sensory and motor functions following traumatic spinal cord injury (SCI) is dependent on injury severity. Here we identified 49 proteins from cerebrospinal fluid (CSF) of SCI patients, eight of which were differentially abundant among two severity groups of SCI. It was observed that the abundance profiles of these proteins change over a time period of days to months post SCI. Statistical analysis revealed that these proteins take part in several molecular pathways including DNA repair, protein phosphorylation, tRNA transcription, iron transport, mRNA metabolism, immune response and lipid and ATP catabolism. These pathways reflect a set of mechanisms that the system may adopt to cope up with the assault depending on the injury severity, thus leading to observed physiological responses. Apart from putting forward a picture of the molecular scenario at the injury site in a human study, this finding further delineates consequent pathways and molecules that may be altered by external intervention to restrict neural degeneration.

Editor: Naren L. Banik, Medical University of South Carolina, United States of America

Funding: Grant Number: 12-R&D-SIN-5.04-0101, Project Title: Integrative Biology on Omics Platform (IBOP), Department of Atomic Energy (DAE), Government of India, author receiving funding: DM. MBS acknowledges Council of Scientific and Industrial Research (CSIR), Government of India, for her fellowship. The funders had no role in study design, data collection and analysis, decision to publish, or preparation of the manuscript.

Competing Interests: The authors have declared that no competing interests exist.

* Email: debashis.mukhopadhyay@saha.ac.in

Introduction

Spinal cord injury (SCI) is one of the leading causes of disability and morbidity worldwide [1] although epidemiological studies are limited in India [2]. In the present study we included a cohort of East Indian population.

SCI due to trauma has two stages: the primary and the secondary injuries [3]. As the acute primary phase is over by seconds to minutes, the secondary injury gives a valuable time window to explore events before interventions are done for stabilizing the patient. Although there are a few well established pathways of secondary injury, most of these are not readily known or accessible for clinical practice.

Right after the initial mechanical damage inflicted by the primary injury, a plethora of molecular changes set in, initiating the secondary injury processes [4]. Various processes like hypoperfusion in the grey matter, glutamate excitotoxicity, plasma membrane failure, ionic perturbation, energy failure, ATP catabolism, inflammatory pathways, demyelination, apoptosis, cell and tissue damage and lipid peroxidation [5] become predominant. Although some of these mechanisms overlap with acute primary injury, myelin associated inhibitory factors (MAIF) [6, 7, and 8] and glial scar formation [9], are known to act in conjunction and limit axonal growth severely, leading to collapse of growth cones.

The processes mentioned above vary in extent depending on the injury severity and hence it is imperative to study human CSF of spinal cord injured patients during secondary phase. Proteins thus found can help speculating on various molecular pathways and their perturbation at the backdrop of neuronal injury. Severity dependent biomarker studies based on American Spinal Injury Association (ASIA) Impairment Scale (AIS) classification [10] have been conducted in human CSF samples [11] where it has been shown that inflammatory cytokine levels are elevated in AIS grade A (complete) injury and an inflammatory profile of CSF from cervical SCI rats [12] has revealed MMP-8 as a biomarker. Other studies have also documented several biomarkers in SCI of rodents [13].

The objective of the present study is to survey the intracellular molecular pathways that are perturbed in severe SCI during the secondary phase. Towards this, we compared CSF from AIS A (complete injury) and AIS C or D (incomplete injury) patients at an early time period after injury to identify proteins having differential abundance among the two severity groups. This is because regeneration outcomes vary widely among the two groups. We further compared their differential abundance at a

Table 1. Study details.

Type of study	Cohort study
Period of study	December 2011-July 2014
No of participants	45
Total sample drawn	45 ml
Included samples	20

later time-period post injury as it is presumed that CSF undergoes substantial molecular alteration as the secondary phase progresses. Additionally, a protein-protein interaction network (PPIN) was constructed taking proteins identified from CSF and their interactors as nodes. The network analysis revealed a number of vulnerable molecular pathways which may be regarded as soft targets for further exploration in severe SCI.

Materials and Methods

Ethics Statement

The study was conducted as a collaboration of SINP and NRSMC&H, Kolkata, India, after it was approved by 'Institutional Ethical Committee, NRS Medical College, Kolkata' and 'Institutional Ethics Committee, SINP, Kolkata'. An informed written consent was obtained from the subjects as per Helsinki Declaration, 2013.

Patient selection and scoring

The study was conducted in two patient groups with CSF drawn at two time periods (1–8 days and 15–60 days) post injury respectively. Patients with traumatic spinal cord injury in the secondary phase admitted in the spinal injury ward under the Dept. of Orthopaedic Surgery were enrolled in the two study groups (Table 1), after screening by an orthopaedist and a physiatrist from Dept. of Orthopaedic Surgery and Dept. of Physical Medicine & Rehabilitation respectively. Patients were evaluated according to the International Standards for Neurological Classification of SCI (ISNC SCI). Patients who conformed to the set inclusion and exclusion criteria were selected for study (Table 2). Any patient with factors that have the possibility to alter the regenerative and degenerative process in the injured area as mentioned in Table 2 was excluded from the study. First we determined if it was a complete injury with loss of anal sensation and contraction. Then tests for sensory perception (pin prick and feather touch) and motor activity for upper and lower limbs were done to ascertain the ASIA grade of injury. Motor and sensory levels were determined and scored clinically. Clinical level was matched with radiological level determined with non contrast MRI and X-rays. MRI showing oedema in the cord was considered for complete injury. In incomplete injuries of lower grade where MRI did not show oedema, we considered X-ray for determining radiological level. In case of different sensory and motor levels on clinical examination we fixed the highest clinical level that matched with MRI or X-ray. It was this spinal segment we considered for collecting CSF.

Before collection of CSF a complete hemogram, ESR, CRP, serum fasting sugar, post prandial sugar, electrolyte, calcium, urea, creatinine, total protein, albumin and globulin were done along with a lipid profile, liver function test and thyroid profile. A routine urine examination with ultrasound check of lower abdomen was done to assess the bladder and to look out for hidden injury because infection, metabolic disorder, electrolyte imbalance and bladder abnormality could have potential effect on the environment of injured spine under study.

CSF collection and processing for proteomics experiments

All the vital parameters were checked. The patient's heart rate and ECG recording were noted. Patient's blood pressure, oxygen saturation and signs of postural hypotension were noted in a sterile operation theatre with all resuscitation equipment. This is considered vital because hemodynamic alteration can affect the internal environment of the injured site under study.

CSF was drawn by thecal puncture with 23 G spinal needle (Spinocaine 23/G) to minimize injury. Adequate flow of CSF on spinal tapping suggested normal flow of CSF through the central nervous system bathing the spinal cord, thereby giving us CSF sample that adequately represented the deranged process in the spine we were attempting to study. The patient was made to lie on one side with spine flexed in crouched hand to knee position. This flexed position ensures easy access into thecal space. Median or paramedian approach was taken as per convenience of the procedurist. Sample was only taken when the patient was comfortable with all parameters mentioned in acceptable physiological level. CSF was collected in sterile vials and protease inhibitor cocktail preparation (Roche Diagnostics, USA) was added.

As there might be a breach in blood brain barrier at the injury site, blood infiltration in the CSF was a common occurrence. We tried to deplete albumin but lost most of the other proteins along with it, and moreover our aim was to look at the actual protein scenario for the two injury conditions so we chose not to deplete any abundant protein. Therefore the first few drops of CSF were discarded and the CSF was centrifuged to remove any RBCs and cellular debris. Protein content of the CSF was determined by Bradford (Biorad, CA, USA) reagent, using BSA (Sigma Aldrich, St. Louis, MO, USA) as standard.

We did not pool CSF samples for any study. All proteomics work was conducted using individual samples as per selection criteria. CSF aliquots containing 50 μg and 25 μg protein were acetone precipitated and dissolved in 20 μl and 10 μl DIGE buffer (7 M urea, 2 M thiourea, 4% CHAPS, 30 mM Tris pH 8.8, PI cocktail, Roche diagnostics, USA) respectively and 1500 μg protein containing CSF aliquot was dissolved in 330 μl rehydration buffer (7 M urea, 2 M thiourea, 2% chaps, 60 mM DTT, 0.2% pH 3–10 ampholyte, Biorad, CA, USA). Isoelectric focussing was done with IPG strips (Biorad, CA, USA) of pH gradient 5–8 and 12% SDS-polyacrylamide gels were used for the second dimension separation.

Differential expression analysis by DIGE

Each AIS A CSF sample was randomly paired with an AIS C or D CSF sample and Difference Gel Electrophoresis (DIGE) was

Table 2. Patient inclusion and exclusion criteria.

No	Inclusion criteria
1	Patient with SCI due to fall or crush with AIS-A, C and D grade injuries
2	Patient should be at 24 hrs to eight days post injury for the first study group
3	Patient should be at 15–60 days post injury for the second study group
	Exclusion criteria
1	Patient in spinal shock stage
2	Other neurodegenerative diseases
3	SCI with lacerated cord or due to electrical injury
4	Associated poly trauma
5	Prior surgical stabilization of spine
6	Infectious diseases
7	Metabolic disorders
8	Patients on molecules that may inhibit Rho-ROCK pathways

conducted. 50 µg of protein for DIGE experiments, was labelled with 200 nM DMF reconstituted Cy5 dye (GE Healthcare, USA). The counterpart sample was similarly labelled with Cy3 dye. The samples were reverse labelled in half of the total number of DIGE experiments. Internal standard was made for each experiment by pooling 25 µg of protein from two samples followed by Cy2 labelling. DeCyder 2D Differential In-gel Analysis (version 6.5) software (GE Healthcare, USA) was used for the differential in gel analysis (DIA), where a threshold of 1.5 (volume ratio of Cy3 and Cy5 spots) was set and non-protein gel features were excluded manually. The gels were then analysed using the biological variance analysis (BVA) software (DeCyder 6.5). For BVA analysis, intensive repeated landmarking was performed for the gels selected in Cy2 filter. Automated gel to gel spot matching was applied, Student's t-test was performed by the software and spots that showed a particular trend of increase or decrease in three or more gels out of seven, with a p-value$<$0.1 was taken into consideration during analysis.

Protein identification using MALDI-MS

For identification of CSF proteins, we used AIS A grade CSF sample. AIS A sample encompasses CSF proteins as well as serum proteins, due to higher serum permeation in complete injury cases. This factor does not confound our analysis because all proteins identified from incomplete injury (AIS C and D) CSF samples are also present in AIS A samples.

1500 µg of protein was separated on a 2D gel and stained with blue-silver stain (10% v/v orthophosphoric acid; Merck, India, 10% w/v ammonium sulphate; SRL, India, 20% v/v methanol; SRL, India, 0.12% Coomassie brilliant blue G-250; SRL, India) and spots were picked using the Proteome works spot cutter (Biorad, CA, USA). Spots were de-stained, processed for MALDI sample preparation using the processing kit (Thermo Scientific, IL, USA), overnight trypsin digested (Thermo Scientific, IL, USA) and lyophilised in Heto Vacuum Centrifuge (Thermo). α-Cyano-4-hydroxycinnamic acid (CHCA) matrix (Thermo Scientific, IL, USA) was mixed in 1:1 ratio with 50% ACN (Thermo Scientific, IL, USA), 0.1% TFA reconstituted lyophilised spots and spotted on 192 well tungsten MALDI plates (AB Sciex, MA, USA). 4700 MALDI TOF/TOF Analyser, (AB Sciex, MA, USA) was used for matrix assisted laser desorption ionisation (MALDI) mass spectrometry.

Peptide mass fingerprint was obtained in positive MS reflector mode with fixed laser intensity of 5500, 2000–3000 laser hits in the range of 800–4000 Da. Signal to noise ratio was set at 10 and mass exclusion tolerance at 150 ppm [14]. For internal calibration, minimum signal to noise ratio was set at 20 and a mass tolerance of ±300 ppm was set which included monoisotopic peaks only. Peptides of interest were isolated at a relative resolution of 50 (full width at half maximum) and data from 3000 to 5000 laser shots were collected [14]. GPS Explorer version 3.6 (Applied Biosystems, MA, USA) was used for analysis of spectral data. MASCOT database scoring algorithm and NCBI and Swiss-Prot protein databases were used for peptide identification. Search settings: single missed tryptic cut, fixed carbamidomethylation, variable methionine oxidation, N-terminal acetylation and 150 ppm mass accuracy. Autolytic tryptic peaks were excluded in the MASCOT search parameter and p$<$0.05 was considered significant during identification.

Validation by western blot

50 µg protein was dissolved in co-ip buffer (50 mM Tris, pH 7.5, 15 mM EDTA, pH 8.0, 100 mM NaCl, 0.1% Triton X 100, PMSF 100 µg/µl) and used for western blot for validation. The protein was transferred from polyacrylamide gel onto polyvinyledene difluoride (PVDF) membrane (Millipore, Billerica, MA, USA) and primary antibodies were added and kept overnight at 4°C. We validated our DIGE results for Zinc alpha 2 glycoprotein (Mouse anti human, Santa Cruz Biotechnology, TX, USA) and Haptoglobin (Mouse anti human, Santa Cruz Biotechnology, TX, USA) and used Transferrin (Mouse anti human, Abcam, Cambridge, MA, USA), as a loading control, since the total amount of this abundant protein showed little variance from patient to patient and we did not find a suitable conventionally used protein as a loading control due to very low abundance of GAPDH and possible involvement of α-Tubulin in cytoskeletal rearrangements post SCI. Goat anti mouse Ig-HRP conjugate secondary antibody (Genei, Bangalore, India) was used for two hours at room temperature after TBST wash after the removal of primary antibody. SuperSignal West Pico Chemilu-

Table 3. Clinical details of the 14 CSF samples collected at 1-8 days post injury.

No	Age	Sensory level of injury	Motor level of injury	Days post injury	DIGE pair	AIS grade	Cause of injury
1	22	T9	L2	3	DIGE 1	A	fall
2	36	none	L2	2	DIGE 1	D	fall
3	45	none	L2	4	DIGE 2	D	crush
4	20	T6	L2	8	DIGE 2	A	crush
5	30	none	L2	1	DIGE 3	C	fall
6	23	T12	L2	2	DIGE 3	A	fall
7	45	L4	L2	5	DIGE 4	C	fall
8	28	L1	L2	7	DIGE 4	A	fall
9	30	T12	L2	2	DIGE 5	A	fall
10	55	L1	L2	2	DIGE 5	C	fall
11	19	none	L2	3	DIGE 6	C	fall
12	50	T7	L2	8	DIGE 6	A	fall
13	25	L1	L2	6	DIGE 7	A	fall
14	38	L2	L2	4	DIGE 7	C	fall

Table 4. Clinical details of six CSF samples collected at 15–60 days post injury.

No	Age	Sensory level of injury	Motor level of injury	Days post injury	DIGE pair	AIS grade	Cause of injury
1	55	T8	L1	27	DIGE 1	A	fall
2	23	none	L1	25	DIGE 1	D	fall
3	28	T11	L1	15	DIGE 2	A	fall
4	26	none	L1	60	DIGE 2	C	fall
5	20	T9	L1	16	DIGE 3	A	fall
6	25	none	L3	30	DIGE 3	D	fall

Table 5. Identified proteins from AIS A CSF.

Sl no	Spot No	Protein name	Gene name
1	1	Alpha 1B glycoprotein precursor	A1BG
2	4	Serine (or cysteine) proteinase inhibitor, clade C (antithrombin), member 1	SERPINC1
3	12	Alpha-1-antitrypsin	SERPINA1
4	13	Vitamin D-binding protein precursor	GC
5	14	Hemopexin precursor	HPX
6	16	Fibrinogen gamma	FGG
7	20	Fibrinogen beta chain precursor	FGB
8	26	Haptoglobin	HP
9	28	Zinc alpha 2 glycoprotein	AZGP1
10	32	Apolipoprotein E precursor	APOE
11	32	Glial fibrillary acidic protein, astrocyte (GFAP)	GFAP
12	34	Transthyretin precursor	TTR
13	38	Clusterin precursor	CLU
14	42	Ig kappa chain C region	IGKC
15	42	Prostaglandin H2 D-isomerase	PTGDS
16	46	Apolipoprotein A-I precursor	APOA1
17	51	Peroxiredoxin 2	PRDX2
18	52	Complement C4 precursor	CO4
19	54	AMBP protein precursor	AMBP
20	60	Protein N-terminal asparagine amidohydrolase	NTAN1
21	61	Apolipoprotein A-IV precursor	APOA4
22	62	Carbonic anhydrase I	CA1
23	66	Hemoglobin beta chain	HBB
24	71	Ficolin 3 precursor	FCN3
25	73	Creatine kinase, M chain	CKM
26	76	SH3-domain kinase binding protein 1	SH3KBP1
27	81	WD-repeat protein 37	WDR37
28	81	Nonspecific lipid-transfer protein, mitochondrial precursor	SCP2
29	83	Transferrin	TF
30	85	Ig mu chain C region	IGHM
31	86	Gelsolin isoform b	GSN
32	94	Ig alpha-1 chain C region	IGHA1
33	96	Glypican-1 precursor	GPC1
34	96	Phenylalanine-4-hydroxylase	PAH
35	96	Pro-neuregulin-3 precursor (Pro-NRG3)	NRG3
36	97	Heat shock 70 kDa protein 4L (Osmotic stress protein 94)	HSPA4L
37	99	Retinoic acid receptor gamma-1	RARG
38	99	3-hydroxyanthranilate 3,4-dioxygenase	HAAO
39	99	Protein C20orf151 (RBBP8 N-terminal-like protein)	RBBP8NL
40	100	Astrotactin 1 (Fragment)	ASTN1
41	103	Heat shock 70 kDa protein 4L (Osmotic stress protein 94)	HSPA4L
42	104	Beta-2-glycoprotein I precursor (Apolipoprotein H)	APOH
43	104	General transcription factor 3C polypeptide 5	GTF3C5
44	107	Serum albumin precursor	ALB
45	112	Ig gamma-2 chain C region	IGHG2
46	116	TBC1 domain family member 15	TBC1D15
47	119	Ig gamma-1 chain C region	IGHG1
49	121	Ig gamma-3 chain C region	IGHG3
49	126	Ig gamma-4 chain C region	IGHG4
50	128	Serum paraoxonase/arylesterase 1	PON1

L-R: serial number, spot number (the spot number here and in subsequent tables corresponds to Figure S1 and Table S1), protein name and gene name.

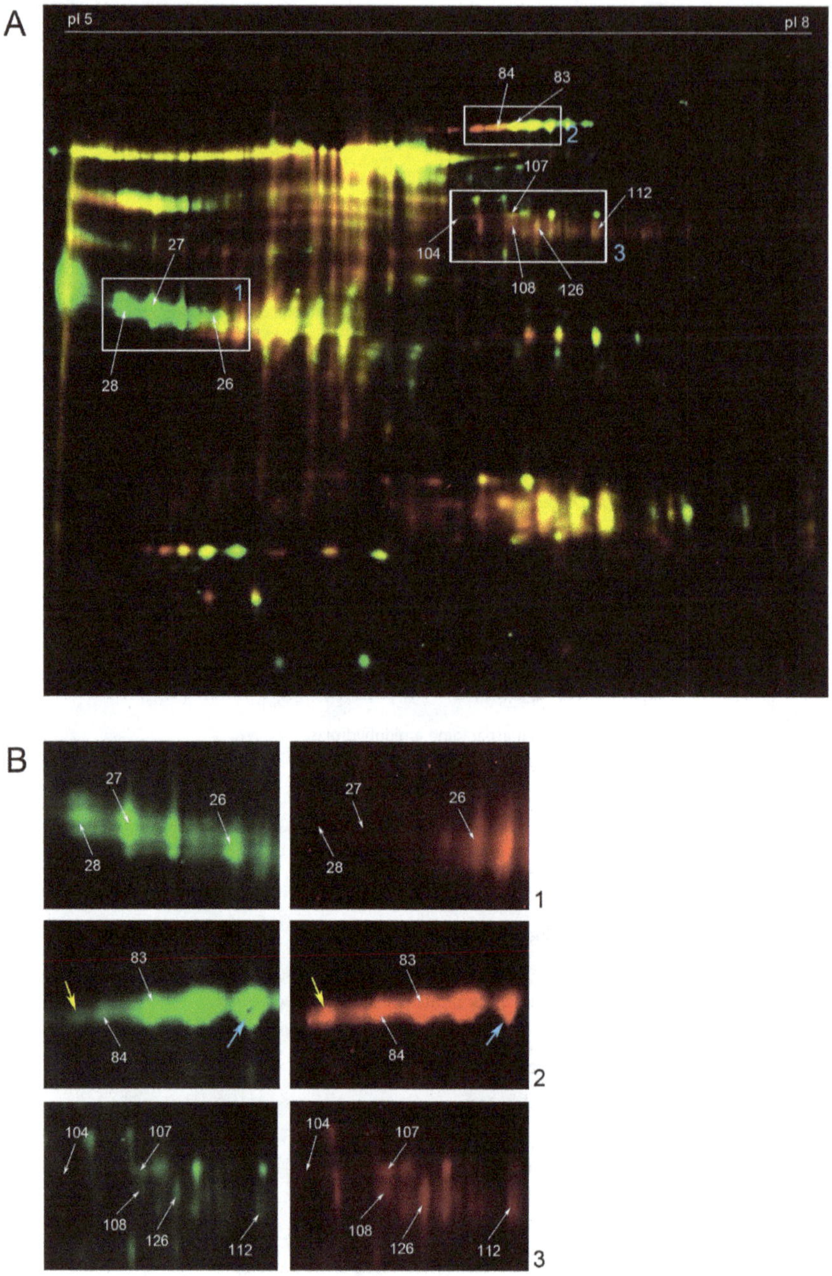

Figure 1. Differential abundance pattern by DIGE at 1–8 days post injury. A. A representative merged image of DIGE experiment with numbers indicating spot numbers. Complete injury CSF sample is labelled with Cy5 and incomplete injury CSF sample is labelled with Cy3. Proteins that show significant differential abundance are marked with white arrows and are boxed. B. Boxes 1, 2 and 3 with significant differential abundance of proteins are enlarged. Left hand panels show incomplete injury (Cy3 channel) image and the right hand panels show complete injury (Cy5 channel) image. Expression patterns of Transferrin are marked with yellow (acidic isoform) and blue (basic isoform) arrows in box 2.

minescent Substrate kit (Thermo Scientific, IL, USA) was used for X ray film (Kodak, Colorado, USA) exposure.

Construction of the protein-protein network (PPIN)

We constructed the protein-protein interaction network (PPIN) of spinal cord injury in human subjects (denoted as SCI-PPIN) taking the proteins identified by MALDI-MS and their interacting partners listed in BioGrid (version 3.2.103, Oct 2013) as nodes. For this analysis we had to drop 4 proteins (NTAN1, NRG3, as RBBP8NL and IGHG4) whose interacting partners were not listed in BioGrid and replaced CO4 by two of its aliases namely C4A and C4B. Thus SCI-PPIN had 866 nodes comprising of 45 proteins identified by MALDI-MS and their 821 interacting partners. The nodes were then connected pair-wise when the concerned proteins were interacting partners of each other. In total the network had 7121 links (interactions). For details of the network properties, see Text S1.

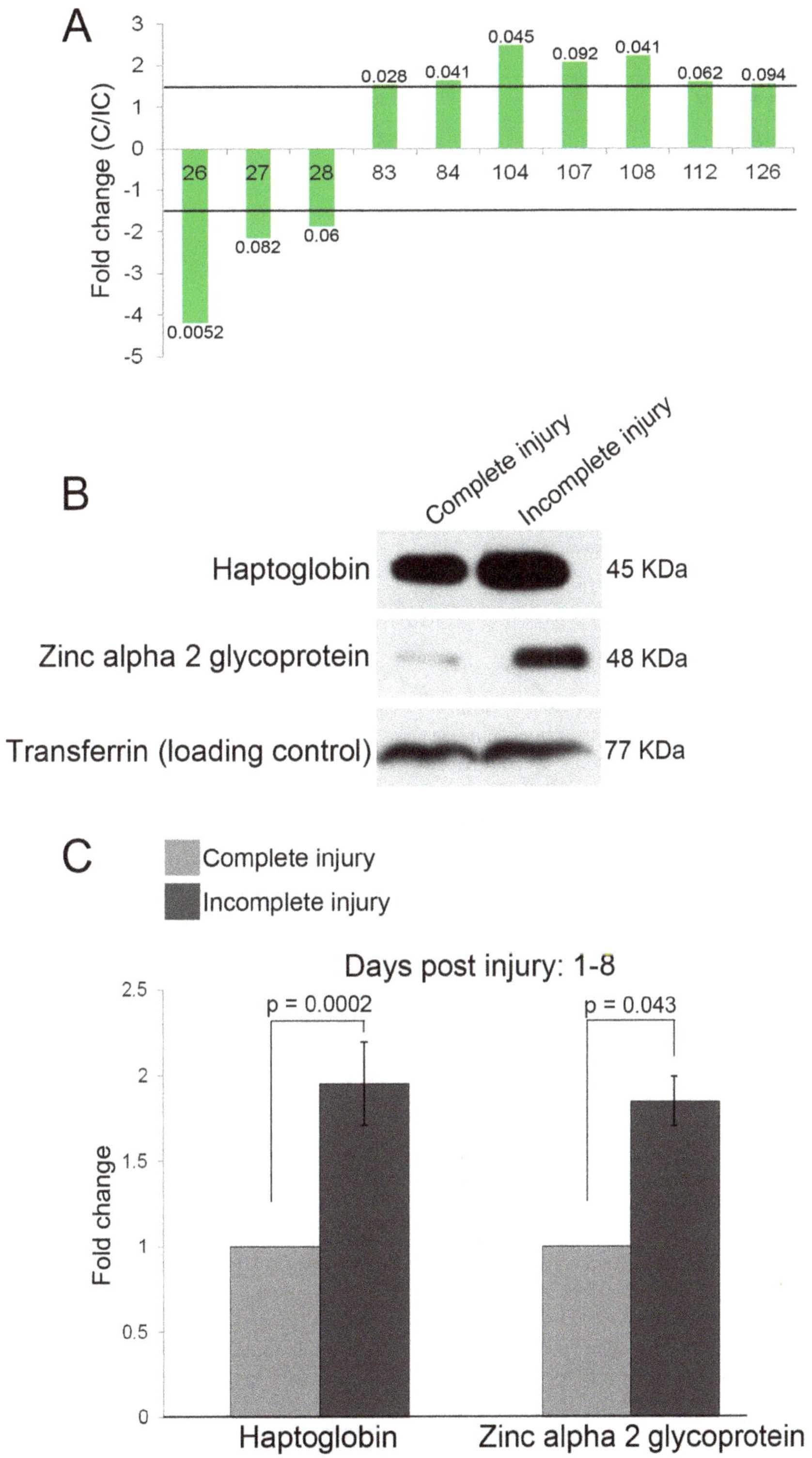

Figure 2. Differentially expressed proteins in complete and incomplete injury at 1–8 days post injury. A. Representation of fold changes (complete injury to incomplete injury) of differentially expressed proteins ($\geq \pm 1.5$ fold; outside the range between the lines) with p-values ($n = 7$) for each spot calculated by BVA (see Figure S3). B. Scanned Western Blot images for validation of fold changes of HP and AZGP. The observed band for AZGP was obtained a few kilo Daltons above the expected region and has been observed (as a possible result of glycosylation) by the manufacturers of the antibody. C. Quantification of the western blot ($n = 6$) showing significant difference in expressions.

Table 6. List of proteins showing differential expression by DIGE.

Spot no	Protein name	Average fold change (1–8 DPI)	Average fold change (15–60 DPI)
26	Haptoglobin	−4.21	0.49
27	Haptoglobin	−2.15	1.37
28	Zinc alpha 2 glycoprotein	−1.88	0.66
83	Transferrin	1.52	0.52
84	Transferrin	1.63	0.45
104	Beta-2-glycoprotein I-precursor (Apolipoprotein H)	2.47	−0.6[A]
104	General transcription factor 3C polypeptide 5	2.47	−0.6[A]
107	Serum albumin precursor	2.07	2.23[A]
108	Serum albumin precursor	2.23	1.2[A]
112	Ig gamma-2 chain C region	1.58	1.47[A]
126	Ig gamma-4 chain C region	1.52	2.13[A]

L-R: Spot number, protein name, average fold change of differential abundance at 1–8 days post injury (DPI) (Complete injury/Incomplete injury, n = 7, BVA algorithm used; Figure 2A and Figure S3), average fold change at 15–60 DPI (n = 3, manually calculated; Figure 3C).
[A]These spots were obtained in two out of three experiments.

Module Detection

Modules are partitions of a network such that nodes within a partition would have large number of connections among themselves compared to nodes in other partitions. In context of protein interaction network, proteins within a module have more interacting partners and thus it is expected that they would form a complex to work together and achieve some well-defined biological function [15] fairly independently from the rest of the system. Thus, study of modularized set of proteins is relatively less noisy and enhances the significance of enrichment analysis. To find the modules of SCI-PPIN we adopted the commonly used Newman-Girvans modularization (NGM) algorithm [16,17,18].

Enrichment analysis

To identify possible biological function(s) associated with a protein complex [19], we utilized GeneCodis3 [20] for enrichment analysis, where the proteins (or corresponding genes) belonging to each module of SCI-PPIN were taken as different query sets. GeneCodis would take a set of genes as the query field and associate GO terms/pathway ID/cellular component ID for each gene and calculate whether the fraction of genes in a particular item among the input gene list is over-represented compared to the background frequency (the total number of genes involved in that GO term/pathway ID/cellular component ID over the total number gene in the organism). For example, if K genes are involved in a particular GO term out of total N genes of *Homo sapiens* and if the query set has n genes with k of them associated with the concerned GO terms, we would evaluate the p-value using the hypergeometric distribution:

$$Hyp = \binom{N}{n}^{-1} \sum_{i=k}^{n} \binom{K}{i} \binom{N-K}{n-i}$$

This p-value Hyp was further corrected for False Discovery Rate (FDR) and denoted as Hyp^*. In our analysis, proteins belonging to any particular module of the SCI-PPIN were taken as input to GeneCodis3 [20] to obtain significantly enriched Gene Ontology (GO) terms for Biological Processes (BPs), KEGG pathways and cellular components. To ensure robustness we used a conservative cut-off $Hyp^* < 0.001$.

Results

Patient details

- *Group I (1–8 days post injury)*

The mean age of patients participating in this study group was 33.3 years with a standard deviation of 11.7 years (Table 3). All patients were male and hemiplegic. The most reported cause of injury among the participants was fall from trees. For all the participants, the upper limb motor activity was fully retained and the motor level of injury was L2.

- *Group II (15–60 days post injury)*

The mean age of patients participating in this study group was 29.5 years with a standard deviation of 12.8 years (Table 4). All patients were male and the cause of injury was fall.

Eight CSF proteins show differential abundance in complete and incomplete SCI at 1–8 days post injury

On proteome analysis of AIS A grade CSF, we could identify 49 proteins (Table 5) from 129 spots in 2D gel (with identical proteins in multiple spots; see Table S1 and Figure S1). Proteomics data for all identified spots have been provided in Figure S2A and Figure S2B. The set of proteins identified from complete injury were not distinct from those identified from incomplete injury CSF proteome. Only the abundance levels of several proteins differed, as we have found from our DIGE results.

We identified eight proteins which showed differential abundance (Figure 1A) among the two injury severities at 1–8 (average: 4.07 days) days post injury by DIGE and subsequent BVA analysis (n = 7). These eight proteins belonged to ten spots (Figure S3). Two proteins have been identified from spot 104. Three proteins, namely, Haptoglobin (26 and 27), serum albumin precursor (spots 107 and 108) and Transferrin (spots 83 and 84) were present in two different spots each as isoforms (Figure 1B). Curiously, a bias was observed in the isoform distribution of Transferrin (Figure 1B,

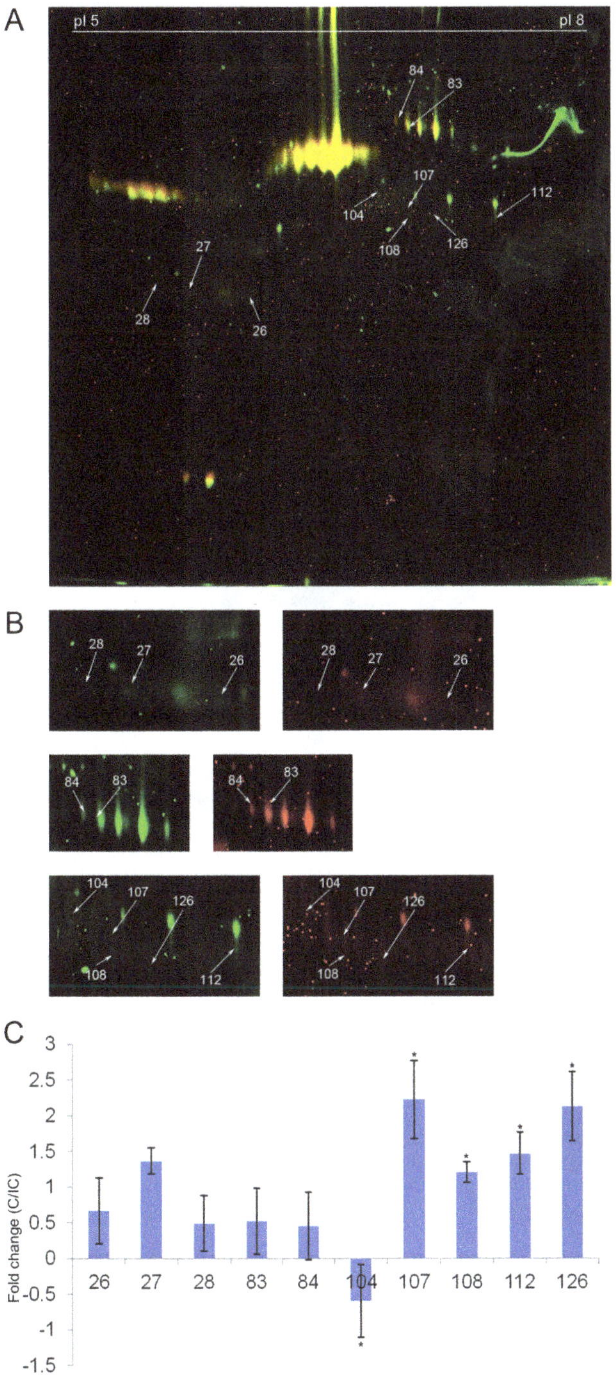

Figure 3. Differential abundance pattern by DIGE at 15–60 days post injury. A. Representative image with spot numbers. Complete injury CSF sample is labelled with Cy3 and incomplete injury CSF sample is labelled with Cy5. B. Enlarged areas of the gel showing the differentially abundant spots in detail. Left hand panel represents complete injury (Cy3 channel) image and right hand panel represents incomplete injury (Cy5 channel) image. C. Average fold change (complete/incomplete injury) for each protein (n = 3). Starred values have been obtained from 2 experiments.

panel 2), where, a lower pI isoform was more abundant in complete injury CSF whereas a higher pI isoform showed greater abundance in incomplete injury CSF.

The proteins that were more abundant in complete injury CSF at 1–8 days post injury were Transferrin (acidic isoforms, spots 83 and 84), Beta-2 glycoprotein I precursor and General transcription factor 3C polypeptide 5 (spot 104), Serum albumin precursor (spots 107 and 108), Immunoglobulin gamma-2 chain C region (spot 112) and Immunoglobulin gamma-4 chain C region (spot 126) (Figure 2A, Table 6 and Figure S3) and those less abundant in complete injury CSF were Haptoglobin (spots 26 and 27) and Zinc alpha 2 glycoprotein (spot 28). The total content of Transferrin encompassing all its isoforms was constant, as seen by western blot (Figure 2B and C) and subsequent laser scanning.

Abundance levels of the eight proteins at 15–60 days post injury

We looked at the levels of the eight proteins in CSF drawn at 15-60 days post injury (average: 28.83 days). Haptoglobin (spots 27 and 28) and Zinc alpha 2 glycoprotein (spot 26) showed a reversal in their abundance profiles. Both proteins were found to be more abundant in complete injury CSF during this time period as seen by DIGE (n = 3) (Figure 3A and B, Table 6). Transferrin levels showed similar abundance (within the threshold of ±1.5 fold) in complete injury CSF (Figure 3C, Table 6). Unlike the findings for Transferrin at 1–8 days post injury, the bias in abundance between different isoforms was not observed among the two severity groups at 15–60 days post injury. Serum albumin precursor (spots 107 and 108), Immunoglobulin gamma 2 chain C region (spot 112) and Immunoglobulin gamma 4 chain C region (spot 126) continued to be more abundant in complete injury CSF, while the spot pertaining to General transcription factor 3 C polypeptide 5 and Beta 2 glycoprotein 1 precursor (spot 104) showed marginal reduction in abundance for complete injury CSF (within the threshold of ±1.5 fold). Western blot for Haptoglobin and Zinc alpha 2 glycoprotein corroborated the findings by DIGE (Figure 4A and B).

Temporal changes in abundance of Haptoglobin and Zinc alpha 2 glycoprotein in both injury severities

We observed that the overall abundance level of Haptoglobin and Zinc alpha 2 glycoprotein decreased at 15–60 days post injury as compared with their levels at 1–8 days post injury. This trend was observed for both complete injury (Figure 4C and D) and incomplete injury (Figure 4E and F) by western blot.

Enrichment analysis revealed six functional modules with perturbed members

The constructed SCI-PPIN was unweighted and dense having about 25% of the total connections possible. The visual presentation of the SCI-PPIN was done using Cytoscape [21] (Figure 5A). We found 31 modules of different sizes in SCI-PPIN with number of members varying in the range 2 to 91 (Figure 5B, Table S2 and Table S3). The enrichment analysis revealed several statistically significant biological processes, cellular components and KEGG pathways, the major ones being those of protein transport and metabolism, DNA repair, cell division, migration and adhesion, immune response, apoptosis, lipid and cholesterol metabolism, transcription, complement activation, vesicle endocytosis, tRNA metabolism, iron transport and axon growth (Table 7). We focussed on 6 out of 31 modules where the differentially expressed proteins from DIGE experiments belonged (Figure 5B, Table 7). These pathways were assumed to be perturbed in the event of severe SCI, as their protein components showed altered abundance in a severe injury scenario.

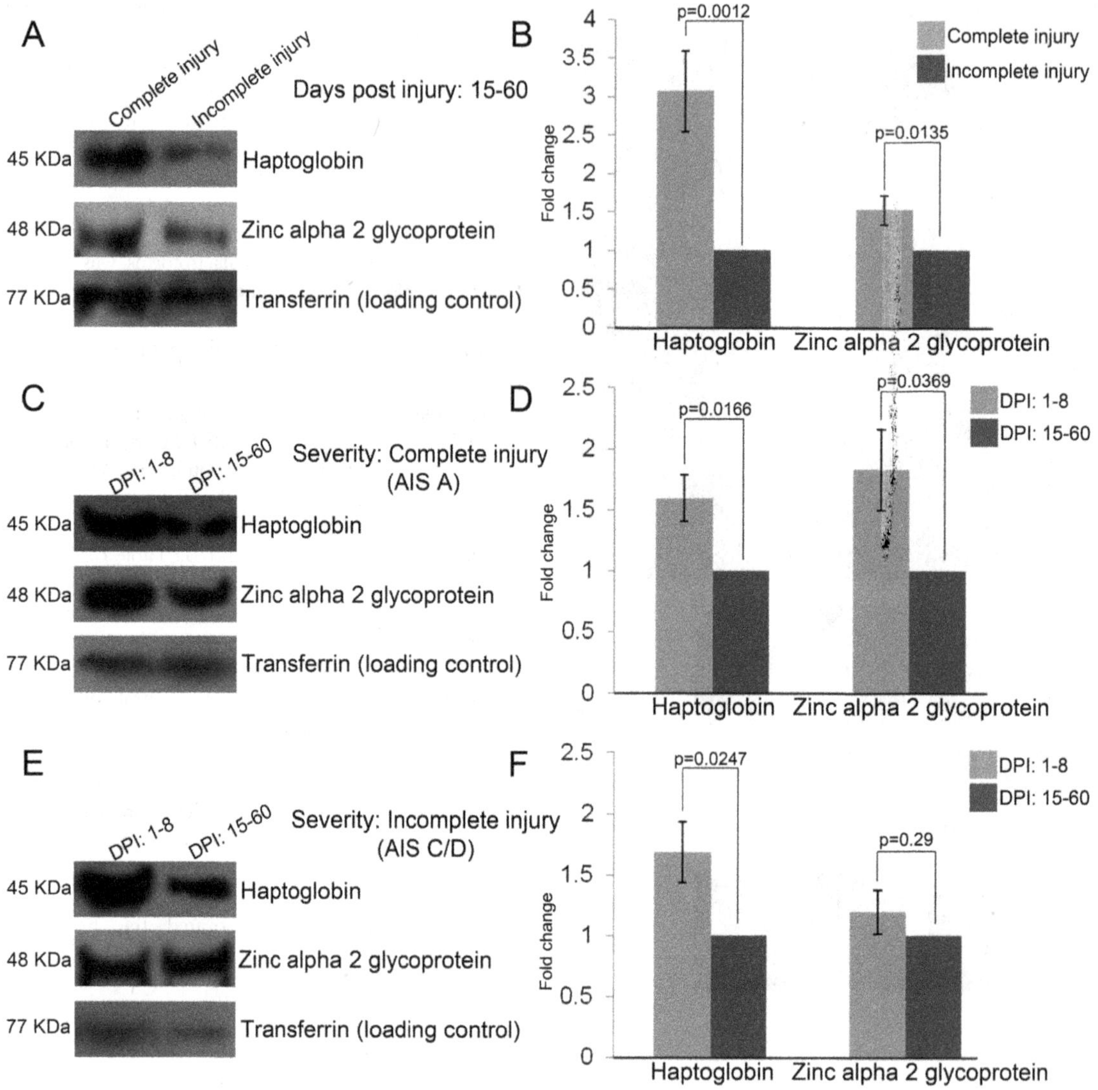

Figure 4. Changes in abundance levels of HP and AZGP on a temporal manner. A. Scanned blot images for these proteins at 15–60 days post injury (DPI) for the two severity groups. B. Quantification of the blots showing significant difference in expression. Comparison of abundance for HP and AZGP in complete injury (C) and incomplete injury (E), between two time periods. Quantification for the same (D, F) respectively (n = 4).

Discussion

SCI typically throws the normal functioning of Central Nervous System (CNS) and adjoining tissues into a haywire, as is evident from our study and several others [3,4,22–29,36]. Two perspectives emerge in this scenario: the off-balance situation of the CNS pathophysiology and the start and progression of efforts to bring back homeostasis and repair. The analysis of protein interaction network constructed from proteins associated with SCI reveals that both categories of pathways are altered.

Starting with the initial impact on the spinal cord, a breach of blood brain barrier may occur along with extensive cell and tissue damage. Consequences are myelin membrane disruption, DNA damage and iron toxicity. Transcriptomics studies of SCI in rodents and humans [22,23] have reported the involvement of cholesterol biosynthesis, myelination, transcription regulation and apoptosis pathways. Especially cholesterol biosynthesis would be predominant in the post injury scenario as myelination is necessary to replace the damaged axon membranes. In this context, PPAR-α has been shown to be over-expressed at the lesion site [24] mediating anti-inflammatory properties of drugs like Simvastatin [25]. DNA damage is another major consequence of cell disruption after trauma. It necessitates the activation of p53, which minimises inflammatory processes initiated by microglia and promotes DNA repair, cell division and axon genesis [26]. Microglial activation also initiates release of a number of beneficial trophic factors like BDNF following MAPK signalling pathway [27]. Iron homeostasis [28] and blood coagulation pathways are also active during this phase. Administration of Resveratrol in SCI rats has shown upregulation of IGF-1 and Wnt1 mRNA indicating the involvement of insulin receptor signalling and Wnt pathways in post SCI pathophysiology [29]. tRNA transcription, which is a perturbed pathway in our study, probably points towards increased protein synthesis and has not been reported so far.

An interesting finding from our proteomics study is the higher abundance of Zinc alpha 2 glycoprotein (AZGP) and Haptoglobin (HP) in incomplete injury CSF at 1–8 days post injury. Both being serum proteins, they can be presumed to have higher abundance

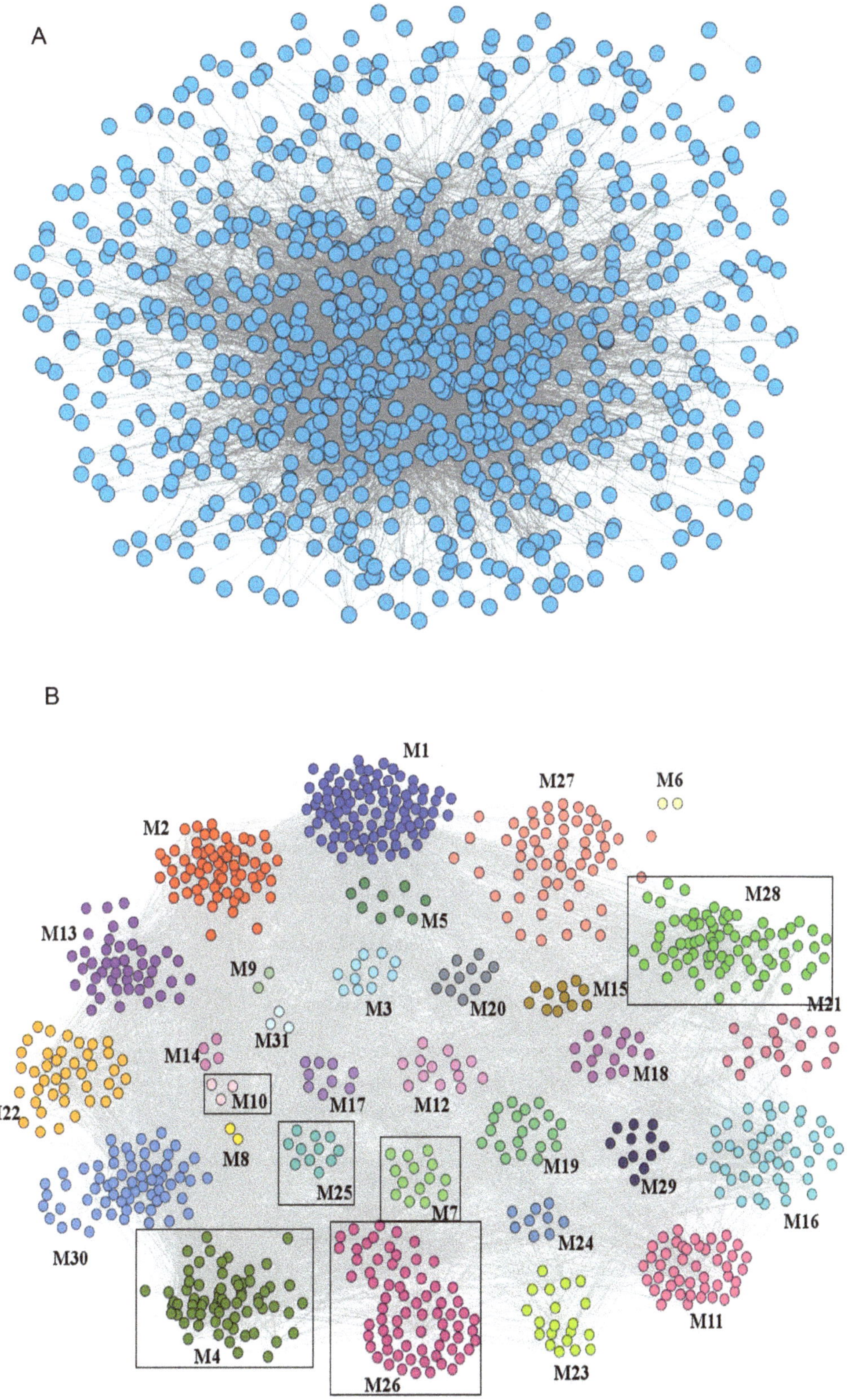

Figure 5. The spinal cord injury protein-protein interaction network. A. SCI-PPIN representation of 866 proteins (blue dots) and 7121 interactions (grey lines). B. Modularised SCI-PPIN consisting of 31 modules, dots representing proteins and coloured differently to demarcate different modules. Module numbers correspond to Table S2. The modules which contain proteins having differential abundance and detected by DIGE are boxed.

Table 7. Details of 31 modules generated through enrichment analysis.

Module ID	No. of proteins	Enriched Biological process	Enriched Kegg pathways	Enriched Cellular components
M1	91	Protein transport, fatty acid oxidation	Peroxism, PPAR signalling pathway[B]	Peroxism and cytoplasm
M2	65	RNA metabolism, epidermis development	RNA dynamics, ubiquitin mediated proteolysis	Nucleus and cytoplasm
M3	11	mRNA metabolism and transport	mRNA surveillance and transport	Nucleus and cytoplasm
M4[A]	68	Protein phosphorylation, mRNA metabolism	MAPK and Wnt signalling, meiosis	Nucleus and cytoplasm
M5	9	Glucocorticoid receptor signalling[B]	Wnt signalling[B]	Nucleus
M6	2	Complement activation	No annotations	Extracellular region
M7[A]	14	Iron transport, insulin receptor signalling[B]	P53 signalling[B]	Insulin like growth factor binding protein complex
M8	2	Meiotic sister chromatid cohesion, cell division[B]	No annotations	Mitotic cohesion complex
M9	2	No annotations	No annotations	No annotations
M10[A]	3	Lipid and ATP catabolism, immune response[B]	ABC transporters[B]	MHC class I protein complex[B]
M11	45	Vesicle endocytosis	Endocytosis	Cytoplasm and cytoskeleton
M12	13	Cell shape, migration and adhesion	Chemokine signalling and axon guidance	Plasma membrane, cytoskeleton, cytoplasm, membrane rafts
M13	44	NGF and T cell receptor signalling, axon guidance	Cancer	Cytoplasm and plasma membrane
M14	4	Axogenesis, NGF and Rho signalling	Actin cytoskeleton and chemokine signalling	Cytoplasm
M15	11	Lipoprotein metabolism and transport	No annotations	Coated pit
M16	45	Mitosis, blood coagulation, platelet activation	Regulation of actin cytoskeleton[B]	Cytoplasm, cytoskeleton
M17	9	Cerebellum development[B], meiosis[B]	Type II diabetes, dialeted cardiomyopathy[B]	Cytoplasm[B]
M18	15	Protein metabolism in the ER	Protein processing in the ER	Endoplasmic reticulum
M19	20	Complement activation and Cu ion homeostasis	Complement and immune response	Trans golgi network, membrane attack complex, extracellular space
M20	11	Apoptosis	Neurological disorders, cancer and apoptosis	Mitochondria and cytoplasm
M21	18	Removal of superoxide radicals[B]	Amylotropic lateral sclerosis[B]	Cytoplasm
M22	41	Sarcomere organisation[B]	Cardiomyopathy	Cytoplasm and nucleus
M23	20	Cellular component movement, brain morphogenesis	Adherens junctions	Z disc and ciliary rootlet
M24	9	Mitosis and protein ubiquitination	Cell cycle and ubiquitination	Nucleus and cytoplasm
M25[A]	11	tRNA and rRNA transcription	RNA polymerase[B]	Nucleus
M26[A]	71	DNA repair	P53 pathway and basal transcription factor	Nucleus
M27	58	Lipid and cholesterol metabolism	Complement, coagulation, PPAR signalling	Extracellular space
M28[A]	74	Organ regeneration[B]	E. coli infection	Cytoplasm and extracellular space
M29	12	Apoptosis[B]	Apoptosis and cancer	Cytoplasm and cell membrane
M30	65	Transcription, NGF receptor signalling	Cancer, TGF-beta and PPAR signalling	Nucleus and cytoplasm
M31	3	B and T cell tolerance induction[B]	TGF-beta signalling[B]	TGF-beta receptor complex

[A]Modules containing the proteins which show differential abundance in DIGE, and therefore, thought to represent perturbed biological pathways. [B]Biological processes, KEGG pathways and cellular components that are non-significant according to Hyp*<0.001, but are still listed here as they are known to be significant in other modules. For details of enrichment analysis of Biological Process, see Table-S3.

in more severe injury because of serum contamination of CSF. Contrary to this expectation, their predominance in incomplete injury CSF at an early phase of secondary injury suggests possible role in facilitation of recovery process after tissue injury. Furthermore, the revelation of changed abundance pattern of these non inflammatory proteins at a later time period, suggests that the possibility in their likely involvement post injury cannot be ruled out. We also noticed that over the period of weeks during which the secondary injury process progresses, the levels of these proteins decline in the CSF of both injury types. This observation allows us to further hypothesize the involvement of HP and AZGP in an early secondary injury phase.

Many of the proteins identified in CSF do not show significantly different abundance in AIS severity groups despite having roles in neuronal regeneration. Retinoic acid receptors can initiate neurite outgrowth in retinal degeneration cell models [30] and direct the transformation of fibroblasts into neurons [31]. There is increased secretion of ApoE and increased recruitment of ApoA1 by injured peripheral nerves [32] during their regenerative phase. In CSF from complete SCI, we identified several immune response proteins like Glial fibrillary acidic protein (GFAP), an inflammatory biomarker in SCI [11], complement precursors and Ficolin 3 precursor which substantiate the role of immune response post SCI [3]. Ficolin 3, Haptoglobin, Alpha-1-antitrypsin, Hemopexin precursor and IgM chain also showed increased expression in plasma of rheumatoid arthritis patients [33] as an indication of immune response.

A non-sialated version of Transferrin, called Beta-2 Transferrin, is more predominant in CSF than in blood [34] and has been used as a diagnostic biomarker for CSF leakage. This carbohydrate free Beta-2 Transferrin is less acidic than the sialated isoforms and suggests that the preponderance of a higher pI isoform in incomplete injury (Figure 1B, panel 2) is a result of lesser blood infiltration.

In this work we have constructed the protein interaction network comprising of proteins that were identified from CSF of complete injury SCI patients. It turns out that the network has strong underlying modular structure and keeping the proteins which exhibit differential abundance in CSF (complete versus incomplete SCI) in view, several modules were highlighted (Figure 5B). As proteins essentially act in conjunction with one another in the form of pathways, we could identify the molecular pathways that are perturbed in complete SCI.

The modularisation reveals that mRNA metabolism, tRNA and rRNA transcription, protein phosphorylation, lipid catabolism, immune response, iron transport, DNA repair and ATP catabolism pathways are the predominant pathways being perturbed in complete SCI. The picture that emerges here is of the system switching on certain very basic molecular mechanisms on the event of trauma. Chronologically placed, a lot of protein synthesis would have been initiated for repair and regeneration as manifested in our study by mRNA metabolism pathways being perturbed. tRNA and rRNA synthesis should get upregulated to initiate protein synthesis on a larger scale. A number of signalling pathways must follow suit and we see protein phosphorylation pathways emerging. The damaged myelin membrane has to be repaired or replaced necessitating lipid metabolism. It may be noted here that the cholesterol transport protein ApoA1 has shown differential abundance in several of the DIGE experiments (although statistically insignificant in our final analysis) and there have been reports linking ApoA1 to activation of Cdc42 [35] and F-actin polymerisation further downstream. How could these pathways be involved in regenerative mechanisms is worth looking into.

We have also seen that the breach of blood brain barrier during the mechanical trauma elicits immune response [3,36]. On the damage control front, excess free iron released by RBC rupture is being sequestered and transported away from the damaged site. Damaged cellular DNA repair mechanisms are also being initiated. Finally, as a cumulative effect, the traumatized system initiates these biological processes in expense of energy (ATP catabolism).

This combinatorial analysis therefore creates a picture of the real time molecular map around the injury site in the secondary phase. External intervention by manipulating the potentially important of these pathways could usher in greater regenerative efforts, though such an extrapolation is futuristic at this moment. CSF being a circulating fluid rather than a solid tissue, it is highly likely that the highlighted pathways are not only predominant at the injury site but are general consequences of the SCI trauma. Considering the limitations to obtain solid tissue from living human subjects and the methodology adopted, this study, to the best of our knowledge, is first of its kind in that it reflects the pathophysiological situation in the milieu of the injured cord by means of protein expression and abundance and a statistical analysis rather than by transcriptome analysis.

Conclusions

Traumatic SCI debilitates thousands of people worldwide every year. There have been many studies to decipher the molecular scenarios in the injured spinal cord and we have approached this problem as an analysis of differentially expressed proteins in complete and incomplete injury forms. Because the prognosis of incomplete injury cases is much better than those of the complete injury types, pathways perturbed among these two scenarios directly point to the molecular processes that may be responsible for the recovery patterns. Consequently, as the study has been conducted in the human system, the results could be attempted to be translated to animal models.

Supporting Information

Figure S1 Representative 2D gel of SCI (AIS A) CSF. Identified protein spots are numbered.

Figure S2 Mass spectrometry analysis details of all identified spots. A. MS and MSMS spectra. B. Probability based Mowse scores for each spot.

Figure S3 Differential abundance ratios of the eight differentially abundant proteins from complete and incomplete injury SCI CSF.

Table S1 Details of identified spots. L-R: Spot number (corresponds to Figure S1), protein name, NCBI/Swiss Prot accession numbers, pI, molecular weight, Mowse score, expect value, sequence coverage, peptide count, peptides matched.

Table S2 Composition of the modules. Each module is mentioned per column followed by the number of members in that module. The member proteins are listed in each column. Proteins identified in this study have been highlighted in grey and red. Among these, proteins that show differential abundance in DIGE have been highlighted in red. Note that "module" has been referred to as "group".

Table S3 Details of the modules. Protein id, GO annotations, annotation details and component genes for each module per sheet. GO annotations highlighted in green are statistically significant ($Hyp^{*}<0.001$) and those highlighted in yellow are not statistically significant but included for their significant biological roles in the current perspective.

Text S1 Properties and parameters of the SCI-PPIN.

Author Contributions

Conceived and designed the experiments: DM KKM BA. Performed the experiments: MBS KPS. Analyzed the data: MBS MB PKM SI. Contributed reagents/materials/analysis tools: SI KPS KKM BA. Wrote the paper: MBS PKM DM.

References

1. Furlan JC, Sakakibara BM, Miller WC, Krassioukov AV (2013) Global Incidence and Prevalence of Traumatic Spinal Cord Injury. Can J Neurol Sci 40: 456–464.
2. Razdan S, Kaul RL, Motta A, Kaul S, Bhatt RK, et al. (1994) Prevalence and pattern of major neurological disorders in rural Kashmir (India) in 1986. Neuroepidemiology 13: 113–119.
3. Oyinbo CA (2011) Secondary injury mechanisms in traumatic spinal cord injury: a nugget of this multiply cascade. Acta Neurobiol Exp (Wars) 71: 281–299.
4. McDonald JW, Sadowsky C (2002) Spinal-cord injury. Lancet 359: 417–25.
5. Beattie MS, Farooqui AA, Bresnahan JC (2000) Apoptosis and secondary damage after experimental spinal cord injury. Top Spinal Cord Inj Rehabil 6: 14–26.
6. Sandvig A, Berry M, Barret LB, Butt A, Logan A (2004) Myelin-, reactive glia-, and scar-derived CNS axon growth inhibitors: expression, receptor signalling, and correlation with axon regeneration. Glia 46: 225–251.
7. Schwab ME (2010) Functions of Nogo proteins and their receptors in the nervous system. Nat Rev Neurosci 11: 799–811.
8. Filbin MT (2003) Myelin-associated inhibitors of axonal regeneration in the adult mammalian CNS. Nat Rev Neurosci 4: 1–11.
9. Yiu G, He Z (2006) Glial inhibition of CNS axon regeneration. Nat Rev Neurosci 7: 617-627.
10. Maynard FM Jr, Bracken MB, Creasey G, Ditunno JF Jr, Donovan WH, et al. (1997) International standards for neurological and functional classification of spinal cord injury. Spinal Cord 35: 266–274.
11. Kwon BK, Stammers AMT, Belanger LM, Bernardo A, Chan D, et al. (2010) Cerebrospinal fluid inflammatory cytokines and biomarkers of injury severity in acute human spinal cord injury. J Neurotrauma 27: 669–682.
12. Light M, Minor KH, DeWitt P, Jasper KH, Davies SJ (2012) Multiplex array proteomics detects increased MMP-8 in CSF after spinal cord injury. J Neuroinflammation 9: 1–10.
13. Lubieniecka JM, Streijger F, Lee JHT, Stoynov N, Liu J, et al. (2011) Biomarkers for severity of spinal cord injury in the cerebrospinal fluid of rats. PLoS One 6: 1–13.
14. Chakrabarti A, Mukhopadhyay D (2012) Novel adaptors of Amyloid Precursor Protein intracellular domain and their functional implications. Genomics Proteomics Bioinformatics 10: 208–216.
15. Spirin V, Leonid A, Mirny LA (2003) Protein complexes and functional modules in molecular networks. Proc Natl Acad Sci USA 100: 12123–12128.
16. Fortunato S (2010) Community detection in graphs. Phys Rep 486: 75–174.
17. Clauset A, Newman MEJ, Moore C (2004) Finding community structure in very large networks. Phys Rev E Stat Nonlin Soft Matter Phys 70 (6 Pt 2): 066111.
18. Newman MEJ (2006) Modularity and community structure in networks. Proc Acad Sci USA 103: 8577–8582.
19. Huang da W, Sherman BT, Lempicki RA (2009) Bioinformatics enrichment tools: paths toward the comprehensive functional analysis of large gene lists. Nucleic Acids Res 37: 1–13.
20. Tabas-Madrid D, Nogales-Cadenas R, Pascual-Montano A (2012) GeneCodis3: a non-redundant and modular enrichment analysis tool for functional genomics. Nucleic Acids Res 40: W478–483.
21. Shannon P, Markiel A, Ozier O, Baliga NS, Wang JT, et al. (2003) Cytoscape: a software environment for integrated models of biomolecular interaction networks. Genome Res 13: 2498–2504.
22. Tachibana T, Noguchi K, Ruda MA (2002) Analysis of gene expression following spinal cord injury in rat using complementary DNA microarray. Neurosci Lett 327: 133–137.
23. Rabert D, Xiao Y, Yiangou Y, Kreder D, Sangameswaran L, et al. (2004) Plasticity of gene expression in injured human dorsal root ganglia revealed by GeneChip oligonucleotide microarrays. J Clin Neurosci 11: 289–299.
24. Fandela D, Wasmuhta D, A'vila-Martin G, Taylor JS, Galan-Arriero I, et al. (2013) Spinal cord injury induced changes of nuclear receptors PPARα and LXRα and modulation with oleic acid/albumin treatment. Brain Res 1535: 89–105.
25. Esposito E, Rinaldi B, Mazzon E, Donniacuo M, Impellizzeri D, et al. (2012) Anti-inflammatory effect of simvastatin in an experimental model of spinal cord trauma: involvement of PPAR-a. J Neuroinflammation 9: 1–17.
26. Floriddia EM, Rathore KI, Tedeschi A, Quadrato G, Wuttke A, et al. (2012) p53 Regulates the Neuronal Intrinsic and Extrinsic Responses Affecting the Recovery of Motor Function following Spinal Cord Injury. J Neurosci 32: 13956–13970.
27. Yang H, Feng GD, Liang Z, Vitale A, Jiao XY, et al. (2012) In vitro beneficial activation of microglial cells by mechanically-injured astrocytes enhances the synthesis and secretion of BDNF through p38MAPK. Neurochem Int 61: 175–186.
28. Koszyca B, Manavis J, Cornish RJ, Blumbergs PC (2002) Patterns of immunocytochemical staining for ferritin and transferrin in the human spinal cord following traumatic injury. J Clin Neurosci 9: 298–301.
29. Wang HD, Shi YM, Li L, Guo JD, Zhang YP, et al. (2013) Treatment with resveratrol attenuates sublesional bone loss in spinal cord-injured rats. Br J Pharmacol 170: 796–806.
30. Lin Y, Jones BW, Liu A, Tucker JF, Rapp K, et al. (2012) Retinoid receptors trigger neuritogenesis in retinal degenerations. FASEB J 26: 81–92.
31. Shi Z, Shen T, Liu Y, Huang Y, Jiao J (2014) Retinoic acid receptor gamma (Rarg) and nuclear receptor subfamily 5, group A, member 2 (Nr5a2) promote conversion of fibroblasts to functional neurons. J. Biol. Chem 289: 6415–6428.
32. Boyles JK, Zoellner CD, Anderson LJ, Kosik LM, Pitas RE, et al. (1989) A Role for Apolipoprotein E, Apolipoprotein A-I, and Low Density Lipoprotein Receptors in Cholesterol Transport during Regeneration and Remyelination of the Rat Sciatic Nerve. J. Clin. Invest 83: 1015–1031.
33. Roy S, Biswas S, Saroha A, Sahu D, Das HR (2013) Enhanced expression and fucosylation of ficolin3 in plasma of RA patients. Clin Biochem 46: 160–163.
34. Chan DTM, Poon WS, Ip CP, Chiu PWY, Goh KYC (2004) How Useful is Glucose Detection in Diagnosing Cerebrospinal Fluid Leak? The Rational Use of CT and Beta-2 Transferrin Assay in Detection of Cerebrospinal Fluid Fistula. Asian J Surg 27: 39–42.
35. Zhao GJ, Yin K, Fu YC, Tang CK (2012) The Interaction of ApoA-I and ABCA1 Triggers Signal Transduction Pathways to Mediate Efflux of Cellular Lipids. Mol Med 18: 149–158.
36. Anderson AJ, Robert S, Huang W, Young W, Cotman CW (2004) Activation of complement pathways after contusion-induced spinal cord injury. J Neurotrauma 21: 1831–1846.

7

Differential Effects of 670 and 830 nm Red near Infrared Irradiation Therapy: A Comparative Study of Optic Nerve Injury, Retinal Degeneration, Traumatic Brain and Spinal Cord Injury

Marcus K. Giacci[1,2,3], Lachlan Wheeler[1,3], Sarah Lovett[1,3], Emma Dishington[1,3], Bernadette Majda[1,3], Carole A. Bartlett[1,2], Emma Thornton[4], Elizabeth Harford-Wright[4], Anna Leonard[4], Robert Vink[4], Alan R. Harvey[1,3], Jan Provis[5], Sarah A. Dunlop[1,2], Nathan S. Hart[2,6¶], Stuart Hodgetts[1,3¶], Riccardo Natoli[5¶], Corinna Van Den Heuvel[4¶], Melinda Fitzgerald[1,2]*

1 Experimental and Regenerative Neurosciences, The University of Western Australia, Crawley, Australia, **2** School of Animal Biology, The University of Western Australia, Crawley, Australia, **3** School of Anatomy, Physiology and Human Biology, The University of Western Australia, Crawley, Australia, **4** School of Medical Sciences, The University of Adelaide, Adelaide, Australia, **5** ANU Medical School and John Curtin School of Medical Research, The Australian National University, Canberra, Australia, **6** Neuroecology Group, The Oceans Institute, The University of Western Australia, Crawley, Australia

Abstract

Red/near-infrared irradiation therapy (R/NIR-IT) delivered by laser or light-emitting diode (LED) has improved functional outcomes in a range of CNS injuries. However, translation of R/NIR-IT to the clinic for treatment of neurotrauma has been hampered by lack of comparative information regarding the degree of penetration of the delivered irradiation to the injury site and the optimal treatment parameters for different CNS injuries. We compared the treatment efficacy of R/NIR-IT at 670 nm and 830 nm, provided by narrow-band LED arrays adjusted to produce equal irradiance, in four *in vivo* rat models of CNS injury: partial optic nerve transection, light-induced retinal degeneration, traumatic brain injury (TBI) and spinal cord injury (SCI). The number of photons of 670 nm or 830 nm light reaching the SCI injury site was 6.6% and 11.3% of emitted light respectively. Treatment of rats with 670 nm R/NIR-IT following partial optic nerve transection significantly increased the number of visual responses at 7 days after injury ($P \leq 0.05$); 830 nm R/NIR-IT was partially effective. 670 nm R/NIR-IT also significantly reduced reactive species and both 670 nm and 830 nm R/NIR-IT reduced hydroxynonenal immunoreactivity ($P \leq 0.05$) in this model. Pre-treatment of light-induced retinal degeneration with 670 nm R/NIR-IT significantly reduced the number of Tunel+ cells and 8-hydroxyguanosine immunoreactivity ($P \leq 0.05$); outcomes in 830 nm R/NIR-IT treated animals were not significantly different to controls. Treatment of fluid-percussion TBI with 670 nm or 830 nm R/NIR-IT did not result in improvements in motor or sensory function or lesion size at 7 days ($P > 0.05$). Similarly, treatment of contusive SCI with 670 nm or 830 nm R/NIR-IT did not result in significant improvements in functional recovery or reduced cyst size at 28 days ($P > 0.05$). Outcomes from this comparative study indicate that it will be necessary to optimise delivery devices, wavelength, intensity and duration of R/NIR-IT individually for different CNS injury types.

Editor: Cesar V. Borlongan, University of South Florida, United States of America

Funding: This work was supported by the Neurotrauma Research Program (Western Australia) (http://www.nrp.org.au/). This project is funded through the Road Trauma Trust Account, but does not reflect views or recommendations of the Road Safety Council. NSH was funded by The University of Western Australia and The Western Australian State Government as part of a Western Australian Premiers Fellowship to Prof. Shaun Collin. No individuals employed or contracted by the funders (other than the named authors) played any role in study design, data collection and analysis, decision to publish, or preparation of the manuscript.

Competing Interests: The authors have declared that no competing interests exist.

* Email: lindy.fitzgerald@uwa.edu.au

¶ These authors contributed equally to this work.

Introduction

Oxidative stress occurs when the production of reactive oxygen (ROS) and nitrogen (RNS) species overwhelms the endogenous antioxidant reducing enzymes, and is considered a hallmark of injury to the central nervous system (CNS) [1–6]. The high rate of oxidative metabolic activity and associated reactive oxygen metabolites, low antioxidant capacity, and high content of polyunsaturated fats render CNS neurons and glia particularly prone to the deleterious effects of oxidative stress. Furthermore, during secondary degeneration, mitochondrial dysfunction and oxidative stress occur soon after injury [4,7,8]. As such, the alleviation of oxidative stress is an important therapeutic strategy for the treatment of neurotrauma. However, despite encouraging pre-clinical assessments of numerous antioxidants, there are currently no effective antioxidant strategies for attenuation of ROS production in clinical use following neurotrauma [9].

Irradiation in the red/near infrared spectrum (R/NIR, 630–1000 nm) has been developed as a therapeutic strategy to treat a range of injuries and diseases. Improvements following R/NIR-IT have been reported both in animals and humans in a wide range of injuries and disease including cardial infarct [10], renal and hepatic complications during diabetes [11,12], and oral mucositis [13]. In addition, conditions specific to the nervous system have shown improved recovery following R/NIR-IT, including retinal degeneration [14,15], CNS injury and stroke [16–22]. Clinical trials are currently underway assessing R/NIR-IT for stroke, with NeuroThera Effectiveness and Safety Trial (NEST)-1 and NEST-2 already completed with some clinical improvement shown [23,24]. This has led to the commencement of a third trial (NEST-3). However, the trial was halted following an interim futility analysis [25], perhaps due to a failure to employ effective treatment parameters [17].

While there is substantial controversy regarding the mechanism of action of R/NIR-IT, one widely supported hypothesis is that it acts by improving oxidative metabolism and reducing oxidative stress. The enzyme cytochrome *c* oxidase, complex IV of the electron transport chain, is proposed to act as a photoacceptor for irradiation at R/NIR wavelengths, with peaks in its absorption spectrum matching known efficacious treatment wavelengths. Irradiation is thought to lead to improvements in oxidative metabolism *via* changes in the oxidation-reduction state of the enzyme [26,27]. Increases in cytochrome *c* oxidase activity with R/NIR-IT are associated with increases in adenosine triphosphate (ATP) content and oxygen consumption *in vitro* and *in vivo*, indicating increased flux through the electron transport chain [28–30]. This may lead to lower concentrations of reactive species and reduced oxidative stress, due to maintenance of the mitochondrial permeability transition [31].

Other potential mechanisms of action of R/NIR-IT have been suggested, including effects downstream of cytochrome *c* oxidase activation. Photo-activation of the chromophores haemoglobin, myoglobin, flavins and metal free porphyrins may play a role *via* as yet unknown mechanisms [32–34]. Nitric oxide catalysed from cytochrome *c* oxidase may lead to downstream vasodilatation [35,36] and signal transduction, potentially contributing to functional improvements. R/NIR-IT has also been shown to modulate gene expression [14], reduce apoptosis [29,37], alter cytokine release and modulate immune responses [20,38–40]; outcomes perhaps independent of modulation of cytochrome *c* oxidase activity. Nevertheless, R/NIR-IT has been shown to reduce indicators of oxidative stress following CNS injury *in vivo* [8,22], and may serve as an effective first line antioxidant as part of a combinatorial strategy to reduce oxidative stress following neurotrauma.

R/NIR-IT is usually delivered using either lasers or light-emitting diodes (LEDs). LEDs are an increasingly accepted source for R/NIR-IT [41]. It was originally thought that the coherence of laser light was essential to achieve the therapeutic effects of R/NIR-IT, resulting in the widespread use of HeNe lasers (which emit light at a wavelength of 632.8 nm) [41]. More recently, therapeutic benefits of R/NIR-IT have been observed using non-coherent light sources such as LEDs [37,42,43], giving credence to the concept of using cheaper and more convenient LED devices to administer treatment. However, very few studies have reported the efficacy of R/NIR-IT delivered by LED for treatment of TBI or SCI *in vivo*. Furthermore, few studies have quantitatively compared the therapeutic effects of different wavelengths of light [20,29,44–47] and, to our knowledge, none of these compared different wavelengths of R/NIR-IT, delivered by LED, in more than one *in vivo* model of CNS injury. The therapeutic dose can be defined by the number of photons interacting with the photoacceptor (chromophore). As the energy of a photon varies with its wavelength, intensities of irradiation can be adjusted to ensure delivery of equal numbers of photons to provide an effective comparison of the efficacy of R/NIR-IT of different wavelengths [48]. We have conducted a multi-centre study designed to compare efficacy of equal numbers of photons of 670 nm and 830 nm R/NIR-IT, delivered to the surface of the skin overlying injury sites using LED arrays, in four models of CNS injury, each of mild to moderate severity: 1) in a model of secondary degeneration following partial injury to the optic nerve; 2) in light-induced retinal degeneration; 3) in traumatic brain injury (TBI) induced by fluid percussion impact; and 4) following a moderate contusion spinal cord injury (SCI). The R/NIR-IT treatment parameters were kept constant for the three traumatic injury models. Because previous experiments had established the approximate parameters for effective treatment of the retina, a 10-fold lower dose, delivered prior to light damage, was used in the retinal degeneration model. Penetrance of R/NIR-IT to the eye is greater than to the other CNS injury sites [22]. As such, delivery of the full dose to the retina that was used in the other CNS injury models would have resulted in unnecessary exposure to excess irradiation. We have already determined that there is no benefit in delivering this tenfold greater dose in the retinal degeneration model (unpublished). Although we delivered equal numbers of photons of each light source (670 and 830 nm) to the surface of the body, it is possible that any differences in the spectral transmission properties of the intervening tissue(s) could affect the relative irradiance actually received at the injury site. However, given the difficulties in measuring these transmission properties *in vivo*, especially in thick highly-scattering tissues, we attempted to equate quantal irradiance as far as practicable. We have assessed treatment outcomes of behavioural function or neuroprotection, of lesion volume, and of oxidative stress, as appropriate for each model system, and demonstrated differential effects dependent on wavelength used and injury type.

Materials and Methods

All procedures involving animals complied with the "Principles of Laboratory Animal Care" (National Institutes of Health publication no. 86–23, revised 1985) and were approved by the relevant institutional Animal Ethics Committee (The University of Western Australia approvals: RA3/100/673, RA3/100/1247; Australian National University approval A2011/029; University of Adelaide approval M-2013-160).

R/NIR-IT delivery, calibration and treatment

The spectral transmittance (300–890 nm) of an excised block of skin and muscle (plus the skin and muscle separately for information purposes) lying dorsal to the spinal column of a Fischer rat cadaver was measured to assess the degree to which light penetrates to the site of injury in the contusion SCI rat model. Broadband 'white' light from a 175 W xenon lamp (Spectral Products, CT, USA) was delivered to the dorsal surface of excised tissue via a 600 μm diameter quartz fibre optic fitted with a quartz collimating lens. Light transmitted by the tissue was collected via a cosine-corrector (CC-3-UV, Ocean Optics, Dunedin, FL, USA; covered with a thin layer of 'cling-wrap') connected to a 1000 μm diameter quartz fibre optic that delivered the light to an Ocean Optics USB4000 CCD spectroradiometer. Data acquisition was controlled through SpectraSuite software (Ocean Optics). The irradiance of R/NIR-IT received at the spinal cord was calculated by multiplying the spectral irradiances produced by the 670 and 830 nm devices at a surface of the skin, by the measured spectral transmittance of the skin and muscle.

R/NIR-IT was delivered to live rats using two different LED arrays: 670 nm R/NIR-IT from a commercially available device (VET75, Quantum Devices Inc, Barneveld, WI, USA) or 830 nm R/NIR-IT from a custom built device. The custom built adjustable intensity 830 nm LED array was constructed from infra-red LEDS and had a similar emission cross sectional area to the Vet75 device (70 cm^2). The light output of the custom built 830 nm LED array was adjusted to produce an equal photon irradiance (5.33×10^{16} photons cm^{-2} s^{-1}) to the VET75 670 nm LED array, at the surface of the skin (3 cm from the LED array). Because of the difference in photon energy at these two wavelengths, this equal quantal dose equates to an energy dose of 28.4 J cm^{-2} for the 670 nm array and 22.6 J cm^{-2} for the 830 nm array. Treatment of all rats with R/NIR-IT delivered by LED array was conducted using consistent procedures for each model of CNS injury. Rats were either gently held by hand or within a clear perspex box such that the LED arrays delivered irradiation at a distance of 3 cm above the surface of the skin overlying the injury, or 2.5 cm from the eye for the retinal degeneration model. Rats were conscious throughout treatment except for the first treatment after surgery, for which they were still anaesthetised. For the traumatic injury models, treatment duration was 30 minutes, delivered once per day, commencing immediately following surgical injury and continuing until euthanasia; control, sham-treated rats were similarly handled, but the overlying LED array was not turned on (referred to as control). For the retinal degeneration model, treatment duration was 3 minutes (resulting in lower doses of 3.4 J cm^{-2} for the 670 nm array or 2.7 J cm^{-2} for the 830 nm array at the eye, in this model) and occurred daily, for the 5 days prior to 24 hours' exposure to bright light.

Partial optic nerve injury animals and surgery

Adult, female Piebald-Virol-Glaxo (PVG) hooded rats were procured from the Animal Resources Centre (Murdoch, WA), and housed under temperature controlled conditions on a 12 hour light/dark cycle, with access to standard rat chow and water *ad libitum*. The partial optic nerve transection procedure was conducted as described elsewhere [4]. Briefly, PVG rats were anaesthetized (i.p. injection of 50 mg/kg ketamine hydrochloride and 10 mg/kg xylazil hydrochloride, Troy Laboratories, NSW, Australia), the right optic nerve exposed surgically and a diamond keratotomy knife (Geuder, Germany) used to make a controlled dorsal incision in each ON, to a depth of 200 μm. Post-operative analgesia was provided once (subcutaneous injection of 2.8 mg/kg Carprofen; Norbrook Australia, Pty. Ltd., VIC, Australia). Each treatment or control group consisted of 12 rats, and the groups were control, 670 nm or 830 nm R/NIR-IT treated, i.e. a total of 36 rats for this model, all animals experienced partial optic nerve transection.

Optokinetic nystagmus visual reflex was assessed in all rats 7 days after injury and daily R/NIR-IT using established procedures [22], by an investigator blinded to animal identity and treatment. Following behavioural assessments, under anaesthesia as described above, the injured optic nerves in 6 rats/treatment group were dissected from the ocular cavity, collected onto a microscope slide maintained at −20°C over a bed of dry ice, mounted in O.C.T. (optical cutting temperature compound) (Tissue-Tek, Sakura, Japan) then snap-frozen in eppendorf tubes in liquid nitrogen. Rats were then euthanased with Lethabarb© (800–1000 mg/kg i.p, Virbac, Australia Pty. Ltd., NSW, Australia). Immediately following euthanasia, the remaining 6 rats per treatment group were transcardially perfused with 0.9% saline followed by 4% paraformaldehyde (PFA) (0.1 M phosphate buffer; pH 7.2) for immunohistochemical assessments of optic nerves.

Partial optic nerve injury outcome measures

Fresh-frozen optic nerves were cryosectioned longitudinally at −20°C and free floating tissue sections (20 μm thickness) from each rat were labelled with 10 μM dihydroethidium (DHE) (Life Technologies, VIC, Australia) in phosphate buffered saline (PBS) for 10 minutes, for detection of reactive species. Optic nerves for immunohistochemical analyses were cryosectioned and processed according to established procedures [4], using primary antibodies recognising: manganese superoxide dismutase (MnSOD) (1:500, Stressgen); heme oxygenase-1 (HO-1) (1:200; Abcam); glutathione peroxidase 1 (GPx1) (1:250; Abcam); 3-nitrotyrosine (3NT) (1:500; Abcam); 4-hydroxynonenal (HNE) (1:200; Jomar Bioscience); 8-hydroxyguanosine (8OHDG) (1:500; Abcam); NG2 (1:250, Invitrogen) and olig2 (1:500, Abcam) to recognise oligodendrocyte precursor cells as well as Hoechst nuclear stain (1:1000; Invitrogen, VIC, Australia). Secondary antibodies were species-specific AlexaFluor 555- and 488-conjugated antibodies (1:500; Invitrogen, VIC, Australia).

Reactive species and immunohistochemical labelling were visualized in a single section of ventral optic nerve directly below the primary injury site for each animal, and photographed using a Leitz Diaplan fluorescence microscope (Leica, Germany). All images for each outcome measure were captured at constant exposures and in a single session. Image analysis was conducted on a single image using Image J/Fiji analysis software, setting constant arbitrary threshold intensities for all images in an analysis and semi-quantifying mean intensities and areas above that threshold. Data shown are either mean areas or intensities above threshold, with choice of analysis dependent on the pattern of staining and the most pronounced increases observed with injury compared to normal optic nerve (unpublished data).

Retinal degeneration animals and light damage

Albino Sprague-Dawley rats were born and reared in dim cyclic light conditions (12 hr:12 hr, light:dark) with an ambient light level of approximately 5 lux. Between post-natal days (P) 90–120, and following 5 days of R/NIR-IT pre-treatment, photochemical damage to the retina (light damage, LD) was induced in some groups of rats by 24 hours' exposure to a cold-white fluorescent light source positioned above the cages (18 W, Cool White; TFC), at an intensity of approximately 1000 lux at the cage floor. The six treatment or control groups consisted of 6 rats (n = 6), - control, 670 nm or 830 nm R/NIR-IT treated, LD, 670 nm+LD and 830 nm+LD - a total of 36 rats. At the end of the LD period, rats were euthanized with an overdose of barbiturate (60 mg/kg bodyweight i.p., Valabarb; Virbac, Milperra, Australia).

Retinal degeneration outcome measures

The eyes from the animals was marked at the superior surface for orientation, enucleated and then processed for cryosectioning by immersion fixation in 4% PFA in 0.1 M PBS (pH 7.3) for 3 h at room temperature. The fixed eyes were then washed in PBS (3×5 minutes) and placed in 30% sucrose overnight. Eyes were oriented and embedded in O.C.T. compound, snap frozen in dry ice cooled acetone and cryosectioned at 16 μm. The sections were mounted on superfrost-plus glass slides and dried overnight at 37°C. Sections were stained for histological examined using either immunohistochemistry or TUNEL.

TUNEL staining was used to quantify photoreceptor apoptosis/death following LD in frozen sections using our published method [49]. Counts of TUNEL positive cells in the outer nuclear layer (ONL) were carried out along the retinal sections cut in the parasagittal plane (superoinferior), including the optic disc. The final count from each animal was then averaged at comparable locations in two non-sequential sections. Sections adjacent, or close, to those used for TUNEL analysis were used for immunohistochemistry. Sections were rehydrated in graded ethanols and then placed in 10% normal goat serum (Sigma) for 1 h to block non-specific binding. Primary antibodies were GFAP (1:700 Dako); and 8OHDG (1:500; Abcam) incubated overnight at 4°C. Secondary antibodies were anti-mouse IgG-alexa 594 or anti-rabbit IgG-alexa 488 (1:1000, Life Technologies) incubated overnight at 4°C. Sections were washed in 0.1 M PBS and coverslipped in a ProLong Gold Antifade (Life Technologies). Primary antibodies were omitted for controls assessing non-specific binding of the secondary antibody. Images were visualised and captured using a LSM5 Confocal microscope (Zeiss), Pascal (Zeiss, v4.0) and prepared using Photoshop CS5 (Adobe). No manipulation to the intensity or gain was performed using either software.

TBI animals and surgery

A total of 21 adult male Sprague-Dawley rats (weighing between 300–330 grams) were randomly assigned into 4 groups: sham uninjured animals (n = 5), injured untreated controls (n = 6), 670 nm R/NIR-IT treated (n = 5), 830 nm R/NIR-IT treated (n = 5). To administer TBI (n = 16) we used the lateral fluid percussion model (LFP), which has been co-developed by our laboratory in collaboration with others [50] This focal model of TBI produces extensive oxidative stress, inflammation, ion changes, mitochondrial damage and energy crisis, along with both motor and cognitive deficits [51]. Briefly, rats were obtained one to two weeks prior to injury and group housed with unrestricted access to food and water. On the day of trauma, rats were initially anaesthetised via nose cone induction by inhalation of 3–4% isoflurane in 1.5 L/min O_2, subsequently intubated and then mechanically ventilated to a surgical level by inhalation of 1–2% isoflurane in 1.5 L/min O_2.

Under anaesthesia, a midline incision was made on the skin overlaying the skull and the bone exposed. Lignocaine (local anaesthetic) was injected prior to incision. After exposing the skull, a 4 mm craniotomy centered over the parietal cortex between the midline and the temporal ridge was performed using a trephine drill. Care was taken not to damage the dura which was left intact at the opening. A female luer loc was then cemented over the craniotomy using polyacrylamide adhesive. The injury device was connected to the female luer loc using a male luer loc fitting. The device then induced injury by generating a 25 msec saline pressure pulse which was transmitted to the brain. This pressure pulse results in a transient deformation of brain tissue at the site of the craniotomy. The amplitude of the pressure pulse was measured using a pressure transducer. In our experience, a 2.5 atmosphere pressure pulse results in moderate injury. Throughout this procedure the rats remained anaesthetized. After confirming that the condition of the rat was stable, the luer loc fitting was removed, the craniotomy was sutured, the skin sutured and the animals removed from anaesthesia to permit recovery. Throughout all procedures, temperature of rats was maintained at 37°C using a heating pad. Rats usually woke within 15 minutes of injury and were exhibiting normal exploratory behaviour within 60 minutes.

TBI outcome measures

Rats motor abilities were assessed by their ability to remain on a rotarod, according to established procedures [52]. Rats were trained on the rotarod for 5 days prior to injury unless they recorded the maximum time of 120 seconds for 2 consecutive days, in which case they were deemed trained. The final day of the training day was used as the pre-injury score. Rats were assessed at the same time each day for the 7 R/NIR-IT treatment days following injury. The Bilateral Asymmetry Test was used to assess sensory function. Forepaw latency was assessed according to established procedures [53], on both the ipsilateral and contralateral forepaws prior to induction of injury. Latency of both forepaws was then assessed on days 1, 3 and 7 post-injury. Due to the individual variability between animals, each rat's contralateral forepaw latency (forepaw which is affected) was compared to their ipsilateral forepaw latency to give a percentage of latency score.

Following perfusion fixation at 7 days after injury with 10% formalin, a 10 mm section of whole brain (Bregma; 1.0 mm to − 9.0 mm AP) (Paxinos and Watson Rat brain stereotaxic atlas) was processed and embedded in paraffin. Serial sections were taken at every 250 um interval for the entire described brain region. Sections were stained with Haematoxylin and Eosin stain, scanned using the Hamamatsu Nanozoomer and viewed with the associated software. The area of the lesion was circumscribed using this software, with the area recorded for each section. The following equation was then used to determine lesion volume (mm^3): $= \sum$ (lesion volume of each section) * 0.25 (250 um): this method has been used routinely within our laboratory, modified from Corrigan et al., (2012) [54].

SCI animals and surgery

Adult female Fischer rats (F344, 160–190 g) were bred at the Animal Resources Center (Animal Research Center, Murdoch, W.A.), housed under a standard 12 h light/dark cycle, fed wet and dry rat chow and water ad libitum. Each treatment group consisted of 7 or 8 rats, groups were control, 670 nm or 830 nm R/NIR-IT treated, total n = 22 for this model, all rats received the SCI. Moderate contusion SCI was performed as described in [55] and in brief as follows; rats were anaesthetised by i.p. injection of xylazine in combination with ketamine (50 mg/kg ketamine hydrochloride and 10 mg/kg xylazil hydrochloride, Troy Laboratories, NSW, Australia). Amacin ophthalmic eye ointment (Provet, Queensland, Australia) was applied after the rats were placed under anaesthetic. A longitudinal incision and partial laminectomy were performed at vertebral level T9–T10 to expose the underlying thoracic spinal cord without disrupting the dura. Rats were positioned on a surgical plate for spinal cord impact using flexible armatures and Adson forceps (spinal cord stabilizing forceps). All rats received a moderate contusion injury (200KDyne) using an Infinite Horizon impactor device on the dorsal surface of the exposed spinal cord. Rats were maintained in a temperature and humidity controlled chamber until recovery from anaesthetic. Rehydrating saline (2 mL) in conjunction with Buprenorphine Hydrochloride (Provet) (Temgesic, 0.01 ml/100 g body weight, 300 U/ml) and intramuscular injection of Benicillin (Provet) (0.02 mL/100 g body weight, 300 U/mL) was administered immediately after surgery and every 12 h thereafter to hydrate and act as an analgesic respectively. Bladders were manually expressed every 12 h until function was recovered and total volumes of given saline were adjusted for rat bladder size. Frequency of saline - Temgesic injections was reduced to every 24 h when animals were able to drink unassisted, and generally ceased around day 7–10 after SCI. 50 uL of Benicillin (Provet, 0.02 ml/100 g body weight, 300 U/mL, (150 mg/ml procaine penicillin, 150 mg/ml benzathine penicillin, 20 mg/ml procaine hydrochloride; Troy Laboratories Pty. Ltd., Glendenning, NSW, Australia)) was administered intramuscularly immediately after surgery and at 2, 4 and 6 days to prevent wound and bladder infections.

SCI outcome measures

Functional assessments were performed on days 1, 2, 3, 7, 14, 21 and 28 following surgery and daily R/NIR-IT, and consisted of open field locomotion assessment, quantitative gait analysis (Ratwalk) and ladder walking. The Basso, Beattie, Bresnahan (BBB) locomotor rating scores were used to assess the range and type of open field spontaneous forward locomotion [56]. Rats were recorded in an open field for 4–5 minutes on days 7, 14, 21 and 28-post injury. Video recordings were made on the left, right and posterior views of the animal. Scoring was by 3 independent assessors blinded to animal treatments: assessors had to score animals within 1 point of each other or animals were re-assessed. Quantitative gait analysis using Ratwalk was performed at days 14, 21 and 28-post injury under red light, according to established procedures [57] and assessed using Ratwalk software. The stride length was obtained by measuring the distance (in pixels) between successive placements of an individual paw. Ladder walking was also assessed at days 14, 21 and 28 days post-injury. All rats were recorded walking the length of the ladder walk apparatus 3 times per session. Analysis was performed using video recordings, analysed frame-by-frame by 3 independent scorers. The foot faults for both the left and right limbs were recorded over the total distance travelled [58].

At day 28-post injury, animals were euthanized by lethal injection of sodium pentobarbitone (Provet; 50 mg/100 g) and perfused with approximately 200 mL of 1% (v/v) Heparin (Prover) in PBS, followed by approximately 250 mL of 4% (w/v) paraformaldehyde pH 7.2 (Sigma) in PBS. Spinal cords were dissected and cryosectioned longitudinally (40 μm). Sections were stained with toluidine blue for assessment of cyst size and for immunohistochemical analysis according to established procedures [55] ($n = 4$/group), using antibodies to: glial fibrillary acidic protein (GFAP) (1:400, Dakopatts); β-III tubulin (1:400, Covance); neuronal doublecortin (DcX) (1:400, Novex); GAP43 (1:400, Invitrogen) and activated macrophage ED1 (CD68) (1:400, Serotec). Secondary antibodies were species specific AlexaFluor 555- and 488-conjugated antibodies (1:500; Invitrogen).

Toluidine blue sections were scanned at high power magnification (40x) using a ScanScope digital slide scanner with Aperio Software. Analysis of the cyst area was carried out using the software Image-Pro Plus (Image-Pro version 3.0 for Windows, Media Cybemetics Image-Pro, Rockville MD) where the total area of cystic structures within ±5 mm (rostral-caudal axis) from the epicenter of the lesion was calculated as a percentage of total tissue. Immunohistochemical labelling was visualized in sections taken within the central part of the lesion ($n = 4$) in each treatment group (repeated 2x), and photographed using a Nikon Eclipse E800 microscope. All images for each outcome measure were captured at constant exposures and in a single session.

Statistical analyses

All data were expressed as mean ± SEM: statistical analyses were conducted using SPSS statistical software (IBM) or PRISM (GraphPad Software). Data were analyzed using two-tailed Student's t test, one- or two-way ANOVA and Bonferroni Dunn or Dunnett's post-hoc tests as appropriate (F values, degrees of freedom (dF) and post-hoc test p values given). In the case of the open field locomotion test, the Kruskal Wallis post-hoc test for non-parametric data was used. Ladder walk analysis was performed using two-way ANOVAs comparing identical treatment groups over days 14, 21 and 28, and experimental conditions at each time point. Probabilities ≤0.05 were considered significant.

Results

Penetrance of light including R/NIR to a CNS injury site

The effect of wavelength of light on penetrance of R/NIR light through skin and/or muscle was assessed by measuring the spectral transmittance (300 nm to 890 nm) of the tissue overlying the spinal cord in a Fischer rat cadaver, allowing calculation of the irradiation doses received at the injury site in the SCI model. Transmittance was higher through skin than muscle, and was greatest between 750–890 nm, with a minor secondary peak at around 500 nm (Fig. 1A). Unlike lasers, LEDS are not monochromatic and instead are narrowband light sources that emit significant amounts of light either side of the specified emission peak (Fig. 1A, B). Thus, measured irradiances produced by the LED devices are integrated over the wavelength range 400–890 nm. The total irradiance of R/NIR-IT received at the surface of the skin, 3 cm from the emission surface of the 670 nm device, was 5.3×10^{16} photons cm^{-2} s^{-1} (peak irradiance at 670 nm was approximately 2×10^{15} photons cm^{-2} s^{-1}) and this was calculated to drop to 3.5×10^{15} photons cm^{-2} s^{-1} (6.6%) at the SCI injury site, below the overlying skin and muscle (Fig. 1B). Similarly, the total irradiance of R/NIR-IT received at the surface of the skin, 3 cm from the surface of the 830 nm device, was 5.3×10^{16} photons cm^{-2} s^{-1} (peak irradiance at 830 nm was approximately 1.2×10^{15} photons cm^{-2} s^{-1}) and this dropped to 6.0×10^{15} photons cm^{-2} s^{-1} (11.3%) at the SCI injury site (Fig. 1C).

Effects of R/NIR-IT following partial optic nerve injury

Partial dorsal optic nerve transection leaves the remaining ventral optic nerve vulnerable to secondary degeneration, and provides a model to assess efficacy of therapeutic strategies to prevent spreading damage following injury to the CNS [59]. Analysis of functional behaviour following partial optic nerve transection and R/NIR-IT was assessed using the optokinetic nystagmus visual reflex at 7 days after injury. R/NIR-IT delivered at 670 nm led to a significantly increased number of smooth pursuits and fast reflexes compared to numbers of responses by injured, control animals ($F = 12.8$ and 3.9 respectively, $dF = 2$, $P \leq 0.05$), indicating improved visual function and confirming previous findings [22]. R/NIR-IT at 830 nm resulted in significantly more smooth pursuits compared to control ($F = 12.8$, $dF = 2$, $P \leq 0.05$), but there was no significant improvement in the number of fast resets ($F = 3.9$, $dF = 2$, $P > 0.05$, Fig. 2A). There were no significant differences between either numbers of smooth pursuits or fast reset responses by rats treated with 670 nm R/NIR-IT, compared to rats treated with 830 nm R/NIR-IT ($P > 0.05$) (Fig. 2A).

DHE fluoresces upon oxidation by a range of reactive species and was used to semi-quantify increases in ROS/RNS, in fresh frozen tissue sections. Note that data shown here and throughout are either mean areas or mean intensities above threshold, with choice of analysis dependent on the pattern of staining and the most consistent or pronounced increases observed with injury compared to normal optic nerve (unpublished data). In ventral optic nerve vulnerable to secondary degeneration, there was a small but significant decrease in the mean fluorescence intensity of DHE, when animals were treated with 670 nm R/NIR-IT ($F = 5.3$, $dF = 2$, $P \leq 0.05$) (Fig. 2B), indicating that 670 nm R/NIR-IT reduced ROS/RNS in CNS tissue vulnerable to

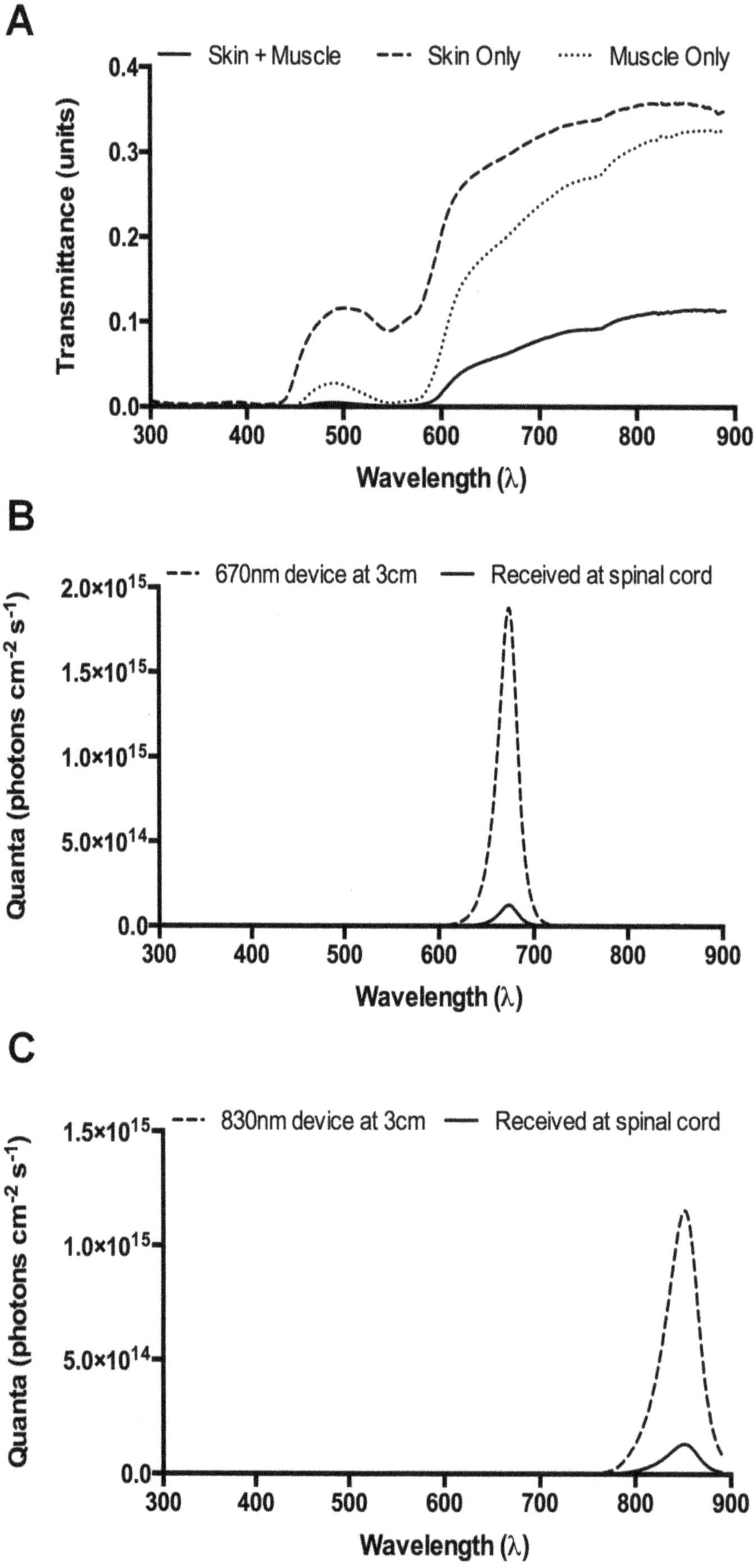
A
Skin + Muscle
Skin Only
Muscle Only
Transmittance (units)
0.4
0.3
0.2
0.1
0.0
300
400
500
600
700
800
900
Wavelength (λ)
B
670nm device at 3cm
Received at spinal cord
Quanta (photons cm-2 s-1)
2.0×10^15
1.5×10^15
1.0×10^15
5.0×10^14
0.0
300
400
500
600
700
800
900
Wavelength (λ)
C
830nm device at 3cm
Received at spinal cord
Quanta (photons cm-2 s-1)
1.5×10^15
1.0×10^15
5.0×10^14
0.0
300
400
500
600
700
800
900
Wavelength (λ)

Figure 1. Penetrance of light through rat skin and muscle and irradiance delivered by the 670 nm and 830 nm R/NIR-IT LED arrays. (A) Spectral transmittance of light from 300 nm to 890 nm through skin (red), muscle (green), and skin plus muscle combined (blue), taken from the area overlying the SCI injury site in a Fischer rat cadaver (n = 1). Spectral irradiance (300–890 nm) received at the surface of the skin from the 670 nm (B) or 830 nm (C) LED arrays at a distance of 3 cm (blue lines) and calculated numbers of photons reaching the SCI injury site (red line).

spreading damage at 7 days. There was no effect of R/NIR-IT delivered at 830 nm on DHE fluorescence at this time (F = 5.3, dF = 2, P>0.05) (Fig. 2B).

The intensities of immunoreactivity of the antioxidant enzymes MnSOD, HO-1 and GPx1 were quantified in ventral optic nerve vulnerable to secondary degeneration at 7 days following injury. We observed no significant change in immunoreactivities when animals were treated with either 670 nm or 830 nm R/NIR-IT, compared to control at this time (F = 4.6, 4.5 and 1.7 respectively, dF = 2, P>0.05) (Figs. 2C–E), in contrast to our reported reductions in MnSOD following 670 nm R/NIR-IT at 1 day after injury[22]. MnSOD and HO-1 immunoreactivities in animals treated with 830 nm R/NIR-IT were significantly lower than in rats treated with 670 nm R/NIR-IT (F = 4.6 and 4.5 respectively, dF = 2, P≤0.05) (Figs. 2C–E). Similarly, there was no change in the immunoreactivity of the indicator of protein nitration 3NT or the indicator of oxidized DNA 8OHDG in ventral optic nerve, when rats were treated with either 670 nm or 830 nm R/NIR-IT, compared to control at 7 days (F = 5.0 and 4.6 respectively, dF = 2, P>0.05) (Figs. 2F, G). However, immunoreactivities of both 3NT and 8OHDG in rats treated with 830 nm R/NIR-IT were significantly lower than in rats treated with 670 nm R/NIR-IT (F = 5.0 and 4.6 respectively, dF = 2, P≤ 0.05) (Figs. 2F, G). Importantly, the immunoreactivity of the indicator of lipid oxidation HNE, was significantly reduced relative to control, when animals were treated with either 670 nm or 830 nm R/NIR-IT (F = 15.0, dF = 2, P≤0.05) (Fig. 2H), indicating reduced oxidative stress. There was no significant difference in HNE immunoreactivity between the two wavelengths of R/NIR-IT at this time (F = 15.0, dF = 2, P>0.05) (Fig. 2H).

Effects of R/NIR-IT on light-induced retinal degeneration

Light damage induces cell death, indicated by large numbers of TUNEL positive (+) cells in rat retina from as early as 6 hours after injury, particularly in the photoreceptor layers, as described previously [60,61]. We detected no effect of pre-treatment with 830 nm R/NIR-IT on numbers of TUNEL+ cells relative to controls (F = 1.417, dF = 5, P>0.05) (Fig 3A). In contrast, we observed a significant decrease in the total number of TUNEL$^+$ photoreceptors in the outer nuclear layer of LD retinae pre-treated with 670 nm R/NIR-IT compared with controls, confirming previous findings (F = 1.678, dF = 5, P≤0.05) [62,63]. The lower numbers of TUNEL+ cells in retinas treated with 670 nm R/NIR-IT were significant in samples taken from both superior retina and inferior retina (F = 3.423, dF = 2, P≤0.05) (Fig. 3B). Immunoreactivity for 8OHDG, indicative of oxidised DNA and therefore oxidative stress, was significantly reduced in LD retinae treated with 670 nm R/NIR-IT (F = 1.632, dF = 4, P≤0.05), but not those treated with 830 nm R/NIR-IT (F = 3.267, dF = 4, P>0.05) (Fig. 3C). While there was a trend towards reduced GFAP immunoreactivity following treatment of light damaged retinae with 670 nm R/NIR-IT, this was not significant (F = 1.867 dF = 4, P>0.05) (Figs. 3C, D).

Effects of R/NIR-IT following TBI

The fluid percussion model was used to assess efficacy of 670 nm and 830 nm R/NIR-IT at improving motor and sensory outcomes as well as decreasing lesion volume following TBI. Motor ability of injured rats was assessed daily by quantifying the length of time rats could remain on a rotarod. As expected [64], there was a substantial decrease in rotarod score relative to pre-injury in control animals (significant for the first 3 days following injury, P≤0.05), which gradually improved during the 7 days following injury (Fig. 4A). R/NIR-IT at 670 nm or 830 nm did not affect motor outcomes during the 7 days following TBI, relative to control (F = 0.5, dF = 2, P>0.05) (Fig. 4A). Sensory ability was assessed using the bilateral asymmetry test as has been described [53], at 1, 3 and 7 days following injury, compared to pre-injury performance. However, somewhat unexpectedly, there was no significant difference in contralateral *vs* ipsilateral latency in control (sham treated) rats when comparing pre- and post-injury outcomes for the first 7 days after injury (F = 0.4, dF = 2, P>0.05) (Fig 4B). Sensory abilities in rats treated with R/NIR-IT at 670 nm or 830 nm were not different to control rats or pre-injury levels (F = 0.4, dF = 2, P>0.05) (Fig. 4B). Lesion volume at 7 days following TBI was also not altered by R/NIR-IT at either 670 nm or 830 nm (F = 0.1, dF = 2, P>0.05) (Fig. 4C).

Effects of R/NIR-IT following SCI

Analysis of functional recovery following moderate contusion SCI and R/NIR-IT was conducted, assessing open field locomotion (BBB), quantitative gait analysis (Ratwalk) and ladder walking. Rats were scored for their performance on the BBB test at 7, 14, 21 and 28 days following SCI [56]. All animals exhibited a steep recovery from day 0 to 7 and were able to weight support by day 14 (BBB score of 9). At day 21, the scores began to plateau and the average score across all groups was 10. At day 28 the average score for all groups was 11 - characterised by frequent to consistent weight-supported plantar steps and no forelimb - hindlimb coordination. There were no significant differences in BBB scores of rats treated with either wavelength of R/NIR-IT compared to control rats (Fig. 5A, F = 0.5, dF = 2, P>0.05). Although no significance was recorded, it is important to note that even though the applied Kruskal-Wallis test is an analysis of variance for non-parametric data, the BBB scale is neither linear nor exponential. Higher BBB values represent a score comprised of increasing numbers of variables that are often unrelated to previous (lower) scores. Careful interpretation should always be exercised when equating biological significance with statistical significance in such cases [65].

The gait of rats in the treatment groups was analysed using Ratwalk computer software at days 14, 21 and 28 following SCI and R/NIR-IT, and stride lengths were quantified. Data generated from animals pre-injury were used to illustrate 'normal' locomotor patterns (baseline) and as a reference point for comparison to R/NIR-IT treated rats following SCI. Data generated from left and right limbs of the fore-and hindquarters were compared and no significant differences were found (P> 0.05). Therefore, data generated from left and right forelimbs and left and right hindlimbs were averaged and referred to as forelimbs and hindlimbs respectively. The stride length of forelimbs following SCI was significantly reduced in all treatment groups and time-points following injury, compared to scores generated from pre-injury animals (Fig. 5B, 28 day data shown, F = 15.4, dF = 3, P≤0.05). This indicated that there was some compensatory change in forelimb movement following SCI, most likely as

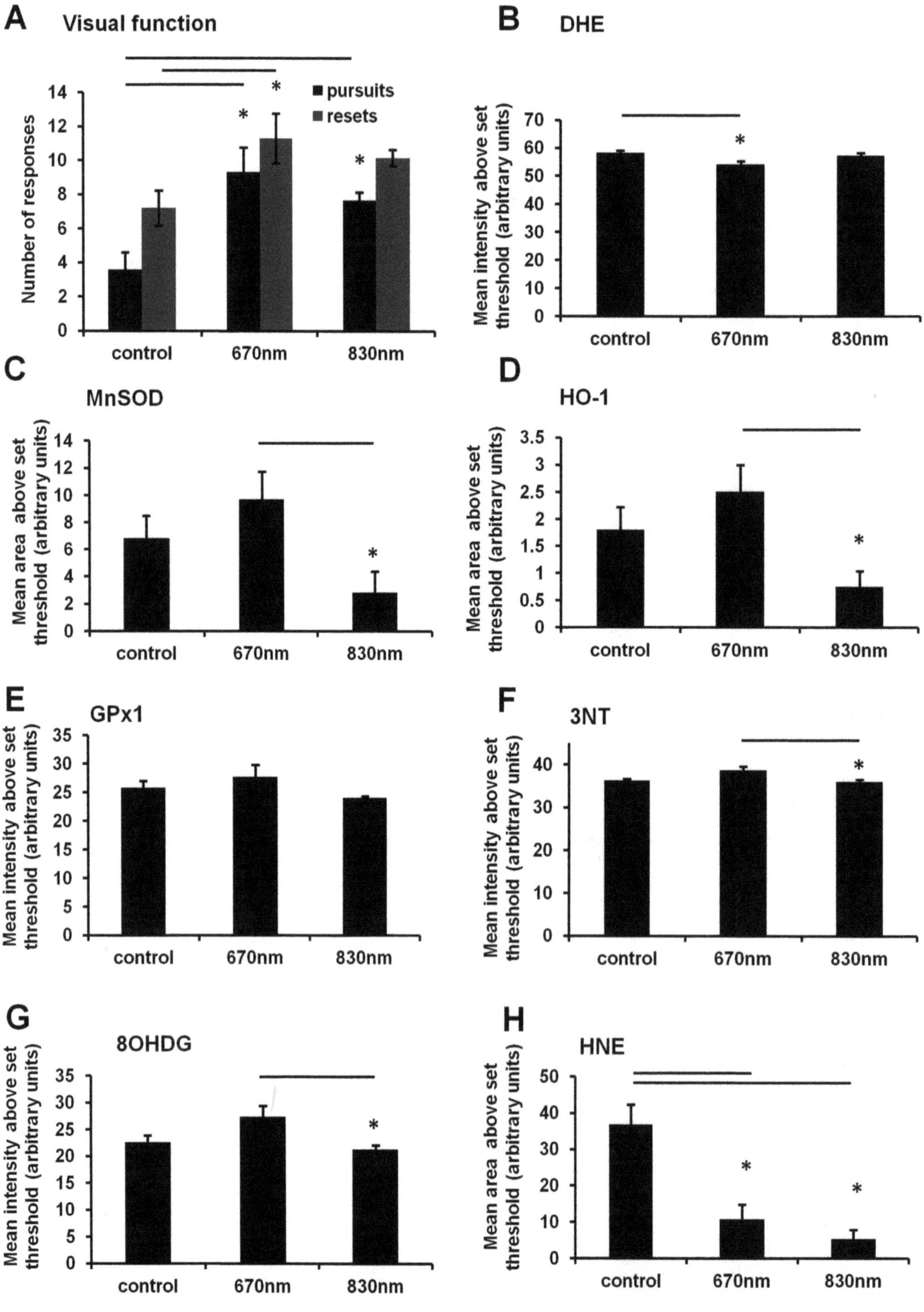
A
Visual function
Number of responses
14
12
10
8
6
4
2
0
pursuits
resets
control
670nm
830nm
B
DHE
Mean intensity above set threshold (arbitrary units)
70
60
50
40
30
20
10
0
control
670nm
830nm
C
MnSOD
Mean area above set threshold (arbitrary units)
14
12
10
8
6
4
2
0
control
670nm
830nm
D
HO-1
Mean area above set threshold (arbitrary units)
3.5
3
2.5
2
1.5
1
0.5
0
control
670nm
830nm
E
GPx1
Mean intensity above set threshold (arbitrary units)
35
30
25
20
15
10
5
0
control
670nm
830nm
F
3NT
Mean intensity above set threshold (arbitrary units)
40
30
20
10
0
control
670nm
830nm
G
8OHDG
Mean intensity above set threshold (arbitrary units)
35
30
25
20
15
10
5
0
control
670nm
830nm
H
HNE
Mean area above set threshold (arbitrary units)
50
40
30
20
10
0
control
670nm
830nm

Figure 2. Visual behaviour, reactive species, antioxidant enzymes and indicators of oxidative damage 7 days following partial optic nerve transection and treatment with 670 nm or 830 nm R/NIR-IT compared to sham treated control. Number of responses in the optokinetic nystagmus visual reflex task (A) were quantified as smooth pursuits (black) or fast resets (grey), n = 12/group. Mean ± SEM DHE fluorescence (B), MnSOD (C), HO-1 (D), GPx1 (E), 3NT (F), 8OHDG (G) or HNE (H) immunoreactivity in ventral ON vulnerable to secondary degeneration were semi-quantified: *indicates significant differences (P≤0.05), n = 6/group.

hindlimb function is impaired. The animals use their forelimbs to propel their body forward, a movement which would not otherwise be possible if the stride length of the forelimb remained at its original pre-injury distance. However, there were no significant differences in forelimb stride length of rats treated with either wavelength of R/NIR-IT compared to control sham-treated rats (Fig. 5B, F = 15.4, dF = 3, P>0.05). The stride length of the hindlimbs did not change with SCI (Fig. 5B, F = 1.6, dF = 3, P> 0.05).

There were significantly more hindlimb missteps following SCI at each time point assessed, for both R/NIR-IT treated and control groups (F = 3.4, dF = 6, Fig. 5C, P≤0.05), compared to pre-injury performance. The total number of missteps at 21 and 28 days after injury, for the control and 670 nm R/NIR-IT

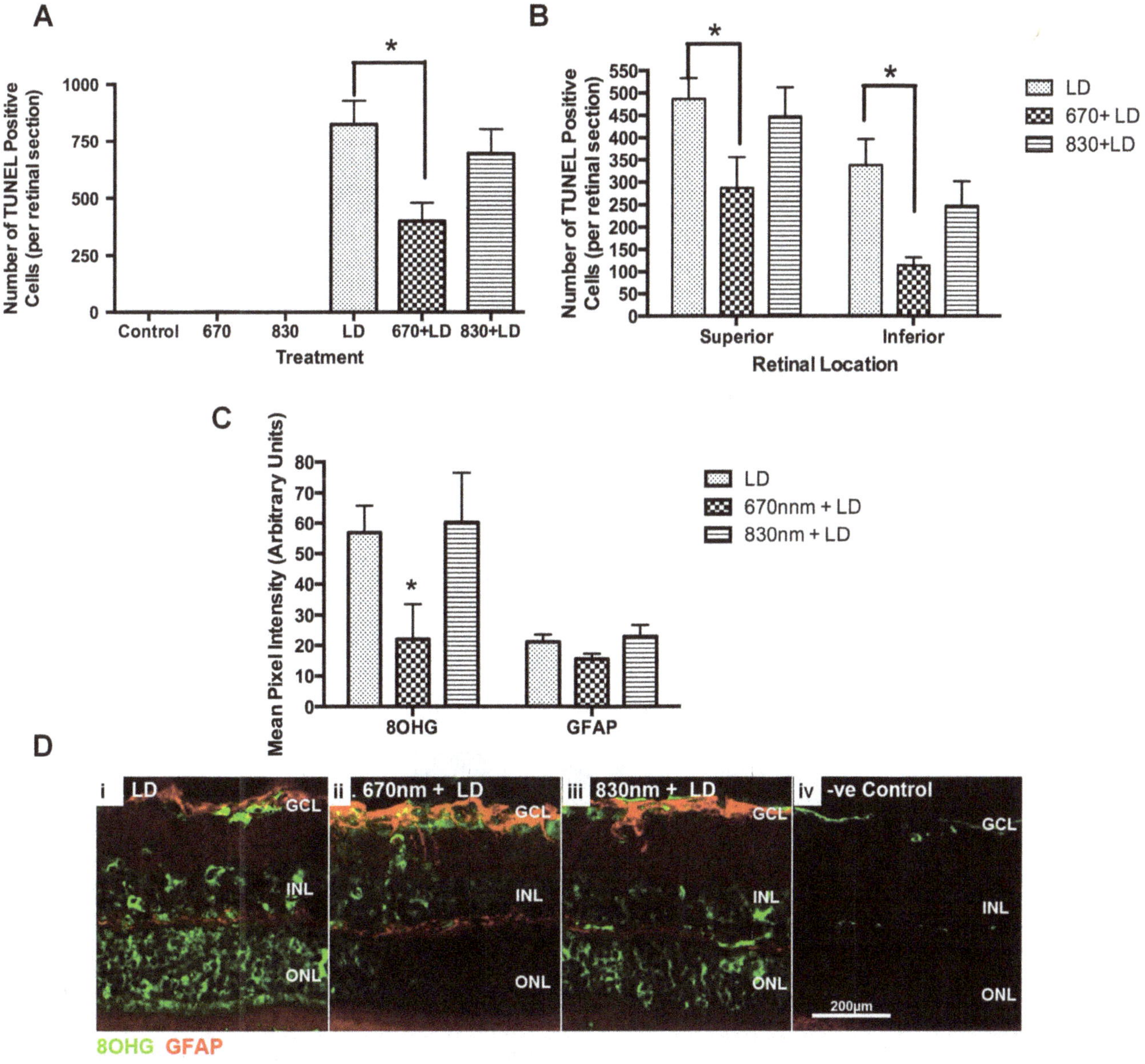

Figure 3. Number of Tunel+ cells, 8OHDG and GFAP immunoreactivity following pre-treatment with 670 nm or 830 nm R/NIR-IT or sham treatment and light induced retinal degeneration, compared to uninjured animals. Mean ± SEM total number of Tunel+ cells/ retinal section (A) and number of Tunel+ cells in superior and inferior retina (B) were quantified. Mean ± SEM 8OHDG and GFAP immunoreactivities in retinal sections were semi-quantified (C): *indicates significantly different from injured control (P≤0.05), n = 6/group. Representative images of 8OHDG (green) and GFAP (red) immunofluorescence from control and R/NIR-IT treated animals are shown (D) (scale = 200 μm).

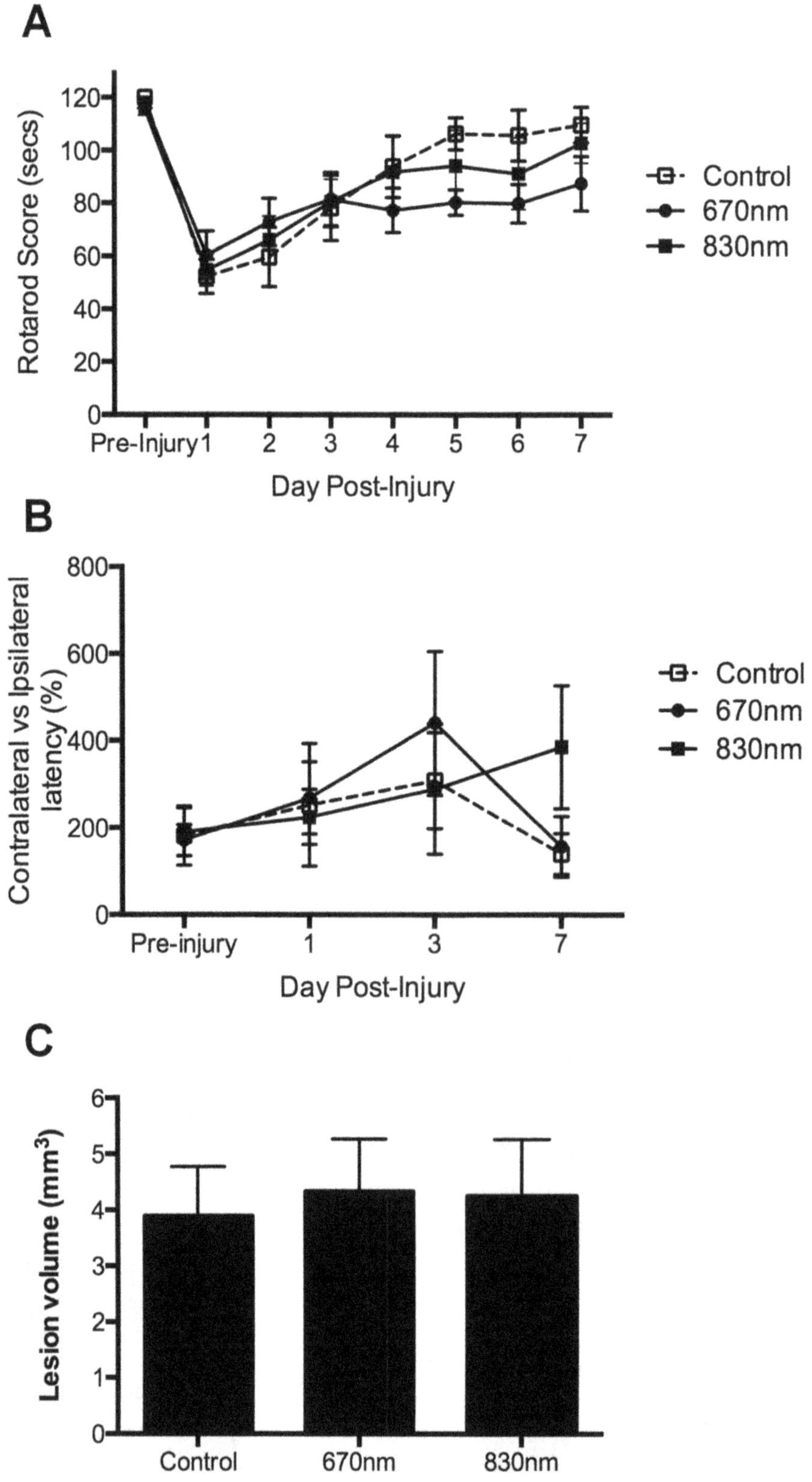

Figure 4. Motor and sensory function as well as lesion size following fluid percussion TBI and treatment with 670 nm or 830 nm R/NIR-IT compared to sham treated control. Mean ± SEM length of time animals remained on a rotarod (A), and contralateral vs ipsilateral latency (B) were quantified as measures of motor and sensory function respectively over the 7 days following TBI. Lesion volumes were also quantified at 7 days following injury (C): there were no significant differences relative to control at each time point ($P>0.05$), $n = 5$ or 6/group.

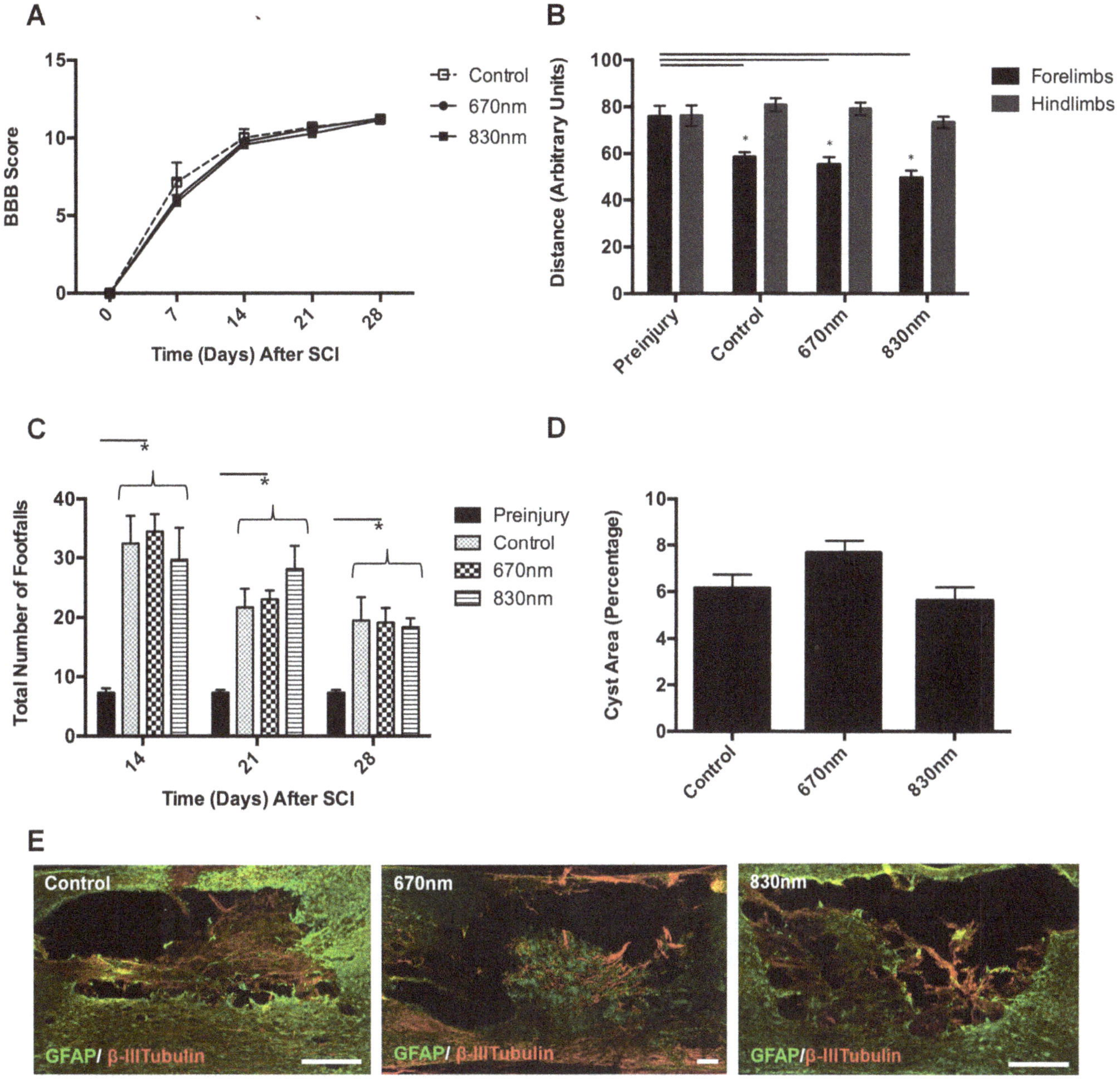

Figure 5. Analysis of functional recovery and lesion size following SCI and treatment with 670 nm or 830 nm R/NIR-IT compared to sham treated control. Functional recovery was quantified for 28 days using BBB scores (A), Ratwalk gait analysis (B) and ladder walking (C) (n = 7 or 8/group). Semi-quantification of lesion size from toluidine blue stained sections (D), and representative images of GFAP and β-III tubulin immunoreactivity (E) are shown at 28 days following SCI (n = 4/group), scale = 400 μm. Data are mean ± SEM, * indicates significant differences from pre-injury (P≤0.05).

groups, was significantly lower than the number of missteps at 14 days (F = 3.4, dF = 6, Fig. 5C, P≤0.05), whereas treatment with 830 nm R/NIR-IT only resulted in significant decreases in the total number of missteps at 28 days, compared to 14 days (F = 3.4, dF = 6, Fig. 5C, P≤0.05). However, there were no significant differences between R/NIR-IT treatment and control groups at any of the time points assessed (F = 3.4, dF = 6, P>0.05).

Cyst size and morphological parameters, including the amount of degenerative tissue immediately surrounding the cyst, were assessed in toluidine blue stained sections and using immunohistochemical assessments of GFAP, β-III tubulin, DcX and GAP43 immunoreactivity at 28 days following SCI. The borders of larger cysts stained with toluidine blue were well defined, whereas smaller cysts were present within spared tissues to varying degrees in all R/NIR-IT treatment and control groups. Semi-quantitative analysis of cyst size revealed no significant differences between 670 nm or 830 nm R/NIR-IT and control groups (Fig. 5D, F = 3.9, dF = 2, P>0.05). In all groups GFAP immunoreactivity was present around the lesion site and occasionally appeared within "spared" bridges of tissue within the lesion site, whilst β-III tubulin was present both in and around the lesions site (Fig. 5E). In some sections β-III tubulin positive fibres were seen to traverse across the lesion site within spared tissue, but this did not appear to be specific for any particular group, and was therefore not quantitated. Small numbers of DcX and GAP43 positive fibres penetrated into tissue located within the cyst region, although these tended to be located immediately at the periphery of the cyst walls, and the number of fibres did not appear to differ between groups (data not shown). Infiltrating macrophage numbers (ED1+) remained high within and around the lesion area and projected several mm beyond the lesion epicentre, with no effect of R/NIR-IT observed (data not shown).

Discussion

R/NIR-IT has the potential to be a clinically relevant, cost-effective and easy-to-administer treatment to reduce oxidative stress and preserve function following traumatic injury. However, R/NIR-IT has not been widely adopted in clinical practice for CNS injury, in part due to the large range of treatment fluences, irradiation time, wavelengths and devices cited in the literature making comparisons between studies difficult. As such, a consensus paradigm for treatment has not yet been established[48]. Here we report the outcomes of a multi-centre comparative study which shows that delivery of a defined number of photons at the surface of the skin overlying a CNS injury has differential effects on function and neuroprotection (as indicated by Tunel staining), depending upon the wavelength used to deliver the R/NIR-IT and the injury type.

Our study design allows the first direct comparison of efficacy of 670 nm and 830 nm R/NIR-IT, delivered by LED array, in four models of CNS injury. We demonstrate that the most effective wavelength for treatment depends upon the type of injury. Specifically, 830 nm R/NIR-IT is beneficial following partial optic nerve transection but not following light-induced retinal degeneration. Given the greater penetrance of R/NIR-IT to the retina than to the optic nerve, and our demonstration of efficacy of 670 nm R/NIR-IT for treatment of retinal degeneration, our data indicate that the nature of the tissue being treated dictates the potential efficacy of different wavelengths of irradiation. Further, our study design allows us to demonstrate that wavelengths and dosages of R/NIR-IT that are effective in one model of CNS injury (e.g. partial optic nerve transection) are not necessarily effective in another. The demonstrated penetrance of R/NIR-IT to the site of SCI in the current study was greater than that to the optic nerve injury site, yet there was no positive effects on function following SCI [22]. We conclude therefore that delivery of equivalent or greater dosages of R/NIR-IT does not guarantee beneficial effects across different CNS injury models.

670 nm R/NIR-IT delivered by LED was generally more effective at improving function or protecting neurons than 830 nm R/NIR-IT, but this only applied in models involving the visual system. The greater efficacy of 670 nm R/NIR-IT was apparent despite a greater percentage of delivered photons of 830 nm than 670 nm R/NIR-IT penetrating through skin and muscle, leading to a likely greater dose of 830 nm R/NIR-IT at the injury site. Neither 670 nm nor 830 nm R/NIR-IT delivered by LED array were effective at improving outcomes following TBI or SCI at the dosages and time points assessed. Our data could be interpreted to indicate that R/NIR-IT delivered by LED array is more effective in the visual system than in other CNS injuries, but it is important to note that the beneficial effects observed in the retinal degeneration model may have been enhanced due to the pre-treatment paradigm employed. Nevertheless, our study indicates that effective R/NIR-IT treatment parameters including wavelength and dosage do not necessarily apply in different CNS injuries. Efficacy does not appear to be directly proportional to the numbers of photons reaching the injury site, but may instead be a function of the number of photons absorbed by the photoacceptor responsible for any beneficial effects. For example, the absorbance of cytochrome *c* oxidase is much greater at 670 nm than 830 nm [66], which may explain why the 670 nm light was more effective, despite the injury site receiving a lower fluence at this wavelength compared to 830 nm. Furthermore, analysis of the absorption spectra of cytochrome *c* oxidase within cell monolayers indicates that the enzyme is oxidised by irradiation at 670 nm, whereas it is reduced at 830 nm [26], perhaps also contributing to differential efficacies.

To date, few studies have compared R/NIR-IT in CNS at two or more wavelengths. Wong-Riley et al., 2005 assessed ATP production by visual cortex neurons treated with 670, 728, 770, 830 or 880 nm R/NIR-IT (*via* LED) emitting 4 J cm^{-2} over 80 sec *in vitro*, demonstrating a positive correlation with the known absorption spectra of cytochrome *c* oxidase, the postulated photoacceptor for R/NIR-IT [29]. Comparison of efficacy of 665, 730, 810 or 980 nm R/NIR-IT delivered by laser emitting 36 J cm^{-2} over 4 min *in vivo* following acute contusion TBI resulted in significant improvements in Neurological Severity Scores in animals treated with 665 nm and 810 nm R/NIR-IT [45]. Although these studies did not appear to standardise the dosages for the numbers of photons delivered at different wavelengths, our choices of wavelengths to assess in the current study were based on those comparative assessments.

The penetrance of irradiation at a given wavelength is determined by the optical properties of the tissue being treated. Irradiation between 600 and 1000 nm has better penetration because of reduced absorption at these wavelengths [48]. We demonstrate here that while the 830 nm R/NIR-IT array delivered an equal quantal dose to the surface of the skin (5.33×10^{16} photons cm^{-2} s^{-1}), the number of photons received at the SCI injury site was greater due to the increased penetrance of the longer wavelength R/NIR-IT through tissue (6.0×10^{15} photons cm^{-2} s^{-1} for the 830 nm device compared to 3.5×10^{15} photons cm^{-2} s^{-1} for the 670 nm device). To our knowledge, two published studies have quantified the penetrance of R/NIR irradiation in animal specimens. Byrnes et al., 2005 used power transmission and spectrophotometric analyses to show that 6% (9 mW) of the radiant power of an 810 nm laser irradiation with a nominal power output of 150 mW, was transferred from the dorsal surface of the skin to the ventral side of the spinal cord [16]. We have also previously shown that irradiation directed at the dorsal surface of the head of the rat (R/NIR irradiance 252 W m^{-2} 550–750 nm, WARP10, Quantum Devices), resulted in 0.1% (0.3 W m^{-2}) reaching the ventral surface of the braincase and 0.7% (1.75 W m^{-2} or 0.32 J cm^{-2}) reaching the ventral surface of the optic nerve[22]. These light levels achieved therapeutic benefits and were significantly lower than the doses used in the superficial wound healing studies (8 J cm^{-2}) [67] implying that relatively low doses of light can have therapeutic benefits.

Nevertheless, delivery of doses of 28.4 J cm^{-2} of 670 nm R/NIR-IT or 22.6 J cm^{-2} of 830 nm R/NIR-IT (equal quantal doses) in the current study, equating to 1.9 J cm^{-2} and 2.6 J cm^{-2} respectively at the SCI injury site, did not result in improvements following SCI. The doses we administered fall within the lower end of the range of doses of R/NIR-IT delivered by laser and shown to have beneficial effects in SCI (9.6–250 J cm^{-2} [68,69] emitted from the treatment devices). Importantly however, previous studies demonstrating functional improvements with R/NIR-IT following SCI utilised a substantially higher dosage of 1589 J cm^{-2} day^{-1} [16,21]. It remains a possibility that beneficial effects of R/NIR-IT delivered by laser for SCI are dependent on the coherence, narrow beam profile or some other physical aspect of laser light. However, a comprehensive assessment of the effects of an increased dosage of R/NIR-IT delivered using LED arrays would be necessary before such a conclusion could be drawn. Alternatively, the time points at which efficacy of R/NIR-IT for SCI were assessed may have been too early after injury to reveal improvements, although efficacy has been demonstrated at 21 days in other SCI studies [21,69], indicating that we conducted our assessments within an appropriate time-scale. Further, it is possible that the handling of animals required for the 30 minute treatments using the LED arrays, increased stress levels such that improvements following SCI and/or TBI were masked. However, given that efficacy was demonstrated in visual system models where animals were handled similarly, we consider this to be unlikely. It is perhaps more likely that the degree of inflammatory involvement, vascular changes, cyst formation, oedema and myelination [70–72] are likely to alter penetrance of the R/NIR-IT [48,73] and may explain the lack of efficacy following SCI at the current comparatively low dosage. The moderate contusion SCI may be too severe an injury to enable detection of modest improvements at the doses of R/NIR-IT employed in the current study. Other spinal cord injury types such as hemisection, or injuries targeting limited demyelination of specific tracts (e.g. corticospinal), may prove more effective at revealing modest improvements.

The doses of R/NIR-IT delivered by LED in the current study also did not result in significant improvements in the tested model of TBI. Previous assessments of efficacy of R/NIR-IT for TBI in rodents have predominantly used lasers and have delivered doses ranging from 1.2–268 J cm^{-2} [74]. Improved neurobehavioural function and reduced lesion size have been reported at four weeks after acute, relatively severe cortical impactor injuries [45,75,76]. However, approximately equivalent dosages of R/NIR-IT, also delivered by laser, were not effective at improving motor function or lesion volume following a less severe cortical piston TBI, assessed at 1 week after injury [77]. Similarly, the lack of positive effect may be due to the relatively mild nature of the focal TBI delivered in the current study, resulting in lack of a sufficient window of opportunity in which to detect improvements. Spontaneous return of function was observed by seven days after injury in our model, rendering longer term assessments irrelevant in this model. However, beneficial effects on function in TBI may require a longer time scale to become apparent. Importantly, our demonstration of lack of efficacy highlights the need to optimise R/NIR-IT with regard to injury severity.

Our demonstration of greater efficacy of 670 nm than 830 nm R/NIR-IT in models of injury to the visual system was unexpected, given that more photons are likely to have been delivered to the injury site with the 830 nm irradiation (given calculations for the SCI injury site). It is possible that there is a biphasic effect, with higher numbers of photons less effective than lower numbers [41,78], such that dosage needs to be carefully titrated for each CNS injury model to ensure the most effective treatment protocol. Importantly however, the cellular targets in the various CNS injury models are different. 670 nm R/NIR-IT pre-treatment protected photoreceptors and reduced oxidative damage to DNA in the retinal degeneration model; 830 nm R/NIR-IT pre-treatment had no effect, with the caveat of a lower dosage of irradiation (shorter time of exposure) delivered in this model. It is possible that 670 nm R/NIR-IT readily penetrates to the retina and so the dosage received is greater and thus, more effective, than the 830 nm R/NIR-IT. In contrast, in the optic nerve damage model, both 670 and 830 nm R/NIR-IT reduced HNE immunoreactivity, indicative of lipid oxidation, in lipid rich ventral optic nerve white matter vulnerable to secondary degeneration. Furthermore, both wavelengths resulted in improved visual function in this model. The types of cells that are damaged or vulnerable in the different CNS injuries may be critical in determining the number of photons required to modulate disrupted cellular functions such as oxidative metabolism, given differential sensitivities to oxidative stress of different cell types [79,80]. Whether it is the neuronal somata or the lipid-rich myelinated axons as opposed to unmyelinated axons that are vulnerable may also influence efficacy of R/NIR-IT.

The outcomes of the study indicate that comprehensive optimisation of the dosages, wavelengths and delivery mechanisms (laser vs LED) of R/NIR-IT appear to be required in each model of CNS injury, to provide an indication of effective treatment protocols. These must then be confirmed and refined in human clinical trials that draw upon these rationally designed pre-clinical studies. Only then will we know whether R/NIR-IT can provide an effective, cheap and convenient first-line treatment strategy for CNS injury.

Acknowledgments

We thank Dr Krisztina Valter Kocsi for helpful advice regarding assays and treatment conditions in the retinal light damage model.

Author Contributions

Conceived and designed the experiments: MF SAD JP RV ARH SH NSH CVDH RN. Performed the experiments: MG NSH RN CVDH SH CAB LW ED SL BM ET EHW AL. Analyzed the data: MG NSH RN SH CVDH MF ET EHW AL. Contributed reagents/materials/analysis tools: MF NSH RN CVDH RV JP SAD AH SH. Contributed to the writing of the manuscript: MG ET EHW AL RV AH JP SAD NSH RN SH CVDH MF.

References

1. Park E, Velumian AA, Fehlings MG (2004) The Role of Excitotoxicity in Secondary Mechanisms of Spinal Cord Injury: A Review with an Emphasis on the Implications for White Matter Degeneration. Journal of Neurotrauma 21: 754–774.
2. Tator CH, Fehlings MG (1991) Review of the secondary injury theory of acute spinal cord trauma with emphasis on vascular mechanisms. Journal of Neurosurgery 75: 15–26.
3. Lu J, Ashwell KWS, Waite P (2000) Advances in Secondary Spinal Cord Injury: Role of Apoptosis. Spine 25: 1859–1866.
4. Fitzgerald M, Bartlett CA, Harvey AR, Dunlop SA (2010) Early events of secondary degeneration after partial optic nerve transection: an immunohistochemical study. Journal of Neurotrauma 27: 439–452.
5. Wells J, Kilburn MR, Shaw JA, Bartlett CA, Harvey AR, et al. (2012) Early in vivo changes in calcium ions, oxidative stress markers, and ion channel immunoreactivity following partial injury to the optic nerve. Journal of Neuroscience Research 90: 606–618.
6. Carrico KM, Vaishnav R, Hall ED (2009) Temporal and spatial dynamics of peroxynitrite-induced oxidative damage after spinal cord contusion injury. J Neurotrauma 26: 1369–1378.
7. Cummins N, Bartlett CA, Archer M, Bartlett E, Hemmi JM, et al. (2013) Changes to mitochondrial ultrastructure in optic nerve vulnerable to secondary degeneration in vivo are limited by irradiation at 670 nm. BMC Neurosci 14: 98.
8. Szymanski CR, Chiha W, Morellini N, Cummins N, Bartlett CA, et al. (2013) Paranode Abnormalities and Oxidative Stress in Optic Nerve Vulnerable to Secondary Degeneration: Modulation by 670 nm Light Treatment. PLoS One 8: e66448.
9. Hall ED, Vaishnav RA, Mustafa AG (2010) Antioxidant therapies for traumatic brain injury. Neurotherapeutics 7: 51–61.
10. Oron U, Yaakobi T, Oron A, Hayam G, Gepstein L, et al. (2001) Attenuation of infarct size in rats and dogs after myocardial infarction by low-energy laser irradiation. Lasers Surg Med 28: 204–211.

11. Lim J, Ali ZM, Sanders RA, Snyder AC, Eells JT, et al. (2009) Effects of low-level light therapy on hepatic antioxidant defense in acute and chronic diabetic rats. J Biochem Mol Toxicol 23: 1–8.
12. Lim J, Sanders RA, Snyder AC, Eells JT, Henshel DS, et al. (2010) Effects of low-level light therapy on streptozotocin-induced diabetic kidney. J Photochem Photobiol B 99: 105–110.
13. Eells JT, Wong-Riley MT, VerHoeve J, Henry M, Buchman EV, et al. (2004) Mitochondrial signal transduction in accelerated wound and retinal healing by near-infrared light therapy. Mitochondrion 4: 559–567.
14. Natoli R, Zhu Y, Valter K, Bisti S, Eells J, et al. (2010) Gene and noncoding RNA regulation underlying photoreceptor protection: microarray study of dietary antioxidant saffron and photobiomodulation in rat retina. Mol Vis 16: 1801–1822.
15. Albarracin RS, Valter K (2012) Treatment with 670-nm light protects the cone photoreceptors from white light-induced degeneration. Adv Exp Med Biol 723: 121–128.
16. Byrnes KR, Waynant RW, Ilev IK, Wu X, Barna L, et al. (2005) Light promotes regeneration and functional recovery and alters the immune response after spinal cord injury. Lasers Surg Med 36: 171–185.
17. Lapchak PA (2012) Transcranial near-infrared laser therapy applied to promote clinical recovery in acute and chronic neurodegenerative diseases. Expert Rev Med Devices 9: 71–83.
18. Detaboada L, Ilic S, Leichliter-Martha S, Oron U, Oron A, et al. (2006) Transcranial application of low-energy laser irradiation improves neurological deficits in rats following acute stroke. Lasers Surg Med 38: 70–73.
19. Oron A, Oron U, Chen J, Eilam A, Zhang C, et al. (2006) Low-level laser therapy applied transcranially to rats after induction of stroke significantly reduces long-term neurological deficits. Stroke 37: 2620–2624.
20. Moreira MS, Velasco IT, Ferreira LS, Ariga SK, Barbeiro DF, et al. (2009) Effect of phototherapy with low intensity laser on local and systemic immunomodulation following focal brain damage in rat. J Photochem Photobiol B 97: 145–151.
21. Wu X, Dmitriev AE, Cardoso MJ, Viers-Costello AG, Borke RC, et al. (2009) 810 nm Wavelength light: an effective therapy for transected or contused rat spinal cord. Lasers Surg Med 41: 36–41.
22. Fitzgerald M, Bartlett CA, Payne SC, Hart NS, Rodger J, et al. (2010) Near infrared light reduces oxidative stress and preserves function in CNS tissue vulnerable to secondary degeneration following partial transection of the optic nerve. J Neurotrauma 27: 2107–2119.
23. Lampl Y, Zivin JA, Fisher M, Lew R, Welin L, et al. (2007) Infrared laser therapy for ischemic stroke: a new treatment strategy: results of the NeuroThera Effectiveness and Safety Trial-1 (NEST-1). Stroke 38: 1843–1849.
24. Zivin JA, Albers GW, Bornstein N, Chippendale T, Dahlof B, et al. (2009) Effectiveness and safety of transcranial laser therapy for acute ischemic stroke. Stroke 40: 1359–1364.
25. Hacke W, Schelinger, PD, Albers, GW, Bornstein, NM, Dahlof, BS, Kasner, S, Howard, G, Shuaib, A, Richieri, SP, Dilly, SG, Zivin, J Transcranial laser therapy (TLT) for acute ischemic stroke. Results of NEST3, a pivotal phase III randomized clinical trial (RCT); 2013; London, UK.
26. Karu TI, Pyatibrat LV, Kolyakov SF, Afanasyeva NI (2005) Absorption measurements of a cell monolayer relevant to phototherapy: reduction of cytochrome c oxidase under near IR radiation. J Photochem Photobiol B 81: 98–106.
27. Karu TI, Pyatibrat LV, Kolyakov SF, Afanasyeva NI (2008) Absorption measurements of cell monolayers relevant to mechanisms of laser phototherapy: reduction or oxidation of cytochrome c oxidase under laser radiation at 632.8 nm. Photomed Laser Surg 26: 593–599.
28. Lapchak PA, De Taboada L (2010) Transcranial near infrared laser treatment (NILT) increases cortical adenosine-5'-triphosphate (ATP) content following embolic strokes in rabbits. Brain Res 1306: 100–105.
29. Wong-Riley MT, Liang HL, Eells JT, Chance B, Henry MM, et al. (2005) Photobiomodulation directly benefits primary neurons functionally inactivated by toxins: role of cytochrome c oxidase. J Biol Chem 280: 4761–4771.
30. Gkotsi D, Begum R, Salt T, Lascaratos G, Hogg C, et al. (2014) Recharging mitochondrial batteries in old eyes. Near infra-red increases ATP. Exp Eye Res 122C: 50–53.
31. Kowaltowski AJ, de Souza-Pinto NC, Castilho RF, Vercesi AE (2009) Mitochondria and reactive oxygen species. Free Radic Biol Med 47: 333–343.
32. Sutherland JC (2002) Biological effects of polychromatic light. Photochem Photobiol 76: 164–170.
33. Karu T (1989) Photobiology of Low-Power Laser Effects. Health Physics 56: 691–704.
34. Peoples C, Shaw VE, Stone J, Jeffery G, Baker GE, et al. (2012) Survival of Dopaminergic Amacrine Cells after Near-Infrared Light Treatment in MPTP-Treated Mice. ISRN Neurol 2012: 850150.
35. Mason MG, Nicholls P, Wilson MT, Cooper CE (2006) Nitric oxide inhibition of respiration involves both competitive (heme) and noncompetitive (copper) binding to cytochrome c oxidase. Proc Natl Acad Sci U S A 103: 708–713.
36. Ball KA, Castello PR, Poyton RO (2011) Low intensity light stimulates nitrite-dependent nitric oxide synthesis but not oxygen consumption by cytochrome c oxidase: Implications for phototherapy. J Photochem Photobiol B 102: 182–191.
37. Liang HL, Whelan HT, Eells JT, Wong-Riley MT (2008) Near-infrared light via light-emitting diode treatment is therapeutic against rotenone- and 1-methyl-4-phenylpyridinium ion-induced neurotoxicity. Neuroscience 153: 963–974.
38. Albarracin R, Valter K (2012) 670 nm Red Light Preconditioning Supports Muller Cell Function: Evidence from the White Light-induced Damage Model in the Rat Retina(dagger). Photochem Photobiol.
39. Kokkinopoulos I, Colman A, Hogg C, Heckenlively J, Jeffery G (2013) Age-related retinal inflammation is reduced by 670 nm light via increased mitochondrial membrane potential. Neurobiol Aging 34: 602–609.
40. Rutar M, Natoli R, Albarracin R, Valter K, Provis J (2012) 670-nm light treatment reduces complement propagation following retinal degeneration. J Neuroinflammation 9: 257.
41. Chung H, Dai T, Sharma SK, Huang YY, Carroll JD, et al. (2012) The nuts and bolts of low-level laser (light) therapy. Ann Biomed Eng 40: 516–533.
42. Eells JT, Henry MM, Summerfelt P, Wong-Riley MT, Buchmann EV, et al. (2003) Therapeutic photobiomodulation for methanol-induced retinal toxicity. Proc Natl Acad Sci U S A 100: 3439–3444.
43. Rojas JC, Lee J, John JM, Gonzalez-Lima F (2008) Neuroprotective effects of near-infrared light in an in vivo model of mitochondrial optic neuropathy. J Neurosci 28: 13511–13521.
44. Naeser MA, Saltmarche A, Krengel MH, Hamblin MR, Knight JA (2011) Improved cognitive function after transcranial, light-emitting diode treatments in chronic, traumatic brain injury: two case reports. Photomed Laser Surg 29: 351–358.
45. Wu Q, Xuan W, Ando T, Xu T, Huang L, et al. (2012) Low-level laser therapy for closed-head traumatic brain injury in mice: effect of different wavelengths. Lasers Surg Med 44: 218–226.
46. Demidova-Rice TN, Salomatina EV, Yaroslavsky AN, Herman IM, Hamblin MR (2007) Low-level light stimulates excisional wound healing in mice. Lasers Surg Med 39: 706–715.
47. Gupta A, Dai T, Hamblin MR (2014) Effect of red and near-infrared wavelengths on low-level laser (light) therapy-induced healing of partial-thickness dermal abrasion in mice. Lasers Med Sci 29: 257–265.
48. Fitzgerald M, Hodgetts S, Van Den Heuvel C, Natoli R, Hart NS, et al. (2013) Red/near-infrared irradiation therapy for treatment of central nervous system injuries and disorders. Rev Neurosci 24: 205–226.
49. Maslim J, Valter K, Egensperger R, Hollander H, Stone J (1997) Tissue oxygen during a critical developmental period controls the death and survival of photoreceptors. Invest Ophthalmol Vis Sci 38: 1667–1677.
50. McIntosh TK, Vink R, Noble L, Yamakami I, Fernyak S, et al. (1989) Traumatic brain injury in the rat: characterization of a lateral fluid-percussion model. Neuroscience 28: 233–244.
51. Thompson HJ, Lifshitz J, Marklund N, Grady MS, Graham DI, et al. (2005) Lateral fluid percussion brain injury: a 15-year review and evaluation. J Neurotrauma 22: 42–75.
52. Hamm RJ, Pike BR, O'Dell DM, Lyeth BG, Jenkins LW (1994) The rotarod test: an evaluation of its effectiveness in assessing motor deficits following traumatic brain injury. J Neurotrauma 11: 187–196.
53. Modo M, Stroemer RP, Tang E, Veizovic T, Sowniski P, et al. (2000) Neurological sequelae and long-term behavioural assessment of rats with transient middle cerebral artery occlusion. J Neurosci Methods 104: 99–109.
54. Corrigan F, Vink R, Blumbergs PC, Masters CL, Cappai R, et al. (2012) Evaluation of the effects of treatment with sAPPalpha on functional and histological outcome following controlled cortical impact injury in mice. Neurosci Lett 515: 50–54.
55. Hodgetts SI, Simmons PJ, Plant GW (2013) Recombinant Decorin Does Not Improve Behavioral or Anatomical Outcomes by Itself or in Combination with Human Mesenchymal Precursor Cell Transplantation following Acute and Chronic Contusive Spinal Cord Injury. Exp Neurol 248: 343–359.
56. Basso DM, Beattie MS, Bresnahan JC (1995) A sensitive and reliable locomotor rating scale for open field testing in rats. J Neurotrauma 12: 1–21.
57. Godinho MJ, Teh L, Pollett MA, Goodman D, Hodgetts SI, et al. (2013) Immunohistochemical, ultrastructural and functional analysis of axonal regeneration through peripheral nerve grafts containing Schwann cells expressing BDNF, CNTF or NT3. PLoS One 8: e69987.
58. Metz GA, Whishaw IQ (2009) The ladder rung walking task: a scoring system and its practical application. J Vis Exp.
59. Fitzgerald M, Bartlett CA, Evill L, Rodger J, Harvey AR, et al. (2009) Secondary degeneration of the optic nerve following partial transection: the benefits of lomerizine. Exp Neurol 216: 219–230.
60. Abler AS, Chang CJ, Ful J, Tso MO, Lam TT (1996) Photic injury triggers apoptosis of photoreceptor cells. Res Commun Mol Pathol Pharmacol 92: 177–189.
61. Aonuma H, Yamazaki R, Watanabe I (1999) Retinal cell death by light damage. Jpn J Ophthalmol 43: 171–179.
62. Albarracin R, Eells J, Valter K (2011) Photobiomodulation protects the retina from light-induced photoreceptor degeneration. Invest Ophthalmol Vis Sci 52: 3582–3592.
63. Qu C, Cao W, Fan Y, Lin Y (2010) Near-infrared light protect the photoreceptor from light-induced damage in rats. Adv Exp Med Biol 664: 365–374.
64. Thornton E, Vink R, Blumbergs PC, Van Den Heuvel C (2006) Soluble amyloid precursor protein alpha reduces neuronal injury and improves functional outcome following diffuse traumatic brain injury in rats. Brain Res 1094: 38–46.
65. Hodgetts SI, Simmons PJ, Plant GW (2013) Human mesenchymal precursor cells (Stro-1(+)) from spinal cord injury patients improve functional recovery and

tissue sparing in an acute spinal cord injury rat model. Cell Transplant 22: 393–412.

66. Moody DJ (2005) Specific extinction spectrum of oxidised cytochrome c oxidase (520 nm - 999 nm) h Biomedical Optics Research Laboratory UCL Department of Medical Physics and Bioengineering.
67. Whelan HT, Smits RL, Jr., Buchman EV, Whelan NT, Turner SG, et al. (2001) Effect of NASA light-emitting diode irradiation on wound healing. J Clin Laser Med Surg 19: 305–314.
68. Medalha CC, Amorim BO, Ferreira JM, Oliveira P, Pereira RM, et al. (2010) Comparison of the effects of electrical field stimulation and low-level laser therapy on bone loss in spinal cord-injured rats. Photomed Laser Surg 28: 669–674.
69. Ando T, Sato S, Kobayashi H, Nawashiro H, Ashida H, et al. (2013) Low-level laser therapy for spinal cord injury in rats: effects of polarization. J Biomed Opt 18: 098002.
70. Sykova E, Vargova L (2008) Extrasynaptic transmission and the diffusion parameters of the extracellular space. Neurochem Int 52: 5–13.
71. Iwamura A, Taoka T, Fukusumi A, Sakamoto M, Miyasaka T, et al. (2012) Diffuse vascular injury: convergent-type hemorrhage in the supratentorial white matter on susceptibility-weighted image in cases of severe traumatic brain damage. Neuroradiology 54: 335–343.
72. Lenz P (1999) Fluorescence measurement in thick tissue layers by linear or nonlinear long-wavelength excitation. Appl Opt 38: 3662–3669.
73. Hebeda KM, Menovsky T, Beek JF, Wolbers JG, van Gemert MJ (1994) Light propagation in the brain depends on nerve fiber orientation. Neurosurgery 35: 720–722; discussion 722–724.
74. McCarthy TJ, De Taboada L, Hildebrandt PK, Ziemer EL, Richieri SP, et al. (2010) Long-term safety of single and multiple infrared transcranial laser treatments in Sprague-Dawley rats. Photomed Laser Surg 28: 663–667.
75. Oron A, Oron U, Streeter J, de Taboada L, Alexandrovich A, et al. (2007) Low-level laser therapy applied transcranially to mice following traumatic brain injury significantly reduces long-term neurological deficits. J Neurotrauma 24: 651–656.
76. Ando T, Xuan W, Xu T, Dai T, Sharma SK, et al. (2011) Comparison of therapeutic effects between pulsed and continuous wave 810-nm wavelength laser irradiation for traumatic brain injury in mice. PLoS One 6: e26212.
77. Khuman J, Zhang J, Park J, Carroll JD, Donahue C, et al. (2012) Low-level laser light therapy improves cognitive deficits and inhibits microglial activation after controlled cortical impact in mice. J Neurotrauma 29: 408–417.
78. Huang YY, Sharma SK, Carroll J, Hamblin MR (2011) Biphasic dose response in low level light therapy - an update. Dose Response 9: 602–618.
79. Back SA, Gan X, Li Y, Rosenberg PA, Volpe JJ (1998) Maturation-dependent vulnerability of oligodendrocytes to oxidative stress-induced death caused by glutathione depletion. J Neurosci 18: 6241–6253.
80. Back SA, Luo NL, Mallinson RA, O'Malley JP, Wallen LD, et al. (2005) Selective vulnerability of preterm white matter to oxidative damage defined by F2-isoprostanes. Ann Neurol 58: 108–120.

8

Traumatic Brain Injury in the Netherlands: Incidence, Costs and Disability-Adjusted Life Years

Annemieke C. Scholten[1]*, Juanita A. Haagsma[1], Martien J. M. Panneman[2], Ed F. van Beeck[1], Suzanne Polinder[1]

1 Department of Public Health, Erasmus University Medical Center, Rotterdam, The Netherlands, **2** Research Department, Consumer and Safety Institute, Amsterdam, The Netherlands

Abstract

Objective: Traumatic brain injury (TBI) is a major cause of death and disability, leading to great personal suffering and huge costs to society. Integrated knowledge on epidemiology, economic consequences and disease burden of TBI is scarce but essential for optimizing healthcare policy and preventing TBI. This study aimed to estimate incidence, cost-of-illness and disability-adjusted life years (DALYs) of TBI in the Netherlands.

Methods: This study included data on all TBI patients who were treated at an Emergency Department (ED - National Injury Surveillance System), hospitalized (National Medical Registration), or died due to their injuries in the Netherlands between 2010–2012. Direct healthcare costs and indirect costs were determined using the incidence-based Dutch Burden of Injury Model. Disease burden was assessed by calculating years of life lost (YLL) owing to premature death, years lived with disability (YLD) and DALYs. Incidence, costs and disease burden were stratified by age and gender.

Results: TBI incidence was 213.6 per 100,000 person years. Total costs were €314.6 (USD $433.8) million per year and disease burden resulted in 171,200 DALYs (on average 7.1 DALYs per case). Men had highest mean costs per case (€19,540 versus €14,940), driven by indirect costs. 0–24-year-olds had high incidence and disease burden but low economic costs, whereas 25–64-year-olds had relatively low incidence but high economic costs. Patients aged 65+ had highest incidence, leading to considerable direct healthcare costs. 0–24-year-olds, men aged 25–64 years, traffic injury victims (especially bicyclists) and home and leisure injury victims (especially 0–5-year-old and elderly fallers) are identified as risk groups in TBI.

Conclusions: The economic and health consequences of TBI are substantial. The integrated approach of assessing incidence, costs and disease burden enables detection of important risk groups in TBI, development of prevention programs that target these risk groups and assessment of the benefits of these programs.

Editor: Subhra Mohapatra, University of South Florida, United States of America

Funding: These authors have no support or funding to report.

Competing Interests: The authors have declared that no competing interests exist.

* Email: a.scholten@erasmusmc.nl

Introduction

Traumatic brain injury (TBI) – defined as an alteration in brain function, or other evidence of brain pathology, caused by an external cause [1] – is a leading cause of morbidity, disability, and mortality worldwide. In Europe, the annual incidence rate of hospitalized and fatal TBI is about 235 per 100,000 person years [2]. TBI survivors almost all experience some level of impairment or disability [2], which drastically reduces their health-related quality of life (HRQL) [3,4].

In addition to the often long-term impact of TBI on a person's life, the economic consequences of TBI for both individuals and society are substantial [5,6]. TBI patients require specialized pre-hospital care, transport, in-hospital (emergency) care, and often long-term rehabilitation. Survivors of more severe TBI are often unable to return to full employment [7,8]. TBI therefore leads to significant direct healthcare costs in terms of pre-hospital care, emergency care, hospitalization, long-term outpatient care and rehabilitation, and indirect costs due to loss of productivity. The total direct and indirect costs of TBI occurring in Europe were estimated to €33 billion (approximately USD $45.4 billion) [9].

Most efforts on assessing the impact of TBI have been limited to either its epidemiology [2,10,11], costs [5,6,9,12–18] or disease burden [17,19,20]. Integrated knowledge on epidemiology, economic consequences and disease burden of TBI is scarce but essential for optimizing healthcare policy, allocating scarce resources, preventing TBI, and developing effective healthcare and rehabilitation services. Up till now, an insight of the total population impact of TBI is lacking. The purpose of this study was to estimate the incidence, cost-of-illness and disability-adjusted life years (DALYs) of TBI in the Dutch population, and to detect important risk groups in TBI.

Methods

Data sources

This surveillance-based study included data on all patients with TBI treated at an ED and/or admitted to hospital in the Netherlands in the period 2010–2012. TBI cases were extracted from the Dutch Injury Surveillance System (LIS) [21] and the National Hospital Discharge Registry (LMR) [22], to include data of TBI patients treated at the ED and hospitalized TBI patients respectively.

LIS is an ongoing monitoring system which records data of all unintentional and intentional injured patients who attend the ED. LIS is based upon the registration of 13 hospitals in the Netherlands (12–15% coverage) that are considered to be representative for the total Dutch injury-related ED visits. To generate national estimates of the injury-related ED visits in the Netherlands, an extrapolation factor was calculated in which the number of ED treatments due to injury registered by the participating hospitals is multiplied by the quotient of the number of hospital admissions due to injury in the Netherlands divided by the number of hospital admissions due to injury registered in the participating hospitals [23]. The required data on the number of hospital admissions due to TBI in the Netherlands is obtained from the LMR, which collects data from all Dutch hospitals regarding patient information from hospital admission to discharge. In this study, data from LIS was used to assess socio-demographic (age at injury and sex), injury (type of injury, external cause of injury, multiple injury), and healthcare related characteristics (hospitalization and length of stay). To avoid double counting, only the LMR was used to obtain data of hospitalized patients on the type of injury (ICD-9-codes) and for costs calculations.

Definition of TBI

For patients treated at the ED, TBI was defined as having a "Concussion" or "Other skull – brain injury" in at least one of the three injuries that can be recorded in LIS. This study therefore included all cases in which TBI was registered as first, second or third injury. In case of multiple injuries, an hierarchy derived from the literature was used to determine the most severe injuries [24]. This hierarchy prioritized spinal cord injury over skull or brain injury (except concussions), hip fracture, and other lower extremity fractures, respectively. For hospitalized patients, TBI was defined using the International Classification of Diseases, ninth revision (ICD-9-CM). This study included ICD-9-codes related to concussion (850), fractures (800–801, 803, 804), lesion (851–854), late effects (905, 907), nerve injury (950), and unspecified head injury (959).

Cost-of-illness

Short- and long-term direct costs (e.g., healthcare costs) and indirect costs (e.g., productivity loss) of TBI were calculated with use of the incidence-based Dutch Burden of Injury Model [23,25]. This model calculates patient numbers, healthcare consumption, and related costs for predefined patient groups that are homogenous in terms of health service use. Data on healthcare consumption was obtained from the LIS and LMR database, rehabilitation centers (LIVRE), nursing homes (SIVIS), and a patient follow-up survey conducted in 2007–2008 [23,26,27].

Direct healthcare costs of TBI were calculated by multiplying incidence by healthcare volumes (e.g., length of stay), transition probabilities (e.g., probability of hospital admission), and unit costs (e.g., costs per day in hospital). All unit costs were estimated according to national guidelines for healthcare costing [28], reflecting real resource use (Table 1). Indirect costs of TBI were calculated for all TBI patients in the working age 15 to 64 years treated at the ED or hospitalized, based on information on work absence and return to work from the patient follow-up questionnaire conducted in 2007–2008 [23,26,27].

In order to compare the costs of TBI in the Netherlands with previous cost studies conducted in other countries and at varying points in time, all costs estimates were adjusted for inflation with use of the Consumer Price Index [29–31] and converted into 2012 Euros (as at 31 December 2012 €1.00 = USD $1.3203).

Burden of TBI

The national disease burden of TBI was measured using the disability-adjusted life year (DALY), a summary measure of population health [32]. To calculate the burden of disease, information on premature mortality, and morbidity and disability due to non-fatal health outcome is combined into one single number. This number represents the health gap between the current state of a population's health compared to an ideal situation where individuals would live to the standard life expectancy in full health, i.e., free of disease and disability. DALYs are the sum of the years of life lost due to premature mortality (YLLs) and years lived with disability (YLDs). YLLs were calculated by multiplying the number of deaths at each age by a standard life expectancy at that age. The number of deaths at each age were calculated with use of the average European case-fatality rate of 11%; about 3% in-hospital and 8% out-of-hospital [2,33]. To allow for international comparisons, the life expectancy was calculated using the Coale-Demeny model West life tables, with a life expectancy at birth of 80 years for males and 82.5 years for females [34].

YLDs were calculated in three steps [35]. First, data was gathered on the incidence, age and sex distribution of patients treated at the ED or hospitalized due to TBI. Second, the incidence data was divided into the injury categories "Concussion" and "Skull-brain injury" of the EUROCOST classification system [36]. Finally, the grouped incidence data was combined with the disability weights and durations developed within the framework of the European INTEGRIS (Integration of European Injury Statistics) study [35]. Registered cases were multiplied with the 1-year disability weight, the proportion of lifelong consequences (Concussion: 4% ED, 21% hospitalized; Skull-brain injury: 13% ED, 23% hospitalized) and the duration (life expectancy at age of injury, by sex). The mean 1-year disability weights included the temporary and lifelong consequences for cases seen in EDs and those recorded in hospital discharge registers for both concussions (Temporary: 0.015 ED, 0.100 hospitalized; Lifelong: 0.151) and skull-brain injuries (Temporary: 0.090 ED, 0.241 hospitalized; Lifelong: 0.323).To compare the impact of TBI with that of other injuries, YLDs for the other injuries were also calculated with disability weights obtained from the INTEGRIS study. The disability weights were derived from empirical follow-up data on the health-related quality of life of individual trauma patients, and adjusted for population norms, age and gender [35].

Data and statistical analysis

All statistical analyses were carried out using the statistical package SPSS for Windows, version 21 (IBM SPSS Statistics, SPSS Inc, Chicago, IL). Descriptive statistics were used to provide insight in the characteristics of TBI patients. Continuous variables were described by presenting the median and interquartile range. Incidence rates per 100,000 person years were calculated using population data from Statistics Netherlands [37]. A value of $p < 0.05$ was used to determine statistical significance. All data reported in this article are national estimates.

Table 1. Unit costs (2012).

Resource	Unit costs
General Practitioner	
Practice consultation	€33.70
Consultation by telephone	€16.90
Home visit	€67.40
Referral patient treated at the ED	€35.00
Referral hospitalized patient	€44.00
Follow-up care patient treated at the ED	€33.70
Follow-up care hospitalized patient	€37.80
Ambulance	
Emergency journey	€538.20
Scheduled journey	€206.20
Hospital	
Attendance of emergency department	Injury specific fees[1]
Hospitalization general hospital	€460.40/day
Hospitalization academic hospital	€629.00/day
Intensive care	€1,751.50/day
Day care	€310.30/day
Outpatient department visit	€178.10/visit
Medical procedures	Reimbursement fees
Long term care	
Nursing home	€264.60/day, 138.80/day care
Rehabilitation	€469.10/day
Physiotherapy	€38.00/treatment
Home care	
Domestic care	€30.60/h
Care	€39.10/h
Nursing	€67.60/h
Nursing & care	€46.40/h
Labor costs (including VAT)	
15–19 year	€13.50/hour
20–24 year	€24.70/hour
25–29 year	€32.80/hour
30–34 year	€39.30/hour
35–39 year	€43.30/hour
40–44 year	€45.40/hour
45–49 year	€46.80/hour
50–54 year	€48.50/hour
55–59 year	€49.70/hour
60–64 year	€50.70/hour
Overall mean	€40.90/hour

[1]Unit costs for attendance of emergency department are calculated per type of injury in an annually unit cost study indexing the tariffs per minute of nurses, physicians and specialists.
ED: emergency department; VAT: value added tax.

Results

Incidence

In the period 2010–2012, annually 34,681 patients visited the ED due to TBI (Table 2), comprising about 4% of the total injury-related ED visits per year in the Netherlands. The overall incidence rate of ED visits due to TBI was 213.6 per 100,000 person years, 241.9 for males and 175.3 for females respectively. Incidence rates were highest in children (268.2), young adults (271.6) and older patients in the age of 75–84 years (307.6) or 85 and older (578.2). The majority of patients sustained a TBI because of a home and leisure injury (47.9%) or traffic injury (33.5%).

Table 2. Incidence and characteristics of traumatic brain injuries in the Dutch population (2010–2012)[1].

	Dutch Injury Surveillance System N = 3,762 (%)	National estimate N = 34,681 (%)	Incidence (per 100,000) Total: 213.6
Gender			
Male	2,162 (57.5)	19,937 (57.5)	241.9
Female	1,600 (42.5)	14,744 (42.5)	175.3
Age			
0–14	846 (22.5)	7,793 (22.5)	268.2
15–24	601 (16.0)	5,538 (16.0)	271.6
25–44	714 (19.0)	6,584 (19.0)	148.7
45–64	789 (21.0)	7,281 (21.0)	156.1
65–74	332 (8.8)	3,062 (8.8)	211.4
75–84	287 (7.6)	2,648 (7.6)	307.6
85+	192 (5.1)	1,775 (5.1)	578.2
Accident category and type of road user			
Home and leisure	1,806 (48.0)	16,628 (47.9)	
Traffic	1,256 (33.4)	11,616 (33.5)	
Pedestrian	*66 (5.3)*	*613 (5.3)*	
Bicyclist	*706 (56.9)*	*6,522 (56.9)*	
Moped occupant	*151 (12.2)*	*1,406 (12.3)*	
Motor vehicle/scooter occupant	*63 (5.1)*	*575 (5.0)*	
Passenger vehicle occupant	*205 (16.5)*	*1,898 (16.5)*	
Other	*49 (4.0)*	*455 (4.0)*	
Unknown	*16*	*148*	
Sport	307 (8.2)	2,824 (8.1)	
Occupational	109 (2.9)	1,003 (2.9)	
Assault	247 (6.6)	2,269 (6.5)	
Self-mutilation	18 (0.5)	171 (0.5)	
Other	19 (0.5)	172 (0.5)	
Type of brain injury[2,3]			
Concussion		8,983 (44.7)	
Fracture			
Vault		317 (1.6)	
Base		1,319 (6.6)	
Other/unqualified		330 (1.6)	
Multiple fractures		130 (0.6)	
Lesion			
Cerebral laceration/contusion		1,977 (9.8)	
Subarachnoid/sub-/extradural hemorrhage		1,598 (7.9)	
Other/NFS intracranial hemorrhage		262 (1.3)	
Intracranial injury, other/NFS nature		5,116 (25.5)	
Late effects			
Musculoskeletal and connective tissue		46 (0.2)	
Nervous system		18 (0.1)	
Nerve injury			
Optic nerve and pathways		3 (<0.1)	
Unknown		14,581 (42.0)	
Number of injuries			
1 injury	1,065 (28.3)	9,766 (28.2)	
2 injuries	2,033 (54.0)	18,773 (54.1)	
≥3 injuries	664 (17.7)	6,142 (17.7)	
Hospitalization			

Table 2. Cont.

	Dutch Injury Surveillance System N = 3,762 (%)	National estimate N = 34,681 (%)	Incidence (per 100,000) Total: 213.6
Not admitted	1,633 (43.5)	15,024 (43.4)	
Unknown	8	70	
1–3 days	1,424 (70.4)	13,146 (70.4)	
≥4 days	597 (29.6)	5,529 (29.6)	
N days unknown	106	982	

[1]Mean number per year in the period 2010–2012.
[2]Traumatic brain injury diagnoses (ICD-9 codes): *Concussion:* Concussion (850): *Cranial fracture:* Fracture of vault of skull (800); Fracture of base of skull (801); Other and unqualified skull fractures (803); Multiple fractures involving skull or face with other bones (804): *Lesion:* Cerebral laceration and contusion (851); Subarachnoid, subdural, and extradural hemorrhage after injury (852); Other and unspecified intracranial hemorrhage after injury (853); Intracranial injury of other and unspecified nature (854): *Late effects:* Late effects of musculoskeletal and connective tissue injuries (905); Late effects of injuries to the nervous system (907): *Nerve injury:* Injury to optic nerve and pathways (950): *Head injury, unspecified* (959, N = 0).
[3]Data on injury type (ICD) only known for hospitalized patients in the LMR database (National estimate: N = 20,100).

Patients that sustained a TBI due to a traffic accident often concerned bicyclists (56.9%) and passenger vehicle occupants (16.5%). Home and leisure injuries often concerned a fall among 0–5-year-olds and elderly patients (aged 60 years and older). ED visits due to TBI often included the diagnoses concussion (44.7%), intracranial injury of other or unspecified nature (25.5%) and cerebral laceration or contusion (9.8%). Almost one in three TBI patients were treated for more than one injury and more than half of the patients were hospitalized, most frequently for 1 or 2 days (61.7% of the hospitalized patients).

Cost-of-illness

The estimated total costs of TBI in the Netherlands was €314.6 million per year (Table 3). Total direct healthcare costs (€158.6 million) were comparable to indirect costs (€155.9 million), whereas in the working population per case mean direct healthcare costs were more than 3 times lower than the indirect costs. Overall, the mean total costs per case were €18,030, and were higher for men (€19,540) than for women (€14,940). This difference is mostly driven by the difference in indirect costs per TBI patient (males €15,416; females €10,257; $p<0.001$). The estimated total amount of omitted work days among TBI patients with paid employment was 44 days per case, and significantly differed between men (mean 46 days) and women (mean 38 days) ($p<0.001$). Both direct and indirect costs per TBI patient increased with the length of hospital stay.

The average direct costs per case increased with age (Figure 1). Mean direct costs per case were higher (up to €950) for men than for women in the ages up to 74 years, while in individuals aged over 75 years women had much higher mean direct costs per case (up to € 3,210) than men. Indirect costs (applicable to individuals aged 15–64 years old) also increased with age, and were higher (up to €6,280) for men than for women.

Disability-adjusted life years

TBI resulted in 52,998 YLD and 118,207 YLL respectively, amounting to 171,205 DALYs (on average 7.07 DALYs per TBI patient, Table 4). Overall, 69% of the total burden was caused by premature mortality. The burden due to permanent (lifelong) disability was high compared with temporary (short-term) disability. Men were responsible for 59% of the total burden of TBI, and had higher YLDs, YLLs and DALYs per case than women (YLD per case: 2.29 in men vs 2.05 in women; YLL per case: 4.97 vs 4.76; DALY per case: 7.27 vs 6.81). Mean YLD decreased with age in both men and women, and was highest among 0–14-years-olds (Figure 2).

Table 3. Cost-of-illness by hospitalization and gender (2010–2012).

	Hospitalization	Direct costs per case[1]	Indirect costs per case[1]	Total costs per case[1]	Total costs (€)
Total	0–7 days	3,584	12,454	16,040	234,259,230
	>7 days	9,854	21,431	31,280	64,608,290
	Total	**4,361**	**13,668**	**18,030**	**314,592,930**
Men	0–7 days	3,413	14,116	17,530	149,815,870
	>7 days	8,809	22,216	31,020	41,805,590
	Total	**4,128**	**15,416**	**19,540**	**202,953,300**
Women	0–7 days	3,812	9,479	13,290	84,443,360
	>7 days	11,433	18,638	30,070	22,802,690
	Total	**4,680**	**10,257**	**14,940**	**111,639,630**

[1]Mean costs per case: indirect costs per case are presented as an average of only the working population (15 to 65 years).

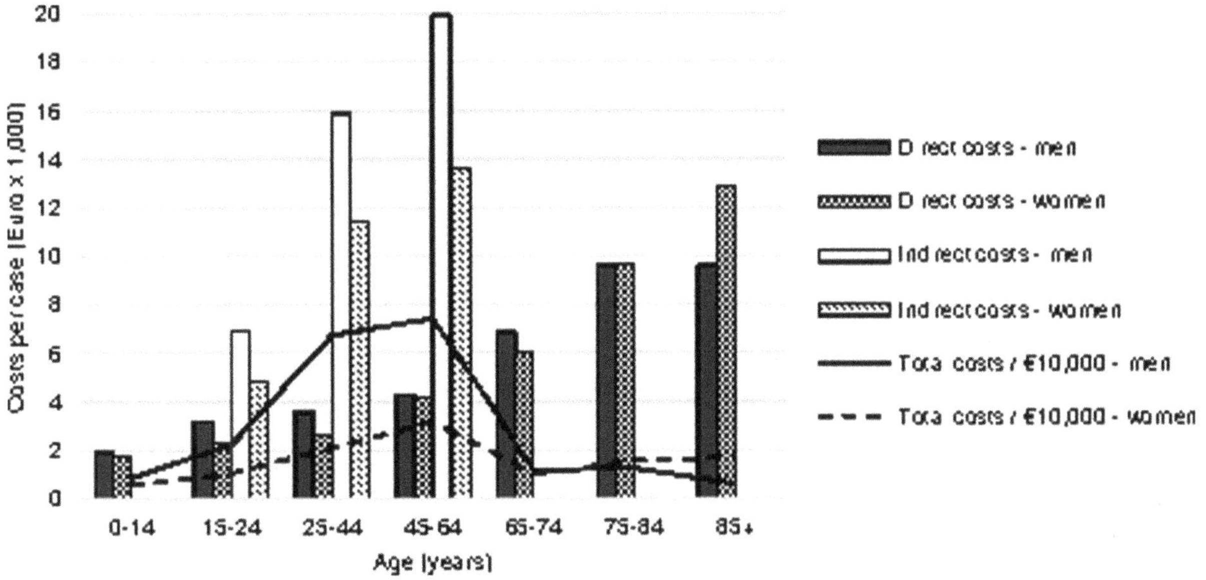

Figure 1. Mean direct and indirect costs per case and total costs by age and gender (2010–2012).

TBI in comparison to other injury categories

In the period 2007–2011, TBI accounted 10% of the total YLDs and 12% of the lifelong YLDs caused by all injuries in the Netherlands (data not shown). Concussion and skull-brain injury both were ranked in the top 5 of injuries with highest total YLDs, after fractures of the knee or lower leg, ankle, and foot or toes (Table 5). Skull-brain injury accounted for the highest YLDs per case after spinal cord injury: 2.89 and 14.68 respectively (data not shown).

Discussion

The purpose of this paper was to estimate the incidence, cost-of-illness and disability-adjusted life years (DALYs) of TBI in the Netherlands. Our study revealed that TBI imposes a substantial economic and disease burden (on average 7.1 DALYs per TBI patient) on the Dutch population, accounting for more than 4% of injury-related ED visits, 9% of the injury-related costs and 10% of the injury-related YLDs in the Netherlands.

The integrated approach of our study showed that the incidence and burden of disease among children and young adults aged 0–24 years is high, whereas the economic consequences for this group were low due to relatively shorter hospitalization and almost no indirect costs (Figure 3). The reverse is shown in the 25–64-year-olds, who have relatively low incidence and high economic costs, driven by loss of productivity. Older patients aged 65+ had highest

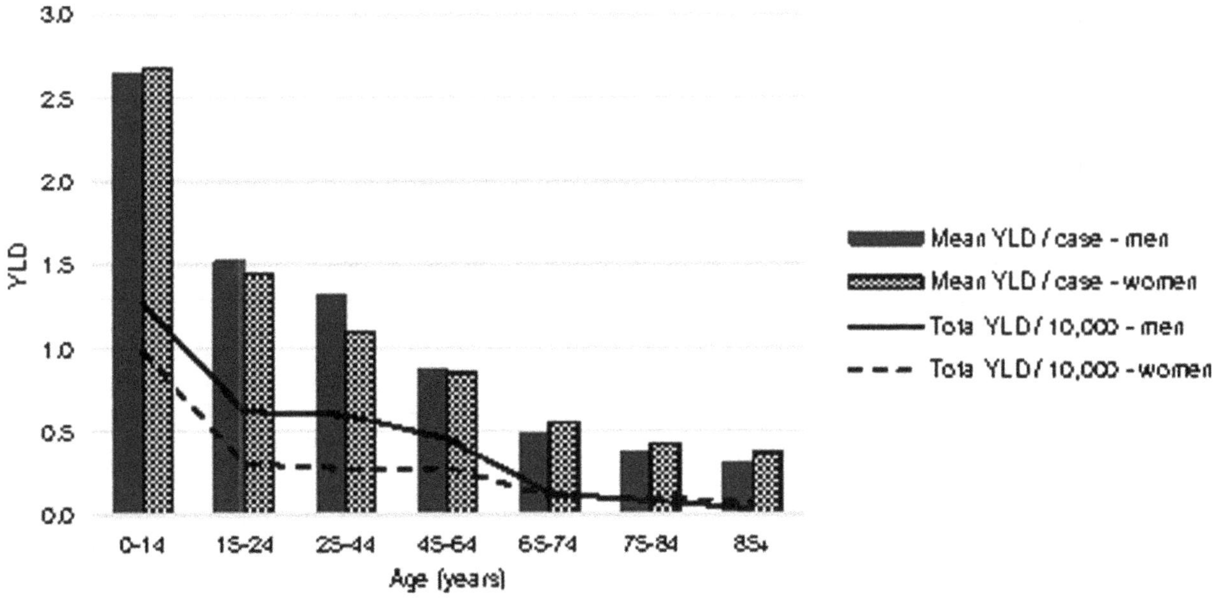

Figure 2. Mean years lived with disability by age and gender (2010–2012). YLD: years lived with disability.

Table 4. Total temporary and lifelong years lived with disability, years of life lost and disability-adjusted life-years per 1-year interval (2010–2012).

		YLD ED visits		YLD hospital admission				
	N	Temporary	Lifelong	Temporary	Lifelong	YLL	Total DALYs[1]	DALYs per case
Men	13,877	56	1,077	2,098	28,603	69,022	100,856	7.27
Women	10,330	47	941	1,470	18,706	49,185	70,348	6.81
Concussion	12,580	54	1,023	897	13,540	118,207	171,205	7.07
Skull-brain injury	11,631	50	995	2,670	33,769			
Total	**24,211**	**104**	**2,018**	**3,567**	**47,309**	**118,207**	**171,205**	**7.07**

[1]Disability-adjusted life-years (DALYs) per year.
YLD: years lived with disability; ED: emergency department; YLL: years of life lost.

incidence of TBI, leading to considerable direct healthcare costs, and a relatively low disease burden.

Comparison of results to other studies

Incidence. Our estimated incidence rate of ED treated, hospitalized and fatal TBI for the Netherlands of about 214 per 100,000 person years was lower than the estimated rate of hospitalized and fatal TBI for Europe of about 235 per 100,000 persons years [2]. This difference may partly be explained by the time period covered in the studies. The European rate was derived from studies with data over 1974 to 2000, with incidence rates ranging from 150 to 300 per 100,000 person years [2], whereas our study included data from 2010 to 2012. Compared to the US, the Dutch estimated incidence rates of ED visits, hospital admissions and deaths are considerably lower. It is estimated that the incidence of TBI in the US is 577 per 100,000 person years in 2006 [38], comprising about 1,365,000 ED visits (81%), 275,000 hospitalizations (16%) and 52,000 deaths (3%). However, other population-based studies suggest that the incidence of TBI in the US is somewhat lower, between 180 to 250 per 100,000 person years in 1965 to 1996 [2,11].

Consistent with prior research [2,38], TBI incidence was higher among men than women, and highest among children and older people. Whereas motor vehicle accidents and falls were the most common mechanisms of injury in previous studies in Europe [2] and the US [6,17,38], our sample showed a high number of ED treatments among bicyclists in the traffic setting. Cycling is a very popular form of transport and recreation in the Netherlands, as up to 28% of all trips nationwide are made by bicycle [39]. The popularity of cycling however also imposes a high burden on society, due the large number of (brain) injuries among cyclist [40–42]. Bicycle helmets are not compulsory in the Netherlands and are only commonly used among road cyclist, mountain bikers and young children.

Cost-of-illness. TBI accounted for 9% of total costs of all injuries in the Netherlands (about €3.5 billion). The direct healthcare costs of TBI are on average €4,300 per case. This is in line with the outcomes of a previous study on the costs of all types of injuries in the Netherlands in 2004 that estimated the average direct healthcare costs of skull and brain injury cases at €3,100 [12]. This is approximately €4,100 when converting 2004 Euros to 2012 Euros using consumer price index.

Compared to other European countries our estimation of direct healthcare costs of TBI are somewhat higher [5]: from €2,700 in whole Europe, to €2,930 in Germany, €3,490 in Spain and €3,453 in Sweden after adjustment for inflation up to 2012. Estimates from the US are however more than two times the estimates in our present study: about €23,500 acute hospital charges per TBI [15], €6,200 per TBI in Missouri [17], and €8,500 to €35,000 for mild to severe hospitalized patients [6] - all scaled to 2012 price levels and 2012 Euro. These differences can partly be explained by differences in cost calculations. The European cost calculations were limited to inpatient costs while the current study included also extramural healthcare costs, and most US studies used charges instead of unit costs. Although the methodology of cost calculations varied considerably, our study confirms that indirect costs of TBI are far higher than direct healthcare costs of TBI [9,17,43,44], costs of TBI are higher among men than women and increase with age [5] and that the costs increase with the length of hospital stay [6]. The latter suggests that the economic burden of TBI varies considerably by TBI severity.

Overall, TBI imposes a high economic burden on society and, together with hip fracture, is a leading source of hospital costs [13]

Table 5. Top ten injuries with highest disability in the Netherlands by accident category (2007–2011)[1].

Rank	Home and leisure	Traffic	Sport	Occupational	Total
1	Fracture ankle	Fracture knee/lower leg	Fracture knee/lower leg	Fracture foot/toes	Fracture knee/lower leg
2	Fracture foot/toes	**Skull-brain injury**	Fracture ankle	Fracture knee/lower leg	Fracture ankle
3	Fracture knee/lower leg	**Concussion**	Fracture foot/toes	Fracture ankle	Fracture foot/toes
4	**Concussion**	Fracture ankle	Lux/dist ankle/foot	Spinal cord injury	**Skull-brain injury**
5	**Skull-brain injury**	Spinal cord injury	Lux/dist knee	**Skull-brain injury**	**Concussion**
6	Hip fracture	Fracture foot/toes	**Concussion**	Complex soft tissue arm/hand	Spinal cord injury
7	Spinal cord injury	Hip fracture	Fracture wrist	Lux/dist ankle/foot	Hip fracture
8	Fracture upper arm	Fracture shoulder	**Skull-brain injury**	**Concussion**	Lux/dist ankle/foot
9	Lux/dist ankle/foot	Fracture upper arm	Fracture upper arm	Lux/dist knee	Fracture upper arm
10	Fracture wrist	Fracture upper leg	Fracture shoulder	Open wound	Lux/dist knee

[1]Ranked by total years lived with disability (YLD) for short- and long-term disability.
Lux/dist: luxation/distortion.

and direct healthcare costs [12] in the Netherlands due to high healthcare costs per patient.

Disability-adjusted life years. TBI accounted for 10% of total YLD and 12% of the lifelong YLD caused by all injuries in the Netherlands, due to lifelong consequences in a relative young patient group. TBI resulted in both high temporary and lifelong YLD among road traffic injuries and home and leisure injuries, as confirmed in the literature [19,45]. TBI is one of the leading causes of disease burden compared to other injuries and diseases in the Netherlands. TBI imposes a disease burden comparable to that of depression, diabetes, and lung cancer, which are all in the top 10 diseases with highest total DALY in the Netherlands [46]. Mean YLD decreased with age and was highest among children (0–14 years). This can partly be explained by the use of the expected number of years of life remaining as the duration of TBI in the YLD calculation. This method assumes that a proportion of the TBI patients will live with disability outcomes for the remainder of their expected lifetime. Therefore the duration used in the YLD calculation equaled the life expectancy at age based on the Coale-Demeny model West life tables [34]; in our sample on average 45 years in men and 43 in women. This may have led to a higher estimate of the years lived with disability after TBI in comparison to the use of a fixed average duration for TBI.

Limitations

The number of deaths due to TBI in the Netherlands could not be generated from national death statistics, because these are only available for specific diseases (e.g., type of cancer, cardiovascular diseases) or injuries specified by cause (e.g., traffic accidents, falls, drowning, self-mutilation). Therefore, the YLL component of the total DALY was estimated with use of the European average case fatality rate of TBI, derived from 18 studies. This overall case fatality rate was on average about 11 per 100 persons with TBI; about 3% in-hospital and 8% out-of-hospital deaths among patients with TBI [2,33]. Due to the use of the average European overall case fatality rate, the number of YLLs and thereby the

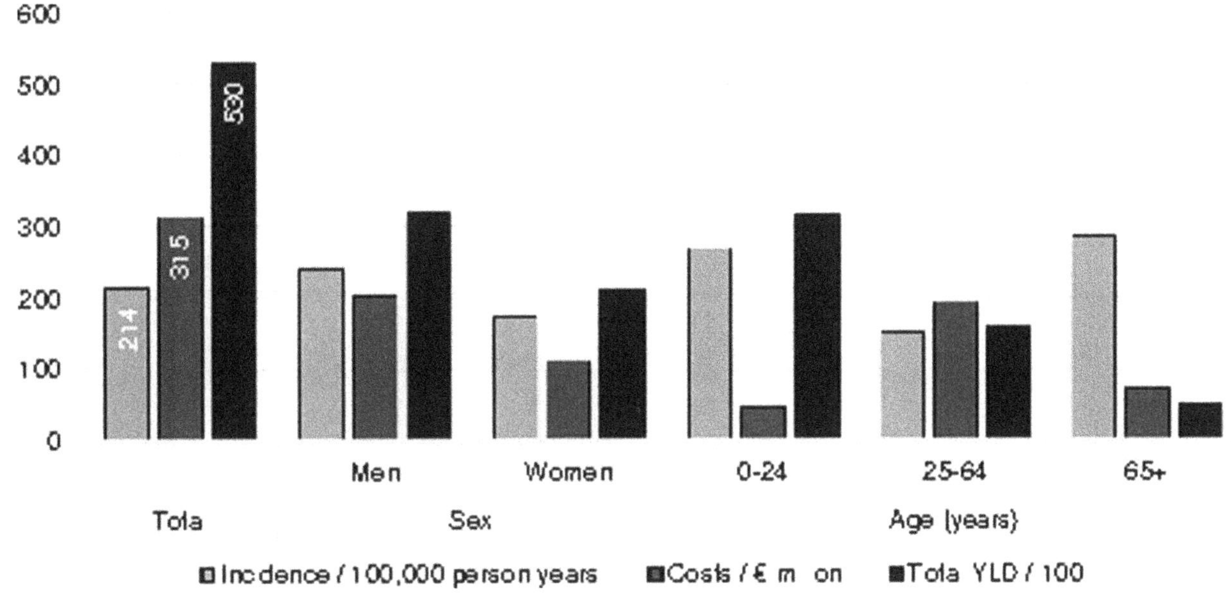

Figure 3. Economic and disease burden of traumatic brain injury in the Netherlands (2010–2012). YLD: years lived with disability.

disease burden of TBI may be over- or underestimated. However, actual case fatality rates and disease burden of TBI may be even higher due to higher excess mortality in the long-term [47–49]. In order to improve the YLL and disease burden estimates of TBI and other injuries and diseases in the Netherlands, specific (long-term) mortality data should be registered and available for future research.

Other limitations concern the classification of TBI and the calculation of costs. TBI patients treated at the ED were registered as having a "Concussion" or "Other skull – brain injury". No additional data was available on ICD-codes, AIS-codes or a Glasgow Outcome Scale to uniformly determine TBI; data that was available for the majority of the hospitalized patients.

The ICD-9 codes used to determine the type of TBI among hospitalized patients slightly differed from those recommended by the Center for Disease Control (CDC) [50], in that this study also included the late effects of TBI (ICD-9 codes 905, 907, 950). These late effects however comprise far less than 1% of all hospitalized traumatic brain injuries in the Netherlands, and therefore will not complicate comparison of our results to those of other studies in which the CDC ICD-9 codes for TBI were used.

The cost-of-illness of TBI may have been overestimated because of the use of a patient follow-up survey to obtain information on healthcare consumption and labor status. Comparison of the hospital discharge data and the patient follow-up data indicated that there is a higher response among the more severe injured patients. This may lead to an overestimation of the costs and disease burden of TBI.

On the other hand, our estimation of indirect costs of TBI comprised only costs of lost work productivity for TBI patients of working age. Other potential sources of indirect costs, such as the work productivity and finances of families and caregivers were not incorporated in this study. Previous research showed that TBI imposes a significant level of financial burden on families and caregivers [51,52], which is directly related to the severity of TBI [51]. Total indirect costs of TBI will therefore be far higher than estimated in this study, particularly among children and elderly with caregivers in the working age.

Our study is limited to TBI patients that were treated at the ED or admitted to hospital. Patients who consulted a GP were not included in our overview. Hence, incidence rates, cost-of-illness and burden of TBI may be even higher [53]. According to registries from Dutch general practice, in 2012 about 7,600 persons contacted their General Practitioner (GP) or after-hours General Practitioner Co-operation (GPC) due to TBI [54]. Assuming that direct healthcare costs of GP visits are on average €39 per contact (Table 1; mean costs for practice or telephone consultation, and home visit), and the indirect costs and disease burden of TBI will not be larger than that of ED-treated patients, they will add about 7–8% only to our cost estimate and about 1–2% only to our DALY estimate.

Recommendation for future research

The results of our study reveal that TBI imposes a relatively high economic and health impact compared to all injuries and diseases in the Netherlands. TBI is a growing worldwide problem, as recent reports suggest a rapid increase in ED visits and hospitalizations resulting from traumatic brain injury, especially fall-related TBI in older adults [55–57] and traffic-related TBI [58,59]. There is a need for prevention programs targeting on the reduction of incidence and severity of TBI. On the bases of our study, we conclude that especially children and young adults aged 0–24 years, men aged 25–64 years and traffic injury victims (in the Netherlands especially bicyclists) and home and leisure injury victims are an important target for intervention. In the working population, screening for risk of problems to return to work and immediate rehabilitation after TBI may help to minimize lost productivity [60].

Future research should examine how helmet use among cyclists can be increased. Bicycle helmets have shown to be highly effective in preventing head, brain, and facial injuries to cyclist [61,62]. Previous research in Canada showed that helmet legislation may be an effective tool in the prevention of childhood bicycle-related head injuries [63]. Overall, future research on the population impact of TBI in terms of costs and disease burden should also include patients who receive no treatment or out-of-hospital treatment (e.g., from a GP or by sports trainers).

Conclusions

This study provided comprehensive population-based estimates on the epidemiology, costs and disease burden (in DALYs) of ED-treated and hospitalized persons with TBI over 2010–2012 in the Netherlands. The study included all age groups, all TBI severities, and both patients treated at the ED and hospitalized patients. The economic and health consequences of TBI are substantial. Prevention programs are needed to reduce incidence and severity of TBI. The integrated approach of assessment of incidence, costs and disease burden (in DALYs) of TBI enables the detection of all important risk groups in TBI.

Author Contributions

Analyzed the data: AS MP. Contributed reagents/materials/analysis tools: MP. Wrote the paper: AS JH SP EvB.

References

1. Menon DK, Schwab K, Wright DW, Maas AI (2010) Demographics and Clinical Assessment Working Group of the International Interagency Initiative toward Common Data Elements for Research on Traumatic Brain Injury Psychological Health. Position statement: definition of traumatic brain injury. Arch Phys Med Rehabil 91: 1637–1640.
2. Tagliaferri F, Compagnone C, Korsic M, Servadei F, Kraus J (2006) A systematic review of brain injury epidemiology in Europe. Acta Neurochir (Wien) 148: 255–268; discussion 268.
3. Andelic N, Hammergren N, Bautz-Holter E, Sveen U, Brunborg C, et al. (2009) Functional outcome and health-related quality of life 10 years after moderate-to-severe traumatic brain injury. Acta Neurol Scand 120: 16–23.
4. Dijkers MP (2004) Quality of life after traumatic brain injury: a review of research approaches and findings. Arch Phys Med Rehabil 85: S21–35.
5. Berg J, Tagliaferri F, Servadei F (2005) Cost of trauma in Europe. Eur J Neurol 12 Suppl 1: 85–90.
6. McGarry LJ, Thompson D, Millham FH, Cowell L, Snyder PJ, et al. (2002) Outcomes and costs of acute treatment of traumatic brain injury. J Trauma 53: 1152–1159.
7. Radford K, Phillips J, Drummond A, Sach T, Walker M, et al. (2013) Return to work after traumatic brain injury: cohort comparison and economic evaluation. Brain Inj 27: 507–520.
8. Holtslag HR, Post MW, van der Werken C, Lindeman E (2007) Return to work after major trauma. Clin Rehabil 21: 373–383.
9. Olesen J, Gustavsson A, Svensson M, Wittchen HU, Jönsson B, et al. (2012) The economic cost of brain disorders in Europe. Eur J Neurol 19: 155–162.
10. Feigin VL, Theadom A, Barker-Collo S, Starkey NJ, McPherson K, et al. (2013) Incidence of traumatic brain injury in New Zealand: a population-based study. Lancet Neurol 12: 53–64.
11. Bruns J, Hauser WA (2003) The epidemiology of traumatic brain injury: a review. Epilepsia 44 Suppl 10: 2–10.
12. Meerding WJ, Mulder S, van Beeck EF (2006) Incidence and costs of injuries in The Netherlands. Eur J Public Health 16: 272–278.
13. Polinder S, Meerding WJ, van Baar ME, Toet H, Mulder S, et al. (2005) Cost estimation of injury-related hospital admissions in 10 European countries. J Trauma 59: 1283–1290; discussion 1290–1281.
14. McGregor K, Pentland B (1997) Head injury rehabilitation in the U.K.: an economic perspective. Soc Sci Med 45: 295–303.

15. Schootman M, Buchman TG, Lewis LM (2003) National estimates of hospitalization charges for the acute care of traumatic brain injuries. Brain Inj 17: 983–990.
16. Humphreys I, Wood RL, Phillips CJ, Macey S (2013) The costs of traumatic brain injury: a literature review. Clinicoecon Outcomes Res 5: 281–287.
17. Kayani NA, Homan S, Yun S, Zhu BP (2009) Health and economic burden of traumatic brain injury: Missouri, 2001–2005. Public Health Rep 124: 551–560.
18. Farhad K, Khan HM, Ji AB, Yacoub HA, Qureshi AI, et al. (2013) Trends in outcomes and hospitalization costs for traumatic brain injury in adult patients in the United States. J Neurotrauma 30: 84–90.
19. Polinder S, Meerding WJ, Mulder S, Petridou E, van Beeck E, et al. (2007) Assessing the burden of injury in six European countries. Bull World Health Organ 85: 27–34.
20. Olesen J, Leonardi M (2003) The burden of brain diseases in Europe. Eur J Neurol 10: 471–477.
21. Meerding WJ, Polinder S, Lyons RA, Petridou ET, Toet H, et al. (2010) How adequate are emergency department home and leisure injury surveillance systems for cross-country comparisons in Europe? Int J Inj Contr Saf Promot 17: 13–22.
22. Van der Stegen RHM, Ploemacher J (2009) Discription of methods for statistics by diagnoses in time by using the LMR (1981–2005). The Hague: Statistics Netherlands.
23. Consumer and Safety Institute (2005) The Dutch Burden of Injury Model. Amsterdam: Consumer and Safety Institute.
24. MacKenzie EJ, Siegel JH, Shapiro S, Moody M, Smith RT (1988) Functional recovery and medical costs of trauma: an analysis by type and severity of injury. J Trauma 28: 281–297.
25. Mulder S, Meerding WJ, Van Beeck EF (2002) Setting priorities in injury prevention: the application of an incidence based cost model. Inj Prev 8: 74–78.
26. Polinder S, van Beeck EF, Essink-Bot ML, Toet H, Looman CW, et al. (2007) Functional outcome at 2.5, 5, 9, and 24 months after injury in the Netherlands. J Trauma 62: 133–141.
27. Haagsma JA, Polinder S, Olff M, Toet H, Bonsel GJ, et al. (2012) Posttraumatic stress symptoms and health-related quality of life: a two year follow up study of injury treated at the emergency department. BMC Psychiatry 12: 1.
28. Oostenbrink JB, Koopmanschap MA, Rutten FF (2002) Standardisation of costs: the Dutch Manual for Costing in economic evaluations. Pharmacoeconomics 20: 443–454.
29. Eurostat (2014) HICP - inflation rate.
30. Statistics Netherlands (CBS) (2014) [Consumer prices; inflation from 1963]. The Hague: Statistics Netherlands.
31. US Inflation Calculator (2014) US Inflation Calculator.
32. Murray CJL, Lopez AD, Harvard School of Public Health, World Health Organization, World Bank. (1996) The global burden of disease: a comprehensive assessment of mortality and disability from diseases, injuries, and risk factors in 1990 and projected to 2020. Cambridge, MA: Published by the Harvard School of Public Health on behalf of the World Health Organization and the World Bank; Distributed by Harvard University Press. xxxii, 990 p. p.
33. World Health Organization (2006) Neurological disorders: public health challenges: World Health Organization.
34. Murray CJ (1994) Quantifying the burden of disease: the technical basis for disability-adjusted life years. Bull World Health Organ 72: 429–445.
35. Haagsma JA, Polinder S, Lyons RA, Lund J, Ditsuwan V, et al. (2012) Improved and standardized method for assessing years lived with disability after injury. Bull World Health Organ 90: 513–521.
36. Polinder S, Meerding W, Toet H, van Baar M, Mulder S, et al. (2004) A surveillance based assessment of medical costs of injury in Europe: phase 2. Amsterdam: Consumer and Safety Institute.
37. Statistics Netherlands (CBS) (2014) [Population data]. The Hague: Statistics Netherlands.
38. Faul M, Xu L, Wald MM, Coronado VG (2010) Traumatic brain injury in the United States: emergency department visits, hospitalizations and deaths 2002–2006. Atlanta, GA: Centers for Disease Control and Prevention, National Center for Injury Prevention and Control. 2–70 p.
39. Statistics Netherlands (CBS) (2014) [Mobility in the Netherlands]. The Hague: Statistics Netherlands.
40. Consumer and Safety Institute (2011) [Fact sheet: bicycle accidents]. Amsterdam.
41. Consumer and Safety Institute (2011) [Fact sheet: sports injuries]. Amsterdam.
42. Consumer and Safety Institute (2012) [Fact sheet: sports injuries]. Amsterdam.
43. Schulman J, Sacks J, Provenzano G (2002) State level estimates of the incidence and economic burden of head injuries stemming from non-universal use of bicycle helmets. Inj Prev 8: 47–52.
44. Gustavsson A, Svensson M, Jacobi F, Allgulander C, Alonso J, et al. (2011) Cost of disorders of the brain in Europe 2010. Eur Neuropsychopharmacol 21: 718–779.
45. Hyder AA, Wunderlich CA, Puvanachandra P, Gururaj G, Kobusingye OC (2007) The impact of traumatic brain injuries: a global perspective. NeuroRehabilitation 22: 341–353.
46. Gommer A, Poos M, Hoeymans N (2010) [Years of life lost, morbidity and disease burden for 56 selected disorders]. Bilthoven: Rijksinstituut voor Volksgezondheid en Milieu (RIVM).
47. McMillan TM, Teasdale GM (2007) Death rate is increased for at least 7 years after head injury: a prospective study. Brain 130: 2520–2527.
48. Baguley IJ, Nott MT, Howle AA, Simpson GK, Browne S, et al. (2012) Late mortality after severe traumatic brain injury in New South Wales: a multicentre study. Med J Aust 196: 40–45.
49. Flaada JT, Leibson CL, Mandrekar JN, Diehl N, Perkins PK, et al. (2007) Relative risk of mortality after traumatic brain injury: a population-based study of the role of age and injury severity. J Neurotrauma 24: 435–445.
50. Thurman DJ SJE, Johnson D., Greenspan A., Smith S.M. (1995) Guidelines for surveillance of central nervous system injury. Atlanta, GA: US Department of Health and Human Services, Public Health Service, CDC.
51. Hoang HT, Pham TL, Vo TT, Nguyen PK, Doran CM, et al. (2008) The costs of traumatic brain injury due to motorcycle accidents in Hanoi, Vietnam. Cost Eff Resour Alloc 6: 17.
52. Hall KM, Karzmark P, Stevens M, Englander J, O'Hare P, et al. (1994) Family stressors in traumatic brain injury: a two-year follow-up. Arch Phys Med Rehabil 75: 876–884.
53. Consumer and Safety Institute (2013) [Fact sheet: traumatic brain injury]. Amsterdam.
54. Nielen M, Spronk I, Davids R, Zwaanswijk M, Verheij R, et al. (2014) [Incidence and prevalence rates of health problems in Dutch general practice in 2012]. NIVEL Zorgregistraties eerste lijn: Netherlands institute for health services research (NIVEL).
55. Hartholt KA, Van Lieshout EM, Polinder S, Panneman MJ, Van der Cammen TJ, et al. (2011) Rapid increase in hospitalizations resulting from fall-related traumatic head injury in older adults in The Netherlands 1986–2008. J Neurotrauma 28: 739–744.
56. Kannus P, Niemi S, Parkkari J, Palvanen M, Sievänen H (2007) Alarming rise in fall-induced severe head injuries among elderly people. Injury 38: 81–83.
57. Coronado VG, McGuire LC, Sarmiento K, Bell J, Lionbarger MR, et al. (2012) Trends in Traumatic Brain Injury in the U.S. and the public health response: 1995–2009. J Safety Res 43: 299–307.
58. World Health Organization (2004) World report on road traffic injury prevention Geneva: World Health Organization.
59. Murray CJ, Vos T, Lozano R, Naghavi M, Flaxman AD, et al. (2012) Disability-adjusted life years (DALYs) for 291 diseases and injuries in 21 regions, 1990–2010: a systematic analysis for the Global Burden of Disease Study 2010. Lancet 380: 2197–2223.
60. Boake C, McCauley SR, Pedroza C, Levin HS, Brown SA, et al. (2005) Lost productive work time after mild to moderate traumatic brain injury with and without hospitalization. Neurosurgery 56: 994–1003; discussion 1994–1003.
61. Thompson RS, Rivara FP, Thompson DC (1989) A case-control study of the effectiveness of bicycle safety helmets. N Engl J Med 320: 1361–1367.
62. Rivara FP, Thompson DC, Patterson MQ, Thompson RS (1998) Prevention of bicycle-related injuries: helmets, education, and legislation. Annu Rev Public Health 19: 293–318.
63. Macpherson AK, To TM, Macarthur C, Chipman ML, Wright JG, et al. (2002) Impact of mandatory helmet legislation on bicycle-related head injuries in children: a population-based study. Pediatrics 110: e60.

9

Spinal Cord Transection-Induced Allodynia in Rats – Behavioral, Physiopathological and Pharmacological Characterization

Saïd M'Dahoma[1,2]*, Sylvie Bourgoin[1,2], Valérie Kayser[1,2], Sandrine Barthélémy[1,2], Caroline Chevarin[1,2], Farah Chali[3], Didier Orsal[3], Michel Hamon[1,2]

1 Centre de Psychiatrie et Neurosciences, Institut National de la Santé et de la Recherche Médicale, INSERM U894, Université Paris Descartes, Paris, France, **2** Neuropsychopharmacologie, Faculté de Médecine Pierre et Marie Curie, site Pitié-Salpêtrière, Paris, France, **3** Laboratoire de Neurobiologie des Signaux Intercellulaires, Centre National de la Recherche Scientifique, CNRS UMR 7101, Université Pierre et Marie Curie, Paris, France

Abstract

In humans, spinal cord lesions induce not only major motor and neurovegetative deficits but also severe neuropathic pain which is mostly resistant to classical analgesics. Better treatments can be expected from precise characterization of underlying physiopathological mechanisms. This led us to thoroughly investigate (i) mechanical and thermal sensory alterations, (ii) responses to acute treatments with drugs having patent or potential anti-allodynic properties and (iii) the spinal/ganglion expression of transcripts encoding markers of neuronal injury, microglia and astrocyte activation in rats that underwent complete spinal cord transection (SCT). SCT was performed at thoracic T8–T9 level under deep isoflurane anaesthesia, and SCT rats were examined for up to two months post surgery. SCT induced a marked hyper-reflexia at hindpaws and strong mechanical and cold allodynia in a limited (6 cm^2) cutaneous territory just rostral to the lesion site. At this level, pressure threshold value to trigger nocifensive reactions to locally applied von Frey filaments was 100-fold lower in SCT- versus sham-operated rats. A marked up-regulation of mRNAs encoding ATF3 (neuronal injury) and glial activation markers (OX-42, GFAP, P2×4, P2×7, TLR4) was observed in spinal cord and/or dorsal root ganglia at T6-T11 levels from day 2 up to day 60 post surgery. Transcripts encoding the proinflammatory cytokines IL-1β, IL-6 and TNF-α were also markedly but differentially up-regulated at T6–T11 levels in SCT rats. Acute treatment with ketamine (50 mg/kg i.p.), morphine (3–10 mg/kg s.c.) and tapentadol (10–20 mg/kg i.p.) significantly increased pressure threshold to trigger nocifensive reaction in the von Frey filaments test, whereas amitriptyline, pregabalin, gabapentin and clonazepam were ineffective. Because *all* SCT rats developed *long lasting, reproducible and stable* allodynia, which could be alleviated by drugs effective in humans, thoracic cord transection might be a reliable model for testing innovative therapies aimed at reducing spinal cord lesion-induced central neuropathic pain.

Editor: Mohammed Shamji, Toronto Western Hospital, Canada

Funding: This research has been supported by grants from Institut National de la Santé et de la Recherche Médicale (INSERM), University Pierre and Marie Curie (UPMC), Agence Nationale de la Recherche (Contract ANR 11BSV4 017 04, TrkBDNFarmod), and Institut pour la Recherche sur la Moelle Epinière et l'Encéphale (IRME, Contract "M.Hamon, 2010–2011"). Saïd M'Dahoma was supported by fellowships from the Ministère de la Recherche et de l'Enseignement Supérieur (France) during performance of this work. The funders had no role in study design, data collection and analysis, decision to publish, or preparation of the manuscript.

Competing Interests: The authors have declared that no competing interests exist.

* Email: said.mdahoma@yahoo.fr

Introduction

Spinal cord injury (SCI) is a debilitating state which causes not only severe motor dysfunctions, loss of bladder control and impairment of sexual function, but also chronic pain, especially neuropathic pain [1,2]. Pain can be so severe that some SCI patients would be ready to privilege pain relief at the expense of further deficits in bladder control or sexual function. SCI-induced central neuropathic pain can be localized above-, at- or below- the level of injury and is mostly characterized by allodynia refractory to conventional treatments [2,3].

Several animal models of SCI-induced neuropathic pain have been developed (through spinal cord contusion, compression, ischemia, section; see [4]), each of them displaying different characteristics in terms of localization, duration, type of pain and even responses to drugs. Although some studies did provide relevant data regarding treatment efficacy and underlying molecular mechanisms [5–7], they focused mostly on pain below the lesion produced by contusion or clip compression of the spinal cord. Yet, despite the fact that these SCI models reproduce adequately some types of spinal cord injuries seen in humans, they suffer from limitations because of unavoidable, large, interindividual variations in the extent and severity of evoked lesions [8,9]. Furthermore, lesion-induced neuroinflammatory processes could be highly variable among SCI rats which underwent the very same lesion procedure [10], so that characterization of actual physiopathological mechanisms underlying neuropathic pain might be a real challenge in, at least, some SCI models.

In contrast to these models, complete transection of the spinal cord would be cleared of such limitations due to unavoidable interindividual variations in the extent and severity of the lesion. Indeed, spinal cord transection (SCT) has already been widely used to study the mechanisms of subsequent locomotor recovery [11–13] and reorganization of the somatosensory system [14–15] in medullary lesioned rats. However, to date, only few studies showed that the SCT model could be used to investigate spinal lesion-induced neuropathic pain [16], and, indeed, some authors even reported that no neuropathic pain develops in rats with complete SCT [17,18].

These discrepant data led us to reinvestigate whether or not the rat model consisting of complete SCT at the thoracic level could be a relevant model of central neuropathic pain, allowing studies of underlying physiopathological mechanisms and responses to drugs with patent or potential alleviating properties. Nocifensive responses to mechanical and thermal stimulations were assessed using the validated von Frey filaments test and the paw immersion and acetone drop tests, respectively. We then investigated whether responses to these tests could be affected by acute treatments with various drugs (opioids, antidepressants, anticonvulsants and others) known to alleviate neuropathic pain in SCI patients. Finally, we analyzed by real time quantitative RT-PCR, at different times after thoracic cord transection, the expression of mRNAs encoding proteins implicated in neuroinflammation and neuroplasticity, with particular focus on markers of microglia and astrocyte activation, pro- and anti-inflammatory cytokines (Interleukins IL-1β, IL-6 and IL-10, Tumor Necrosis Factor alpha, TNF-α), Brain-Derived Neurotrophic Factor (BDNF) and nociceptive signaling pathways in dorsal root ganglia (DRG) and spinal cord tissues, for comparison with previous studies aimed at unveiling physiopathological mechanisms associated with neuropathic pain in other SCI models.

Materials and Methods

Animals and Ethics Statements

Male Sprague–Dawley rats, weighing 225–250 g (7–8 weeks old) on arrival in the laboratory, were purchased from Janvier Breeding Center (53940 Le Genest Saint Isle, France). They were housed under standard controlled environmental conditions (22±1°C, 60% relative humidity, 12:12 h light–dark cycle, lights on at 7:00 am), on ground corn cobs (GM-12, SAFE, 89290, Augy, France), with complete diet for rats/mice/hamster (105, SAFE, 89290, Augy) and tap water available *ad libitum.* Before surgery, rats were housed 5 per cage (40×40 cm, 20 cm high) and allowed to habituate to the housing facilities without any handling for at least 1 week before being used. After surgery, all efforts were made to minimize suffering. In particular, SCT rats were housed under the very same conditions, except that each cage was for only two operated rats, so as to avoid as much as possible allodynic contacts between them. All animals were thoroughly examined each day, and in case of any sign of abnormal physiological alterations or suffering appeared, they were immediately sacrificed by a lethal dose of pentobarbital (150 mg/kg i.p.), strictly following the recommendations of the Ethical Committee of the French Ministry of Research and High Education (articles R.214–124, R.214–125). Both the Ethics and Scientific Committee of the French *Institut pour la Recherche sur la Moelle Epinière et l'Encéphale* (IRME; contract to M.H., 2010–2011) and the national (French) Committee for Animal Care and Use for Scientific Research (registration nb.01296.01; official authorization B75-116 to M.H., 31 December 2012) specifically approved the study.

In addition, the Ethical Guidelines of the Committee for Research and Ethical Issues of the International Association for the Study of Pain [19] and the Institutional Guidelines in compliance with French and international laws and policies (Council directive 87–848, October 19, 1987, *Ministère de l'Agriculture et de la Forêt, Service vétérinaire de la santé et de la protection animale*, permissions nb A752128 to S.M., 006228 to S.B., nb 00482 to V.K.) were strictly followed.

Spinal Cord Transection

Animals underwent surgery under deep isoflurane anaesthesia (3%). Paravertebral muscles were cut bilaterally and the T8 vertebra was opened using a gouge-forceps. Local anaesthesia was made by cooling the spinal cord with cryoflurane (Promedica, France) a few seconds before the lesion. Complete transverse section with ophthalmic scissors at the T8–T9 spinal cord segments level was performed following the procedure described by Antri et al. [11], then sterile absorbable haemostatic gel foam (Surgicel; Ethicon, Somerville, NJ, USA) was inserted into the lesion. Sham-operated animals underwent laminectomy only. At the last step of surgery, muscles were sutured and the skin was closed up by skin clips. Both SCT and sham-operated rats then received antibiotic treatments to prevent staphylococcic infection (oxacillin, Bristol Myers Squibb S.P.A., Italy, 0.3 mg/100 g s.c. once a day during 7 days) and urinary infection (gentamicin, Panpharma, France, 0.2 mg/100 g s.c., immediately after the surgery). No further treatment was administered to operated animals, to avoid potential interference with the development of allodynia and hyperalgesia. For recovery, SCT and sham rats were housed two per cage. The bladder of SCT rats was emptied manually once daily until reappearance of the voiding reflex (usually before the 10th day post surgery) (see Results).

Tests with Von Frey Filaments

Assessment of At-Level Mechanical Allodynia. For assessment of SCT-induced neuropathic-like pain in the cutaneous territory bordering surgery scar, rats were placed individually into a plastic cage (42×24×15 cm) and allowed to adapt to this environment for 1 hour before any stimulation. Tactile allodynia was then looked for with a graded series of von Frey filaments (Bioseb, 92370 Chaville, France) producing a bending force ranging between 0.008 g and 100 g. The threshold pressure to trigger a response (see below) was determined using the "up-down" method [20]. The stimuli were applied 3 times (3 seconds apart) for each filament, within a cutaneous territory of about 6 cm^2 just rostral to the lesion (see Results). When positive nociceptive behaviors, consisting of either a shake, an attack (filament biting), or an escape reaction [5,20], occurred, the next lower pressure-von Frey filaments were tested down to the filament producing no response. Then, the next higher pressure-filaments were applied back to the one triggering a response. The minimal force filament causing at least one of these responses (usually biting) allowed determination of the mechanical pressure threshold value. The 100 g filament, chosen as cut-off to prevent tissue injury, induced no nociceptive behavior in the majority (> 90%) of naïve rats. To avoid nonspecific responses, only these "non-reactive" rats were selected for surgery and included in the study.

Assessment of Mechanical Sensitivity in Body Territories Outside the Allodynic Area. SCT and sham-operated rats were also subjected to mechanical stimulation with von Frey filaments to assess evoked responses at the level of forepaws, hindpaws, vibrissae pad and other body territories outside the allodynic 6 cm^2 area just rostral to the surgery scar. For these tests, each rat was placed on a wire grid platform (5×5 mm mesh) under a small plastic (35×20×15 cm) cage for 2 hours, and mechanical sensitivity was determined with a graded series of 9 von Frey filaments (bending force of 4, 6, 8, 10, 12, 15, 26, 60 and 100 g). The "up-down" method [20] was also used at all of these sites. At paw level, stimuli were applied onto the lateral plantar surface of the right forepaw or hindpaw 3 times (3 seconds apart) for each filament. The minimal force filament for which animals presented either a brisk paw withdrawal and/or an escape attempt allowed determination of the mechanical pressure threshold [21]. Usually, the mechanical pressure threshold value to trigger a (non nocifensive) response in naïve healthy rats was around 60 g. Because SCT rats presented large time-dependent changes in mechanical sensitivity (see Fig. 1), higher pressures were also tested, with cut-off fixed at 100 g to avoid any tissue injury.

Assessment of Thermal Sensitivity

Paw Immersion Test. Because variations in skin temperature can affect the responses in nociceptive tests [22], we systematically performed control experiments that consisted of measuring hindpaw skin temperature just before the paw immersion test. The rat was left in its cage and a thermistor probe (Thermocouple thermometer Digi-Sense, Model N°8528-10; Cole-Parmer Instrument Company, Chicago, IL; 15 mm in diameter) was applied onto the plantar surface of hindpaw. Stable temperature readings were obtained after 10 sec with a precision measure of 0.1°C [23].

Thermal sensitivity at the hindpaw level was determined using the paw immersion test in both SCT and sham-operated rats [24]. Briefly, the right hindpaw was immersed into a water bath maintained at 46°C (Polystat, Bioblock Scientific, Illkirch-Graffenstaden, France) for heat stimulation or at 10°C (Ministat, Bioblock Scientific) for cold stimulation, and the latency to struggle reaction (paw withdrawal) was measured to the nearest 0.1 sec.

At-Level Cold Allodynia. Cold allodynia in SCT rats was assessed at day 15 post-surgery using a procedure slightly adapted from the acetone drop test described by Baastrup et al. [5]. Four drops of 10 μL acetone were gently deposited within two seconds all around the surgery scar in SCT and sham-operated rats. The number of trunk shakes and the time spent in escape or licking behavior were determined for one min after acetone drops application.

Pharmacological Treatments

Gabapentin and pregabalin were purchased from Sequoia (Pangbourne, UK). Amitriptyline, baclofen, ketamine and 8-OH-DPAT [(±)-8 hydroxy-2-dipropylamino-tetralin] were from Sigma-Aldrich (Saint-Quentin Fallavier, France). Other compounds

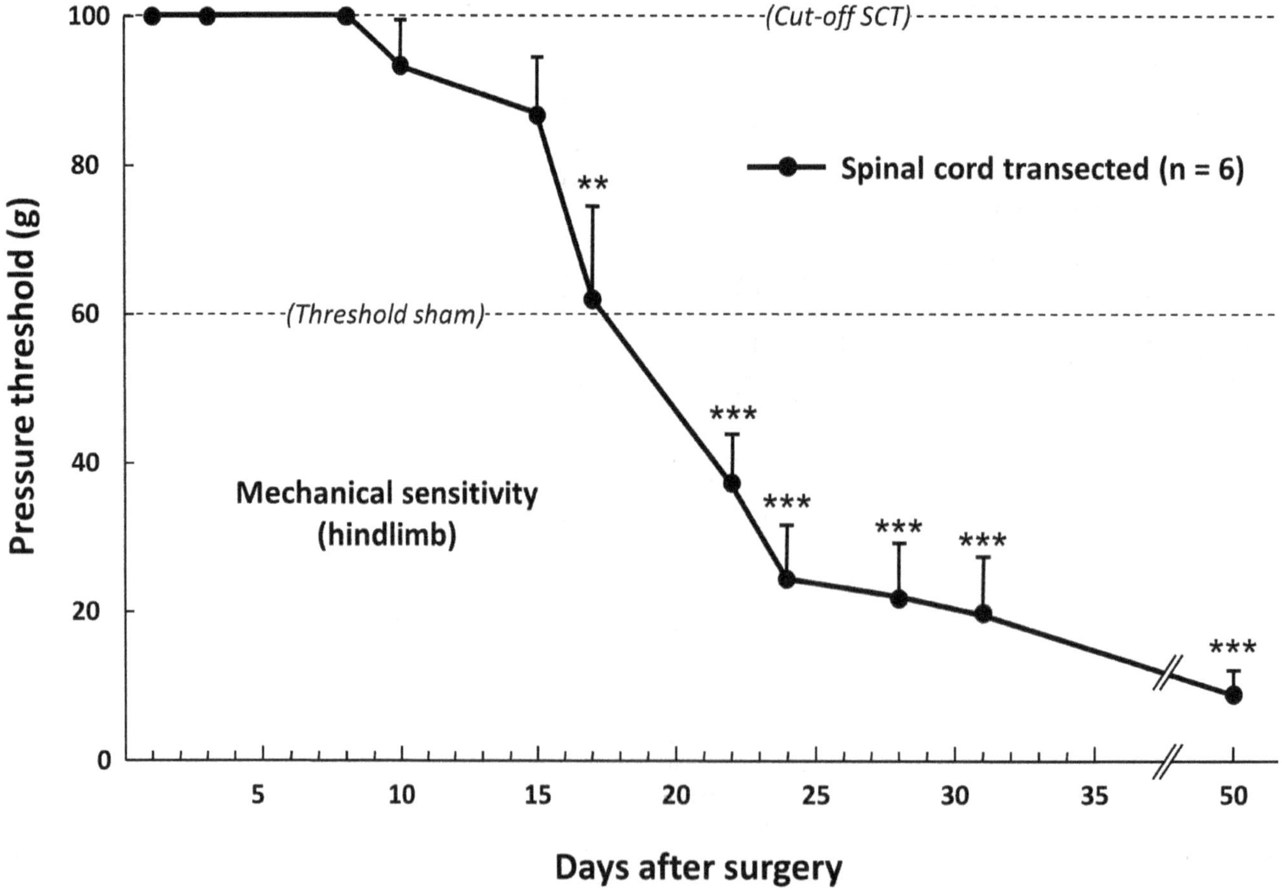

Figure 1. Time-course changes in the pressure threshold value to trigger hindpaw withdrawal in spinal cord-transected rats. Pressure threshold values were determined using a graded series of von Frey filaments applied onto hindpaw. Each point is the mean + S.E.M. of independent determinations in 6 rats. « Cut-off SCT » corresponded to the maximal pressure tested in spinal cord-transected rats; even at this high pressure level (100 g), no response of hindpaws was evoked for the first 9 days post-surgery. The « Threshold sham » corresponded to the minimal pressure (60 g) to which sham-operated animals start to respond by hindpaw withdrawal. ** P<0.01, *** P<0.001, significantly different from 100 g « cut-off SCT » value. One-way ANOVA for repeated measures followed by Dunnett's test.

were clonazepam (Roche, Basel, Switzerland), cyclotraxin B (BIO S&T, Montreal, Canada), morphine (Pharmacie Centrale des Hôpitaux de Paris, France), tapentadol (Grünenthal, Aachen, Germany), naratriptan and ondansetron (Glaxo Wellcome, Harlow, UK).

All treatments were administered between 2 pm and 4 pm. Routes of administration and doses (as free bases; see Table 1) were chosen according to previous data in the literature (see appropriate references in sections of Results and Discussion). All drugs were dissolved in saline (0.9% NaCl) except baclofen which was dissolved in dimethyl-sulfoxide (DMSO):0.9% NaCl (50:50) and clonazepam in ethanol:water (50:50). Drugs or their vehicles were injected acutely 30 days after thoracic cord transection, when mechanical allodynia had fully developed in the 6 cm^2 area just rostral to the lesion (see Results). For intrathecal injections (of ondansetron), rats were briefly anaesthetized with isoflurane (3% in air), and the needle (26 G) was inserted into the lumbar space between the L5 and L6 vertebrae [25] for administration of the appropriate dose in 20 µL of saline. Von Frey filaments test was then applied (by a skilled experimenter blind to treatments) at various times after acute drugs administration to determine the time course of drug-induced changes in pressure threshold value to trigger nocifensive response (biting of the filament, see Results), until the drug effect completely disappeared. In all experiments, only one treatment was administered per rat.

Real Time Quantitative RT-PCR Measurements

SCT- and sham-operated rats were decapitated at various times, from 2 to 60 days, after surgery. DRG, thoracic cord segments below (T9–T11) and above (T6–T8) the lesion, along with cervical and lumbar enlargements, were rapidly dissected out at 0–4°C, and immediately frozen in liquid nitrogen to be stored at −80°C. In some experiments, spinal cord samples were further sectioned by a medio-vertical cut to separate dorsal and ventral halves. Total RNA was extracted using the NucleoSpin RNA II extraction kit (Macherey-Nagel, 67722 Hoerdt, France) and quantified using NanoDrop. First-stranded cDNA synthesis (from 660 ng total RNA per 20 µL reaction mixture) was carried out using High Capacity cDNA reverse transcription kit (Applied Biosystems, Courtaboeuf, France). PCR amplification, in triplicate for each sample, was performed using ABI Prism 7300 (Applied Biosystems), TaqMan Universal PCR Master Mix No AmpErase UNG (Applied Biosystems) and Assays-on-Demand Gene Expression probes (Applied Biosystems) for targets'genes: *ATF3* (assay ID Rn00563784_m1), *GFAP* (Rn01460868_m1), *OX-42* (Rn00709342_m1), *IL-1β* (Rn00580432_m1), *IL-6* (Rn00561420_m1), *TNF-α* (Rn00562055_m1), *IL-10* (Rn00563409_m1), *BDNF* (Rn02531967_s1), *TLR4* (Rn00569848_m1), *P2×4* (Rn00580949_m1), *P2×7* (Rn00570451_m1). mRNA determinations were made with reference to the reporter gene encoding glyceraldehyde 3-phosphate dehydrogenase (*GaPDH*; Rn99999916_s1). The polymerase activation step at 95°C for 15 min was followed by 40 cycles of 15 s at 95°C and 60 s at 60°C. The validity of the results was checked by running appropriate negative controls (replacement of cDNA by water for PCR amplification; omission of reverse transcriptase for cDNA synthesis). Specific mRNA levels were calculated after normalizing from *GaPDH* mRNA in each sample. Data are presented as relative mRNA units compared to control (sham) values (see [21]).

Statistical Analyses

All values are expressed as means ± S.E.M. For von Frey filaments tests, the data were analyzed by one-way ANOVA for repeated measures (effect of a drug over time) followed by Dunnett's test. Statistical evaluations of SCT-induced changes in behavioral responses to thermal stimulations were made using the Student's t test. For qRT-PCR data, the $2^{-\Delta\Delta C_t}$ method [26] was used for analysis of the relative changes in specific mRNA levels and for graphic representations (RQ Study Software 1.2 version; Applied Biosystems). For analysis of the time course expression of the targets'genes, a two-way ANOVA was performed, followed by Bonferroni test for comparison of SCT rats versus respective

Table 1. Pharmacological treatments tested for potential anti-allodynic effects in spinal cord-transected rats.

Drugs	Pharmacological effect	Dose	Efficacy on biting behavior
Morphine	Opioid receptor agonist	1, 3, 10 mg/kg s.c.	+++
Tapentadol	Opioid receptor agonist and noradrenaline reuptake inhibitor	10, 20 mg/kg i.p.	+++
Ketamine	NMDA receptor antagonist	50 mg/kg i.p.	++
Baclofen	GABA B receptor agonist	10 mg/kg i.p.	+
Clonazepam	Benzodiazepine (agonist)	0.25, 2 mg/kg i.p.	-
Gabapentin	Blockade of calcium channel α2δ subunit	30, 100, 300 mg/kg i.p.	-
Pregabalin	Blockade of calcium channel α2δ subunit	30 mg/kg i.p.	-
Amitriptyline	Tricyclic antidepressant	10 mg/kg i.p.	-
Amitriptyline + Gabapentin	Tricyclic antidepressant + Blockade of calcium channel α2δ subunit	10 mg/kg i.p. +100 mg/kg i.p.	-
Cyclotraxin B	TrkB receptor blocker	20 mg/kg i.p.	-
Naratriptan	$5\text{-}HT_{1B/D}$ receptor agonist	0.1 mg/kg i.p.	-
Ondansetron	$5\text{-}HT_3$ receptor antagonist	20 µg i.t.	-
8-OH-DPAT	$5\text{-}HT_{1A/7}$ receptor agonist	0.25 mg/kg i.p.	-

+++: potent anti-allodynic effect (complete recovery of control mechanical sensitivity);
++: potent but short lasting anti-allodynic effect;
+: modest but significant anti-allodynic effect; -: inactive treatment.

(sham) controls at each time. The critical level of statistical significance was set at $P<0.05$.

Results

Physiological State of Spinal Cord Transected Rats

After full recovery from anaesthesia, SCT rats first showed hindlimb paralysis and flabbiness. Although they moved in their cage without major difficulty and could access food and water as readily as before the surgery, SCT rats stopped gaining weight for the first week after surgery (−6.3±3.8 g, mean ± S.E.M., n = 8), in contrast to sham-operated animals (+43±2 g, mean ± S.E.M., n = 8); but, afterwards, weight gain was parallel in both SCT- and sham-operated rats (+175.4±28.3 g and +171.2±12.5 g from day 7 to day 30 post-surgery, respectively, means ± S.E.M., n = 8 in each group).

Most striking symptoms were urinary retention and/or hematuria. Hematuria disappeared after 3 or 4 days without any specific treatment. To deal with urinary retention, we had to trigger off the miction reflex by rubbing the bladder once a day during 8–9 days on average. Then, the reflex recovered completely. It also happened that some SCT rats had an accelerated gut transit with diarrhea for the first 3 days post surgery. Later on, such gut disorders were only exceptionally observed. On the other hand, SCT rats had their fur a little bit more tousled than sham animals, but it stayed very clean in areas located both rostrally and caudally of the lesion site, most probably through grooming (that we regularly noted) by their cage mate. Abnormal suffering (with signs such as skin scratching) and/or autotomy were never observed when SCT rats were housed two per cage, as always used for these studies.

Immediately after the surgery and during usually 9–10 days, SCT rats showed paraplegia, first characterized by a total absence of reaction when hindlimbs were mechanically stimulated with von Frey filaments exerting pressure up to the cut-off value (100 g) (Fig. 1). This was followed by a hypo-reflexia which progressively vanished up to normal-like response (as in control unoperated rats) to mechanical stimulation which was usually recovered two weeks post surgery. Later on, SCT rats developed a hyper-reflexia with a pressure threshold value to trigger brisk hindpaw withdrawal strikingly lower (−80%) than that determined in sham rats up to at least 7 weeks post-surgery (Fig. 1). All along the observation period, SCT rats had paralyzed hindlimbs with spasticity, rigidity and tonicity. They also had frequent spontaneous movements of the tail and hindlimbs (shaking), and developed uncoordinated flexion and extension movements.

Development and Localization of Mechanical Allodynia

Among all the body areas tested, only the lesion site on the back and the hindlimbs (see above) showed altered behavioral responses in the von Frey filaments test in SCT- compared to sham-operated rats.

Within a few days after SCT, supersensitivity to mechanical stimulation appeared at the lesion site. From day 2 to day 9, such supersensitivity was mostly rostro-lateral to the lesion site within small areas on both sides (Fig. 2). Then, the supersensitive territory extended medially and laterally to cover an approximately 6 cm^2 cutaneous area just rostral to the thoracic cord transection. In contrast, no supersensitivity was detected behind the transection, and, indeed, SCT rats did not react even to a 100 g pressure exerted by von Frey filament applied within the cutaneous territory on the back, caudal to the transection.

Further assessment of supersensitivity to application of von Frey filaments within the 6 cm^2 area just rostral to the lesion led to identify three different aversive reactions: biting, shaking and escape (Fig. 3), in agreement with previous observations in SCI rats [5]. Determinations of pressure threshold values to trigger each of these behaviors showed parallel time-course decreases, down to very low levels that were reached 10–14 days after surgery and remained unchanged for the 7-weeks-observation period (Fig. 3).

Thermal Sensitivity

To make sure that no bias due to possible changes in skin temperature occurred in SCT- versus sham-operated rats, we first measured hindpaw skin temperature just prior performance of the paw immersion test, two weeks post surgery. Under controlled environmental conditions (with ambient temperature at 22±1°C; see Materials and Methods), hindpaw skin temperature was of 30.1±1.0°C and 29.8±0.5°C (means ± S.E.M. of 8 independent determinations in each group) in SCT- and sham-operated rats, respectively, indicating the lack of incidence of SCT on this parameter. However, clear-cut differences between SCT- and sham-operated rats were noted in withdrawal latencies after hindpaw immersion in cold (10°C) as well as hot (46°C) water. As shown in Figure 4A, SCT rats reacted with much shorter latencies compared to sham-operated animals, as expected of increased sensitivity to both cold and hot stimulation two weeks post SCT.

Further evaluation of cold hypersensitivity was made using the acetone drop test applied at the lesion site, where SCT rats developed mechanical allodynia (Fig. 2). As illustrated in Figure 4B, both the number of trunk shakes and the time spent in back licking and escape attempts for the first min after acetone drops application were significantly increased in SCT- compared to sham-operated animals (+67% and +400%, respectively).

Pharmacological Studies

Effects of Opioïdergic Drugs (Morphine and Tapentadol) on At-Level Mechanical Allodynia. As treatments with opioids were shown to reduce pain in humans with spinal cord lesions [27,28], we investigated whether morphine (1, 3 and 10 mg/kg s.c.) was effective to reduce at-level mechanical allodynia in SCT-rats. Acute treatment was performed 30 days after the surgery, when pressure threshold to elicit biting behavior in response to von Frey filament application had reached its minimum value (Fig. 3). As illustrated in Figure 5A, morphine exerted a dose-dependent effect: it was inactive at 1 mg/kg s.c., but increased pressure threshold value at higher doses, with complete suppression of allodynia-like response 30 and 60 min after administration of the highest dose tested (10 mg/kg s.c.). Confirmation of the anti-allodynic efficacy of opiate receptor activation was made with tapentadol, a mixed mu opioid receptor agonist and noradrenaline reuptake inhibitor with potent antalgic properties [29], which also reversed SCT-induced mechanical allodynia in a dose-dependent manner. As shown in Figure 5B, tapentadol at 10 mg/kg i.p. slightly increased the pressure threshold value, but the dose of 20 mg/kg i.p. completely suppressed allodynia-like response 30 and 60 min after its administration to SCT rats.

Effects of Ketamine on At-Level Mechanical Allodynia. Ketamine is well known to reduce pain in humans suffering from spinal cord injury, and its pain alleviating efficacy has also been reported in rat models of SCI, such as the one obtained by spinal cord contusion [30]. In SCT rats, acute administration of ketamine (50 mg/kg i.p.) induced a significant increase in pressure threshold value to trigger nocifensive response to von Frey filament application within the allodynic cutaneous area (Fig. 5C). At its maximum, 30 min after treatment, pressure threshold value reached 77.3±17.6 g (from 0.96 g±0.39 g before

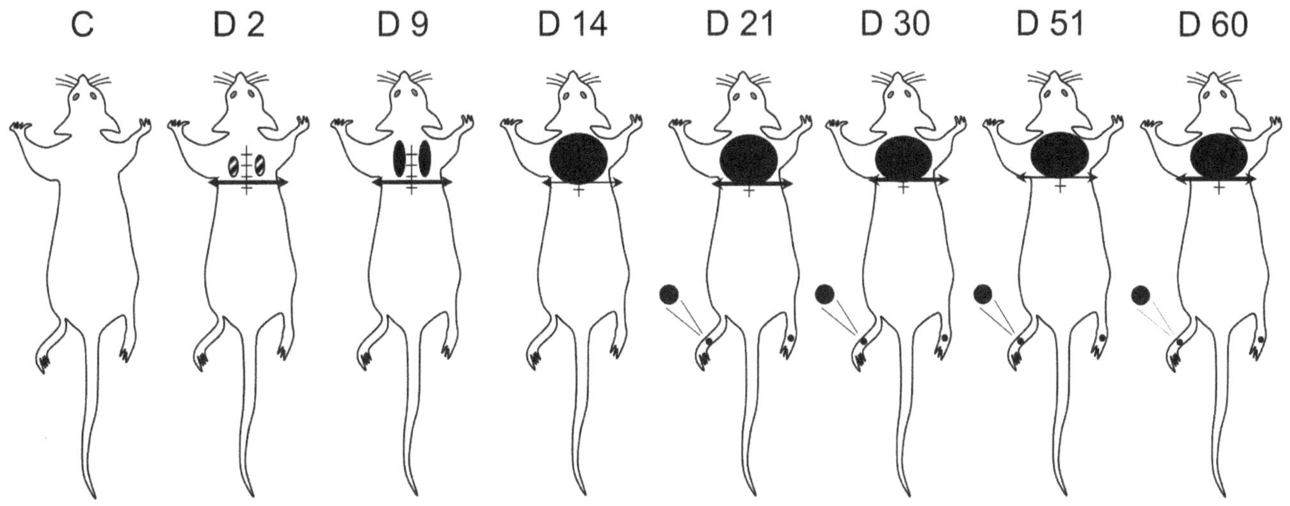

Figure 2. Body territories with increased mechanical sensitivity in spinal cord-transected rats. Pressure threshold values to trigger nocifensive responses were determined using a graded series of von Frey filaments applied throughout the body. Comparison with sham-operated rats (C) showed that pressure threshold values differed in SCT rats only in a limited territory (6 cm^2) bordering rostrally the spinal cord section (at T8–T9, horizontal bar with arrow heads) and in hindpaws (black areas tested), where reactions were obtained for pressure values significantly less than in controls. Time course (day 2 to day 60) changes in spinal cord transected rats showed that supersensitivity (allodynia) in the at-level area just rostral to the lesion was already detected at day 2 (D2) post-surgery, then extended and increased up to a plateau reached at D14 post-surgery. At hindpaw level, supersensitivity developed much later (from D21 post-surgery). Data were obtained in 8–14 rats at each time.

treatment, means ± S.E.M. of 6 determinations), which was not significantly different from the cut-off value corresponding to the non-allodynic state (in naïve rats, before surgery). However, this effect vanished rapidly because mechanical allodynia was completely restored 90 min after ketamine administration (Fig. 5C).

Effects of Baclofen on At-Level Mechanical Allodynia. Because baclofen, a GABA B receptor agonist, is often prescribed to reduce SCI-induced spasticity in humans, and is endowed with anti-neuropathic pain properties [31], we investigated whether this drug could reduce at-level mechanical allodynia in SCT rats. Indeed, baclofen induced a limited and transient increase ($p<0.05$) in pressure threshold value, from 0.6±0.4 g before treatment to 5.0±2.1 g 30 min after i.p. administration of this drug at 10 mg/kg (Fig. 5D).

Effects of Anticonvulsant Drugs on At-Level Mechanical Allodynia. The calcium channel blockers gabapentin and pregabalin and the benzodiazepine clonazepam are anticonvulsants endowed with anti-neuropathic pain properties both in humans [3,27] and in rodent models [32,33], and we tested whether these drugs also exerted anti-allodynic effects in SCT rats. In fact, acute treatments with either gabapentin (30 mg/kg i.p.), pregabalin (30 mg/kg i.p.) or clonazepam (0.25 mg/kg i.p.), at doses devoid of any inhibitory effect on locomotor coordination (as assessed using the rotarod test; not shown), had no significant effect on pressure threshold to trigger nocifensive response in SCT rats (Table 1). Some increase in pressure threshold values was noted with higher doses of clonazepam (2 mg/kg i.p.) and gabapentin

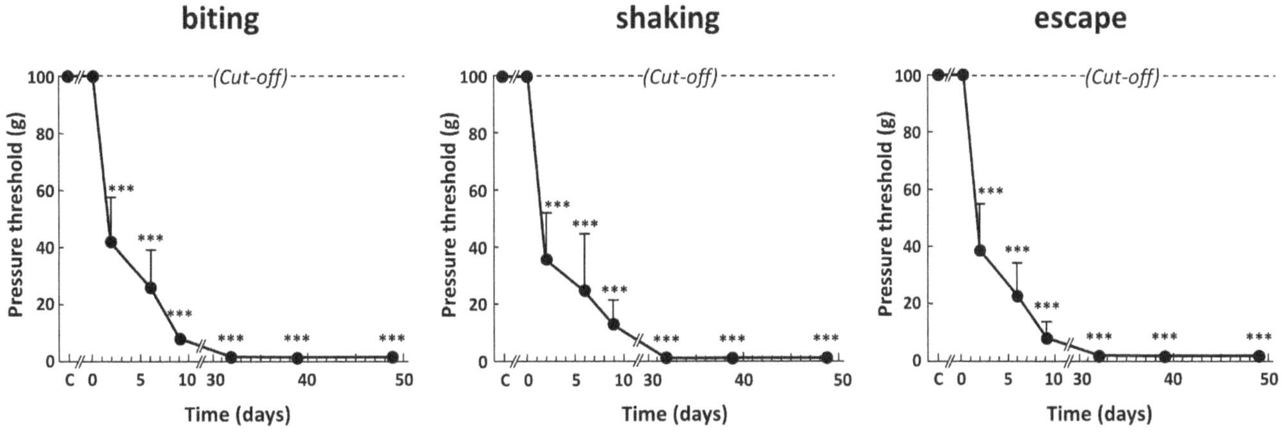

Figure 3. Time-course changes in nocifensive reactions to von Frey filaments application in the « at-level » allodynic territory rostral to the lesion in spinal cord-transected rats. Pressure threshold values to trigger biting (of the filament), shaking or escape were determined using the "up-down" method with a graded series of von Frey filaments applied onto the allodynic at-level area on the back at various times (in days) after surgery (0 on abscissa). Each bar is the mean + S.E.M. of independent determinations in 8 rats. *** $P<0.001$ compared to control (intact) rats (C on abscissa). One-way ANOVA for repeated measures followed by Dunnett's test.

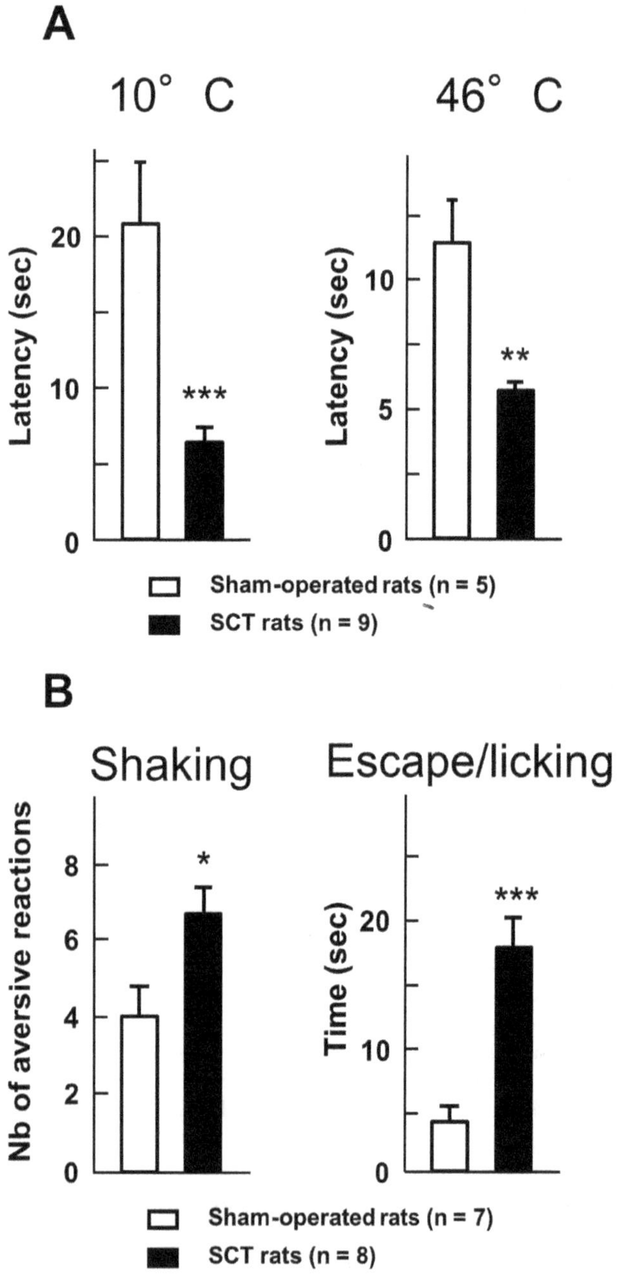

Figure 4. Hyper-responsiveness to thermal stimulation in spinal cord-transected rats. A – Latency (in sec) to hindpaw withdrawal was determined after paw immersion into a bath of hot (46°C) or cold (10°C) water, two weeks after the surgery. Each bar is the mean + S.E.M. of independent determinations in 9 SCT rats and 5 sham-operated rats. ** $P<0.01$, *** $P<0.001$ compared to respective values in sham-operated rats. Student's t test. **B** – Behavioral responses to the acetone drop test applied at the surgical scar two weeks after surgery. The number of shakes and the time (in sec) spent in escape attempts and licking of the back were measured for one minute after acetone drops application. Each bar is the mean + S.E.M. of independent determinations in 8 SCT rats and 7 sham-operated rats. * $P<0.05$, ** $P<0.01$ compared to respective values in sham-operated rats. Student's t test.

(100 and 300 mg/kg i.p.), but rats presented profound ataxia after such treatments (not shown).

Effects of Other Drugs on At-Level Mechanical Allodynia. As detailed in Table 1, the antidepressant amitriptyline, alone or combined with gabapentin, the anti-migraine drug naratriptan, the 5-$HT_{1A/7}$ receptor agonist 8-OH-DPAT, the 5-HT_3 receptor antagonist ondansetron, the BDNF-Trk B receptor blocker cyclotraxin B, at effective doses to reduce pain in validated neuropathic models in rodents [34–39], exerted no anti-allodynic effects up to 3 hours after acute administration in SCT rats.

Neuroinflammatory and Neuroplasticity Markers in Spinal Cord and DRG of SCT rats

Spinal Cord. A first series of determinations consisted of measuring the tissue concentrations of transcripts encoding the neuronal injury marker ATF3, the macrophage-microglial activation marker OX-42 and the astrocytic marker GFAP [21] in the dorsal and ventral halves of spinal cord segments just above (T6–T8) and just below (T9–T11) the surgery level in SCT- compared to sham-operated rats. Measurements were made at day 17 post surgery, when both mechanical (Fig.3) and thermal (Fig.4) allodynia had fully developed. As shown in Figure 6, expression of these three genes was markedly upregulated in both dorsal and ventral halves in segments above and below the section compared to sham-operated rats. Upregulation of ATF3 mRNA was slightly larger in dorsal spinal cord above and below SCT (×20.8- and ×21.1-fold, respectively) than in the corresponding ventral spinal cord segments (×15.7 and ×15.1-fold, respectively). On the other hand, no significant differences were noted between SCT-induced elevation of OX-42 mRNA and GFAP mRNA levels in the dorsal versus the ventral halves of spinal segments above and below SCT. Accordingly, no further distinction between the dorsal and ventral halves was made in subsequent experiments, and whole spinal cord segments were dissected out and processed for investigating the time-course changes in neuroinflammatory and neuroplasticity markers after thoracic cord transection.

As shown in Figure 7, already on day 2 post-surgery, ATF3 mRNA levels were 16.0- and 21.0-fold higher in thoracic spinal cord segments just caudal and rostral to the section, respectively, than in corresponding tissues from sham-operated rats. This up-regulation was long lasting as it persisted, but to a lower extent, up to the last observation day (×7.0 and 6.7 on day 60 post-surgery) (Fig. 7A). As illustrated in Figure 7A, a long lasting up regulation of ATF3 mRNA was also detected in both the cervical and lumbar enlargements of the spinal cord in SCT rats. However, this change was of much lower amplitude than in thoracic segments. OX42 mRNA levels were also markedly increased in thoracic segments of the spinal cord just caudal and rostral to the section on day 2 post-surgery (×6.2 and 4.8, respectively), and remained significantly elevated until day 60 (×2.8 and 2.5, respectively) (Fig. 7B). A long lasting up-regulation of OX-42 mRNA was also noted in both the cervical and lumbar enlargements of the spinal cord. However, it was of lower amplitude than in thoracic segments (Fig. 7B). The time course of SCT-induced changes in GFAP mRNA levels differed from those of the former two transcripts, as the observed up-regulation was delayed and relatively less pronounced (×3 at maximum) (Fig. 7C). However, these changes persisted to similar extents up to the last observation day (day 60 post surgery). In cervical and lumbar enlargements, only slight, generally non significant, increases in GFAP mRNA levels were observed in SCT rats, but they were also of long duration (Fig. 7C).

Concerning pro-inflammatory cytokines, a massive increase in IL-6 mRNA levels was observed as soon as 2 days after the section in thoracic segments bordering caudally (x 76.8 as compared to

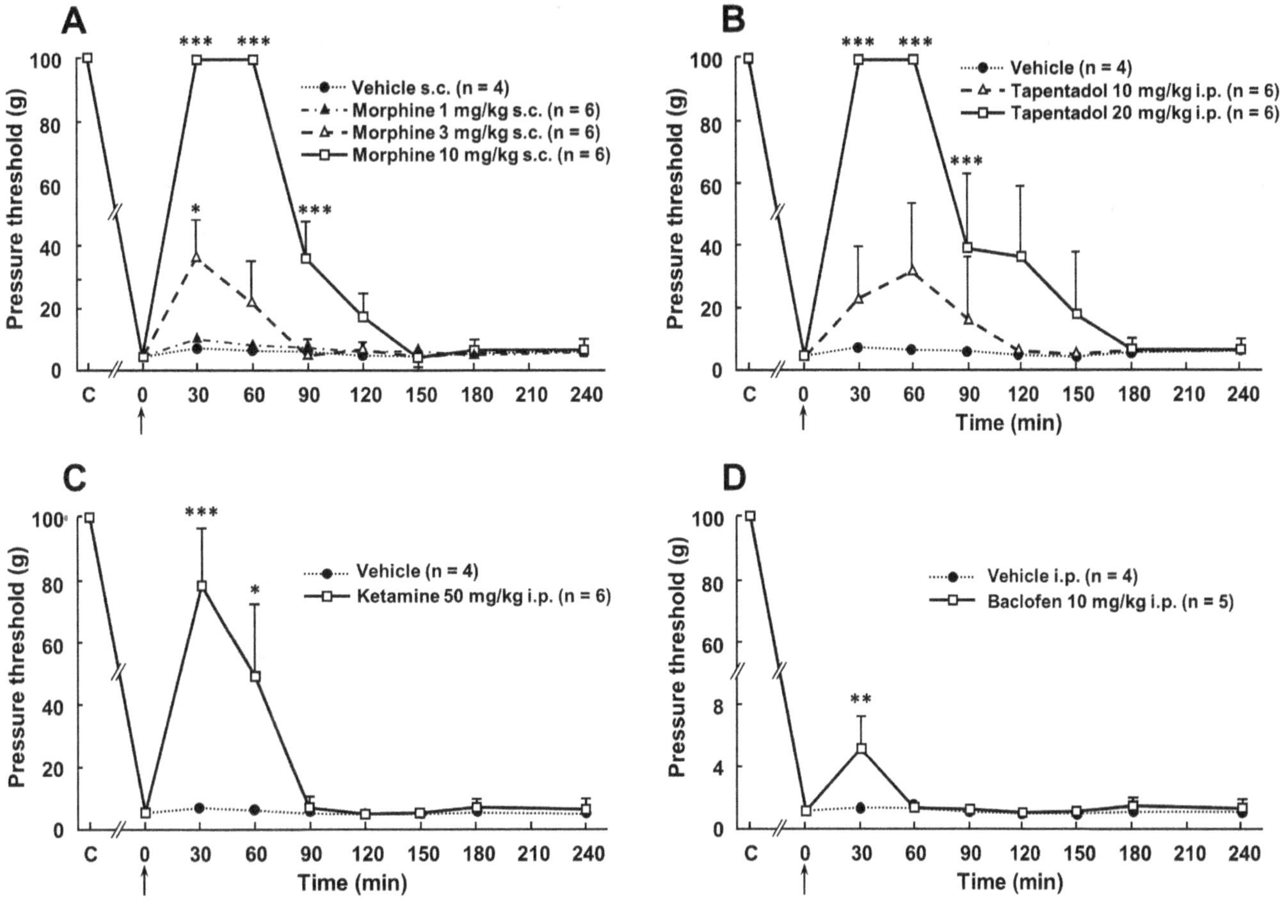

Figure 5. Anti-allodynic effects of acute administration of morphine (A), tapentadol (B), ketamine (C) or baclofen (D) in spinal cord-transected rats. Acute administration of morphine (1, 3 or 10 mg/kg s.c.), tapentadol (10 or 20 mg/kg i.p.), ketamine (50 mg/kg i.p.), baclofen (10 mg/kg i.p.) or their respective vehicle was performed (0 on abscissa, arrow) in rats whose spinal cord had been transected at T8–T9 level one month before. Pressure threshold values to trigger nocifensive biting were determined using von Frey filaments applied within the at-level allodynic territory at various times after treatment. Each point is the mean + S.E.M. of independent determinations in n rats. C on abscissa: Control (naive) rats (prior to surgery). P<0.05, ** P<0.01, *** P<0.001 compared to respective values in vehicle-treated rats. One-way ANOVA for repeated measures followed by Dunnett's test.

sham-operated rats) and rostrally (x 66.4) the section (Fig. 8A). A modest up-regulation was still observed on day 15 but not on day 60 post surgery. In contrast, no significant changes in IL-6 mRNA levels were detected in both the cervical and lumbar enlargements of the spinal cord at any time after SCT as compared to transcript levels measured in the same tissues of sham-operated rats (not shown).

The levels of IL-1β mRNA were also markedly increased 2 days after surgery in thoracic segments bordering caudally (x 172.2 as compared to sham-operated rats) and rostrally (x 98.6) the transection (Fig. 8B). Significant increases in IL-1β mRNA levels still persisted in caudal- and rostral-level segments on day 60 post-surgery, but to a much lower extent than on day 2. Similar but less pronounced changes in TNF-α mRNA levels were noted with a significant up-regulation in thoracic segments on day 2 post surgery (×3.0 caudally and ×1.9 rostrally to the section, respectively) (Fig. 8C). On day 60, a significant increase in TNF-α mRNA levels was still detected principally in thoracic segments rostral to the transection (x 1.9) (Fig. 8C). Finally, tissue concentrations of mRNA encoding the anti-inflammatory cytokine IL-10 were also markedly increased on day 2 after transection in both caudal-level (x 36.3) and rostral-level (x 38.7) thoracic segments, and an up-regulation of much lower amplitude was still detected on day 60 post surgery (Fig. 8D).

In contrast with the aforementioned transcripts, BDNF mRNA levels were reduced in spinal cord tissues of SCT rats, both on days 2 (−49% as compared to sham-operated rats, P<0.05) and 60 (−38%, P<0.05) post surgery in thoracic segments caudal to the section and on day 60 (−23%, P≤0.05) post surgery in thoracic segments rostral to the section (not shown). On the other hand, mRNAs encoding P2×4, P2×7 and TLR4 were upregulated in thoracic segments bordering caudally (×3.2, ×1.8 and ×3.8, respectively) and rostrally (×2.6, ×1.5 and ×3.6, respectively) the transection on day 2 post-surgery. This up-regulation was even more pronounced on post-surgery day 60 (×3.6, ×2.9 and ×4.5 caudal to the section, ×3.8, ×2.9 and ×5.6 rostral to the section, respectively) (Fig. 9A, 9B, 9C).

Dorsal Root Ganglia. Like that observed at spinal level, ATF3 mRNA was strongly up-regulated in DRG at T9–T11 caudal level as well as T6–T8 rostral level for the first two weeks after thoracic cord transection (Fig. 7A). Then, significant increases persisted up to the last observation day, two months after surgery, but to a lower extent, only in T6–T8 DRG (Fig. 7A). Transcripts encoding OX-42 (macrophages) and GFAP (satellite

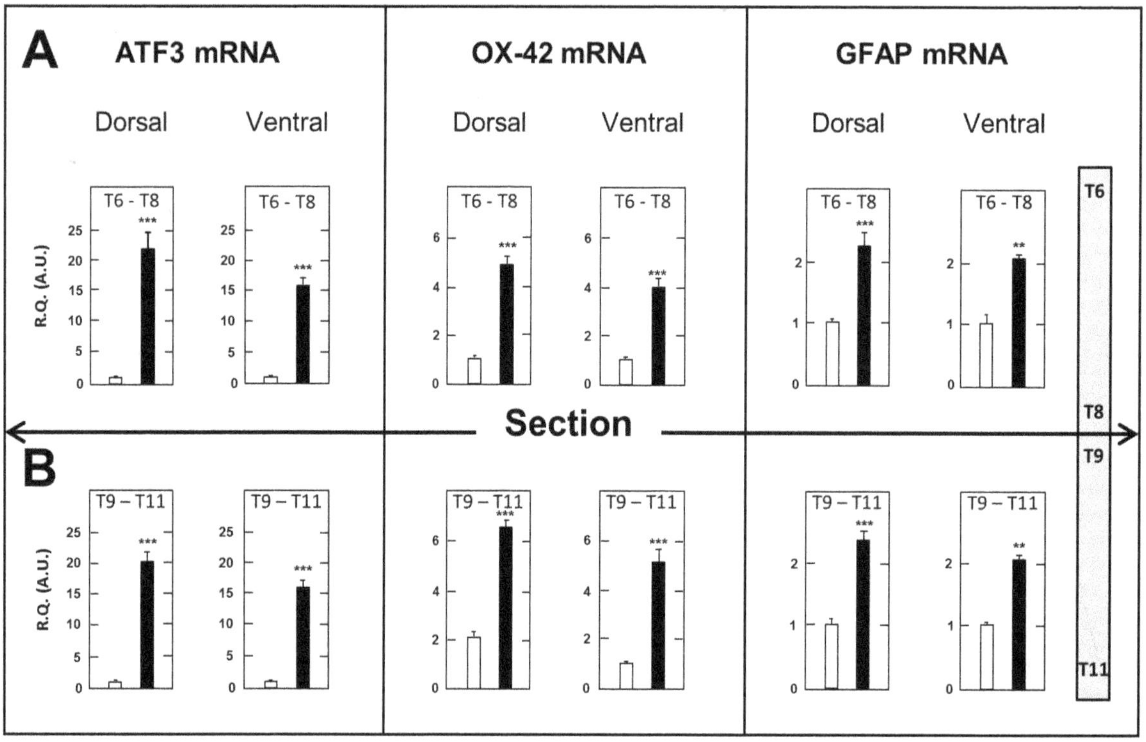

Figure 6. Increased expression of ATF3, OX-42 and GFAP mRNAs in the dorsal and ventral halves of spinal cord segments just above (T6–T8) and below (T9–T11) the surgery level in spinal cord-transected rats. Real time RT-qPCR determinations were made at day 17 after surgery. Data are expressed as the ratio of specific mRNA over GaPDH mRNA [R.Q.(A.U.)]. Each bar is the mean + S.E.M. of 10 independent determinations in both SCT (black bars) and sham-operated (empty bars) rats. *** P<0.001 compared to respective values in sham-operated rats. Two-way ANOVA followed by Bonferroni test.

glial cells) were also markedly up regulated in DRG at spinal cord segments caudal (T9–T11) and rostral (T6–T8) to the transection. However, this effect was transient, especially at rostral level (T6–T8) where significant increases in OX-42 and GFAP transcripts were noted on days 2–4 and up to day 9 post-surgery, respectively. At caudal level (T9–T11), up regulation of these transcripts lasted a few days more, but three weeks post-surgery, both OX-42 and GFAP transcripts no longer differed in thoracic DRG of SCT- versus sham-rats (Figs 7B,7C).

As illustrated in Figure 8A, mRNA encoding IL-6 also showed a dramatic up-regulation (x 65.6) in T9-T11 DRG at day 2 post surgery. Its levels then decreased rapidly, but remained significantly higher than in sham-operated rats up to day 9 post surgery (x 4.4; not shown). Interestingly, up-regulation of IL-6 mRNA was even larger at day 2 (x 145.0) and remained significant for a longer period (up to day 50 post surgery: ×1.6) in rostral level T6–T8 DRG (Fig. 8A, and data not shown). An up regulation of IL-1β mRNA was also noted in thoracic DRG at day 2 post-surgery (but not at day 60) in SCT rats (Fig. 8B), but this change was of much lower amplitude than that noted at spinal level. Also in sharp contrast with that previously noted at spinal level, TNF-α mRNA was not up-regulated in thoracic DRG of SCT rats, neither at day 2 nor at day 60 post-surgery (Fig. 8C). Finally, the levels of mRNA encoding the anti-inflammatory cytokine IL-10 were found to be slightly increased (x 3.1), but only in DRG caudal to the section (T9–T11) on day 2 post surgery, and at a markedly lower extent than in thoracic cord segments (Fig. 8D).

Further transcripts quantifications confirmed the existence of marked differences between DRG and spinal cord tissues. In particular, BDNF mRNA levels were significantly increased in caudal level T9–T11 DRG at both days 2 (×5.6, P<0.01) and 55 (×1.6, P≤0.05) post-surgery, but only at day 2 (×4.3, P<0.01) in rostral level T6–T8 DRG (not shown). On the other hand, mRNAs encoding P2×4, P2×7 and TLR4, which are all expressed by activated macrophages and satellite glial cells [40–42], showed no modification of their expression levels in T9–T11 DRG of SCT rats whatever the time after surgery. Similar negative results were noted in T6–T8 DRG except a modest but significant increase in P2×7 mRNA levels observed on day 2 post surgery (Fig. 9A, 9B, 9C).

Discussion

Spinal cord transection is a model widely used for the study of induced spasticity, hyper-reflexia and subsequent functional and structural plasticity underlying locomotor recovery under the control of the Central Pattern Generator [11–13]. Although neuropathic pain concerns a high proportion of SCI patients, only few investigations have been dedicated to alterations in pain signaling mechanisms in rats with complete SCT. Indeed, a large body of data has already been generated from studies in rodents with partial spinal cord lesion, but unavoidable interindividual variations in the severity and extent of lesion constitute serious limitations of such models (see Introduction). These considerations led us to thoroughly characterize the homogeneous model of complete transection of the spinal cord at thoracic level with regard to its possible relevance for studying central neuropathic pain, associated neuroplasticity changes and responses to drugs used to alleviate pain in SCI patients.

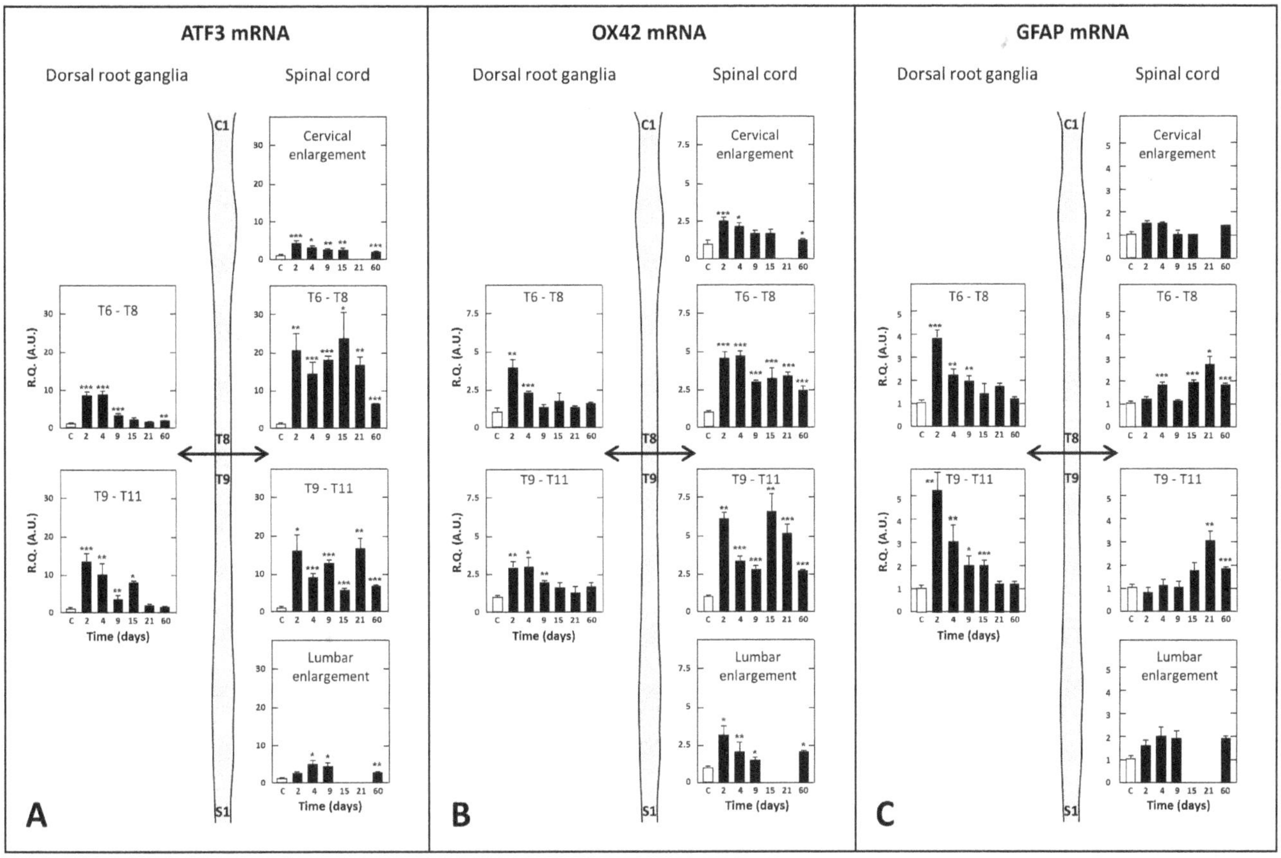

Figure 7. Time-course changes in tissue levels of transcripts encoding ATF3 (A), OX-42 (B) or GFAP (C) in dorsal root ganglia and spinal cord at various times after spinal cord transection. Real-time RT-qPCR determinations were made in T6–T8 and T9–T11 dorsal root ganglia, T6–T8 and T9–T11 spinal cord segments and the cervical and lumbar enlargements at various times (in days, D, abscissa) after spinal cord transection at T8–T9 level. Data are expressed as the ratio of specific mRNA over GaPDH mRNA [R.Q.(A.U.)]. Each bar is the mean + S.E.M. of n independent determinations (D2, D4, D9, D15, D21: n = 6; D60: n = 12). Sham values at every postoperative time are pooled under "C" (control) on abscissa. * P<0.05, * P<0.01, *** P<0.001 compared to respective values in sham-operated rats (C).Two-way ANOVA followed by Bonferroni test.

Clinical State of Spinal Cord Transected Rats

Despite complete transection of the spinal cord, rats showed a relatively good physiological state. The lack of micturition reflex and the hematuria, which are commonly encountered in paraplegic patients [43], usually resolved within 9 days post-surgery. Otherwise, their fur was clean, and very probably because they shared their cage with a congener, autotomia never occurred. Although rats lose weight for the first week after surgery, as a consequence of hindlimb muscles atrophy, they subsequently gained weight at the same rate as sham-operated rats, as expected from animals in good health [44].

Effects of Spinal Cord Transection on Hindlimb Sensitivity

Just after the lesion, hindlimbs no longer responded by a reflex motor reaction to cutaneous mechanical stimulation at high intensity (with the 100 g von Frey filament). Motor reaction then reappeared progressively up to a level corresponding to that found in control (unoperated) animals around the second week post-surgery. A marked hyper-reflexivity subsequently developed, along with spasticity, which reached their maximum approximately 7 weeks post-surgery and were still fully present on the last day (60) of our study. Marked alterations of motor reflexes also occur in humans with complete spinal cord transection, as evidenced by the exacerbated response in the H reflex of hindlimb muscles [45,46]. Such facilitated reflex responses may be due to α-motoneurons hyperexcitability [47]. Indeed, spinal cord transection causes an up-regulation of constitutively active 5-HT_{2C} receptors expressed by motoneurons, and the reinforcement of their membrane depolarizing influence has been demonstrated to contribute to motoneuron hyperexcitability in lesioned rats [48]. On the other hand, spasticity could also be accounted for by a down regulation of the potassium-chloride cotransporter KCC2 within the lumbar spinal cord below transection [12]. Although spasticity can be painful in humans, and below-level pain exists in patients with extensive spinal cord injury [2,49], hyper-reflexivity and spasticity at hindlimb level could not be related to pain behavior in SCT rats because completeness of the lesion prevented the nociceptive messages to reach the sensory cortex where they can generate pain sensation.

Along with mechanical hypersensitivity, SCT rats also developed heat and cold hypersensitivity as shown by the reduced latency of hindpaw withdrawal after immersion in water at 46°C or 10°C (Fig.4). Heat hypersensitivity has already been described in mice after spinal cord contusion and transection [50], and cold hypersensitivity at hindpaw level has been well documented in rats with contused spinal cord [51]. Whether or not similar neuroplasticity mechanisms underlay thermal and mechanical hypersensitivity at hindpaw level in SCT rats is a pending question to be addressed in future studies. In particular, because thermal hypersensitivity was evidenced from a motor response (hindpaw

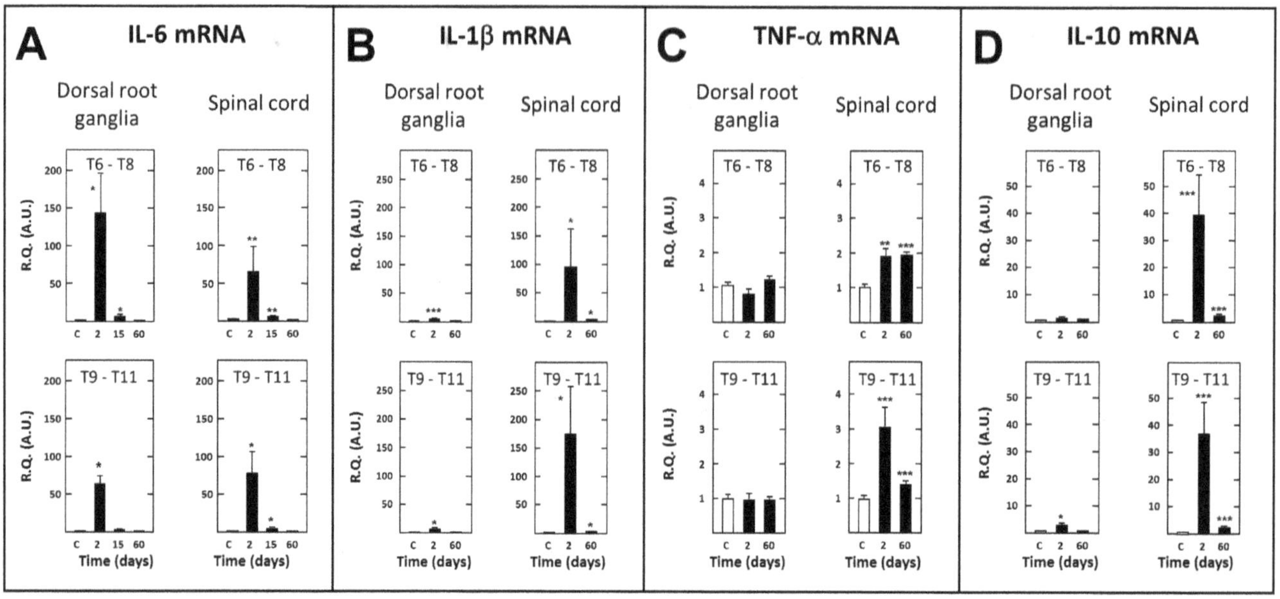

Figure 8. Short- and long-term changes in levels of transcripts encoding IL-6 (A), IL-1β (B), TNF-α (C) and IL-10 in dorsal root ganglia and spinal tissues in spinal cord-transected rats. Real-time RT-qPCR determinations were made in T6–T8 and T9–T11 dorsal root ganglia and T6–T8 and T9–T11 spinal segments at day (D) 2, 15 or 60 (abscissa) after spinal cord transection at T8–T9 level. Data are expressed as the ratio of specific mRNA over GaPDH mRNA [R.Q.(A.U.)]. Each bar is the mean + S.E.M. of n independent determinations (D2, D15: n = 6; D60: n = 12). Sham values at every postoperative time are pooled under "C" (control) on abscissa. * P<0.05, * P<0.01, *** P<0.001 compared to respective values in sham-operated rats (C). Two-way ANOVA followed by Bonferroni test.

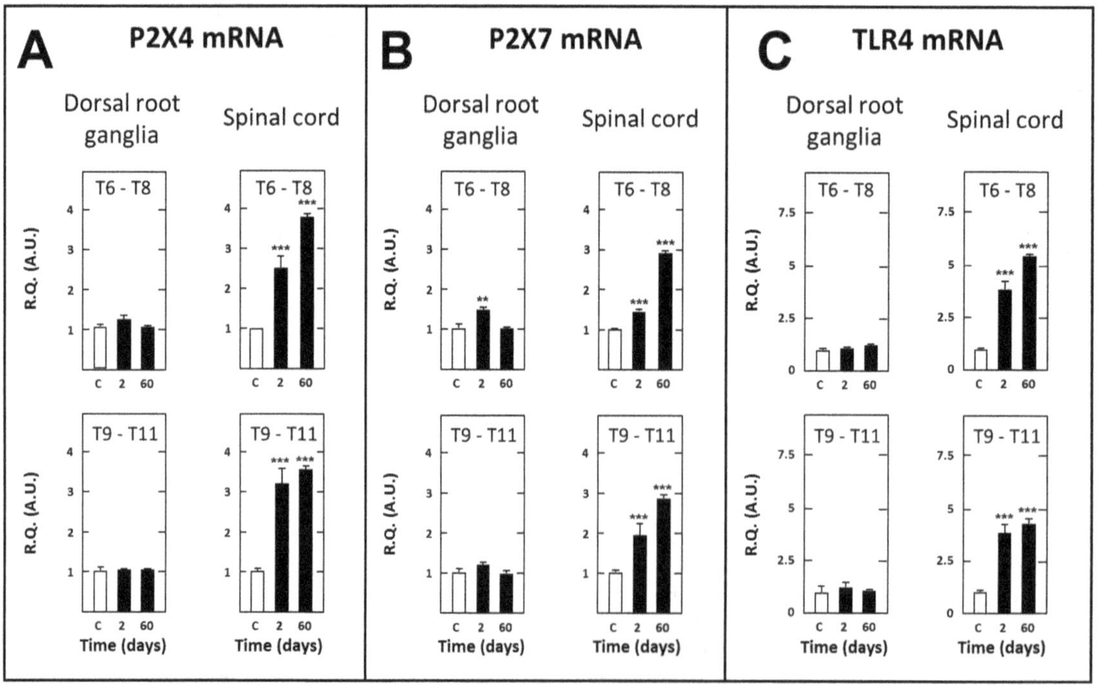

Figure 9. Short- and long-term changes in levels of transcripts encoding P2×4 (A), P2×7 (B) and TLR4 (C) in dorsal root ganglia and spinal tissues in spinal cord-transected rats. Real-time RT-qPCR determinations were made in T6–T8 and T9–T11 dorsal root ganglia and T6–T8 and T9–T11 spinal segments at day 2 or 60 (abscissa) after spinal cord transection at T8–T9 level. Data are expressed as the ratio of specific mRNA over GaPDH mRNA [R.Q.(A.U.)]. Each bar is the mean + S.E.M. of n independent determinations (D2: n = 6; D60: n = 12). Sham values at every postoperative time are pooled under "C" (control) on abscissa. ** P<0.01, *** P<0.001 compared to respective levels in sham-operated rats (C). Two-way ANOVA followed by Bonferroni test.

withdrawal), it might have also involved – at least in part - some α-motoneuron hyperexcitability as discussed above about SCT-induced mechanical hypersensitivity.

At-Level Allodynia

Whereas no behavioral reaction to the application of von Frey filaments within the trunk caudal to the lesion could be elicited in SCT rats, at-level allodynia-like reactions appeared relatively rapidly and reached a maximum 2–3 weeks after surgery. In particular, biting, which is considered as a brainstem response, and escape as a cortical response, were very probably associated with pain in SCT rats [5]. Since sham-operated rats did not develop such behaviors, we can exclude that they might have corresponded to musculoskeletal pain. Instead, at-level mechanical allodynia pain was very probably caused by spinal cord injury itself, as expected of neuropathic pain of central (spinal) origin [2]. Interestingly, 100% of SCT rats developed at-level allodynia, contrary to humans with spinal cord lesion and rats with spinal cord contusion as only a fraction of lesioned subjects suffer from such pain symptoms. Indeed, the prevalence for the rat/human to develop at-level pain depends on the extent of the lesion [52]. Such homogeneous data in SCT rats support the idea that the SCT model might be especially useful to assess the potential effects of drugs aimed at reducing centrally-evoked neuropathic pain and to investigate underlying physiopathological mechanisms.

Even though at-level cold allodynia is frequently seen in SCI patients [53], only few studies have reported this symptom in spinal cord lesioned rodents [5,54]. Indeed, according to Baastrup et al. [5], only 3% of the rats with contusion of the spinal cord exhibit clear-cut cold allodynia. In contrast, in our study, 100% of SCT rats presented at-level cold allodynia further emphasizing the usefulness of this model for improving experimental group homogeneity. A potential at-level heat allodynia could not be assessed in our studies because of the unavailability of appropriate equipment. Nevertheless, it can be recalled that using a Peltier device, Gao et al. [54] were unable to detect any heat allodynia in spinal cord contused rats.

Pharmacological Sensitivity of At-Level Mechanical Allodynia in SCT Rats

Only a few drugs among those tested were found to efficiently reduce at-level allodynia when injected acutely in SCT rats. The efficacy of morphine and tapentadol was probably underlain by the capacity of mu opioid receptor activation to inhibit the activity of wide dynamic range neurons in the dorsal horn of the spinal cord [55]. Interestingly, tapentadol had a somewhat more prolonged effect than morphine, may be because of its additional capacity to inhibit noradrenaline reuptake as this monoamine has been shown to be implicated in descending inhibitory control of neuropathic pain [56].

Ketamine also reversed at-level allodynia in SCT rats, in consistence with human data that demonstrated that this NMDA receptor antagonist is especially efficient to reduce allodynia in SCI patients [57]. This marked effect of ketamine, that may be sustained by a temporary inhibition of astrocyte activation, further supports the key role played by glutamate receptors, particularly NMDA receptors, in physiopathological mechanisms underlying neuropathic pain [58].

Finally, the last drug of the series tested which was found to exert some (but modest) anti-allodynic effects in SCT rats was the GABA B receptor agonist, baclofen, commonly used to suppress spasticity in spinal cord injured patients [59]. Spinal cord injury is known to be associated with a decreased tone of inhibitory GABAergic neurotransmission [7], and it can be proposed that baclofen transiently compensated for this deficit, thereby reducing allodynia in SCT rats. In contrast, clonazepam, which is used to alleviate SCI patients from neuropathic pain [27], was inefficient suggesting that GABA A receptor activation was ineffective to inhibit at-level allodynia in SCT rats.

Serotonin is known to play a major role in pain control via the activation of several receptor types [36]. Thus, F13640, a potent and selective 5-HT$_{1A}$ receptor agonist, appeared to be especially effective to suppress allodynia in spinal cord lesioned rats [60]. In our hands, the prototypical 5-HT$_{1A}$ receptor agonist, 8-OH-DPAT, did not reduce allodynia in SCT rats. Yet, this molecule is also an agonist at 5-HT$_7$ receptors, whose activation can result in effects opposite to that expected from 5-HT$_{1A}$ receptor activation [61]. Further studies with selective 5-HT$_{1A}$ and 5-HT$_7$ receptor ligands have therefore to be performed in order to reach a clear-cut conclusion regarding the potential modulations of at-level allodynia by serotonin acting at these receptors.

Because allodynia-like sensory dysfunctions are associated with migraine [62], we also investigated whether the anti-migraine drug, naratriptan, with potent 5-HT$_{1B/1D}$ receptor agonist properties [36], could alleviate at-level allodynia in SCT rats. Indeed, no effect was observed, possibly because triptans were found to selectively reduce neuropathic pain at cephalic level but not in extra-cephalic territories [35]. Finally, the last 5-HT receptor that we selected for our pharmacological investigations was the 5-HT$_3$ type whose implication in modulatory controls of neuropathic pain has been firmly established [63]. In contrast to the capacity of i.t. injection of ondansetron to attenuate neuropathic pain caused by spinal cord compression [64], this treatment was inactive in SCT rats, probably because complete transection of the spinal cord had suppressed the bulbo-spinal connections involved in 5-HT$_3$ receptor-mediated effects [38].

Under our acute treatment conditions, neither the antidepressant amitriptyline nor the anticonvulsants gabapentin and pregabalin, which are commonly used to reduce neuropathic pain in SCI patients [3], exerted any significant anti-allodynic effect in SCT rats (Table 1). Indeed, numerous studies showed that these drugs are effective only under chronic treatment conditions [39,65], and further experiments consisting of repeated administrations of antidepressants and anticonvulsants have to be performed before concluding about their effectiveness or ineffectiveness in the SCT rat model.

Finally, because BDNF and its receptor TrkB play key roles in physiopathological mechanisms underlying neuropathic pain [66,67], we investigated whether acute TrkB blockade by cyclotraxin B could affect allodynia in SCT rats. Indeed, Constandil et al. [34] reported that this drug can prevent and reverse neuropathic pain caused by peripheral nerve ligation in rats. In contrast, we found that cyclotraxin B was unable to reduce allodynia in SCT rats (Table 1), in line with RT-qPCR determinations which suggested that spinal BDNF expression would not be upregulated (in contrast to that observed in peripheral neuropathic pain models [66,67]) but rather downregulated after thoracic cord transection, as previously reported after other types of SCI in rats [68,69].

Neuroinflammation and Glial Activation in SCT Rats

The transcription factor ATF3 is induced when neurons are injured, and implicated in regeneration and plasticity [21]. Its role in the *maintenance* of central neuropathic pain is the matter of controversy, as it is no longer expressed when pain is still present after spinal cord injury [70]. However, ATF3 implication in the *induction* of central neuropathic pain is supported by data showing that it promotes the expression of the microglial/macrophage marker OX-42 and the astrocyte/satellite glial cell marker GFAP [71,72], two factors closely associated with neural lesion-evoked neuropathic pain [21,70,73–75]. Because ATF3 activation is triggered by cellular damages, and this transcription factor is able to repress its own promoter [71], the long lasting up-regulation of ATF3 transcript that occurred after SCT might reflect an ongoing neuronal damage associated with microglia activation. Convergent data in the literature showed that microglia activation is mediated, among others, by purinergic receptors [76] and Toll-Like Receptors [77]. Consistently, we observed, in thoracic cord segments just caudal (T9–T11) and rostral (T6–T8) to the transection, a long lasting (up to 60 days post-surgery) increase in the expression of mRNAs encoding P2XA, P2×7 and TLR4 receptors.

Numerous reports in the literature ascribe to activated microglia an important role in neuropathic pain consecutive to spinal cord injury [70,73,78], and the marked induction of OX42 mRNA in SCT rats is congruent with these data. In fact, IL-6, IL-1β, and TNF-α cytokines released from activated microglia can induce, by themselves, central (spinal) sensitization, thus maintaining neuropathic pain [79,80]. The huge induction of IL-6 and IL-1β that occurred on day 2 post-surgery suggests that these cytokines were involved more in the *induction* than in the *maintenance* of SCT-evoked neuropathic pain. In contrast, TNF-α would be more concerned by pain *maintenance* as SCT-induced up-regulation of its transcript in spinal T6–T8 segments was as pronounced at day 60 as at day 2 post-surgery. The strong increase in IL-10 mRNA that occurred shortly after the lesion might be linked to some inhibitory control of neuropathic pain for the first days after SCT, through the anti-inflammatory potency of this cytokine [81] and/or its neuroprotective effects in spinal cord injured models [82]. Overall, in contrast to that found in spinal tissues, none of the 11 genes studied were up-regulated beyond two weeks post-surgery in DRG above the lesion, supporting the idea that SCT-induced long lasting at-level allodynia did not involve some peripheral hypersensitivity but corresponded mainly, if not exclusively, to central neuropathic pain. Indeed, the short lasting induction of ATF3, OX-42, GFAP and cytokines encoding genes in DRG might have reflected some limited lesion of T8–T9 dorsal roots possibly occurring during surgery for thoracic cord transection. As a matter of fact, it has to be emphasized that our RT-qPCR determinations of time-course changes in mRNA levels will have to be completed by measurements of corresponding proteins in order to validate the inferences made above about the respective implications of pro-inflammatory cytokines and other neuroinflammatory markers in neuropathic pain-inducing mechanisms in SCT rats.

Within the spinal cord, GFAP mRNA up-regulation after SCT was delayed compared to that of transcripts encoding the pro-inflammatory cytokines IL-1β, IL-6 and TNF-α, in line with the idea that early production and release of these cytokines from microglial activation [83] leads to secondary induction of astrogliosis after injury [84]. That astrogliosis with an up-regulation of GFAP [74] - like that found in SCT rats - contributes to neuropathic pain after spinal cord injury is supported by the fact that pharmacological blockade of astroglia activation reduced pain in spinal cord-lesioned rats [73,85].

Conclusion

Spinal cord transection at thoracic level in rats appeared to generate a highly reproducible model of at-level neuropathic pain, mainly of central origin, suitable for pharmacological studies aimed at testing innovative treatments targeted specifically on spinal lesion-evoked neuropathic pain. Time course changes in mRNA levels of neuroinflammatory markers induced by the lesion supported the idea that both activated microglia and activated astroglia contributed to neuropathic pain in spinally transected rats. However, further investigations of these markers have to be made at protein level in order to determine more precisely the respective roles of both cell types in mechanisms underlying central allodynia in SCT rats.

Acknowledgments

We are grateful to pharmaceutical companies (Glaxo-Wellcome, Grünenthal) for generous gifts of drugs, and to Pr Guglielmo Foffani (Toledo, Spain) for helpful discussions.

Author Contributions

Conceived and designed the experiments: SM S. Bourgoin MH. Performed the experiments: SM S. Bourgoin VK S. Barthélémy CC FC DO. Analyzed the data: SM S. Bourgoin DO MH. Wrote the paper: SM MH.

References

1. Finnerup NB, Johannesen IL, Sindrup SH, Bach FW, Jensen TS (2001) Pain and dysesthesia in patients with spinal cord injury: A postal survey. Spinal Cord 39: 256–262.
2. Bryce TN, Biering-Sørensen F, Finnerup NB, Cardenas DD, Defrin R, et al. (2012) International spinal cord injury pain classification: part I. Background and description. March 6–7, 2009. Spinal Cord 50: 413–417.
3. Attal N, Cruccu G, Baron R, Haanpaa M, Hansson P, et al. (2010) EFNS guidelines on the pharmacological treatment of neuropathic pain: 2010 revision. Eur J Neurol 17: 1113–e1188.
4. Nakae A, Nakai K, Yano K, Hosokawa K, Shibata M, et al. (2011) The animal model of spinal cord injury as an experimental pain model. J Biomed Biotechnol 2011: 939023.
5. Baastrup C, Maersk-Moller CC, Nyengaard JR, Jensen TS, Finnerup NB (2010) Spinal-, brainstem- and cerebrally mediated responses at- and below-level of a spinal cord contusion in rats: evaluation of pain-like behavior. Pain 151: 670–679.
6. Baastrup C, Jensen TS, Finnerup NB (2011) Pregabalin attenuates place escape/avoidance behavior in a rat model of spinal cord injury. Brain Res 1370: 129–135.
7. Yezierski RP (2000) Pain following spinal cord injury: pathophysiology and central mechanisms. Prog Brain Res 129: 429–449.
8. Basso DM, Beattie MS, Bresnahan JC (1996) Graded histological and locomotor outcomes after spinal cord contusion using the NYU weight-drop device versus transection. Exp Neurol 139: 244–256.
9. Onifer SM, Rabchevsky AG, Scheff SW (2007) Rat models of traumatic spinal cord injury to assess motor recovery. ILAR J 48: 385–395.
10. Crown ED, Ye Z, Johnson KM, Xu GY, McAdoo DJ, et al. (2006) Increases in the activated forms of ERK 1/2, p38 MAPK, and CREB are correlated with the expression of at-level mechanical allodynia following spinal cord injury. Exp Neurol 199: 397–407.
11. Antri M, Barthe JY, Mouffle C, Orsal D (2005) Long-lasting recovery of locomotor function in chronic spinal rat following chronic combined pharmacological stimulation of serotonergic receptors with 8-OHDPAT and quipazine. Neurosci Lett 384: 162–167.
12. Boulenguez P, Liabeuf S, Bos R, Bras H, Jean-Xavier C, et al. (2010) Down-regulation of the potassium-chloride cotransporter KCC2 contributes to spasticity after spinal cord injury. Nat Med 16: 302–307.
13. Rossignol S, Frigon A (2011) Recovery of locomotion after spinal cord injury: some facts and mechanisms. Annu Rev Neurosci 34: 413–440.
14. Graziano A, Foffani G, Knudsen EB, Shumsky J, Moxon KA (2013) Passive exercise of the hind limbs after complete thoracic transection of the spinal cord promotes cortical reorganization. PLoS ONE 8(1):e54350.
15. Humanes-Valera D, Aguilar J, Foffani G (2013) Reorganization of the intact somatosensoty cortex immediately after spinal cord injury. PLoS ONE 8(7):e69655.
16. Santos-Nogueira E, Redondo Castro E, Mancuso R, Navarro X (2012) Randall-Selitto test: a new approach for the detection of neuropathic pain after spinal cord injury. J Neurotrauma 29: 898–904.

17. Hubscher CH, Kaddumi EG, Johnson RD (2008) Segmental neurtopathic pain does not develop in male rats with complete spinal transections. J Neurotrauma 25: 1241–1245.
18. Densmore VS, Kalous A, Keast JR, Osborne PB (2010) Above-level mechanical hyperalgesia in rats develops after incomplete spinal cord injury but not after cord transection, and is reversed by amitriptyline, morphine and gabapentin. Pain 151: 184–193.
19. Zimmermann M (1983) Ethical guidelines for investigations of experimental pain in conscious animals. Pain 16: 109–110.
20. Chaplan SR, Bach FW, Pogrel JW, Chung JM, Yaksh TL (1994) Quantitative assessment of tactile allodynia in the rat paw. J Neurosci Methods 53: 55–63.
21. Latrémolière A, Mauborgne A, Masson J, Bourgoin S, Kayser V, et al. (2008) Differential implication of proinflammatory cytokine interleukin-6 in the development of cephalic versus extracephalic neuropathic pain in rats. J Neurosci 28: 8489–8501.
22. Hole K, Tjølsen A (1993) The tail-flick and formalin tests in rodents: changes in skin temperature as a confounding factor. Pain 53: 247–254.
23. Kayser V, Elfassi IE, Aubel B, Melfort M, Julius D, et al. (2007) Mechanical, thermal and formalin-induced nociception is differentially altered in 5-HT1A-/-, 5-HT1B-/-, 5-HT2A-/-, 5-HT3A-/- and 5-HTT-/- knock-out male mice. Pain 130: 235–248.
24. Attal N, Jazat F, Kayser V, Guilbaud G (1990) Further evidence for 'pain-related' behaviours in a model of unilateral peripheral mononeuropathy. Pain 41: 235–251.
25. Mestre C, Pelissier T, Fialip J, Wilcox G, Eschalier A (1994) A method to perform direct transcutaneous intrathecal injection in rats. J Pharmacol Toxicol Methods 32: 197–200.
26. Schmittgen TD, Livak KJ (2008) Analyzing real-time PCR data by the comparative C(T) method. Nat Protoc 3: 1101–1108.
27. Fenollosa P, Pallares J, Cervera J, Pelegrin F, Inigo V, et al. (1993) Chronic pain in the spinal cord injured: statistical approach and pharmacological treatment. Paraplegia 31: 722–729.
28. Norrbrink C, Lundeberg T (2009) Tramadol in neuropathic pain after spinal cord injury: a randomized, double-blind, placebo-controlled trial. Clin J Pain 25: 177–184.
29. Tzschentke TM, Christoph T, Kogel B, Schiene K, Hennies HH, et al. (2007) (-)-(1R,2R)-3-(3-dimethylamino-1-ethyl-2-methyl-propyl)-phenol hydrochloride (tapentadol HCl): a novel mu-opioid receptor agonist/norepinephrine reuptake inhibitor with broad-spectrum analgesic properties. J Pharmacol Exp Ther 323: 265–276.
30. Bennett AD, Everhart AW, Hulsebosch CE (2000) Intrathecal administration of an NMDA or a non-NMDA receptor antagonist reduces mechanical but not thermal allodynia in a rodent model of chronic central pain after spinal cord injury. Brain Res 859: 72–82.
31. Gwak YS, Tan HY, Nam TS, Paik KS, Hulsebosch CE, et al. (2006) Activation of spinal GABA receptors attenuates chronic central neuropathic pain after spinal cord injury. J Neurotrauma 23: 1111–1124.
32. Yasuda T, Iwamoto T, Ohara M, Sato S, Kohri H, et al. (1999) The novel analgesic compound OT-700 (5-n-butyl-7-(3,4,5-trimethoxybenzoyl-amino)pyrazolo[1,5-a]pyrimidine) attenuates mechanical nociceptive responses in animal models of acute and peripheral neuropathic hyperalgesia. Jpn J Pharmacol 79: 65–73.
33. Wallin J, Cui JG, Yakhnitsa V, Schechtmann G, Meyerson BA, et al. (2002) Gabapentin and pregabalin suppress tactile allodynia and potentiate spinal cord stimulation in a model of neuropathy. Eur J Pain 6: 261–272.
34. Constandil L, Goich M, Hernàndez A, Bourgeais L, Cazorla M, et al. (2012) Cyclotraxin-B, a new TrkB antagonist, and glial blockade by propentofylline, equally prevent and reverse cold allodynia induced by BDNF or partial infraorbital nerve constriction in mice. J Pain 13: 579–589.
35. Kayser V, Aubel B, Hamon M, Bourgoin S (2002) The antimigraine 5-$HT_{1B/1D}$ receptor agonists, sumatriptan, zolmitriptan and dihydroergotamine, attenuate pain-related behavior in a rat model of trigeminal neuropathic pain. Br J Pharmacol 137: 1287–1297.
36. Kayser V, Bourgoin S, Viguier F, Michot B, Hamon M (2010) Toward deciphering the respective roles of multiple 5-HT receptors in the complex serotonin-mediated control of pain. In: Beaulieu P, Lussier D, Porreca F, Dickenson AH, editors. Pharmacology of pain. Seattle: IASP Press. pp. 185–206.
37. Kayser V, Latrémolière A, Hamon M, Bourgoin S (2011) N-methyl-D-aspartate receptor-mediated modulations of the anti-allodynic effects of 5-$HT_{1B/1D}$ receptor stimulation in a rat model of trigeminal neuropathic pain. Eur J Pain 15: 451–458.
38. Suzuki R, Rahman W, Hunt SP, Dickenson AH (2004) Descending facilitatory control of mechanically evoked responses is enhanced in deep dorsal horn neurons following peripheral nerve injury. Brain Res 1019: 68–76.
39. Vanelderen P, Rouwette T, Kozicz T, Heylen R, Van Zundert J, et al. (2013) Effects of chronic administration of amitriptyline, gabapentin and minocycline on spinal brain-derived neurotrophic factor expression and neuropathic pain behavior in a rat chronic constriction injury model. Reg Anesth Pain Med 38: 124–130.
40. Fellner L, Irschick R, Schanda K, Reindl M, Klimaschewski L, et al. (2013) Toll-like receptor 4 is required for α-synuclein dependent activation of microglia and astroglia. Glia 61: 349–360.
41. Inoue K (2002) Microglial activation by purines and pyrimidines. Glia 40: 156–163.
42. Inoue K (2006) The function of microglia through purinergic receptors: neuropathic pain and cytokine release. Pharmacol Ther 109: 210–226.
43. Singh R, Rohilla RK, Sangwan K, Siwach R, Magu NK, et al. (2011) Bladder management methods and urological complications in spinal cord injury patients. Indian J Orthop 45: 141–147.
44. Ramsey JB, Ramer LM, Inskip JA, Alan N, Ramer MS, et al. (2010) Care of rats with complete high-thoracic spinal cord injury. J Neurotrauma 27: 1709–1722.
45. Lotta S, Scelsi R, Alfonsi E, Saitta A, Nicolotti D, et al. (1991) Morphometric and neurophysiological analysis of skeletal muscle in paraplegic patients with traumatic cord lesion. Paraplegia 29: 247–252.
46. Calancie B, Broton JG, Klose KJ, Traad M, Difini J, et al. (1993) Evidence that alterations in presynaptic inhibition contribute to segmental hypo- and hyperexcitability after spinal cord injury in man. Electroencephalogr Clin Neurophysiol 89: 177–186.
47. Garrison MK, Yates CC, Reese NB, Skinner RD, Garcia-Rill E (2011) Wind-up of stretch reflexes as a measure of spasticity in chronic spinalized rats: The effects of passive exercise and modafinil. Exp Neurol 227: 104–109.
48. Murray KC, Nakae A, Stephens MJ, Rank M, D'Amico J, et al. (2010) Recovery of motoneuron and locomotor function after spinal cord injury depends on constitutive activity in 5-HT_{2C} receptors. Nat Med 16: 694–700.
49. L, Budh CN, Hultling C, Molander C (2004) Neuropathic pain after traumatic spinal cord injury - relations to gender, spinal level, completeness, and age at the time of injury. Spinal Cord 42: 665–673.
50. Hoschouer EL, Basso DM, Jakeman LB (2009) Aberrant sensory responses are dependent on lesion severity after spinal cord contusion injury in mice. Pain 148: 328–342.
51. Jung JI, Kim J, Hong SK, Yoon YW (2008) Long-term follow-up of cutaneous hypersensitivity in rats with a spinal cord contusion. Korean J Physiol Pharmacol 12: 299–306.
52. Hulsebosch CE, Hains BC, Crown ED, Carlton SM (2009) Mechanisms of chronic central neuropathic pain after spinal cord injury. Brain Res Rev 60: 202–213.
53. Finnerup NB, Norrbrink C, Trok K, Piehl F, Johannesen IL, et al. (2014) Phenotypes and predictors of pain following traumatic spinal cord injury: a prospective study. J Pain 15: 40–48.
54. Gao T, Hao JX, Wiesenfeld-Hallin Z, Xu XJ (2013) Quantitative test of responses to thermal stimulation in spinally injured rats using a Peltier thermode: a new approach to study cold allodynia. J Neurosci Methods 212: 317–321.
55. Wang J, Kawamata M, Namiki A (2005) Changes in properties of spinal dorsal horn neurons and their sensitivity to morphine after spinal cord injury in the rat. Anesthesiology 102: 152–164.
56. Millan MJ (2002) Descending control of pain. Prog Neurobiol 66: 355–474.
57. Kim K, Mishina M, Kokubo R, Nakajima T, Morimoto D, et al. (2013) Ketamine for acute neuropathic pain in patients with spinal cord injury. J Clin Neurosci 20: 804–807.
58. Niesters M, Dahan A (2012) Pharmacokinetic and pharmacodynamic considerations for NMDA receptor antagonists in the treatment of chronic neuropathic pain. Exp Opin Drug Metab Toxicol 8: 1409–1417.
59. Rekand T (2010) Clinical assessment and management of spasticity: a review. Acta Neurol Scand Suppl. 190: 62–66.
60. Colpaert FC, Wu WP, Hao JX, Royer I, Sautel F, et al. (2004) High-efficacy 5-HT_{1A} receptor activation causes a curative-like action on allodynia in rats with spinal cord injury. Eur J Pharmacol 497: 29–33.
61. Amaya-Castellanos E, Pineda-Farias JB, Castaneda-Corral G, Vidal-Cantu GC, Murbartian J, et al. (2011) Blockade of 5-HT_7 receptors reduces tactile allodynia in the rat. Pharmacol Biochem Behav 99: 591–597.
62. Aguggia M, Saracco MG, Cavallini M, Bussone G, Cortelli P (2013) Sensitization and pain. Neurol Sci 34 (Suppl 1): S37–40.
63. McCleane GJ, Suzuki R, Dickenson AH (2003) Does a single intravenous injection of the 5-HT_3 receptor antagonist ondansetron have an analgesic effect in neuropathic pain? A double-blinded, placebo-controlled cross-over study. Anesth Analg 97: 1474–1478.
64. Chen Y, Oatway MA, Weaver LC (2009) Blockade of the 5-HT_3 receptor for days causes sustained relief from mechanical allodynia following spinal cord injury. J Neurosci Res 87: 418–424.
65. Tzellos TG, Papazisis G, Amaniti E, Kouvelas D (2008) Efficacy of pregabalin and gabapentin for neuropathic pain in spinal-cord injury: an evidence-based evaluation of the literature. Eur J Clin Pharmacol 64: 851–858.
66. Merighi A, Salio C, Ghirri A, Lossi L, Ferrini F, et al. (2008) BDNF as a pain modulator. Progr Neurobiol 85: 297–317.
67. Trang T, Beggs S, Salter MW (2011) Brain-derived neurotrophic factor from microglia: a molecular substrate for neuropathic pain. Neuron Glia Biol 7: 99–108.
68. Hajebrahimi Z, Mowla SJ, Movahedin M, Tavallaei M (2008) Gene expression alterations of neurotrophins, their receptors and prohormone convertases in a rat model of spinal cord contusion. Neurosci Lett 441: 261–266.
69. Ying ZI, Roy RR, Edgerton VR, Gomez-Pinilla F (2005) Exercise restores levels of neurotrophins and synaptic plasticity following spinal cord injury. Exp Neurol 193: 411–419.
70. Carlton SM, Du J, Tan HY, Nesic O, Hargett GL, et al. (2009) Peripheral and central sensitization in remote spinal cord regions contribute to central neuropathic pain after spinal cord injury. Pain 147: 265–276.
71. Hai T, Hartman MG (2001) The molecular biology and nomenclature of the activating transcription factor/cAMP responsive element binding family of

transcription factors: activating transcription factor proteins and homeostasis. Gene 273: 1–11.
72. Block ML, Zecca L, Hong JS (2007) Microglia-mediated neurotoxicity: uncovering the molecular mechanisms. Nat Rev Neurosci 8: 57–69.
73. Gwak YS, Crown ED, Unabia GC, Hulsebosch CE (2008) Propentofylline attenuates allodynia, glial activation and modulates GABAergic tone after spinal cord injury in the rat. Pain 138: 410–422.
74. Gwak YS, Kang J, Unabia GC, Hulsebosch CE (2012) Spatial and temporal activation of spinal glial cells: role of gliopathy in central neuropathic pain following spinal cord injury in rats. Exp Neurol 234: 362–372.
75. Kim JY, Choi GS, Cho YW, Cho H, Hwang SJ, et al. (2013) Attenuation of spinal cord injury-induced astroglial and microglial activation by repetitive transcranial magnetic stimulation in rats. J Korean Med Sci 28: 295–299.
76. Marcillo A, Frydel B, Bramlett HM, Dietrich WD (2012) A reassessment of P2×7 receptor inhibition as a neuroprotective strategy in rat models of contusion injury. Exp Neurol 233: 687–692.
77. Kigerl KA, Lai W, Rivest S, Hart RP, Satoskar AR, et al. (2007) Toll-like receptor (TLR)-2 and TLR-4 regulate inflammation, gliosis, and myelin sparing after spinal cord injury. J Neurochem 102: 37–50.
78. Marchand F, Tsantoulas C, Singh D, Grist J, Clark AK, et al. (2009) Effects of etanercept and minocycline in a rat model of spinal cord injury. Pain 13: 673–681.
79. Chen K, Uchida K, Nakajima H, Yayama T, Hirai T, et al. (2011) Tumor necrosis factor-α antagonist reduces apoptosis of neurons and oligodendroglia in rat spinal cord injury. Spine 36: 1350–1358.
80. Guptarak J, Wanchoo S, Durham-Lee J, Wu Y, Zivadinovic D, et al. (2013) Inhibition of IL-6 signaling: A novel therapeutic approach to treating spinal cord injury pain. Pain 154: 1115–1128.
81. Genovese T, Esposito E, Mazzon E, Di Paola R, Caminiti R, et al. (2009) Absence of endogenous interleukin-10 enhances secondary inflammatory process after spinal cord compression injury in mice. J Neurochem 108: 1360–1372.
82. Zhou Z, Peng X, Insolera R, Fink DJ, Mata M (2009) IL-10 promotes neuronal survival following spinal cord injury. Exp Neurol 220: 183–190.
83. John GR, Lee SC, Brosnan CF (2003) Cytokines: powerful regulators of glial cell activation. Neuroscientist 9: 10–22.
84. Tian DS, Dong Q, Pan DJ, He Y, Yu ZY, et al. (2007) Attenuation of astrogliosis by suppressing of microglial proliferation with the cell cycle inhibitor olomoucine in rat spinal cord injury model. Brain Res 1154: 206–214.
85. Cronin M, Anderson PN, Cook JE, Green CR, Becker DL (2008) Blocking connexin43 expression reduces inflammation and improves functional recovery after spinal cord injury. Mol Cell Neurosci 39: 152–160.

10

Delayed Administration of a Bio-Engineered Zinc-Finger VEGF-A Gene Therapy Is Neuroprotective and Attenuates Allodynia Following Traumatic Spinal Cord Injury

Sarah A. Figley[1,2], Yang Liu[1], Spyridon K. Karadimas[1,2], Kajana Satkunendrarajah[1], Peter Fettes[1], S. Kaye Spratt[3], Gary Lee[3], Dale Ando[3], Richard Surosky[3], Martin Giedlin[2], Michael G. Fehlings[1,2,4]*

1 Department of Genetics and Development, Toronto Western Research Institute, and Spinal Program, Krembil Neuroscience Centre, University Health Network, Toronto, Ontario, Canada, **2** Institute of Medical Sciences, University of Toronto, Toronto, Ontario, Canada, **3** Department of Therapeutic Development, Sangamo BioSciences, Pt. Richmond, California, United States of America, **4** Department of Surgery, University of Toronto, Toronto, Ontario, Canada

Abstract

Following spinal cord injury (SCI) there are drastic changes that occur in the spinal microvasculature, including ischemia, hemorrhage, endothelial cell death and blood-spinal cord barrier disruption. Vascular endothelial growth factor-A (VEGF-A) is a pleiotropic factor recognized for its pro-angiogenic properties; however, VEGF has recently been shown to provide neuroprotection. We hypothesized that delivery of AdV-ZFP-VEGF – an adenovirally delivered bio-engineered zinc-finger transcription factor that promotes endogenous VEGF-A expression – would result in angiogenesis, neuroprotection and functional recovery following SCI. This novel VEGF gene therapy induces the endogenous production of multiple VEGF-A isoforms; a critical factor for proper vascular development and repair. Briefly, female Wistar rats – under cyclosporin immunosuppression – received a 35 g clip-compression injury and were administered AdV-ZFP-VEGF or AdV-eGFP at 24 hours post-SCI. qRT-PCR and Western Blot analysis of VEGF-A mRNA and protein, showed significant increases in VEGF-A expression in AdV-ZFP-VEGF treated animals ($p<0.001$ and $p<0.05$, respectively). Analysis of NF200, TUNEL, and RECA-1 indicated that AdV-ZFP-VEGF increased axonal preservation ($p<0.05$), reduced cell death ($p<0.01$), and increased blood vessels ($p<0.01$), respectively. Moreover, AdV-ZFP-VEGF resulted in a 10% increase in blood vessel proliferation ($p<0.001$). Catwalk^{TM} analysis showed AdV-ZFP-VEGF treatment dramatically improves hindlimb weight support ($p<0.05$) and increases hindlimb swing speed ($p<0.02$) when compared to control animals. Finally, AdV-ZFP-VEGF administration provided a significant reduction in allodynia ($p<0.01$). Overall, the results of this study indicate that AdV-ZFP-VEGF administration can be delivered in a clinically relevant time-window following SCI (24 hours) and provide significant molecular and functional benefits.

Editor: Hatem E. Sabaawy, Rutgers-Robert wood Johnson Medical School, United States of America

Funding: This study was supported by Sangamo BioSciences and the Krembil Chair in Neural Repair and Regeneration (held by Dr. Michael G. Fehlings). The funders had no role in data collection, data analysis, or decision to publish; however, they did participate in some aspects of study design and reviewed the manuscript prior to publication.

Competing Interests: The personnel associated with Sangamo Biosciences, Inc. – Kaye Spratt, Gary Lee, Dale Ando, Richard Surosky and Martin Giedlin – fully disclose a conflict of interest related to this research. Each individual is an employee of Sangamo Biosciences, Inc. and receives either a salary and/or ownership interest (stock, stock options, patent or other intellectual property). Sarah Figley, Yang Liu, Spyridon Karadimas and Michael Fehlings disclose that research support (receipt of therapeutics, supplies and equipment) was provided by Sangamo Biosciences, Inc. for the experiments conducted in this manuscript.

* E-mail: michael.fehlings@uhn.on.ca

Introduction

In North America, it is estimated that approximately 1.5 million individuals are currently living with SCI, with over 12,000 traumatic SCI cases occurring each year [1]. Spinal cord injury is divided into two events, to separate the physical and the cellular pathologies. The primary injury, is associated with the initial mechanical trauma that the cord undergoes, whereas the secondary injury refers to the physiological cascade that propagates from 1 minute to 6 months following the initial injury [2]. Although the primary injury is responsible for triggering all of the downstream events, it is widely accepted that the processes that take place in the "secondary injury" phase are predominantly responsible for a significant portion of the damage and degeneration that is associated with SCI, including inflammation, ischemia, lipid peroxidation, production of free radicals, disruption of ion channels, necrosis and programmed cell death [3–5]. Moreover, radical alterations to the spinal microvascular architecture and function occur following SCI and contribute to the secondary injury. Reduction in blood flow, hemorrhage, systemic hypotension, loss of microcirculation, disruption of the blood-spinal cord barrier (BSCB) and loss of structural organization, ultimately enhance the cellular damage post-injury [2,6]. Despite the fact that these secondary events are responsible for the majority of the damage associated with SCI, many of these pathways alternatively provide an opportunity to target with therapeutic interventions.

Recently, research has given much attention to therapies designed at repairing or minimizing vascular damage following injury. Angiogenic factors, such as vascular endothelial growth factor (VEGF)-A, are known to promote the proliferation of endothelial cells and initiate angiogenesis [7]. Emerging evidence suggests that VEGF-A (which will be referred to as VEGF) also has neurotrophic, neuroprotective, and neuroproliferative effects [8]. VEGF is a homodimeric glycoprotein that is expressed as multiple splice variants encoded by a single gene; however, VEGF signals as a homo- or heterodimer via VEGF receptors (VEGFRs) [9]. The predominant isoforms in the central nervous system are $VEGF_{121}$, $VEGF_{165}$ and $VEGF_{189}$. Studies have demonstrated that VEGF and its receptors are upregulated during and after hypoxic/ischemic injury to the brain and spinal cord, which suggests that VEGF likely plays a neuroprotective (or beneficial) role in these pathophysiological processes.

Perhaps the most devastating outcomes of spinal cord injury are paralysis and neuropathic pain. Paralysis is caused by damaged axons and neurons in motor pathways at or above the level of injury. Many models of SCI have been used to model the physical deficits post-injury, and thoracic injuries are among the best-characterized for the targets loss of hindlimb function. Motor impairment following SCI results from damage to and/or loss of both upper and lower motor neurons. Injury to first and second order spinothalamic neurons, or first order neurons from the medial lemniscus pathway, interrupts sensory information processing *at* and *below* the level of injury and prevents normal signal transmission to the brain. Miscommunication in sensory pathways can result in severe complications for patients suffering from SCI. Development of neuropathic pain occurs in many patients, and although the exact mechanism is unknown, it is hypothesized that it is caused by misguided axonal sprouting or abnormal sodium channel excitability in sensory neurons [10].

Previously described approaches using VEGF have relied on the introduction of a single splice isoform of VEGF-A ($VEGF_{165}$), which may not result in optimal neuroprotective or angiogenic effects. In this study, we utilize novel ZFP-VEGF technology – a viral vector encoding a zinc-finger transcription factor protein (ZFP), which activates endogenous VEGF-A expression to produce multiple splice isoforms of VEGF – which has previously demonstrated induced expression of VEGF-A protein, increase vascular counts and significant functional recovery following SCI [11]. Although we have already shown beneficial effects of AdV-ZFP-VEGF when administered immediately following SCI as a proof-of-concept, the current study aims to investigate a clinically-relevant administration of AdV-ZFP-VEGF by ***delaying*** administration by 24 hours post-SCI.

Materials and Methods

All animal experiments were conducted with approval from the Animal Care Committee, University Health Network (Toronto, Canada).

Viral Vector Constructs

The VEGF-A-activating ZFP and controls were provided in viral vectors by Sangamo BioSciences (Pt. Richmond, CA) and have been previously described [12,13]. The VEGF-A-activating ZFP (32E-p65) – referred to as AdV-ZFP-VEGF – is a 378 amino acid multi-domain protein that is composed of three functional regions: (1) the nuclear localization signal (NLS) of the large T-antigen of SV40, (2) a designed 3-finger zinc-fingered protein (32E) that binds to a 9 base-pair target DNA sequence (GGGGGTGAC) present in the human VEGF-A promoter region and (3) the transactivation domain from the p65 subunit of human NFκB, which is identical to VZ+434, subcloned into pVAX1 (Invitrogen, San Diego, CA) with expression driven by the human cytomegalovirus (CMV) promoter. Adenoviral (Ad5-32Ep65 or Ad5- eGFP) vectors, referred to as AdV-ZFP-VEGF and AdV-eGFP, respectively, were packaged by transfecting T-REx-293 cells (Invitrogen, San Diego, CA). T-REx-293 cells in ten-stack cell factories were inoculated with Ad vectors at a multiplicity of infection (MOI) of 50 to 100 particles per cell. When adenoviral mediated cytopathy effect (CPE) was observed, cells were harvested and lysed by three cycles of freezing and thawing. Crude lysates were clarified by centrifugation, and 293 cells were seeded at 4×10^7 PFU and grown 3 days prior to transfection. The calcium phosphate method was used for transfection. Infectious titers of the Ad vectors were quantified using the Adeno-X Rapid Titer kit (Clontech, Mountain View, CA).

SCI and Intraspinal Microinjection

Animals were subject to a compressive spinal cord injury using a modified aneurysm clip, which has been extensively characterized by our laboratory and previously described [14]. Briefly, adult female Wistar rats (250–300 g; Charles River, Montreal, Canada) were deeply anesthetized using 4% isoflurane, and were sedated for the remainder of the surgery under 2% isoflurane. Animals received a two-level laminectomy of mid-thoracic vertebral segments T6–T7. A modified clip calibrated to a closing force of 35 g was applied extradurally to the cord for 1 minute and then removed. The animals were divided into four groups in a randomized and "blinded" manner, (1) Sham control group (laminectomy only – no SCI), (2) Non-injected injured control group (laminectomy and SCI – no injection), (3) AdV -ZFP-VEGF treatment group, and (4) AdV-eGFP control group. Using a stereotaxic frame and glass capillary needle (tip diameter 60 μm) connected to a Hamilton microsyringe, a total of 5×10^8 viral plaque forming units (PFU) were injected into the dorsal spinal cord 24 hours post-SCI. Four 2.5 μl (10 μl total) intraspinal injections were made bilaterally at 2 mm rostral and caudal of the injury site. The injection rate is 0.60 μl/min and when the injection was completed, the capillary needle was left in the cord for at least 1 min to allow diffusion of the virus from the injection site and to prevent back-flow. The incision was closed in layers using standard silk sutures and animals were given a single dose of buprenorphine (0.05 mg/kg). Animals were allowed to recover in their cage under a heat-lamp and, subsequently, were housed in a temperature-controlled warm room (26°C) with free access to food and water. Animals were given buprenorphine (0.05 mg/kg) every 12 hours for 48 hours following surgery, and their bladders were manually voided three times daily. A subcutaneous injection of 10 mg/kg of cyclosporin A was administered daily starting 24 hours prior to the SCI until the end of the experiments for immunosuppression.

Western Blotting

Following deep inhalation anesthetic, animals (n = 4–5/group) were sacrificed at five or ten days post-SCI and a 5 mm length of the spinal cord centered at the injury site was extracted. Samples were mechanically homogenized in 400 μl of homogenization buffer (0.1 M Tris, 0.5 M EDTA, 0.1% SDS, 1 M DTT solution, 100 mM PMSF, 1.7 mg/ml aprotinin, 1 mM pepstatin, 10 mM leupeptin) and centrifuged at 15,000 rpm for 10 minutes at 4°C. Supernatants were extracted and used for western blot analysis, where 20 μg of protein was loaded into 7.5% or 12% polyacrylamide gels (Bio-Rad, Mississauga, Canada). Membranes were probed with either monoclonal anti-NF200 antibody (1:2000; Sigma, Oakville, Canada), rabbit IgG anti-VEGF-A antibody

(1:100; Santa Cruz Biotechnology, Santa Cruz, CA), or rabbit IgG anti-NFκBp65 (1:1000; Santa Cruz Biotechnology, Santa Cruz, CA). NFκBp65 rabbit polyclonal antibody was used to recognize the p65 activation domain in the ZFP-VEGF treated animals. Primary antibodies were labelled with horseradish peroxidase-conjugated secondary antibodies (goat anti-mouse/rabbit IgG, 1:3000; Jackson Immuno Research Laboratories, West Grove, PA), and bands were imaged using an enhanced chemiluminescence (ECL) detection system (Perkin Elmer, Woodbridge, Canada). Mouse monoclonal, beta-actin (Chemicon International, Inc., Temecula, CA) was immunoblotted as a loading control. Quality One detection software (Bio-Rad Laboratories, Hercules, CA) was used for integrated optical density (OD) analysis.

Histochemistry

Histological Processing. Five or 10 days (n = 4–5/group), or 8 weeks (n = 10/group) post-SCI, following deep inhalation anesthetic, animals were transcardially perfused with 4% paraformaldehyde (PFA) in 0.1 M PBS. Then, the tissues were cryoprotected in 20% sucrose in PBS. A 10 mm length of the spinal cord centered at the injury site was fixed in tissue-embedding medium. The tissue segment was snap frozen on dry ice and sectioned on a cryostat at a thickness of 14 μm. Serial spinal cord sections at 500 μm intervals were stained with myelin-selective pigment luxol fast blue (LFB) and the cellular stain hematoxylin-eosin (HE) to identify the injury epicenter. Tissue sections showing the largest cystic cavity and greatest demyelination were taken to represent the injury epicenter.

Immunohistochemistry. The following primary antibodies were used: mouse anti-NeuN (1:500; Chemicon International, Inc., Temecula, CA) for neurons, mouse anti-GFAP (1:500; Chemicon International, Inc., Temecula, CA) for astrocytes, mouse anti-APC (CC1, 1:100; Calbiochem, San Diego, CA) for oligodendrocytes, and mouse anti-RECA-1 (1:25; Serotec Inc., Raleigh, NC) for endothelial cells. The sections were rinsed three times in PBS after primary antibody incubation and incubated with either fluorescent Alexa 568, 647 or 488 goat anti-mouse/rabbit secondary antibody (1:400; Invitrogen, Burlington, Canada) for 1 hour. The sections were rinsed three times with PBS and cover slipped with Mowiol mounting medium containing DAPI (Vector Laboratories, Inc., Burlingame, CA) to counterstain the nuclei. The images were taken using a Zeiss 510 laser confocal microscope.

Quantification of Blood Vessels. Tissue sections – taken from animals sacrificed 10 days post-SCI – were used for immunofluorescence studies with a monoclonal antibody specific for RECA-1 (Rat Endothelial Cell Antibody). Vessels counts were performed on 4 selected fields (ventral horn, dorsal horn, left and right lateral columns) in each section under 25X magnification (0.14 mm^2). The number of RECA-1-positive vessels was calculated at 2 mm and 4 mm, both rostral and caudal from the epicenter, for each animal.

Quantification of Angiogenesis. Tissue sections – taken from animals sacrificed 5 days post-SCI – were used to quantify angiogenesis following SCI and AdV-ZFP-VEGF administration. Angiogenesis was calculated as vessels co-labelled with RECA-1 and Ki67 (cellular proliferation). Angiogenesis quantification was performed on 4 selected fields (ventral horn, dorsal horn, left and right lateral columns) in each section under 25X magnification (0.14 mm^2). The number of angiogenic vessels was calculated at 1, 2 and 3 mm, both rostral and caudal from the epicenter, for each animal. Rostral and caudal values were pooled for each distance.

Quantification of Apoptosis. An *in situ* terminal-deoxytransferase mediated dUTP nick end-labeling (TUNEL) apoptosis kit (Chemicon International, Inc., Temecula, CA) was used to label apoptotic cells in tissues extracted from animals 5 days post-SCI. TUNEL staining was completed as described in the manufacturer's instructions. The numbers of TUNEL positive nuclei were counted at the epicenter, as well as at 1, 2 and 3 mm (rostral and caudal) from the injury epicenter. In each tissue section, the whole section was counted to include all apoptotic nuclei visible.

Quantification of Neurons. Tissue sections – taken from animals sacrificed 5 days post-SCI – were used for immunofluorescence studies with a monoclonal antibody specific for NeuN (Neuronal Nuclei). Neuron quantification was conducted only in the grey matter under 25X magnification (0.14 mm^2), and all cells were counted. The number of NeuN-positive cells was calculated at 1, 2 and 3 mm, both rostral and caudal from the epicenter, as well as at the epicenter.

Assessment of Tissue Sparing and Cavity Formation. Tissue sparing and cavity formation was analyzed 8 weeks after SCI, at the center of the lesion, 2 mm above and 2 mm below the epicenter. Sections were stained with LFB-HE. The measurements were carried out on coded slides using StereoInvestigator® software (MBF Bioscience, Williston, VT). Cross-sectional residual tissue and cavity areas were normalized with respect to total cross-sectional area and the areas were calculated every 500 μm within the rostrocaudal boundaries of the injury site.

Behavioural Testing

Open-field Locomotor Scoring. Locomotor recovery of the animals (n = 8–10/group) was assessed by two independent observers using the 21 point Basso, Beattie, and Bresnahan (BBB) open field locomotor score [15] from 1 to 8 weeks after SCI. The BBB scale was used to assess hindlimb locomotor recovery including joint movements, stepping ability, coordination, and trunk stability. Testing was done every week on a blinded basis and the duration of each session was 4 min per rat. Scores were averaged across both the right and left hindlimbs to arrive at a final motor recovery score for each week of testing.

Automated Gait Analysis (CatWalk). Gait analysis was performed using the CatWalk system (Noldus Information Technology, Wageningen, Netherlands) as described [16,17]. In short, the system consists of a horizontal glass plate and video capturing equipment placed underneath and connected to a PC. In our work, for correct analysis of the gait adaptations to the chronic compression, after standardization of the crossing speed, the following criteria concerning walkway crossing were used: (1) the rat needed to cross the walkway, without any interruption (2) a minimum of three correct crossings per animal were required. Files were collected and analyzed using the CatWalk program, version 7.1. Individual digital prints were manually labeled by one observer blinded to groups. With the CatWalk, a vast variety of static and dynamic gait parameters can be measured during spontaneous locomotion. In the present study, a blinded examiner generated and analyzed data for the following parameters:

- forelimb stride length (expressed in mm): distance between two consecutive forelimb paw placements
- hindlimb print area – maximal area of the paw print in contact with the detection surface of the CatWalk™ (expressed in mm^2)
- hindlimb print width – the maximal distance spanning the medial and lateral contact points of the paw (expressed in mm)
- hindlimb print length – the maximal distance spanning the cranial and caudal contact points of the paw (expressed in mm)

- hindlimb swing speed (expressed in pixels/sec): is the speed of the paw during the swing phase (the duration of no paw contact with the glass plate during a step cycle).

Acclimation and training to the walking apparatus were performed as described by Gensel *et al.* [18]. Since Catwalk quantifies weight support and stepping, only a sub-set of animals exhibiting weight support (BBB scores >9) were used in the CatWalk experiments (n = 5/group). Most AdV-eGFP animals did not reach BBB scores >9; however, animals for this group were subject to CatWalk™ analysis to provide consistency in our experiments.

Mechanical Allodynia. At-level mechanical allodynia was determined at 4 weeks and 8 weeks post-SCI using 2 g and 4 g von Frey monofilaments as previously described [19]. Animals were acclimatized for 30 minutes in an isolated room for 30 minutes prior to pain testing. The von Frey monofilament was applied to the dorsal skin surrounding the incision/injury site 10 times and animals' behavioural response to each was recorded. An adverse response to the application of the monofilament (determined in advance of experiments) included vocalization, licking, biting and immediate movement to the other side of the cage. The proportion of rats to exhibit allodynia in each group is reported, and an increased number of responses was associated with the development of at-level mechanical allodynia. Below-level mechanical allodynia was determined by quantifying the pain threshold of the hindpaws. Animals were placed in stance on a raised grid, allowing von Frey filaments to be applied to the plantar surface of the hindpaw. Increasing monofilaments were used (2, 4, 8, 10, 16, 21, and 26 g) until the animal displayed an adverse response (as described above). The weight of the von Frey filament that elicited the response was recorded as the pain threshold value, with lower threshold values indicating increased sensitivity to mechanical stimuli (and perhaps the development of mechanical allodynia). Finally, below-level thermal allodynia was assessed using the tail flick method. A 50°C thermal stimulus was applied to the distal portion of the animals' tail by a Tail Flick Analgesia Meter (IITC Inc. Life Science, Woodland Hills, California, USA), and the time for the animal to remove its tail from the stimulus was recorded. The latency time is graphed for each treatment group, and decreased latency times were associated with the development of thermal allodynia.

Electrophysiology

Motor Evoked Potentials. Motor evoked potential recordings (MEPs): In addition to the behavioural assessements, MEPs were recorded *in vivo* to assess the physiological integrity of spinal cord. This approach has been extensively used in our laboratory in rodent models of SCI. *In vivo* recordings of motor evoked potentials were recorded from the each of the treatment and control groups at 8 weeks post-injury (n = 6/group). For MEPs, rats were under light isoflurane anaesthesia (<1%), and recordings were obtained from hindlimb biceps femoris muscle. Stainless steel subdermal needle electrodes were inserted into the muscle. Recordings were acquired using Keypoint Portable (Dantec Biomed, Denmark). A reference electrode was placed under the skin between the recording and stimulating electrodes. Stimulation was applied to the midline of the cervical spinal cord using a silver ball electrode (0.13 Hz; 0.1 ms; 2 mA; 200 sweeps). The interlaminar ligaments were removed and a small amount of bone was removed from the vertebra (not a full laminectomy, just enough to create a space for the electrode to reach the cervical cord). The amplitude was determined by the difference between the positive peak and negative peak. Latency was calculated as the time from the start of the stimulus artifact to the first prominent peak. For individual rats, the average of peak amplitude and latency was averaged from 200 sweeps and analyses were undertaken by ANOVA.

H-Reflex. The Hoffmann reflex is one of the most studied reflexes in humans and is the electrical analogue of the monosynaptic stretch reflex. The H-reflex is evoked is evoked by low-intensity electrical stimulation of the afferent nerve, rather than a mechanical stretch of the muscle spindle, that results in monosynaptic excitation of alpha-motorneurons. H-reflex can be used as a tool (in combination with other outcome measures) to examine spasticity and short- and long-term plasticity. Recording electrodes were placed two centimeters apart in the mid-calf region and the posterior tibial nerve was stimulated in the popliteal fossa using a 0.1 ms duration square wave pulse at a frequency of 1 Hz. The rats were tested for maximal plantar H-reflex/maximal plantar M-response (H/M) ratios to determine the excitability of the reflex. The recordings were filtered between 10–10000 Hz.

Statistical Analysis

Data were analyzed with SigmaPlot software (Systat Software Inc., San Jose, California, USA). For data that investigated the percentage of cells, the data were subject to an arcsine transformation prior to statistical analysis to attain a more normal distribution. For comparison of groups sampled at various distances from the injury site (TUNEL, RECA-1, NeuN), a two-way analysis of variance (ANOVA) with repeated measures was used, followed by the post-hoc Holm-Sidak test. For comparisons of multiple groups at a single time point (Western blotting, BBB, Catwalk, Electrophysiology), a one-way ANOVA was performed, followed by the post-hoc Holm-Sidak test.

The Holm-Sidak post-hoc was used, as it is recommended as the best multiple comparisons test following an ANOVA [20,21]. The Holm-Sidak test is more sensitive and powerful compared to Bonferroni or Tukey post-hoc tests, therefore it is more likely to detect all significant results and increases the probability of not committing type II errors (reduces the chance of rejecting something that is true).

In all figures, the mean value ± SEM are used to describe the results. Statistical significance was accepted for p values of <0.05.

Results

AdV-ZFP-VEGF Delivery into the Injured Spinal Cord

To evaluate the transduction efficiency of the adenoviral constructs *in vivo*, AdV-eGFP was injected into animals at 24 hours post-SCI. The AdV-eGFP fluorescent signal was detected in both the white and grey matter of the injured spinal cord five days after SCI (Figure 1A). Figures 1B and 1C demonstrate eGFP expression in neurons, astrocytes, endothelial cells and oligodendrocytes, indicating successful adenoviral transduction into each cell type. Further quantification of co-labelled cells showed that AdV vector non-preferentially transduces all cell types (Neurons – 30.0%±3.6%, Oligodendrocytes – 26.9%±4.2%, Astrocytes – 21.4%±2.9%, Endothelial cells – 17.2%±3.3%). Since the AdV-ZFP-VEGF construct contains the p65 subunit of the human NFκB transcription factor as the activation domain [12], we were able to confirm delivery of AdV-ZFP-VEGF by immunoblotting using an NFκB p65 antibody to detect the presence of the transcription factor (Figure 1D). As a positive control, HEK293 cells were transduced with ZFP-VEGF and cell lysates were processed for immunoblotting using the same NFκB p65 antibody (data not shown). These results demonstrate the successful delivery of a localized gene therapy to the injured spinal cord.

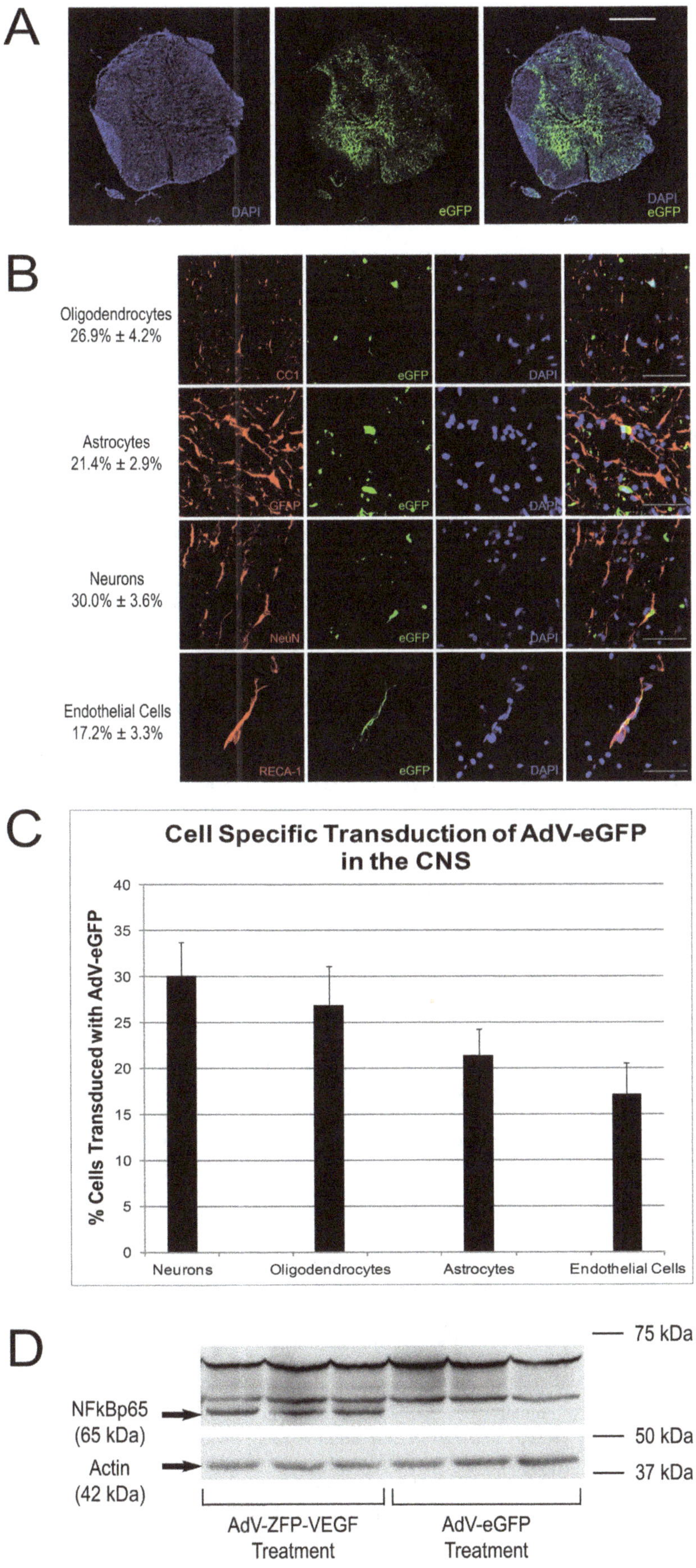
A
DAPI
eGFP
DAPI
eGFP
B
Oligodendrocytes
26.9% ± 4.2%
Astrocytes
21.4% ± 2.9%
Neurons
30.0% ± 3.6%
Endothelial Cells
17.2% ± 3.3%
CC1
GFAP
NeuN
RECA-1
eGFP
DAPI
C
Cell Specific Transduction of AdV-eGFP in the CNS
% Cells Transduced with AdV-eGFP
0
5
10
15
20
25
30
35
40
Neurons
Oligodendrocytes
Astrocytes
Endothelial Cells
D
75 kDa
50 kDa
37 kDa
NFkBp65
(65 kDa)
Actin
(42 kDa)
AdV-ZFP-VEGF
Treatment
AdV-eGFP
Treatment

Figure 1. Transduction of AdV-eGFP/AdV-ZFP-VEGF into the spinal cord. (A) Photomicrographs showing a transverse section of rat spinal cord obtained adjacent to the injury site 10 days after spinal cord injury and AdV-eGFP injection. eGFP signal was detected in both the gray matter and white matter. (B) High-power (63X) confocal images show that the AdV-eGFP vector (green) transfected neurons (NeuN), astrocytes (GFAP), oligodendrocytes (CC1) and endothelial cells (RECA-1). Cells have been counter-stained with DAPI (blue) as nuclear marker. (C) Bar graph displays quantification of transduced cell types ± SEM, as identified by the cell-specific markers NeuN, GFAP, RECA-1 and CC1. (D) Evaluation of AdV-ZFP-VEGF gene transfer. Western blot showed that the NFκB p65 rabbit polyclonal antibody recognizes the p65 activation domain in the AdV-ZFP-VEGF treated animals. The higher molecular weight bands are endogenous NFκBp65 fragments, which are also recognized by the antibody; however, these bands are present in both the control and treatment groups. The lower band (arrow) corresponds to the AdV-ZFP-VEGF and was only present in the treated animals. Lower panel shows actin expression as a protein control. Scale bar: 1000 μm for A; 100 μm for B.

VEGF mRNA and protein expression is increased following 24 hour delayed AdV-ZFP-VEGF administration

Animals were sacrificed 5 days post-SCI and mRNA expression levels of three predominant VEGF isoforms found in the CNS – $VEGF_{120}$, $VEGF_{164}$ and $VEGF_{188}$ – were measured by quantitative real-time PCR (qRT-PCR). Figure 2A shows that 24 hour delayed administration of AdV-ZFP-VEGF resulted in significant increases in VEGF mRNA of isoforms 120 ($p<0.001$), 164 ($p<0.001$), but not isoform 188, when compared with AdV-eGFP control animals and injured control animals (n = 4/sham and injured control; n = 5/AdV-ZFP-VEGF and AdV-eGFP). VEGF-A protein expression was assessed at 10 days following SCI by Western blot using anti-VEGF antibodies, which detect the 42 kDa and 21 kDa bands and are recommended for the detection of the 189, 165 and 121 amino acid splice variants of VEGF. In Figures 2B and 3C, we show that the 42 kDa VEGF-dimer protein was significantly increased by approximately 2.5-fold in AdV-ZFP-VEGF treated animals versus AdV-eGFP and injured control groups ($p<0.02$), and by approximately 1.8-fold in AdV-ZFP-VEGF treated animals compared to sham animals ($p<0.05$) (n = 4/sham, injured control and AdV-eGFP, n = 5/AdV-ZFP-VEGF group). Previous studies using AdV-ZFP-VEGF have shown increases in VEGF mRNA and protein levels [11,22–24]. Consistent with these studies, our results confirm that AdV-ZFP-VEGF increases both mRNA and protein levels of VEGF in the spinal cord following 24 hour delayed administration.

Apoptosis is reduced in animals treated with AdV-ZFP-VEGF 24 hours post-SCI

Our laboratory has previously shown that apoptotic cell death occurs as early as 6 hours following SCI and persists until 14 days post injury [25]. To assess the effects of AdV-ZFP-VEGF treatment on apoptotic cell death, *in situ* terminal-deoxy-transferase mediated dUTP nick end-labeling (TUNEL) staining was performed 5 days after injury (Figure 3). TUNEL-positive cells were found evenly distributed through the gray and white matter in the injured spinal cord, with the greatest apoptosis observed near the injury epicenter. TUNEL-stained nuclei were counted at the injury epicenter, and at 1, 2, and 3 mm from the injury epicenter both rostral and caudal to the lesion site, but rostral and caudal values were pooled. Figure 3B shows that AdV-ZFP-VEGF treatment was associated with an overall significant reduction in the number of TUNEL-positive cells rostral and caudal from the injury epicenter, when conducting a two-way ANOVA for distance from the injury epicenter and treatment group (Two-way ANOVA, Holm-Sidak post-hoc; $p<0.01$; n = 4/sham and injured control groups, n = 5/AdV-eGFP and AdV-ZFP-VEGF groups).

24 hour delayed AdV-ZFP-VEGF administration provides neuroprotection

Neurofilament protein (NF200), a hallmark protein lost following neurodegeneration, was quantified in the injured region of the cord to assess the neuroprotective effects of AdV-ZFP-VEGF after SCI. Previous research from our laboratory indicated a significant loss of NF200 after SCI [26,27]. As shown in Figure 4, the amount of NF200 protein was significantly increased by approximately 2-fold at 10 days following SCI in animals treated with AdV-ZFP-VEGF versus control animals (Figure 4A and 4B) ($p<0.05$).

To further assess the neuroprotective effects of AdV-ZFP-VEGF following SCI, we quantified spared neurons 5 days after injury. NeuN, which recognizes neuronal cell bodies, was used to identify neurons in cross-sections of spinal cord tissue. Figures 4C and 4D demonstrate that AdV-ZFP-VEGF treatment results in a significant sparing of neurons spanning the lesion site, when compared to injured control and AdV-eGFP animals (Two-way ANOVA comparing AdV-ZFP-VEGF with other injured animals across all distances from the epicenter, Holm-Sidak post-hoc; $p<0.02$). AdV-eGFP animals show a significant decrease in NeuN counts compared to injured control animals ($p<0.01$), and the additional loss of cells is likely attributed to the physical damage caused by the intraspinal injections.

24 hour delayed AdV-ZFP-VEGF administration results in an increased number of vessels and promotes angiogenesis

In order to quantify the vascular response to ZFP-VEGF, we conducted immunostaining with RECA-1, a monoclonal antibody specific for endothelial cells, at 10 days following SCI. The severity of the compression injury resulted in considerable disruption to the spinal cord vasculature at the injury epicentre, thus we were unable to quantify the epicenter accurately. Therefore, we assessed spinal cord tissue sections at 2 mm and 4 mm – both caudal and rostral – from the lesion epicenter (Figure 5A). Figures 5B and 5C show that AdV-ZFP-VEGF administration markedly increases the number of RECA-1-positive vessels both rostral and caudal, when compared to control animals ($p<0.01$). These results are consistent with previous findings from our laboratory in studies administering AdV-ZFP-VEGF immediately following injury [11].

To investigate some of the potential mechanisms of AdV-ZFP-VEGF action, we examined the effects of 24 hour delayed AdV-ZFP-VEGF administration on endothelial cell proliferation. One of the most characterized roles of VEGF is promoting angiogenesis in both embryonic development and wound healing [28], therefore we aimed to study if AdV-ZFP-VEGF administration would further promote angiogenesis. Tissues co-labeled with RECA-1 and Ki67 at 5 days following SCI indicated that AdV-ZFP-VEGF administration increased angiogenesis by approximately 10% ($p<0.001$) (Figure 5D and 5E). These results indicate that AdV-ZFP-VEGF administration, which results in an increase in VEGF expression, ultimately promotes angiogenic pathways following SCI. Other research has suggested that VEGF administration results in angiogenesis; however, these studies simply show an increase in the number of vessels present. Here, we demonstrate that VEGF increases endothelial cell proliferation *in*

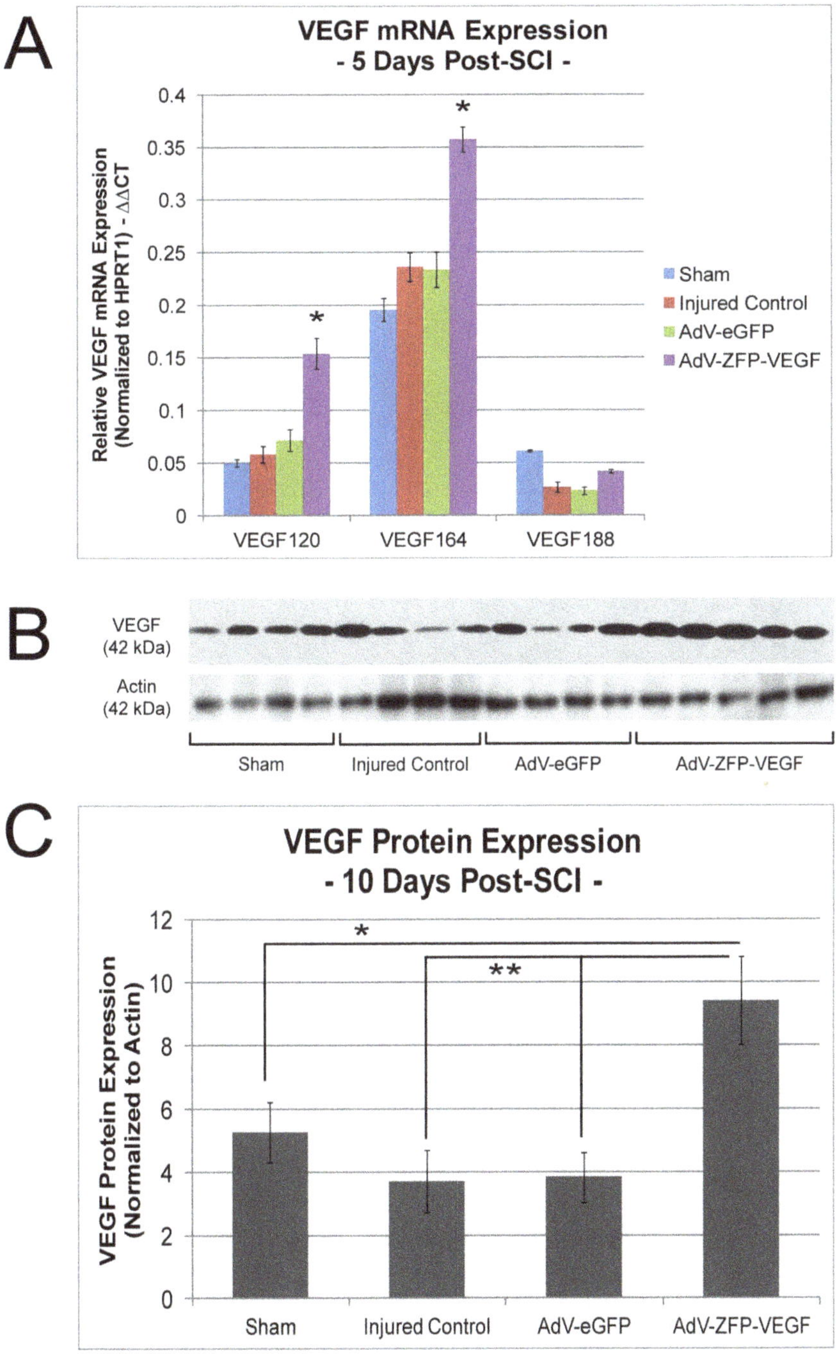

Figure 2. AdV-ZFP-VEGF increases VEGF mRNA and protein. (A) VEGF mRNA levels encoding for $VEGF_{120}$, $VEGF_{164}$ and $VEGF_{188}$ isoforms were measured by quantitative real-time PCR at 5 days post-SCI. The bar graph illustrates that administration of ZFP-VEGF resulted in an increase of VEGF mRNA compared with AdV-eGFP and SCI injured control groups. Relative mRNA levels are expressed as the mean ± SEM, n = 4/sham and injured control groups, n = 5/AdV-eGFP and AdV-ZFP-VEGF groups. One-way ANOVA (Holm-Sidak post-hoc) was completed individually for each isoform $^{**}p<0.001$, $^{*}p<0.01$. (B) Western blot showing administration of AdV-ZFP-VEGF resulted in increased VEGF-A protein levels at 10 days post-SCI, and (C) Quantification shows a significant increase in VEGF-A 42 kD protein in AdV-ZFP-VEGF treated animals compared with control groups. Optical density (OD) of VEGF-A was normalized to actin. Data are presented as mean ± SEM, n = 4/sham, injured control and AdV-eGFP treated groups and n = 5/AdV-ZFP-VEGF treated group. One-way ANOVA (Holm-Sidak post-hoc) $^{**}p<0.02$, $^{*}p<0.05$.

vivo following SCI, and to our knowledge, this is the first study to use a delayed VEGF therapy and demonstrate an increase in vessels, that is likely attributable to angiogenesis.

AdV-ZFP-VEGF results in functional improvement

At the cellular/molecular level, we have observed that AdV-ZFP-VEGF results in beneficial effects. However, in order to assess the viability of any therapy, these effects must be translated into functional gains. In our study, we assessed hindlimb function using

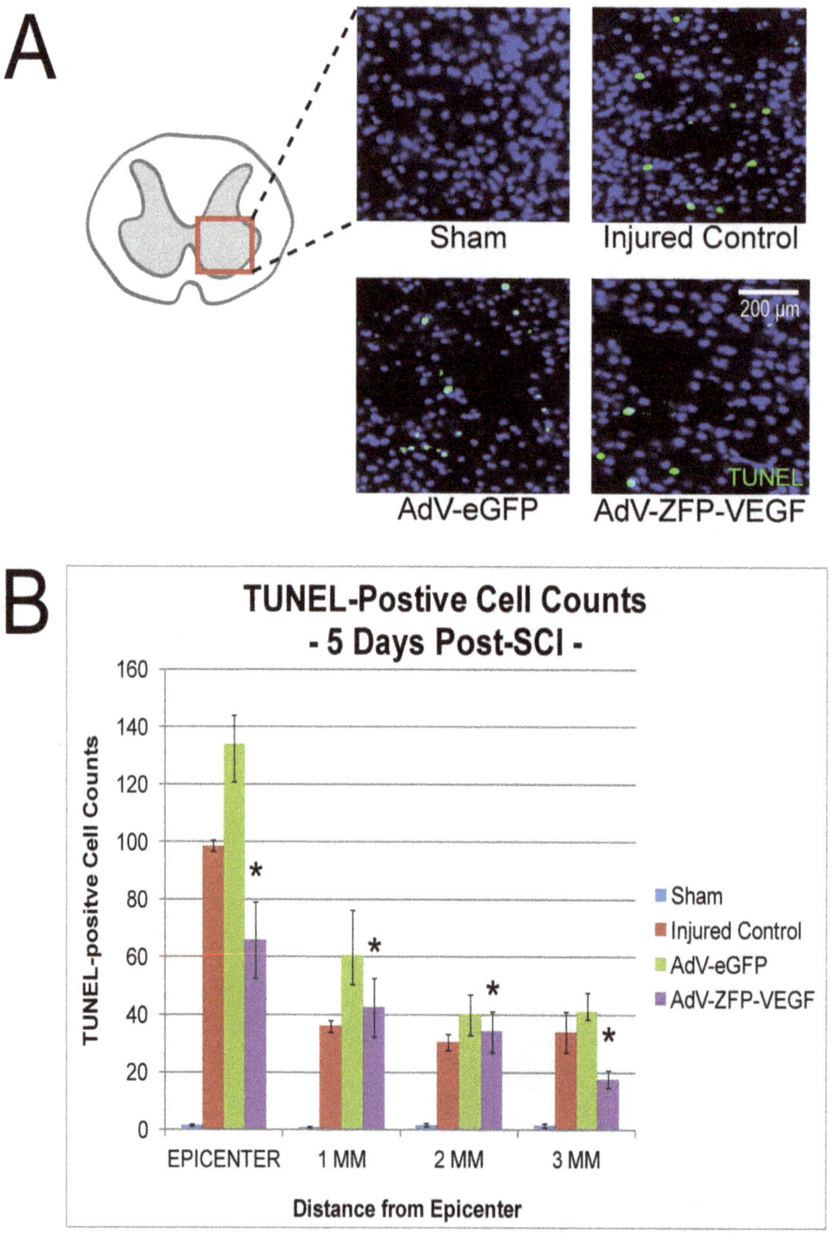

Figure 3. AdV-ZFP-VEGF administration reduces apoptosis after SCI. (A) Representative sections taken 2 mm rostral to the epicenter from animals sacrificed at 5 days post-SCI and tissue processed with TUNEL staining (green); scale 200 μm. An overall reduction of TUNEL-positive cells was observed in the AdV-ZFP-VEGF treated group. Cells have been counter-stained with DAPI (blue) as nuclear marker (B) Bar graph shows quantification of the TUNEL-positive cell counts at 5 days after SCI (pooled values from rostral and caudal counts). There was a significant decrease in TUNEL-positive cells in the AdV-ZFP-VEGF treatment group versus all other injured groups (when compared against other groups and all distances). Values are mean ± SEM, n = 4/sham and injured control groups, n = 5/AdV-eGFP and AdV-ZFP-VEGF groups. Two-way ANOVA (Holm-Sidak post-hoc), *$p < 0.01$.

open-field BBB scoring and Catwalk, between 1-8 weeks following SCI. Analysis of Catwalk data showed that animals treated with AdV-ZFP-VEGF had significantly improved hindlimb weight support ($p<0.05$) (Figure 6), hindlimb swing speed ($p<0.02$) (Figure 7), and forelimb stride length ($p<0.02$) (Figure 7) compared to all other injured control groups. Enhancements in hindlimb weight support and overall gait (hindlimb swing speed, and forelimb stride length) are important changes that may reflect an improved quality of life of individuals suffering with SCI.

AdV-ZFP-VEGF does not result in improved BBB scores

AdV-ZFP-VEGF treated animals did not show improved BBB scores, compared in injured control animals, although they did perform better than AdV-eGFP injected animals ($p<0.01$) (Figure 8). Significant recovery shown by CatWalk (animals analyzed were a sub-set of animals that achieved >8 for BBB scoring) do not correspond with significantly improved BBB scores between injured control and AdV-ZFP-VEGF animals at 8 weeks post-injury. In the discussion we will provide a more detailed explanation that may validate these findings; however, the

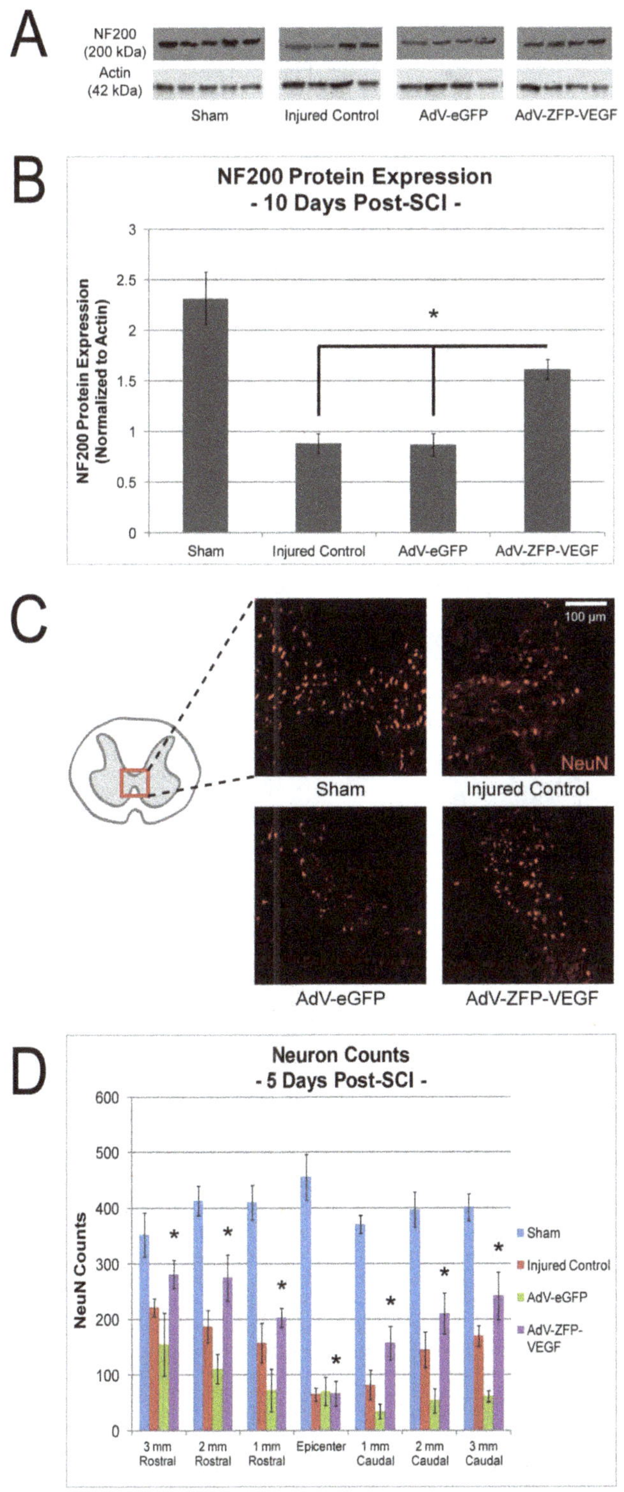

Figure 4. AdV-ZFP-VEGF administration attenuated axonal degradation and increased neuron sparing. (A) Western blot indicates that administration of AdV-ZFP-VEGF resulted in a significant attenuation of NF200 degradation 10 days after injury. Lower panel shows actin protein control. (B) Relative OD value of controls versus AdV-ZFP-VEGF treated animals. Significant NF200 sparing was observed in AdV-ZFP-VEGF-treated animals compared to control groups at 10 days after injury, although all injured groups showed significant NF200 loss following SCI. Optical density of NF200 was normalized to actin. One-way ANOVA (Holm-Sidak post-hoc), *$p<0.05$. (C) Representative sections taken 2 mm rostral to the epicenter from AdV-ZFP-VEGF treated and AdV-eGFP treated animals immunostained with NeuN at 5 days after SCI; scale 200 µm. A greater number of NeuN-positive cells were observed in animals treated with AdV-ZFP-VEGF. (D) Bar graph shows quantification of the NeuN-positive cell counts at 5 days after SCI. There was a significant preservation of neurons overall in the AdV-ZFP-VEGF group compared to all the other injured groups (two-way ANOVA comparing distance from the epicenter and treatment group). Bar graph shows mean OD values ± SEM. Two-way ANOVA (Holm-Sidak post-hoc), *$p<0.02$. n = 5/sham, n = 4/injured control, AdV-eGFP and AdV-ZFP-VEGF groups.

discrepancy between BBB and CatWalk data may be due to the more qualitative nature of the BBB, as opposed to the quantitative gait analysis software.

Delayed AdV-ZFP-VEGF administration does not improve motor evoked potentials or H-reflex following SCI

To further examine the functional changes we performed *in vivo* electrophysiology on the hindlimbs of animals at 8 weeks post-SCI. Our data indicate that although AdV-ZFP-VEGF treated animals show an improved gait via CatWalk™ analysis, we did not observe any significant improvements in axonal conduction in the hindlimbs, as assessed by motor evoked potential recordings (Figure 9A and 9B). We also examined the H-reflex (H/M ratios) following SCI as a measure of spasticity, and observed no electrophysiological differences between groups (Figure 9B).

AdV-ZFP-VEGF administration significantly reduces allodynia

A devastating post-injury condition is neuropathic pain, which affects a significant portion of SCI patients [29,30]. In this study we aimed to investigate the development of thermal and mechanical allodynia in AdV-ZFP-VEGF treated animals: hopeful that we would observe no increases in pain unlike the recent report by Nesic *et al.* [31]. Animals were tested for pain at 4 and 8 weeks following SCI, and here we observe that animals receiving AdV-ZFP-VEGF gene therapy have a significant reduction in allodynia, for both at-level and below-level pain, at 8 weeks post-injury (Figure 10). Testing with calibrated von Frey filaments around the lesion site (on the dorsal skin) showed AdV-ZFP-VEGF animals to have a significant reduction in at-level mechanical allodynia (Figure 10A; $p<0.005$). An increasing application of von Frey filaments to the plantar surface of the hindlimbs demonstrated a marked reduction in below-level alloydnia (Figure 10B), compared to injured control ($p<0.05$) and AdV-eGFP treated animals ($p<0.005$). Furthermore, we examined below-level thermal allodynia (Figure 10C), and observed a significant increase in pain tolerance (increased response time) in animals receiving AdV-ZFP-VEGF ($p<0.05$).

AdV-ZFP-VEGF treatment results in spared grey matter, but not white matter tissue at 8 weeks post-SCI

Eight weeks after SCI, spinal cord cross-sections were stained serially with LFB-HE. Measurements of tissue sparing were calculated using StereoInvestigator software, and are expressed as the average cross-section area. Spinal cords from AdV-ZFP-VEGF treated rats did not show evidence of white matter tissue sparing compared to control injured animals (Figure 11A); however, AdV-ZFP-VEGF administration exhibited an overall increase in residual grey matter in (sections spanning 2 mm rostral and 2 mm caudal to the injury epicenter) when compared to tissue sections from AdV-GFP and injured control rats (Figure 11B; $p<0.001$). The grey matter differences observed in the AdV-ZFP-VEGF group are most

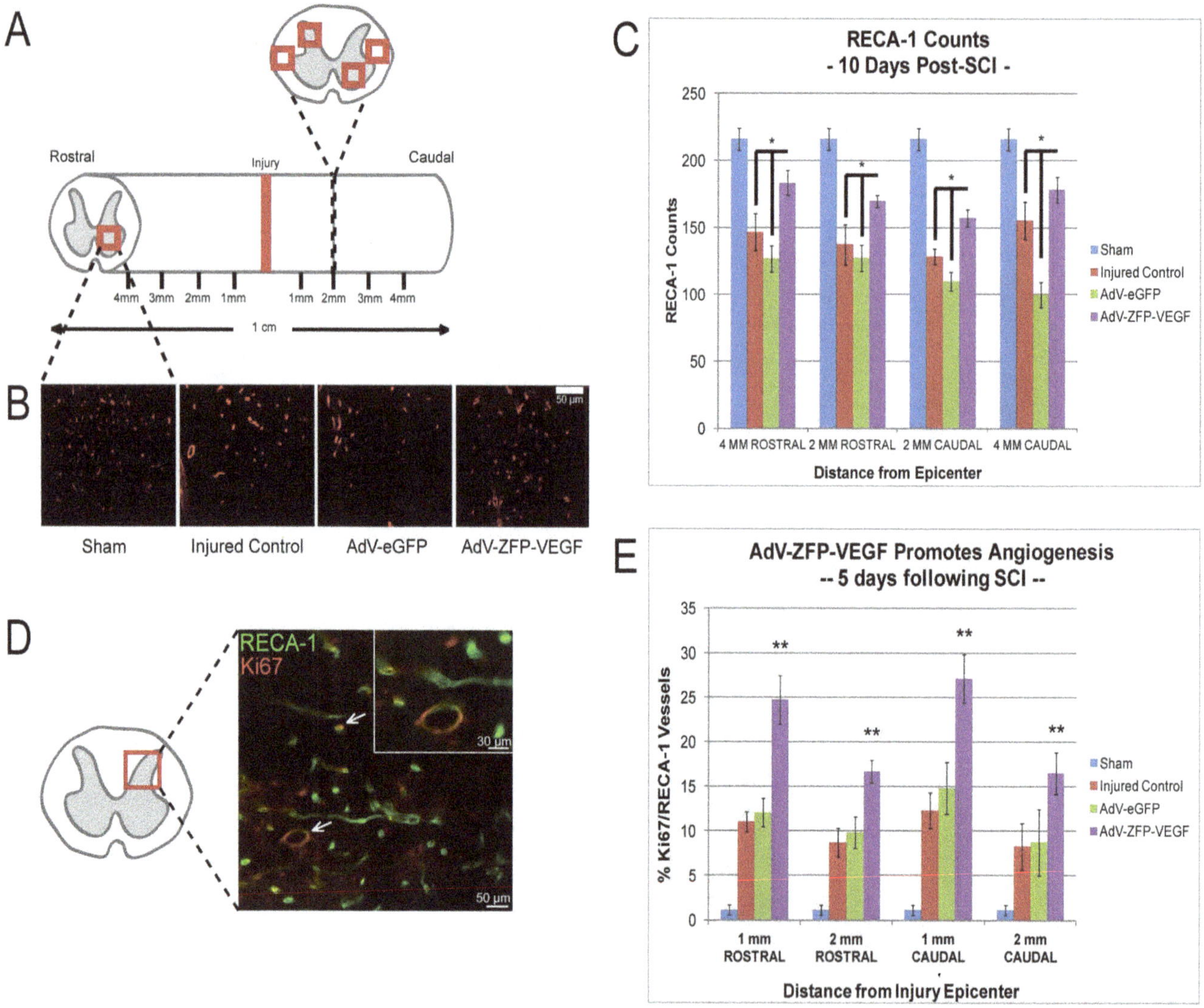

Figure 5. AdV-ZFP-VEGF results in increased vessel counts and angiogenesis. (A) Left panel: Illustration of the area of spinal cord areas used for RECA-1 counting (2 grey matter areas, 2 white matter areas). (B) Representative sections taken 2 mm rostral to the epicenter from a AdV-ZFP-VEGF treated and AdV-eGFP control animal respectively immunostained with RECA-1 at 10 days after SCI; scale 100 µm. An increased number of vessels were observed in the AdV-ZFP-VEGF treated group. (C) Bar graph illustrating the RECA-1 positive cell counts 10 days after SCI. AdV-ZFP-VEGF administration resulted in a significant increase in vascular counts (2 mm and 4 mm away from the epicenter) as compared with the control group. (D) Representative confocal image from an ADV-ZFP-VEGF treated animal at 5 days post-injury. Image was taken at 2 mm rostral from the epicenter, and shows double-labeled cells. Cells were stained for endothelial cells (RECA-1, green) and proliferation (Ki67, red). Scale bar = 50 µm (30 µm for magnified panel). (E) Angiogenesis was assessed by quantifying Ki67/RECA-1 co-labeled vessels. Data is presented at the percentage of RECA-1+ vessels that were also Ki67+, with an overall average increase of 10% vascular proliferation observed in the animals receiving AdV-ZFP-VEGF administration. All data are presented as mean ± SEM, and was analyzed by Two-way ANOVA (Holm-Sidak post-hoc). Angiogenesis data were analyzed by performing an arcsine transformation of the values, prior to Two-way ANOVA and post-hoc testing. *$p<0.01$, **$p<0.001$. n = 4/sham and injured control groups, n = 5/AdV-eGFP and AdV-ZFP-VEGF groups.

notable in the peri-lesional area (1–2 mm rostral caudal to the epicenter). The epicenter of all injured and treated groups showed significant histological damage, and no differences were observed in tissue sparing at the lesion epicenter between the injured groups. Animals treated with AdV-eGFP show significantly reduced grey matter and white matter compared to injured control and AdV-ZFP-VEGF treated groups. As previously mentioned, we attribute the additional damage to the spinal cord in the AdV-eGFP group to the invasive delivery method of the treatment (intraspinal injections).

Discussion

We have shown that AdV-ZFP-VEGF administration can be delayed 24 hours following spinal cord injury, and still provide beneficial effects. To date, we are the first to use AdV-ZFP-VEGF in a delayed fashion, and one of few studies that have used any form of VEGF therapy at a delayed point post-injury [32,33]. In the current research, we chose to investigate the efficacy of 24 hour delayed AdV-ZFP-VEGF administration, which presents a clinically relevant therapeutic window. This form of gene therapy mimics physiological VEGF production, which should result in the production of all VEGF isoforms in the injured spinal

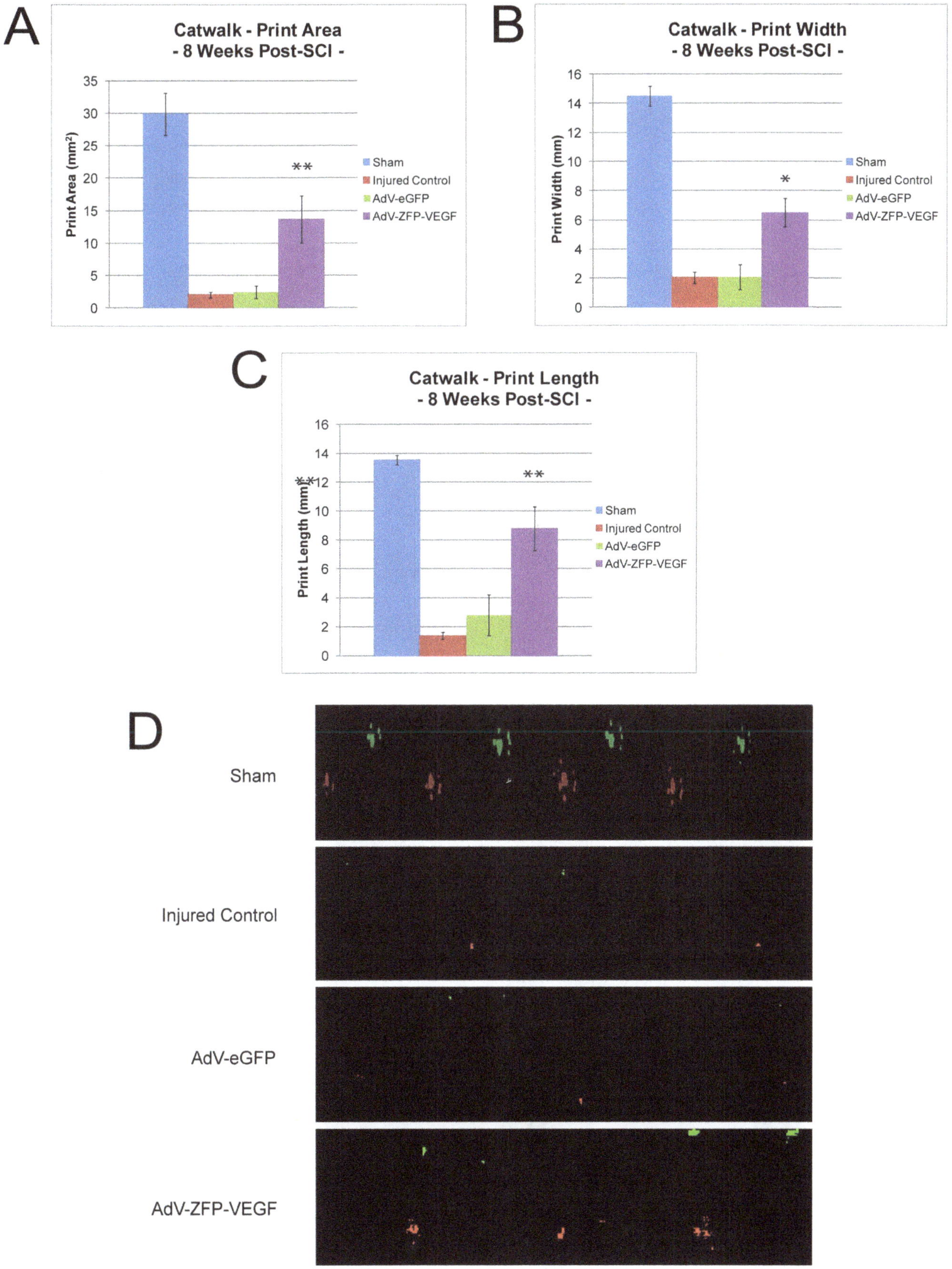
A
Catwalk - Print Area
- 8 Weeks Post-SCI -
Print Area (mm²)
0
5
10
15
20
25
30
35
**
Sham
Injured Control
AdV-eGFP
AdV-ZFP-VEGF
B
Catwalk - Print Width
- 8 Weeks Post-SCI -
Print Width (mm)
0
2
4
6
8
10
12
14
16
*
Sham
Injured Control
AdV-eGFP
AdV-ZFP-VEGF
C
Catwalk - Print Length
- 8 Weeks Post-SCI -
Print Length (mm)
0
2
4
6
8
10
12
14
16
**
Sham
Injured Control
AdV-eGFP
AdV-ZFP-VEGF
D
Sham
Injured Control
AdV-eGFP
AdV-ZFP-VEGF

Figure 6. AdV-ZFP-VEGF improves hindlimb weight support. Catwalk gait analysis was used to assess hindlimb weight support. A sub-set of animals (with BBB scores >9) were assessed every week between 4–8 weeks, and each animal performed a standardized Catwalk run. A blinded observer analyzed the data. (A) Paw area: the maximal area of the paw print in contact with the detection surface of the CatWalk (expressed in mm^2), (B) Paw width: the maximal distance spanning the medial and lateral contact points of the paw (expressed in mm), and (C) Paw length: the maximal distance spanning the cranial and caudal contact points of the paw (expressed in mm). (D) Representative images of CatWalk forelimb (green) and hindlimb (red) prints, which were used to quantify the data presented in Figure 6 and Figure 7. Data presented is the mean ± SEM, n = 5/group, at 8 weeks following SCI. One-way ANOVA (Holm-Sidak post-hoc). *$p<0.05$, **$p<0.005$.

cord: a necessary component for proper and functional angiogenesis. We observed significant improvements at the cellular and molecular levels, including an increased number of vessels, increased angiogenesis, reduced apoptosis and increased neurons. Additionally, we observed improved functional benefits in animals treated with AdV-ZFP-VEGF, including increased hindlimb weight support and significant reductions in allodynia. Collectively, the data suggest that: (i) administration of AdV-ZFP-VEGF results in an increase in VEGF, which may elicit effects through cell survival and angiogenic mechanisms (ii) AdV-ZFP-VEGF has

A

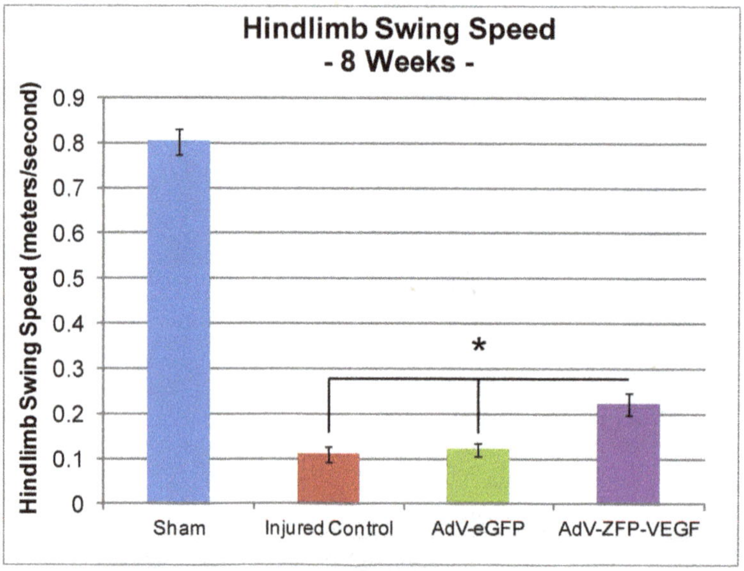

B

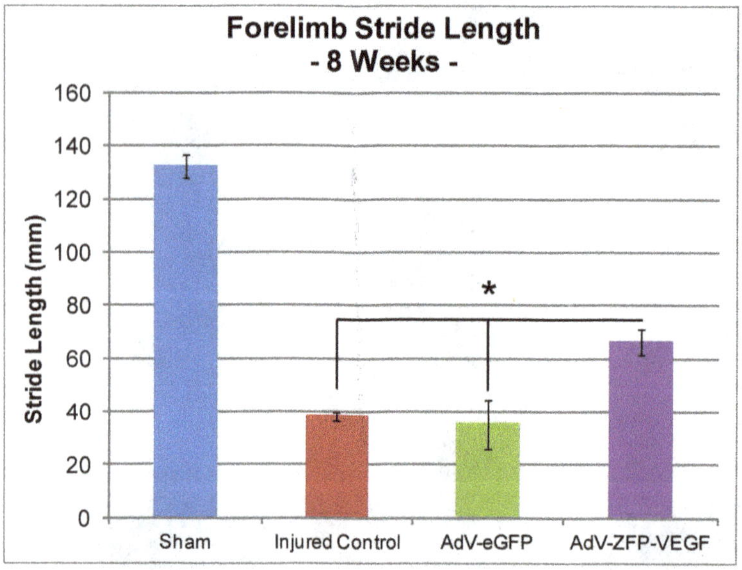

Figure 7. Forelimb and Hindlimb locomotion is improved by AdV-ZFP-VEGF administration. (A) Catwalk gait analysis was used to assess hindlimb swing speed. Animals were assessed every week between 4–8 weeks, and each animal performed a standardized Catwalk run. A blinded observer analyzed the data. Data presented is the mean ± SEM, n = 5/group, at 8 weeks following SCI. One-way ANOVA (Holm-Sidak post-hoc). *$p<0.02$. (B) Catwalk gait analysis was used to assess forelimb stride length. Animals were assessed every week between 4–8 weeks, and each animal performed a standardized Catwalk run. A blinded observer analyzed the data. Data presented is the mean ± SEM, n = 5/group, at 8 weeks following SCI. One-way ANOVA (Holm-Sidak post-hoc). *$p<0.02$.

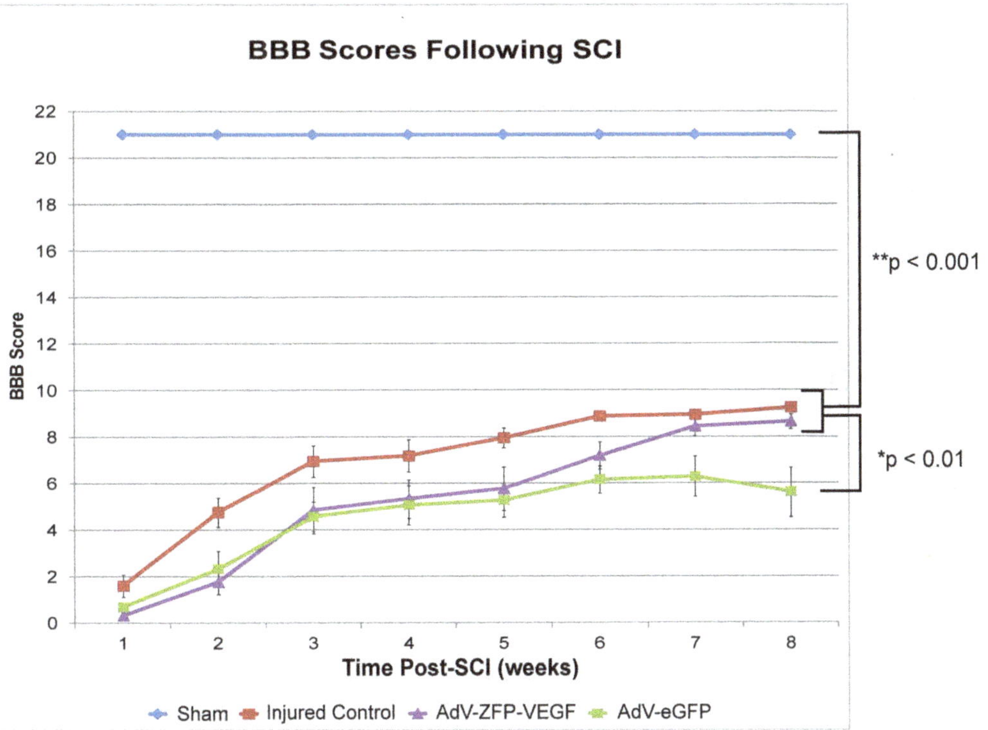

Figure 8. AdV-ZFP-VEGF does not improve open-field walking (BBB) scores following SCI. Open-field locomotion was assessed using the 21-point BBB scale. Animals were assessed weekly for 8 weeks following injury by blinded observers (n = 8/sham and AdV-ZFP-VEGF groups; n = 10/injured control and AdV-eGFP groups). The left and right limbs were scored individually, but the data presented is the average between left and right hindlimb recovery.

a therapeutic time window following SCI which extends at least until 24 hours following injury, (iii) repairing vascular damage following neurotrauma is an important therapeutic target.

Previously, our lab has shown that immediate administration of AdV-ZFP-VEGF following SCI resulted in neuroprotection, increased vascular counts and improved functional recovery [11]. These promising results encouraged us to investigate a more feasible time-window for clinical intervention: 24 hours post-injury administration of AdV-ZFP-VEGF. Moreover, administration 24 hours following injury aimed to target a few important pathophysiological events post-SCI, particularly vascular damage and apoptosis. In a model of spinal cord contusion, Ling and Liu showed that TUNEL-positive cells are maximally observed at 48 hours following injury in both the grey and white matter [34]. Similarly, Crowe *et al.* demonstrated that maximal apoptosis is observed at 48 hours following contusion injury, with apoptosis identified between 6 hours and 3 weeks [35]. Liu *et al.* showed that following contusion injury TUNEL-positive neurons were observed between 4–24 hours, whereas TUNEL-positive glia were seen between 4 hours and 14 days with maximal numbers observed at 24 hours, although another peak of TUNEL-positive glia were observed at 7 days post-injury [36]. With respect to vascular targets, research suggests that angiogenic therapies should be administered to target endogenous vascular repair, which occurs between 3 and 7 days following injury [6,37]. Therefore, by administrating AdV-ZFP-VEGF 24 hours following injury, we aimed to target and reduce apoptosis as well as enhance vascular regeneration. Our data, showing reduced TUNEL and increased endothelial cell proliferation, suggest that AdV-ZFP-VEGF is in fact capable of both neuroprotection and angiogenesis. Although we have not investigated the detailed mechanisms or signaling pathways of AdV-ZFP-VEGF *in vivo*, collectively our data provide strong evidence that increasing VEGF following injury may be beneficial and may stimulate cell survival and angiogenic pathways.

Vasculature is a significant target following SCI

SCI results in significant vascular damage, including disruption of spinal cord blood flow, the onset of spinal cord ischemia, hemorrhage, edema and breakdown of the blood-spinal cord barrier (BSCB). These vascular changes encompass many of the earliest pathological processes following SCI, therefore therapies aimed directly at the vascular disruption or the ensuing downstream consequences of vascular injury are highly attractive; hence, we have chosen to address this therapeutic target in our research. In theory, rapid vascular repair following injury will likely result in the most favourable outcomes. Promoting repair and regeneration of vascular structures would mediate ischemia, hemorrhage and further edema by restoring proper blood-flow and stopping leaky vessels. Moreover, restoring the proper structure and function of the BSCB would likely reduce the influx of inflammatory cells into the spinal cord, thereby reducing the damage caused by reactive microglia [38,39]. Recent reports have shown significant correlations between blood vessel density and improvements in recovery following CNS trauma [40–43]. Rescue and regeneration of the microvasculature within the epicenter and penumbra remains largely unexplored, yet may be a promising therapeutic route to facilitate tissue sparing and functional recovery following SCI. It has been shown that substantial trophic support is provided by CNS microvessels [44] and that microvessels are critical for tissue survival [45].

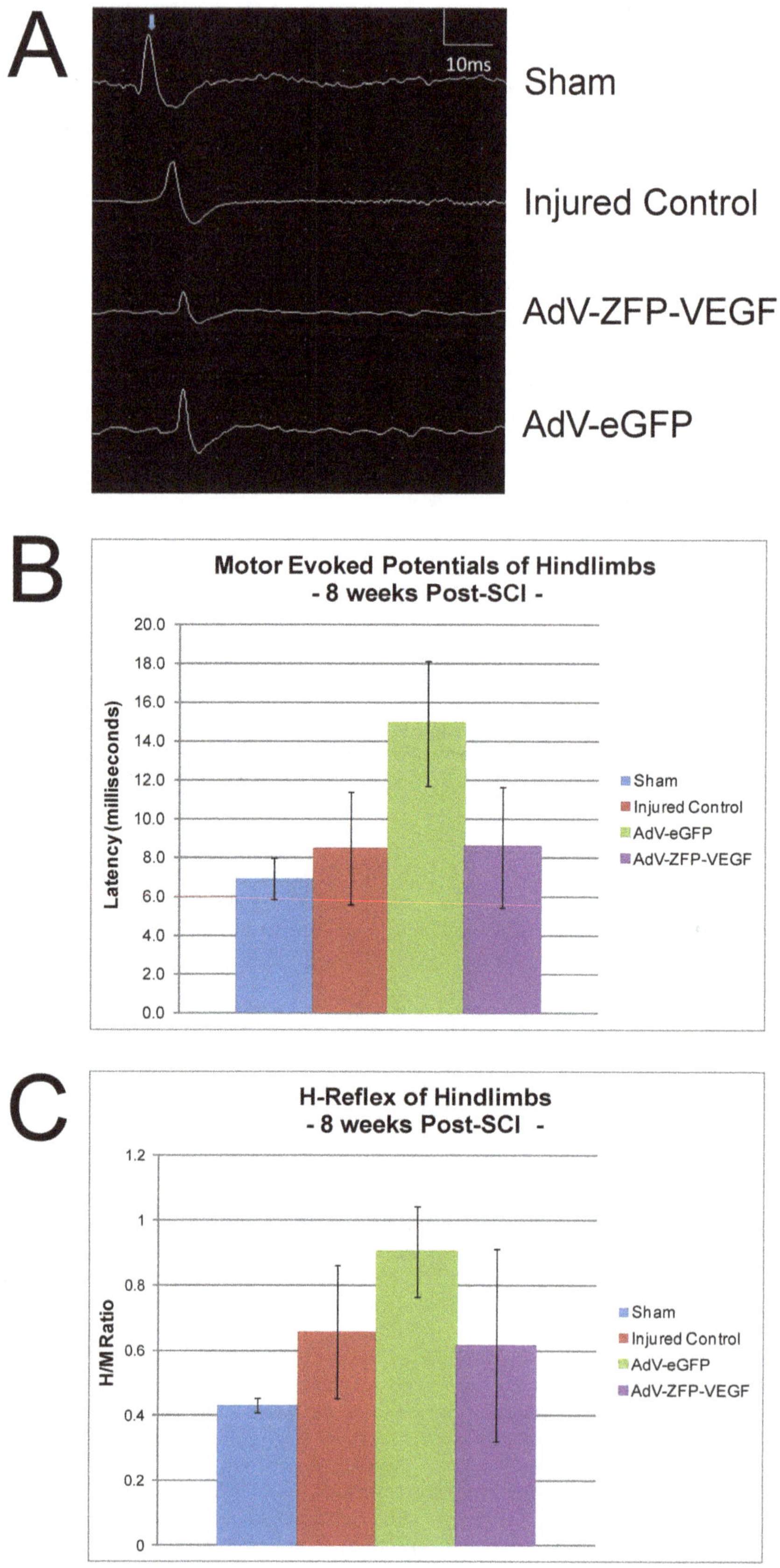

Figure 9. Electrophysiological assessment following AdV-ZFP-VEGF administration. (A) Representative tracings of MEP's recorded from the hindlimb at 8 weeks post-injury. (B) MEP quantification. Recordings were obtained from hindlimb biceps femoris. Stimulation was applied to the midline of the cervical spinal cord (0.13 Hz; 0.1 ms; 2 mA; 200 sweeps). Latency was calculated as the time from the start of the stimulus artifact to

the first prominent peak. AdV-ZFP-VEGF did not result in improved MEP's. (C) H-Reflex quantification. Recording electrodes were placed two centimeters apart in the mid-calf region and the posterior tibial nerve was stimulated in the popliteal fossa using a 0.1 ms duration square wave pulse at a frequency of 1 Hz. The rats were tested for maximal plantar H-reflex/maximal plantar M-response (H/M) ratios to determine the excitability of the reflex. AdV-ZFP-VEGF administration did not significantly alter the H/M ratio. n = 6/group.

VEGF is promising because it targets multiple cellular mechanisms

An immense number of cellular factors are involved in vascular development and repair, and in the pathological processes following SCI, therefore it is often suggested that the best therapy for SCI may involve a combinatorial approach. In the current research, VEGF was specifically selected since it has been shown to support the "neurovascular niche" and appears to play important roles in both vascular and nervous systems: bridging both endogenous systems. Expression of VEGF-R's have been observed in many cell types, including neurons, microglia/macrophages, endothelial cells, smooth muscle cells and astrocytes [46–51]. Through interactions with co-receptors, neuropilins, VEGF is able to influence the function and development of neural cells, which may be a key role for VEGF therapies following neurotrauma [52,53]. Additionally, studies have shown that regenerating axons have a tendency to grow along blood vessels, therefore promoting vascular growth following injury may provide scaffolding for regenerating axons [54,55].

Previous studies using VEGF

In previous research that has used VEGF following SCI, authors have observed varying results. Choi *et al.* used a hypoxia-inducible VEGF-A expression system to treat rats with SCI and observed neuroprotective effects and enhanced VEGF-A expression [56]. Another group used an adenovirus coding for $VEGF_{165}$, delivered via matrigel, in a partial spinal cord transection model. They observed a significant increase in vessel volume and a reduction in the retrograde degeneration of corticospinal tract axons [57]. However, Benton *et al.* [58] reported an exacerbation of lesion size and increased inflammation after the delivery of 2 µg of recombinant $VEGF_{165}$ directly into the contused spinal cord 3 days post SCI. This study highlights several factors which are likely to be critical in the successful application of VEGF-A as a therapy for SCI. The method of VEGF delivery is likely a critical factor. In our study, we injected the ZFP-VEGF adjacent to the injury epicenter as the peri-lesional ischemic penumbra is likely the zone, which would benefit the most from approaches to enhance angiogenesis. Moreover, our delivery technique, using a ZFP-VEGF gene therapy, has the ability to upregulate several isoforms of VEGF-A (specifically we observed an upregulation of the VEGF 120, 164 and 188 isoforms), mimicking endogenous expression. In contrast, most other research has focused on the delivery of a single VEGF isoforms.

Potential pitfalls of VEGF

Although VEGF has many desirable attributes for neuroprotection and vascular repair, it is important to recognize that some of these attributes have the potential to be deleterious and exacerbate damage following SCI. In development or maintenance of vascular structures, VEGF stimulates angiogenesis by signalling matrix-metalloproteinases (MMPs) to breakdown the BSCB and matrix in order to make way for new vascular sprouts. However, following injury, greater amounts of VEGF are released from surrounding cells and vascular remodelling is quickly initiated, which leads to a rapid hyperpermeability of the local vessels. This increase in permeability may contribute to an increased inflammatory response or increased edema following CNS injury. In particular, disruption of the BSCB following injury presents an entry route for inflammatory mediators to enter the CNS without resistance. A previous study reported that VEGF is able to promote monocyte migration *in vitro* and that administration of VEGF therapies may contribute to inflammatory responses following injury [59]. Although we observed no increased inflammatory response in our AdV-ZFP-VEGF animals compared to other injured control groups at 10 days following injury (data not shown), it is possible that VEGF therapies may exacerbate early inflammation.

Disadvantages of intraspinal AdV injections

Although not perfect, direct injection into the spinal cord has some advantages and has been widely used for the delivery of therapeutics and stem cells [60–62]. Firstly, this method allows specific and localized delivery of the ZFP-VEGF gene therapy. We have selected four injections sites directly into the spinal cord, at 1 mm deep into the cord. This depth was selected to administer the vascular therapy close to the highly vascularized grey matter. Injections were administered two-millimeters rostral and caudal to the injury site to target the penumbra of the injury – a site which is more likely to be rescued by a delayed therapeutic intervention compared to the injury epicenter. Additionally, direct injections result in rapid delivery of the therapy, since it is not required to migrate or circulate before reaching the target tissue. In AdV-eGFP treated groups, we observed decreased NeuN counts, increased TUNEL-positive cells, a decrease in RECA-1-positive vessels, and diminished tissue sparing compared to animals which received only a compression injury (injured control group). We hypothesize that these deficits were likely attributed to additional damage caused by the intraspinal injections rather than exacerbated inflammation. Both AdV-eGFP and AdV-ZFP-VEGF groups received cyclosporine-A administration to minimize the inflammatory response, and we have previously shown that there is no difference in inflammation between AdV and control injured groups [11]. AdV-ZFP-VEGF treated animals were able to overcome these additional deficits and still show significant improvement compared to injured control animals, with the exception of white matter sparing. Direct injections (through the dorsal white matter) into the spinal cord may account for the data (Figure 11) that shows reduced white matter sparing for AdV-ZFP-VEGF treated animals compared to injured controls, since the injection likely caused additional physical insult to the spinal cord white matter. The administration of the therapy primarily aimed to rescue the vasculature following SCI, therefore the centrally located grey matter was the initial target and injections were given 1 mm deep into the cord. Although our data (Figure 1) indicate that AdV-ZFP-VEGF is observed in both the grey and white matter, AdV-ZFP-VEGF delivery was perhaps more localized to the deep grey matter tissue, and therefore able to exert the greatest effects on this population of cells (which would be supported by increased neuronal counts and vasculature; Figures 4 and 5, respectively).

In our studies, we believed it was important to include an AdV-eGFP control group to indicate the transduction of the virus *in vivo* (timing and location), and to help elucidate potential adverse effects of administering a gene therapy in an AdV construct. As noted above, the AdV-eGFP control group generally resulted in

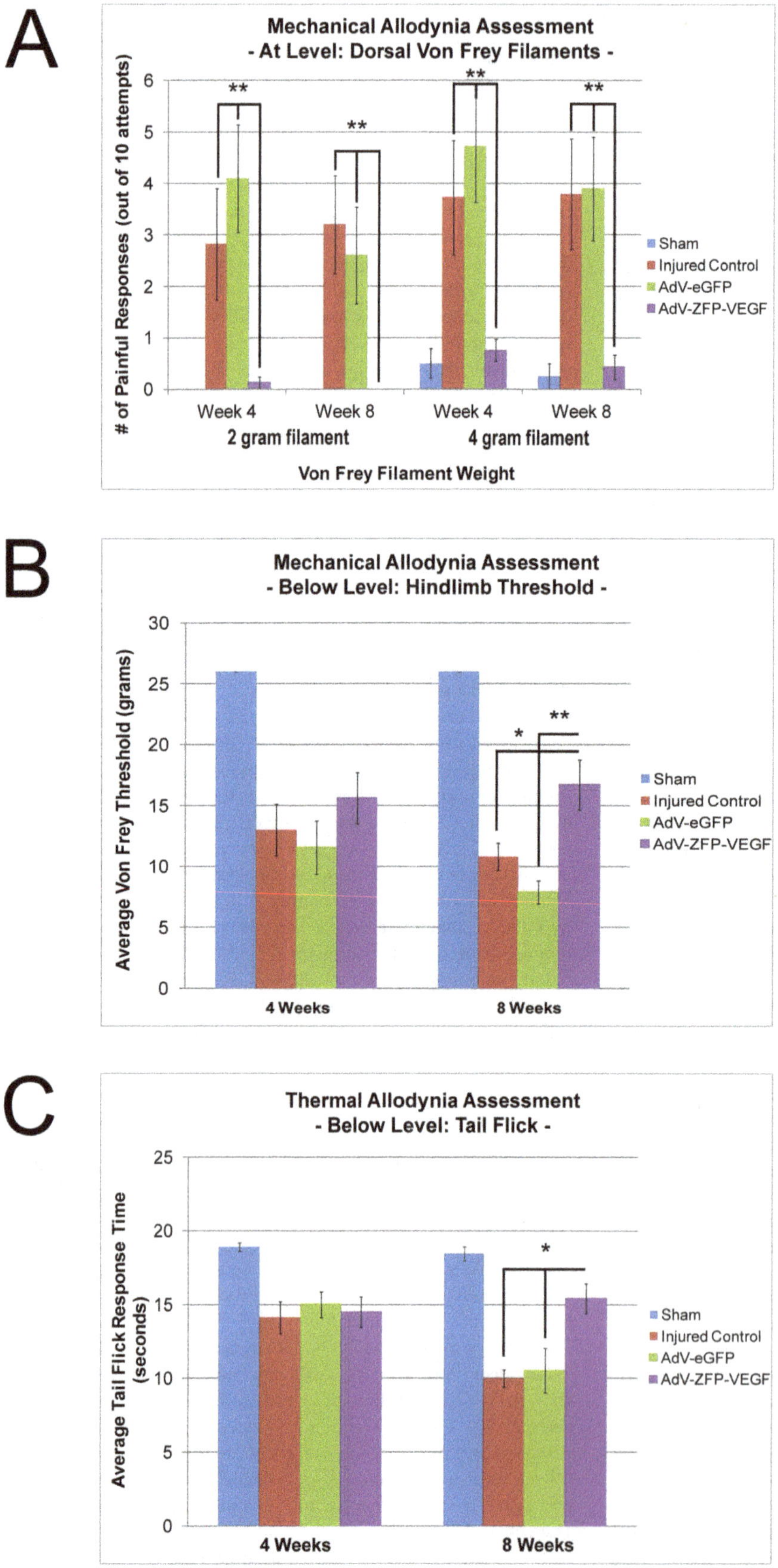

Figure 10. AdV-ZFP-VEGF significantly reduces mechanical and thermal allodynia at 8 weeks post-SCI. Mechanical and thermal allodynia, often used as outcome measures of neuropathic pain, were monitored with von Frey monofilaments and tail-flick tests, respectively. (A) At-level pain. Animals were assessed with 2 g or 4 g von Frey monofilaments around the dorsal incision (above T6–T7 laminectomy and injury). Data are

expressed as the average number of adverse reactions out of 10 applications of the monofilament. There was an overall treatment effect with AdV-ZFP-VEGF using the 2 g and 4 g monofilaments at 4 weeks and 8 weeks post-injury; *$p<0.05$. (B) Below-level pain. Animals were subject to increasing von Frey filaments (2 g–26 g), and the when they elicited a response, this value was taken as the pain threshold value. Data is reported as the average threshold for each group. AdV-ZFP-VEGF increased hindlimb threshold compared to other injured groups; *$p<0.05$, **$p<0.005$. (C) Below-level thermal allodynia. A 50°C thermal stimulus was applied to the distal tip of the tail. The data shown is the average time it took for the animals to withdrawl their tail from the stimulus ("tail flick"). Shorter response times indicate a decreased pain threshold. Animals treated with AdV-ZFP-VEGF showed an increased tolerance/threshold to thermal stimuli at 8 weeks post-injury compared to other injured groups; *$p<0.05$. Data were analyzed by One-way ANOVA. Error bars represent SEM. n = 8/sham and AdV-ZFP-VEGF groups; n = 10/injured control and AdV-eGFP groups.

poorer outcomes compared to injured animals without injections. Future experiments may choose to include a saline-injected control group to more specifically determine the amount of damage caused by the injection verses the potential inflammatory response of an AdV vector. Moreover, additional studies should aim to investigate alternative delivery methods for AdV-ZFP-VEGF, as VEGF-treated animals may display even greater histological improvements over control animals if AdV-ZFP-VEGF were to be administered in a less invasive manner.

Future studies may also wish to examine the use of alternative viral or non-viral delivery methods. The use of AdV may induce a host inflammatory response, although we attempted to reduce these effects by the use of cyclosporine-A. However, AdV infection may result in an increase in inflammation, and increased inflammation may negatively contribute to the secondary injury. On the contrary, inflammation results in expression of cytokines and activation of matrix metalloproteinases, which ultimately drives angiogenesis and re-vascularization [63]. MMPs de-stablize vascular structures, allowing for vascular remodeling, and expression of pro-inflammatory cytokines actively recruits endothelial cells and promotes endothelial cell proliferation. AdV administration may play a role in inducing re-vascularization; however, our data do not indicate that AdV administration results in any substantial vascular benefits. In fact, we observed AdV-eGFP groups showing reduced vascular proliferation and overall vascular counts (Figure 5).

Assessment of Functional Outcomes

We investigated the effects of 24 hour delayed AdV-ZFP-VEGF on the functional recovery and neuroanatomical preservation following thoracic SCI. In the current study, we used BBB locomotor scoring as well as CatWalk analysis to quantify functional outcomes of AdV-ZFP-VEGF therapy. CatWalk analysis is a relatively new method of assessing functional outcomes; however, the methodology has been widely validated for spinal cord injury models and generates data for many parameters of locomotion, which provides a more in-depth evaluation of functional recovery compared to traditional techniques [17]. CatWalk analysis demonstrated that animals treated with AdV-ZFP-VEGF showed improved locomotion as it was demonstrated by the increased forelimb stride length and the hindlimb swing speed. Interestingly, the animals treated with AdV-ZFP-VEGF exhibited improved hindlimb weight support. No differences were observed by BBB testing or electrophysiological assessment. Moreover, results indicated that AdV-ZFP-VEGF drastically reduced the development of mechanical and thermal allodynia in animals at 8 weeks post-injury. Lastly, results showed that AdV-ZFP-VEGF spared a significant amount of grey matter tissue compared to other injured groups.

The Basso Beattie Bresnahan (BBB) scoring scale to assess hindlimb deficits in thoracic SCI has been, and continues to be the "gold standard" for functional assessment [15]. The scoring system evaluates the hindlimb joint movement and the hind-paw orientation/stepping, provides a general indication of the locomotor capabilities of the animal, and establishes if the animal can weight-bear. The major shortcomings of the BBB are two-fold. First, although the BBB is to be conducted by blinded observers, the behavioural assessments are still highly subjective to human errors. Secondly – and perhaps the most confounding factor – the BBB is a qualitative system: simply indicating if the animal is competent of defined movements, providing a relatively subjective score of *how much* or *how well* an animal can perform a task (occasional, frequent or consistent). For detecting major functional differences in animals, the BBB scoring scale is highly effective and easy to conduct; however, more subtle differences between treatment groups may not be observed by BBB assessment. Additionally, since the BBB scale is not a linear relationship between the numerical value and the functional gains associated with them, teasing out meaningful results can become a challenge.

In this research, we used both the BBB and the Catwalk gait analysis software to assess functional recovery post-injury. While scoring animals using BBB, subtle differences between animals were noted (some of them moved more normally, and with greater consistency); however, these variations were not strong enough to increase their BBB score. Overall, we observed no differences in BBB scores between groups. On the other hand, Catwalk data indicated that AdV-ZFP-VEGF treated animals have significant improvements in hindlimb weight support, and hindlimb swing speed. It should be emphasized that CatWalk experiments require weight support, and therefore only a sub-set of animals (n = 5) for each group were tested using the Catwalk system. The average BBB scores for the injured control and AdV-ZFP-VEGF animals used for CatWalk experiments were very similar (injured control = 9.5, AdV-ZFP-VEGF = 9.2), whereas the AdV-eGFP animals had poorer BBB scores and the majority of animals did not reach weight-bearing ability (average BBB score = 7.9). Although the BBB is a valid, widely used method of behavioural evaluation, the Catwalk is a more sensitive and quantitative outcome measure, which may reveal understated changes in recovery not observable using the BBB scoring system. From a clinical perspective, improvements in hindlimb weight support and in overall locomotion may have an important impact on the mobility and independence of an injured individual. Interestingly, Catwalk analysis also revealed that AdV-ZFP-VEGF animals showed improved forelimb stride length, suggesting that AdV-ZFP-VEGF could potentially enhance hindlimb-forelimb coordination; although with BBB scores of 9, we did not observe hindlimb-forelimb coordination in any injured animal group. In the histological examination of grey and white matter post-SCI, we did not investigate sparing of specific pathways or specific neuronal phenotypes (i.e. interneurons vs. motor neurons); however, improvements in both hindlimb and forelimb kinetics could suggest that AdV-ZFP-VEGF may spare propriospinal interneurons, which are located at the grey-white matter interface and are involved in coordination of limb movements [64]. Future experiments involving AdV-ZFP-VEGF should aim to investigate the effects of AdV-ZFP-VEGF on interneuron sparing/survival, since these cells have been attributed to regulating central pattern generators (CPGs) and should therefore be of interest for promoting locomotor recovery following SCI.

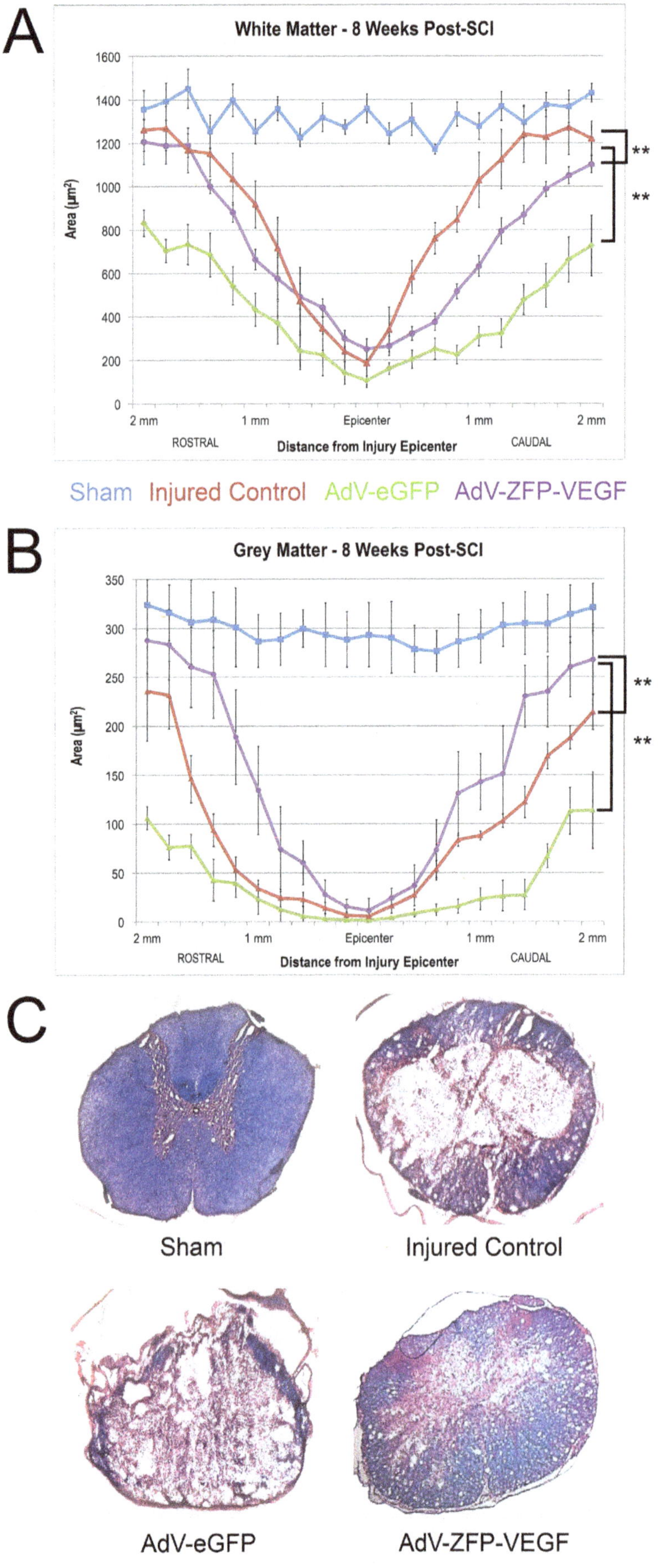
A
White Matter - 8 Weeks Post-SCI
Area (μm²)
1600
1400
1200
1000
800
600
400
200
0
2 mm
1 mm
Epicenter
1 mm
2 mm
ROSTRAL
Distance from Injury Epicenter
CAUDAL
**
**
Sham Injured Control AdV-eGFP AdV-ZFP-VEGF
B
Grey Matter - 8 Weeks Post-SCI
Area (μm²)
350
300
250
200
150
100
50
0
2 mm
1 mm
Epicenter
1 mm
2 mm
ROSTRAL
Distance from Injury Epicenter
CAUDAL
**
**
C
Sham
Injured Control
AdV-eGFP
AdV-ZFP-VEGF

Figure 11. Tissue sparing quantification at 8 weeks post-SCI. (A) Residual white matter quantification. (B) Residual grey matter quantification. AdV-ZFP-VEGF improves spinal cord grey matter preservation. (C) Representative sections are shown from each group. Sections shown are taken 2 mm rostral to the epicenter at 8 weeks after SCI. AdV-ZFP-VEGF treated spinal cord exhibited a larger extent of grey matter spared tissue, but not white matter; **p<0.001. Data are mean ± SEM values. n = 8/sham and AdV-ZFP-VEGF groups; n = 10/injured control and AdV-eGFP groups.

In compliment to our data showing AdV-ZFP-VEGF spares neurons, in this study we quantified residual tissue at 8 weeks post-SCI and our data show that delayed AdV-ZFP-VEGF administration results in improved grey matter sparing, but not white matter sparing. Taken together, these results suggest that AdV-ZFP-VEGF likely acts by promoting survival of neuronal cell bodies. Additionally, we observe that AdV-eGFP animals show notable decreases in both grey and white matter sparing at 8 weeks post-SCI. We do observe the caudal sections to have even less tissue sparing; however, it is often observed that tissue caudal to a traumatic injury is less preserved due to Wallerian degeneration, axonal disruption and reduced vascular flow. In a previous study, we show that AdV administration (in conjunction with cyclosporine-A) does not result in an increased inflammatory response compared to injured control animals [11]. The functional outcomes observed in our study – improved gait, hindlimb weight support and decreased pain – would be consistent with previous research demonstrating improved function and/or sparing of propriospinal tracts (limb coordination) [65], reticulospinal tracts (locomotion and weight-bearing stepping) [66], and spinothalamic tracts (neuropathic pain) [67,68] following SCI. In our study, we did not investigated the sparing of specific spinal tracts via electrophyisiology or dye-tracing experiments; however, an overall increase in residual grey matter likely contributes to improved pain processing pathways (interneurons) and a decrease in aberrant pain [17,69,70]. Varying studies report that 26-96% of human patients experience neuropathic pain following SCI [30]. Research has identified VEGF as one of the potential factors involved in the development of neuropathic pain; however, it is still unclear if VEGF plays a beneficial or detrimental role. Schratzberger *et al.*, found that intramuscular injections of VEGF improved vascularity, blood flow and peripheral nerve function in a rabbit model of diabetic neuropathy [71]. Since it is believed that diabetic neuropathy is caused from microvascular ischemia, their findings reasonably support the use of VEGF for the treatment of neuropathies. Conversely, Nesic *et al.* recently showed that VEGF administration into the spinal cord resulted in an increased number of animals displaying neuropathic pain, as well as an increase in myelinated dorsal horn neurons, suggesting that VEGF results in non-specific axonal sprouting [31]. Regardless of whether VEGF therapies result in favourable or damaging outcomes, it is most important for future research to be aware of potential pitfalls of VEGF administration and to consider the implications they may have on the bench-to-bedside translation of these therapies. Future studies are required to investigate the exact mechanisms of the attenuated allodynia/neuropathic pain observed following AdV-ZFP-VEGF administration.

Conclusions

The present data demonstrate that, similar to the effects seen following immediate administration of AdV-ZFP-VEGF shown by Liu *et al.*, treated animals show increased VEGF mRNA and protein levels, increased vascular counts, increased neuroprotection and reduced apoptosis [11]. Overall, the administration of AdV-ZFP-VEGF shows promise as a therapeutic treatment for SCI, and these findings suggest that AdV-ZFP-VEGF treatment can be delayed up to 24 hours following injury, which presents a feasible time-window for clinical intervention. To the best of our knowledge, we are the first to investigate the delayed administration of AdV-ZFP-VEGF in a model of SCI. Here we observe beneficial effects in a variety of cell populations, and show that these cellular outcomes appear to be translated into improved functional recovery, as well as attenuated allodynia following SCI. Overall, these data suggest that targeting vascular and neuroprotective mechanisms by AdV-ZFP-VEGF administration may be a viable treatment for spinal cord injury. Collectively, this research further supports the use of VEGF as a potential candidate for neurotrauma treatments.

Acknowledgments

The authors would like to express their gratitude to Eunice Cho, Sofia Khan, Ramak Khosravi, Michelle Legasto and Christine Tseng for their help with tissue extraction, tissue processing, immunohistochemistry and cell counting. Thank you to Jared Wilcox and Dr. James Austin for their assistance with data analysis and behavioural techniques. Thank you to Behzad Azad and other members of the Fehlings' lab who assisted with post-operative animal care. The authors thank Philip Gregory and Edward Rebar of Sangamo BioSciences for scientific review.

Author Contributions

Conceived and designed the experiments: SKS GL DA RS MG SAF MGF YL SKK KS. Performed the experiments: SAF YL PF SKS KS. Analyzed the data: SAF YL PF SKK MGF KS. Contributed reagents/materials/analysis tools: SKS GL DA RS MG MGF. Wrote the paper: SAF KS YL SKK MGF.

References

1. Sekhon LH, Fehlings MG (2001) Epidemiology, demographics, and pathophysiology of acute spinal cord injury. Spine 26: S2–S12.
2. Tator CH, Fehlings MG (1991) Review of the secondary injury theory of acute spinal cord trauma with emphasis on vascular mechanisms. J Neurosurg 75: 15–26.
3. Beattie MS (2004) Inflammation and apoptosis: linked therapeutic targets in spinal cord injury. Trends Mol Med 10: 580–583.
4. Fehlings MG, Tator CH, Linden RD (1989) The relationships among the severity of spinal cord injury, motor and somatosensory evoked potentials and spinal cord blood flow. Electroencephalogr Clin Neurophysiol 74: 241–259.
5. Leypold BG, Flanders AE, Schwartz ED, Burns AS (2007) The impact of methylprednisolone on lesion severity following spinal cord injury. Spine 32: 373–378; discussion 379–381.
6. Benton RL, Maddie MA, Minnillo DR, Hagg T, Whittemore SR (2008) Griffonia simplicifolia isolectin B4 identifies a specific subpopulation of angiogenic blood vessels following contusive spinal cord injury in the adult mouse. J Comp Neurol 507: 1031–1052.
7. Shweiki D, Itin A, Soffer D, Keshet E (1992) Vascular endothelial growth factor induced by hypoxia may mediate hypoxia-initiated angiogenesis. Nature 359: 843–845.
8. Greenberg DA, Jin K (2005) From angiogenesis to neuropathology. Nature 438: 954–959.
9. Leung DW, Cachianes G, Kuang WJ, Goeddel DV, Ferrara N (1989) Vascular endothelial growth factor is a secreted angiogenic mitogen. Science 246: 1306–1309.
10. Waxman SG, Cummins TR, Dib-Hajj S, Fjell J, Black JA (1999) Sodium channels, excitability of primary sensory neurons, and the molecular basis of pain. Muscle & Nerve 22: 1177–1187.
11. Liu Y, Figley S, Spratt SK, Lee G, Ando D, et al. (2010) An engineered transcription factor which activates VEGF-A enhances recovery after spinal cord injury. Neurobiology of Disease 37: 384–393.
12. Price SA, Dent C, Duran-Jimenez B, Liang Y, Zhang L, et al. (2006) Gene transfer of an engineered transcription factor promoting expression of VEGF-A protects against experimental diabetic neuropathy. Diabetes 55: 1847–1854.

13. Liu PQ, Rebar EJ, Zhang L, Liu Q, Jamieson AC, et al. (2001) Regulation of an endogenous locus using a panel of designed zinc finger proteins targeted to accessible chromatin regions. Activation of vascular endothelial growth factor A. J Biol Chem 276: 11323–11334.
14. Fehlings MG, Tator CH (1995) The relationships among the severity of spinal cord injury, residual neurological function, axon counts, and counts of retrogradely labeled neurons after experimental spinal cord injury. Exp Neurol 132: 220–228.
15. Basso DM, Beattie MS, Bresnahan JC (1995) A sensitive and reliable locomotor rating scale for open field testing in rats. J Neurotrauma 12: 1–21.
16. Koopmans GC, Deumens R, Honig WM, Hamers FP, Steinbusch HW, et al. (2005) The assessment of locomotor function in spinal cord injured rats: the importance of objective analysis of coordination. J Neurotrauma 22: 214–225.
17. Hamers FP, Koopmans GC, Joosten EA (2006) CatWalk-assisted gait analysis in the assessment of spinal cord injury. J Neurotrauma 23: 537–548.
18. Gensel JC, Tovar CA, Hamers FP, Deibert RJ, Beattie MS, et al. (2006) Behavioral and histological characterization of unilateral cervical spinal cord contusion injury in rats. J Neurotrauma 23: 36–54.
19. Bruce JC, Oatway MA, Weaver LC (2002) Chronic pain after clip-compression injury of the rat spinal cord. Exp Neurol 178: 33–48.
20. Holm S (1979) A simple sequentially rejective multiple test procedure. Scandinavian Journal of Statistics 6: 65–70.
21. Glantz SA (2005) Primer of Biostatistics: McGraw-Hill Companies,Inc. 520 p.
22. Dai Q, Huang J, Klitzman B, Dong C, Goldschmidt-Clermont PJ, et al. (2004) Engineered zinc finger-activating vascular endothelial growth factor transcription factor plasmid DNA induces therapeutic angiogenesis in rabbits with hindlimb ischemia. Circulation 110: 2467–2475.
23. Rebar EJ, Huang Y, Hickey R, Nath AK, Meoli D, et al. (2002) Induction of angiogenesis in a mouse model using engineered transcription factors. Nat Med 8: 1427–1432.
24. Yu J, Lei L, Liang Y, Hinh L, Hickey RP, et al. (2006) An engineered VEGF-activating zinc finger protein transcription factor improves blood flow and limb salvage in advanced-age mice. Faseb J 20: 479–481.
25. Casha S, Yu WR, Fehlings MG (2001) Oligodendroglial apoptosis occurs along degenerating axons and is associated with FAS and p75 expression following spinal cord injury in the rat. Neuroscience 103: 203–218.
26. Schumacher PA, Siman RG, Fehlings MG (2000) Pretreatment with calpain inhibitor CEP-4143 inhibits calpain I activation and cytoskeletal degradation, improves neurological function, and enhances axonal survival after traumatic spinal cord injury. J Neurochem 74: 1646–1655.
27. Karimi-Abdolrezaee S, Eftekharpour E, Fehlings MG (2004) Temporal and spatial patterns of Kv1.1 and Kv1.2 protein and gene expression in spinal cord white matter after acute and chronic spinal cord injury in rats: implications for axonal pathophysiology after neurotrauma. Eur J Neurosci 19: 577–589.
28. Byrne AM, Bouchier-Hayes DJ, Harmey JH (2005) Angiogenic and cell survival functions of Vascular Endothelial Growth Factor (VEGF). Journal of Cellular and Molecular Medicine 9: 777–794.
29. Werhagen L, Budh CN, Hultling C, Molander C (2004) Neuropathic pain after traumatic spinal cord injury—relations to gender, spinal level, completeness, and age at the time of injury. Spinal Cord 42: 665–673.
30. Dijkers M, Bryce T, Zanca J (2009) Prevalence of chronic pain after traumatic spinal cord injury: A systematic review. Journal of Rehabilitation Research & Development 46: 13–30.
31. Nesic O, Sundberg LM, Herrera JJ, Mokkapati VUL, Lee J, et al. (2010) Vascular Endothelial Growth Factor and Spinal Cord Injury Pain. Journal of Neurotrauma 27: 1793–1803.
32. Sun Y, Jin K, Xie L, Childs J, Mao XO, et al. (2003) VEGF-induced neuroprotection, neurogenesis, and angiogenesis after focal cerebral ischemia. The Journal of Clinical Investigation 111: 1843–1851.
33. Widenfalk J, Lipson A, Jubran M, Hofstetter C, Ebendal T, et al. (2003) Vascular endothelial growth factor improves functional outcome and decreases secondary degeneration in experimental spinal cord contusion injury. Neuroscience 120: 951–960.
34. Ling X, Liu D (2007) Temporal and spatial profiles of cell loss after spinal cord injury: Reduction by a metalloporphyrin. Journal of Neuroscience Research 85: 2175–2185.
35. Grossman SD, Rosenberg LJ, Wrathall JR (2001) Temporal-Spatial Pattern of Acute Neuronal and Glial Loss after Spinal Cord Contusion. Experimental Neurology 168: 273–282.
36. Liu XZ, Xu XM, Hu R, Du C, Zhang SX, et al. (1997) Neuronal and Glial Apoptosis after Traumatic Spinal Cord Injury. The Journal of Neuroscience 17: 5395–5406.
37. Loy DN, Crawford CH, Darnall JB, Burke DA, Onifer SM, et al. (2002) Temporal progression of angiogenesis and basal lamina deposition after contusive spinal cord injury in the adult rat. J Comp Neurol 445: 308–324.
38. Kigerl KA, Gensel JC, Ankeny DP, Alexander JK, Donnelly DJ, et al. (2009) Identification of two distinct macrophage subsets with divergent effects causing either neurotoxicity or regeneration in the injured mouse spinal cord. J Neurosci 29: 13435–13444.
39. Mabon PJ, Weaver LC, Dekaban GA (2000) Inhibition of monocyte/macrophage migration to a spinal cord injury site by an antibody to the integrin alphaD: a potential new anti-inflammatory treatment. Exp Neurol 166: 52–64.
40. Glaser J, Gonzalez R, Sadr E, Keirstead HS (2006) Neutralization of the chemokine CXCL10 reduces apoptosis and increases axon sprouting after spinal cord injury. Journal of Neuroscience Research 84: 724–734.
41. Yoshihara T, Ohta M, Itokazu Y, Matsumoto N, Dezawa M, et al. (2007) Neuroprotective Effect of Bone Marrow–Derived Mononuclear Cells Promoting Functional Recovery from Spinal Cord Injury. Journal of Neurotrauma 24: 1026–1036.
42. Kaneko S, Iwanami A, Nakamura M, Kishino A, Kikuchi K, et al. (2006) A selective Sema3A inhibitor enhances regenerative responses and functional recovery of the injured spinal cord. Nature Medicine 12: 1380–1389.
43. Ohab JJ, Fleming S, Blesch A, Carmichael ST (2006) A neurovascular niche for neurogenesis after stroke. Journal of Neuroscience 26: 13007–13016.
44. Raab S, Plate K (2007) Different networks, common growth factors: shared growth factors and receptors of the vascular and the nervous system. Acta Neuropathologica 113: 607–626.
45. Peters KG, De Vries C, Williams LT (1993) Vascular endothelial growth factor receptor expression during embryogenesis and tissue repair suggests a role in endothelial differentiation and blood vessel growth. Proceedings of the National Academy of Sciences 90: 8915–8919.
46. Tsao MN, Li YQ, Lu G, Xu Y, Wong CS (1999) Upregulation of Vascular Endothelial Growth Factor Is Associated with Radiation-Induced Blood-Spinal Cord Barrier Breakdown. Journal of Neuropathology & Experimental Neurology 58: 1051–1060.
47. Skold MK, Gertten CV, Sandbergnordqvist A-C, Mathiesen T, Holmin S (2005) VEGF and VEGF Receptor Expression after Experimental Brain Contusion in Rat. Journal of Neurotrauma 22: 353–367.
48. Jin KL, Mao XO, Nagayama T, Goldsmith PC, Greenberg DA (2000) Induction of vascular endothelial growth factor and hypoxia-inducible factor-1α by global ischemia in rat brain. Neuroscience 99: 577–585.
49. Jin KL, Mao XO, Greenberg DA (2000) Vascular endothelial growth factor: direct neuroprotective effect in in vitro ischemia. Proc Natl Acad Sci U S A 97: 10242–10247.
50. Krum JM, Rosenstein JM (1998) VEGF mRNA and Its Receptor flt-1 Are Expressed in Reactive Astrocytes Following Neural Grafting and Tumor Cell Implantation in the Adult CNS. Experimental Neurology 154: 57–65.
51. Krum JM, Rosenstein JM (1999) Transient Coexpression of Nestin, GFAP, and Vascular Endothelial Growth Factor in Mature Reactive Astroglia Following Neural Grafting or Brain Wounds. Experimental Neurology 160: 348–360.
52. Neufeld G, Kessler O, Herzog Y (2003) The Interaction of Neuropilin-1 and Neuropilin-2 with Tyrosine-Kinase Receptors for VEGF. In: Bagnard D, editor: Springer US. pp. 81–90.
53. Neufeld G, Cohen T, Shraga N, Lange T, Kessler O, et al. (2002) The Neuropilins: Multifunctional Semaphorin and VEGF Receptors that Modulate Axon Guidance and Angiogenesis. Trends in Cardiovascular Medicine 12: 13–19.
54. Bearden SE, Segal SS (2004) Microvessels Promote Motor Nerve Survival and Regeneration Through Local VEGF Release Following Ectopic Reattachment. Microcirculation 11: 633–644.
55. Hobson MI, Green CJ, Terenghi G (2000) VEGF enhances intraneural angiogenesis and improves nerve regeneration after axotomy. Journal of Anatomy 197: 591–605.
56. Choi UH, Ha Y, Huang X, Park SR, Chung J, et al. (2007) Hypoxia-inducible expression of vascular endothelial growth factor for the treatment of spinal cord injury in a rat model. J Neurosurg Spine 7: 54–60.
57. Facchiano F, Fernandez E, Mancarella S, Maira G, Miscusi M, et al. (2002) Promotion of regeneration of corticospinal tract axons in rats with recombinant vascular endothelial growth factor alone and combined with adenovirus coding for this factor. J Neurosurg 97: 161–168.
58. Benton RL, Whittemore SR (2003) VEGF165 therapy exacerbates secondary damage following spinal cord injury. Neurochem Res 28: 1693–1703.
59. Barleon B, Sozzani S, Zhou D, Weich H, Mantovani A, et al. (1996) Migration of human monocytes in response to vascular endothelial growth factor (VEGF) is mediated via the VEGF receptor flt-1. Blood 87: 3336–3343.
60. Karimi-Abdolrezaee S, Eftekharpour E, Wang J, Morshead CM, Fehlings MG (2006) Delayed Transplantation of Adult Neural Precursor Cells Promotes Remyelination and Functional Neurological Recovery after Spinal Cord Injury. The Journal of Neuroscience 26: 3377–3389.
61. Yezierski RP, Liu S, Ruenes GL, Busto R, Dietrich WD (1996) Neuronal Damage Following Intraspinal Injection of a Nitric Oxide Synthase Inhibitor in the Rat. J Cereb Blood Flow Metab 16: 996–1004.
62. Azzouz M, Hottinger A, Paterna J-C, Zurn AD, Aebischer P, et al. (2000) Increased motoneuron survival and improved neuromuscular function in transgenic ALS mice after intraspinal injection of an adeno-associated virus encoding Bcl-2. Human Molecular Genetics 9: 803–811.
63. Naldini A, Carraro F (2005) Role of inflammatory mediators in angiogenesis. Curr Drug Targets Inflamm Allergy 4: 3–8.
64. Flynn JR, Graham BA, Galea MP, Callister RJ (2011) The role of propriospinal interneurons in recovery from spinal cord injury. Neuropharmacology 60: 809–822.
65. Pearse DD, Pereira FC, Marcillo AE, Bates ML, Berrocal YA, et al. (2004) cAMP and Schwann cells promote axonal growth and functional recovery after spinal cord injury. Nature Medicine 10: 610–616.

66. Ballermann M, Fouad K (2006) Spontaneous locomotor recovery in spinal cord injured rats is accompanied by anatomical plasticity of reticulospinal fibers. European Journal of Neuroscience 23: 1988–1996.
67. Defrin R, Ohry A, Blumen N, Urca G (2001) Characterization of chronic pain and somatosensory function in spinal cord injury subjects. Pain 89: 253–263.
68. Österberg A, Boivie J (2010) Central pain in multiple sclerosis – Sensory abnormalities. European Journal of Pain 14: 104–110.
69. Vierck Jr CJ, Siddall P, Yezierski RP (2000) Pain following spinal cord injury: animal models and mechanistic studies. Pain 89: 1–5.
70. Hoheisel U, Scheifer C, Trudrung P, Unger T, Mense S (2003) Pathophysiological activity in rat dorsal horn neurones in segments rostral to a chronic spinal cord injury. Brain Research 974: 134–145.
71. Schratzberger P, Walter DH, Rittig K, Bahlmann FH, Pola R, et al. (2001) Reversal of experimental diabetic neuropathy by VEGF gene transfer. The Journal of Clinical Investigation 107: 1083–1092.

11

Examination of the Combined Effects of Chondroitinase ABC, Growth Factors and Locomotor Training following Compressive Spinal Cord Injury on Neuroanatomical Plasticity and Kinematics

Olivier Alluin[1], Hugo Delivet-Mongrain[1☯], Marie-Krystel Gauthier[2☯], Michael G. Fehlings[3], Serge Rossignol[1], Soheila Karimi-Abdolrezaee[2,4]*

1 Multidisciplinary Team in Locomotor Rehabilitation of the Canadian Institutes of Health Research (CIHR) and Groupe de Recherche sur le Système Nerveux Central (GRSNC) of the Fonds de Recherche du Québec – Santé (FRQS), Department of Physiology, University of Montreal, Montreal, Quebec, Canada, **2** The Department of Physiology and Pathophysiology and the Spinal Cord Research Center, University of Manitoba, Winnipeg, Manitoba, Canada, **3** Department of Surgery and Spinal Program, University of Toronto; Toronto Western Research Institute, University Health Network, Toronto, Ontario, Canada, **4** Regenerative Medicine Program and Manitoba Institute of Child Health, Winnipeg, Manitoba, Canada

Abstract

While several cellular and pharmacological treatments have been evaluated following spinal cord injury (SCI) in animal models, it is increasingly recognized that approaches to address the glial scar, including the use of chondroitinase ABC (ChABC), can facilitate neuroanatomical plasticity. Moreover, increasing evidence suggests that combinatorial strategies are key to unlocking the plasticity that is enabled by ChABC. Given this, we evaluated the anatomical and functional consequences of ChABC in a combinatorial approach that also included growth factor (EGF, FGF2 and PDGF-AA) treatments and daily treadmill training on the recovery of hindlimb locomotion in rats with mid thoracic clip compression SCI. Using quantitative neuroanatomical and kinematic assessments, we demonstrate that the combined therapy significantly enhanced the neuroanatomical plasticity of major descending spinal tracts such as corticospinal and serotonergic-spinal pathways. Additionally, the pharmacological treatment attenuated chronic astrogliosis and inflammation at and adjacent to the lesion with the modest synergistic effects of treadmill training. We also observed a trend for earlier recovery of locomotion accompanied by an improvement of the overall angular excursions in rats treated with ChABC and growth factors in the first 4 weeks after SCI. At the end of the 7-week recovery period, rats from all groups exhibited an impressive spontaneous recovery of the kinematic parameters during locomotion on treadmill. However, although the combinatorial treatment led to clear chronic neuroanatomical plasticity, these structural changes did not translate to an additional long-term improvement of locomotor parameters studied including hindlimb-forelimb coupling. These findings demonstrate the beneficial effects of combined ChABC, growth factors and locomotor training on the plasticity of the injured spinal cord and the potential to induce earlier neurobehavioral recovery. However, additional approaches such as stem cell therapies or a more adapted treadmill training protocol may be required to optimize this repair strategy in order to induce sustained functional locomotor improvement.

Editor: Hatem E. Sabaawy, Rutgers-Robert wood Johnson Medical School, United States of America

Funding: This work was supported by the operating grants from the following: 1) the Craig H. Neilsen Foundation to SKA, MGF and SR; 2) the Christopher and Dana Reeve Foundation to SKA, MGF and SR; 3) the Manitoba Health Research Council (MHRC) to SKA; 4) the Canadian Institutes of Health Research (Sensorimotor Rehabilitation Research Team - SMRRT - grant and Canada Research Chair) to SR; 5) OA was supported by a postdoctoral fellowship from the Fonds de Recherche du Québec - Santé and Sensorimotor Rehabilitation Research Team - SMRRT; and 6) MGF is supported by the Halbert Chair in Neural Repair and Regeneration and by grants from the Krembil and Dezwirek Foundations. The funders had no role in study design, data collection and analysis, decision to publish, or preparation of the manuscript.

Competing Interests: The authors have declared that no competing interests exist.

* Email: soheila.karimi@med.umanitoba.ca

☯ These authors contributed equally to this work.

Introduction

Spinal cord injury (SCI) results in motor deficits below the level of injury that can be temporary or permanent, incomplete or complete depending on the severity of the lesion [1–4]. Recovery of locomotion is generally limited in SCI patients in spite of recent advances in clinical care and rehabilitation medicine [5]. Over the past years, various cellular and neurochemical repair strategies have been evaluated in experimental models of SCI for their efficacy in promoting neuroplasticity, axon regeneration, remyelination, and re-establishment of spinal circuitry to improve motor recovery following such injury [6–13]. Among these treatment strategies, targeting the inhibitory properties of chondroitin sulfate proteoglycans (CSPGs) located in the extracellular matrix of glial scar has shown promising potential in enhancing SCI repair [11,12,14–21].

Chondroitinase ABC (ChABC) facilitates the degradation of CSPGs in the injured spinal cord [12]. Therefore, over the past decade, ChABC has been utilized extensively in different models of SCI and in various combinatorial approaches to evaluate its impact in promoting functional repair and recovery [11,14,16,20,22,23]. Emerging evidence demonstrates that ChABC alone or in conjunction with growth factors, neurotrophins and/or cell-based treatments can promote structural repair and regeneration in the injured spinal cord [11–15,17,21,22,24,25]. ChABC treatment has also shown the potential to enhance locomotion in combination with other therapies in models of transection or compressive/contusive SCI [11,14,21].

ChABC in combination with cell therapies improves moderate recovery of function [11,14]. Studies by Fouad and colleagues showed that ChABC in synergy with a Schwann cell bridge and transplantation of olfactory ensheathing cells allowed recovery of function in rats after complete transection SCI [14]. We have also shown that degradation of CSPGs in the glial scar with ChABC was needed to improve the outcomes of transplanting neural precursor cells (NPCs) in chronic SCI [11] or efficient activation and oligodendrocyte replacement of endogenous spinal cord precursor cells in subacute SCI [15]. Sustained delivery of ChABC in combination with a growth factor (GF) cocktail containing EGF, FGF2 and PDGF-AA significantly increased the long-term survival and migration of transplanted NPCs in chronic compressive SCI [11]. Combined effects of ChABC, GFs and NPCs transplantation attenuated axonal die back in the corticospinal tract (CST) and enhanced sprouting of the CST and serotonergic fibers in the chronically injured spinal cord [11]. Moreover, we have shown that ChABC and GFs synergistically enhances the activation and oligodendrocyte differentiation of endogenous precursor cells after SCI and attenuated astrogliosis [15]. However, our functional testing showed that although ChABC, by itself, allowed substantial structural plasticity in the spinal cord, it was not sufficient to enhance locomotor recovery until it was combined with NPCs transplantation and *in vivo* infusion of GFs [11].

ChABC has been also used in combination with motor training in order to synergistically enhance activity dependent neuroplasticity and the recovery of locomotion in experimental models of SCI [16,20,26]. Current evidence indicates a limited efficiency of motor training in improving function in rodents or cats with incomplete SCI; contusive/compressive or hemisection [26–29]. In our recent work, kinematic analyses showed that regular motor training on treadmill did not improve the quality of spontaneous recovery of locomotion in rats with incomplete compressive SCI, although the rats regained impressive functional locomotion of the hindlimbs [27].

The aim of the present study was to evaluate whether combination of ChABC and growth factors (GFs) with daily treadmill training would synergistically enhance endogenous repair mechanisms and activity dependent functional plasticity, together allowing a significantly better recovery of hindlimb locomotion in rats with compressive SCI. We used neuroanatomical and kinematic analyses to assess neuroplasticity and functional recovery over a 7-week recovery period. Our findings show that this strategy promoted a significant degree of structural plasticity in corticospinal and serotonin-dependent pathways and that our pharmacological treatment mitigated the evolution of chronic peri-lesional astrogliosis and inflammation with a modest synergistic effects of treadmill training. Although an earlier return of locomotion was associated with an overall improvement of hindlimb angular excursions in the group treated with ChABC + GFs, this observation did not reach the statistically significant threshold needed to claim a difference between groups. Additionally, we observed an impressive locomotor recovery at the endpoint of study in all rats; however, the combinatorial approach had no additive long-term beneficial effects on the locomotor parameters studied with our stringent kinematic parameters.

Materials and Methods

All the neurobehavioural and neuroanatomical protocols in this study were performed based on approaches previously described by our group [6,11,15,27,30]. We used appropriate randomization and blinding in all neurobehavioural and histological techniques. Unbiased methodologies were used to undertake the neuroanatomical assessments. A list of abbreviations is provided in Table 1.

Animal care

A total number of 48 adult female Wistar rats (250–275 g) from Charles River Laboratory (Quebec, Canada) were used for different aspects of this study. Animals were housed in standard plastic cages at 22°C before spinal cord injury (SCI) and 25°C after SCI in a 12:12 h light/dark photoperiod. Food (Agribrands Purina, Ontario, Canada) and drinking water were available *ad libitum*. Hardwood sawdust bedding (PWI brand, Quebec, Canada) was used before SCI and then was replaced by soft paper bedding (Diamond Soft Bedding, Harlan Teklad) after SCI to prevent skin lesion. Animals were examined daily. After SCI, the bladder was expressed two times daily until the recovery of spontaneous bladder function occurred (between 7 and 14 days post-injury). All the animal procedures included in the present study were approved by the University of Manitoba and the University of Montreal Research Ethics Board and were conducted according to the Canadian Guide to the Care and Use of Experimental Animals (Canadian Council on Animal Care).

Experimental design and groups

After a one-week period of housing in the animal facility, rats were habituated to walk consistently on the treadmill at different speeds for three weeks. Afterwards, kinematic baselines were recorded for all rats during a second three-week period, and then SCI procedure was performed on each rat. One rat died during the surgery because of respiratory failure. Four days after SCI, rats were randomized into four experimental groups: 1) vehicle/untrained group (n = 12), 2) vehicle/trained group (n = 12), 3) ChABC+GFs/untrained group (n = 11), and 4) ChABC+GFs/trained group (n = 12). All SCI rats from groups 3–4 and 10 SCI rats from groups 1–2 (5 per group) underwent a second surgical procedure to infuse ChABC+GFs or vehicle via an intrathecal catheter connected to an Alzet osmotic minipump. After recovering from the implantation (2–3 days), kinematics was recorded weekly during 7 weeks for all rats of groups 3 and 4 and for 10 rats in groups 1 and 2 (5 per group). Finally, all the spinal cords were harvested for histology. Except for treadmill training sessions and data recording, all rats could move freely in their cage.

Table 1. List of abbreviations.

ChABC	Chondroitinase ABC
GFs	Growth factors (EGF + FGF-2+ PDGF-AA)
SCI	Spinal cord injury
CSPGs	Chondroitin Sulfate Proteoglycans
BBB	Basso, Beattie and Bresnahan rating scale
LFB/HE	Luxol Fast Blue and hematoxylin/Eosin
BDA	Biotin dextran amine
CST	Corticospinal tract
CV	Coefficient of Variation
PBS	Phosphate Buffer Saline
PFA	Paraformaldehyde
GFAP	Glial Fibrillary Acidic Protein
5-HT	Serotonin
ANOVA	Analyse Of Variance
SEM	Standard Error of the Mean
F subphase	First part of the swing phase (Flexion)
E1 subphase	Second part of the swing phase (Extension)

Treadmill apparatus and habituation

The treadmill belt was laid under a Plexiglas box (Length = 41 cm × Depth = 9.3 cm × Height = 14 cm) with a removable top. All rats were progressively familiarized to walk consistently on the treadmill at speeds ranging from 14 $m.min^{-1}$ (low) to 30 $m.min^{-1}$ (high) during the three weeks training program before SCI. Each session lasted 15 minutes and the number of sessions depended on the ability of each rat to perform the task. A soft plastic stick was used when necessary to stimulate the rats and induce appropriate locomotion by touching their hindquarters. Progressively, rats learned to walk freely and regularly in the locomotor device, using all four limbs at each speed of the range defined above.

Surgical procedures

All surgeries were performed in sterile conditions and under general gas anesthesia consisting in a mixture of O_2/isoflurane (2%) given through a mask integrated in a surgical stereotaxic frame. Immediately after surgery, rats were placed under a heating lamp until they fully recovered consciousness. Animals were given postoperative analgesia (50 μg/kg Temgesic, Schering-Plough, Hertfordshire, UK) and saline (3 ml) subcutaneously to prevent pain and dehydration, and then received antibiotics in drinking water (Clavamox drops, Pfizer Animal Health) for 1 week.

Thoracic Spinal Cord Injury. The aneurysm clip spinal compression model has been extensively described previously by our group [6,11,15,27,30–32]. Briefly, a midline incision was made at the thoracic vertebrae (T5-T9) and the skin and superficial muscles were retracted. The rats underwent a T6–T8 laminectomy and then, received a 23.8 g clip (Walsh Inc., Oakville, Ontario, Canada) compression injury for 1 min at the level of T7 of the spinal cord. Next, a piece of sterile absorbable gelatin sponge (1.5 × 1 × 0.7 cm, Gelfoam, Pfizer Inc.) was placed over the dura between T6–T8 and finally, muscles and skin were sutured. This injury produces moderately severe incomplete SCI with neurological outcomes of spastic paraparesis.

Administration of ChABC and Growth Factors. At four days post SCI, all rats were anesthetized using a mixture of O_2/isoflurane (2%) and then the injured spinal cord was carefully re-exposed using microsurgical techniques. ChABC (Seikagaku Corporation, Tokyo, Japan, 5 U/ml in saline plus 0.1% rat serum albumin) plus a cocktail of growth factors [GFs, including PDGF-AA (Sigma, 1 μg/100 μl), bFGF (Sigma, 3 μg/100 μl) and EGF (Sigma, 3 μg/100 μl) in a solution containing saline and 0.1% rat serum albumin] was infused for seven days using a subarachnoid catheter (Alzet, Rat IT, 0007741, 0.36 mm OD; 0.18 mm ID) connected to an osmotic minipump (Alzet pump model No.1007D, 0.5 μl/hr), as we have previously reported [6,33]. The catheter was inserted in the subarachnoid space around the injured area. Five rats in each vehicle group underwent identical surgical procedures but received saline plus 0.1% rat serum albumin). In our previous studies in the same model of SCI [11,15], we have extensively tested the efficacy of ChABC treatment in CSPG degradation. Using quantitative immunohistochemistry and slot blotting for CSPGs as well as 2B6 and C4S (detecting the degraded products of CSPGs), we have confirmed that one week ChABC treatment delivered at 3 days or 6 weeks post SCI can significantly degrade CSPGs after SCI. In our previous studies, our analysis at the end of one-week ChABC delivery with Alzet pump infusion has consistently confirmed a 60–75% reduction in CSPGs deposits and instead an 80% increase in C4S immunoreactivity (by-products of ChABC activity) in the matrix of subacute or chronic SCI [11,15].

BDA Anterograde tracing of the corticospinal tract (CST). Two weeks before the end of experiments, rats underwent anterograde tracing of the corticospinal tract (CST) with biotinylated dextran amine (BDA) (n = 3–6 rats/group). Under isoflurane anesthesia (as above), rats were positioned in a stereotaxic frame. BDA (10%, 10,000 MW; Invitrogen, Eugene, OR) was injected unilaterally into the left sensorimotor cortex at eight sites (0.5 μl per site) using the following coordinates (in reference to Bregma): (1) 1 mm anterior and 1 mm lateral; (2) 0.5 mm anterior and 1 mm lateral; (3) 1 mm posterior and 1 mm lateral; (4) 2.5 mm posterior and 1 mm lateral; (5) 0.5 mm posterior and 2 mm lateral; (6) 1.5 mm posterior and 2 mm lateral, (7) 1 mm anterior and 2.5 mm lateral, (8) 1.5 mm anterior and 2.5 mm lateral. Injections were made 1.2 mm from the surface of the cortex. Our previous studies have shown that the two weeks interval between BDA labeling and animal sacrifice is sufficient for anterograde labelling of the CST in thoracic regions [11,34].

Treadmill training program and kinematic recordings

Rats from groups 2 and 4 were all trained to walk on the motorized treadmill belt from 1 day to 7 weeks following SCI. The training program was performed 5 days/week and consisted in a walking session of 10 min daily on the treadmill at various speeds (from 14 to 26 m.min^{-1}) depending on the locomotor recovery level of each rat. Early after SCI, rats were incapable of autonomous hindlimb stepping, and were therefore stimulated by pinching the perineum. This evoked, in most cases, some hindlimb locomotion adapted to the belt speed but sometimes only flexion/extension alternation without plantar paw placement. During the training session, the belt speed was set at 14 m.min^{-1} and the trunk of the animal was manually maintained to limit the lateral imbalance as long as the animal required perineal stimulation to walk. As soon as the rat was capable to walk without perineal stimulation, the belt speed was incremented in steps of 2 m.min^{-1} every 2 minutes until the maximum speed tolerated by the rat was reached (*i.e.* in the range defined above). Throughout the recovery period, the trunk of the animals was manually supported when necessary.

Kinematic recordings. Kinematic baseline data were recorded at 14, 20 and 26 m.min^{-1} for each rat to obtain control values. After SCI, the locomotor performance was evaluated weekly for 7 weeks until the maximum velocity that the animal could reach in the range defined above. Moreover, the untrained groups were assessed during short sessions to avoid the training effect of the evaluation itself. Kinematic recording method has been previously described in detail by our group [27]. Briefly, after shaving the left hindquarter of the rat, five markers were set on the skin of the lateral side at the level of ilium, greater trochanter, ankle joint, metatarsophalangeal joint and tip of the third toe. During the recording session, a left side view of the rat walking on the treadmill was captured using a high frequency numerical video camera (120 Hz). All the kinematics parameters were generated from the *x*, *y* coordinates of each marker and from the paw contact/lift events. Triangulation was used to extract the knee position from hip and ankle joint markers.

Definition of locomotion on treadmill. Since rats in each group exhibited different locomotor capability on treadmill at the end of the experiment, it was necessary to define simple criteria to include in kinematics analysis only animals capable of producing motor pattern considered as locomotor. Rats capable of performing at least 10 consecutive bilateral flexion-extension alternations of the hindlimbs with paw placement (plantar or dorsal) on the treadmill belt at 14 m.min^{-1} were included in locomotion analysis. Rats that have not reached these criteria were considered not to have recovered locomotion.

Calculation of coordination. The method employed to evaluate the interlimb coordination has been described in detail previously [27] and gives an index of the neuronal coupling between each paw during locomotion. The coordination between fore- and hindlimbs (*i.e.* anteroposterior) as well as limbs from the same girdle (*i.e.* homologous) was calculated using the same method. Briefly, the coordination value of a given limb in a given step cycle represents the temporal position of the ground contact from this limb relative to the whole step cycle duration of the other limb. For instance, left hindlimbs homologous coordination value of 0.5 in a given step cycle means that ground contact of left hindlimb occurs at 50% of the right hindlimb step cycle duration.

Evaluation of individual variability. The method of individual variability assessment has been previously reported in detailed description [27]. Briefly, the coefficient of variation (CV) of every kinematic parameter was used to assess the intrinsic variability of each rat during locomotion. Since the analysis of locomotion of a given rat was based on consecutive sequences of several step cycles, each individual kinematic data at a given time point was an averaged value from the consecutive step cycles associated with a standard deviation. Thus, in the present study, the CV of a given parameter in a given rat at a given time point is the individual standard deviation expressed in percent of the mean of this parameter.

Tissue Processing and Neuroanatomical Analyses

Animal perfusion. At the end of experiments, animals were deeply anesthetized with sodium pentobarbital (80 mg/kg, intraperitoneal.) and then perfused transcardially with cold phosphate buffer saline (PBS, 0.1 M) followed by 4% paraformaldehyde (PFA) in 0.1 M PBS, pH 7.4. A two cm length of the spinal cord centered at the injury center was dissected and processed for different procedures as follows:

Frozen Sections. For cryotomy, the spinal cord were postfixed in the perfusion solution plus 10% sucrose overnight at 4°C, and then cryoprotected in 20% sucrose in PBS for 48 hr at 4°C. Then, the spinal cord centered at the injury site was dissected and embedded in mounting media (HistoPrep, Fisher Scientific) on dry ice. Cryostat sections (25 µm) were cut and stored at –80°C.

Vibratome sectioning. The spinal cords of the rats that underwent BDA anterograde labeling were postfixed in 4% PFA for overnight at 4°C, and then stored in PBS containing 0.1% sodium azide. The spinal cord were embedded in 10% low-temperature gelling agarose (Sigma), and 50 µm free floating serial transverse sections were cut on a vibratome (Leica) and collected in multi-well plates containing PBS plus 0.1% sodium azide.

Morphometric assessment of spinal cord lesion. Serial frozen spinal cord sections at 500 µm intervals were stained with myelin-selective pigment Luxol Fast Blue (LFB) and the tissue stain Hematoxylin-Eosin (HE) to identify the injury epicentre (N = 3–6 rats/group) as we reported previously [27,30]. Tissue sections displaying the largest proportion of cystic cavity compared with total cross-sectional area were taken to represent the epicentre of the injury. For analysis of tissue sparing and cavity formation after SCI, for each rat, we selected the spinal sections at epicentre and 1 mm and 2 mm rostral and caudal to the epicentre. The sections were stained with LFB-HE. We also immunostained the adjacent slide for astrocytes using an antibody against GFAP (rabbit, 1:1000, Dako) to precisely identify the borders of lesion cavity in each section. Reactive astrocytes surround the lesion area that includes the tissue debris and macrophages/microglia. Therefore, we used this criterion to differentiate the damaged tissue/debris within the lesion from the surrounding spared spinal cord tissue. The measurements were carried out in a blinded manner on coded slides using NIH ImageJ software (Media Cybernetics Inc., MD). Spared tissue was measured and normalized as a percentage of the total cross-sectional area of the spinal cord.

Immunohistochemical procedures and image analysis

For all immunohistochemical staining, the blocking solution contained 5% non-fat milk, 1% BSA and 0.3% Triton X-100 in 0.1 M PBS unless otherwise has been mentioned. The specificities of all antibodies were verified with both a negative control, omitting the primary antibody in our immunohistochemistry staining protocol, and a positive control, testing the antibody on tissues or cell preparations known to express the antigen.

GFAP and CD11b (OX42) immunostaining. Five transverse sections at epicentre and 1 mm and 2 mm rostral and caudal to the epicentre from each rat (N = 3–6 rats/group) were immunostained against GFAP and OX42 to assess astrocytic glial scar and macrophages/microglia, respectively. The frozen slides were air-dried at room temperature, and then were washed with PBS for 10 min. The sections were blocked and then incubated with primary antibodies. The following primary antibodies were used overnight at 4°C: rabbit anti-GFAP (1:1000, Dako) for astrocytes and mouse anti-CD11b (OX42, Serotec, 1:50). The slides were washed in PBS three times and then incubated with fluorescent Alexa 568 or 488 goat-anti mouse or anti-rabbit secondary antibodies (Invitrogen, 1:500) for 1 hr. The slides were coverslipped with Mowiol mounting medium containing DAPI to counterstain the nuclei. The images were taken using a Zeiss 710 laser confocal microscope or a Zeiss AxioVision microscope.

BDA visualization. We employed anterograde BDA labeling to study the sprouting of the CST fibers in the spinal gray matter as we described previously [11]. Three transverse vibratome sections (50 μm thickness) per animal at 5, 9 and 11 mm rostral to the injury site were selected for immunohistochemical processing to visualize BDA (N = 3–5/rats per group). One section per distance was processed for immunohistochemistry. Free-floating sections were incubated with the following reagents: 0.3% hydrogen peroxide (H_2O_2) in absolute methanol for 30 min at 4°C (using blocking solution as above), Vectastain AB (ABC Elite Kit, Vector Labs) in PBS containing 0.5% Triton X-10 according to manufacturer instructions for 2 hrs, 0.05% diaminobenzidine and 0.05% H_2O_2 in PBS for about 5 min. Sections were mounted onto slides and air-dried. Then, the slides were dehydrated through an alcohol series, cleared in xylene and coverslipped with Permount (Fisher Scientific).

5-HT immunostaining. Free-floating (50 μm thickness) at the injury epicenter and various distances relative to the injury epicenter: 1.5, 3 and 6 mm both rostrally and caudally were processed for immunohistochemistry for 5-HT (N = 3–6 rats/group). One section per distance was processed for immunohistochemistry. Sections were blocked and then incubated in anti-rabbit 5-HT antibody (1:10,000, ImmunoStar) for overnight at 4°C, and then Alexa 568 goat-anti rabbit secondary antibody (1:400, 2 hrs at room temperature) with three PBS washes after each step.

Image processing and analysis

In all neuroanatomical procedures, quantification was executed in an unbiased fashion by examiners blinded to the treatment groups based on the previously described methods by our group [6,11,15,27,30].

Immunohistochemical assessments of GFAP, CD11b (Ox42) and 5-HT. For immunodensity measurements of GFAP, CD11b (Ox42) and 5-HT, we imaged the entire cross section of the spinal cord at 10× primary objective using Mosaic tiling software (Zeiss). Then, using NIH Image analysis system (Image J), we traced entire cross section of the spinal cord and measured the relative density of GFAP, CD11b or 5-HT immunoreactivity as we performed previously [11] (N = 3–6 rats/group). Furthermore, we performed automatic thresholding for each image using NIH ImageJ software to determine the threshold for specific signal. After setting the threshold, the immunodensity above the threshold was automatically calculated. Background intensity from an area with no positive immunoreactivity was also subtracted from the intensity value to correct for non-specific reactions. Then, we divided the integrated density to the sample area to calculate the mean density per unit area. This calculation was performed to compensate for the different size of the region of interest in the spinal cord as we performed previously [11].

Assessment of axonal sprouting in the corticospinal tract. We performed anterograde BDA labeling to assess the sprouting of the CST fibers in the spinal gray matter as we described previously [11]. We normalized the intensity value of the BDA labeled collaterals in the gray matter to the intensity of BDA labeled fibers in the main CST to correct for inter-animal variation in the BDA labeling efficiency and/or the preservation of CST fibers. We imaged the dorsal columns of the spinal cord at 10×primary magnification using a Zeiss microscope at 5, 9 and 11 mm rostral to injury epicenter (N = 3–5/rats per group). In our SCI model, descending fibers of the CST are directly impacted by the injury and undergo Wallerian degeneration at and caudal to the injury epicenter. The axons in the rostral segment are also subjected to retrograde axonal degeneration or "die-back" as we described before [11].

Therefore, we selected rostral distances at 5 mm and further to the injury epicenter for our assessment of the CST fibers collateral sprouting. Using ImageJ Software, we measured the relative density of BDA immunoreactivity in the CST within the dorsal column. We employed automatic thresholding for each image using ImageJ software to determine the threshold for specific signal. The immunodensity above the threshold was quantified and the mean net density for BDA was calculated by dividing the immunointensity for BDA to the traced area. Background intensity from an area with no BDA positive immunoreactivity was also subtracted from the intensity value to correct for non-specific reactions. For collateral sprouting in spinal gray matter, we undertook the same approach as described above for BDA in the main CST to measure the relative intensity of BDA labeling within a the dorsal and intermediate gray matter. Then, we normalized the intensity value of the BDA labeled collaterals in the gray matter to the intensity of BDA labeled fibers of the main CST [11].

Statistical analysis

For neuroanatomical examinations and statistical intensity measurements, Two-Way ANOVA comparing groups and distances was used followed by post hoc pairwise multiple comparisons testing by the Holm-Sidak post hoc test. For kinematic analysis, individual data from each rat at every time point were averaged from a minimum of 10 consecutive locomotor cycles. Analysis of kinematic and regression data was performed using SigmaPlot program (Systat software Inc., San Jose, USA). Two-way ANOVA Repeated Measures was used to compare the effects of groups and delays on kinematics parameters followed by all pairwise multiple comparison (Holm-Sidak post hoc test) when ANOVA was significant. ANOVA was also used to test the linear regression between kinematic and neuroanatomical data. All the regressions analysis presented in this study have passed the normality test (Shapiro-Wilk) and the equal variance test. Non-parametric χ^2 with Yates correction and power test (α set at 0.05) or Fisher's exact test analysis were used to compare the distribution of rats capable or not to walk on treadmill at the different time points and velocity after SCI. Samples sizes were calculated to allow a 20% chance for a Type II error ($\beta \leq 0.2$). Grouped data are reported as mean ± SEM and the significance threshold for all statistical analysis was $p \leq 0.05$.

Results

Morphometric analysis of the spinal cord lesion

We first studied the effects of the treatments on tissue preservation and lesion following SCI. We quantified the extent of tissue sparing in spinal cord serial sections at five distances along the rostrocaudal length of the injured spinal cord centered at the injury epicenter as we described previously [27,30]. Representative photomicrographs of Luxol Fast Blue, hematoxylin and eosin-Y (LFB/HE) counterstained cross-sectional spinal cord sections are demonstrated for all treatment groups in Fig. 1A. Values representing the mean percentage of spared tissue for each examined distance in all experimental groups are summarized in Table 2. Our quantitative analysis showed no statistically significant difference in tissue sparing across the experimental groups suggesting that ChABC, GFs and training had no beneficial effects on attenuating tissue degeneration following injury.

Effects of ChABC, growth factors and daily exercise on the evolution of chronic astrogliosis and inflammation around the SCI lesion

We further investigated the influence of ChABC, GFs and daily treadmill training on the evolution of chronic reactive astrogliosis and inflammation within the spinal cord lesion. We quantified GFAP immunodensity (marking astrocytes) in spinal cord sections at the injury epicenter and at the peri-lesional areas around 1 mm and 2 mm rostral and caudal points to the epicenter (Fig. 2A–P, images depict representative sections at the epicenter and 1 mm rostral and caudal). Our data showed clear effects of ChABC and GFs attenuating astrogliosis, evident by reduced GFAP immunodensity, at the injury epicenter in the rats that received pharmacological treatments relative to untreated rats (Fig. 2Q, *$p<0.05$, two-way ANOVA, Holm-Sidak *post hoc*). Our analyses of the peri-lesional areas also showed a significantly reduced GFAP immunodensity in ChABC+GFs/trained group compared to the SCI vehicle/untrained group at 1 mm rostral and caudal points and compared to the SCI vehicle/trained group only at the 1 mm rostral distance (Fig. 2Q). These significant peri-lesional effects only present in ChABC+GFs/trained animals suggest a trend of synergy in our combinatorial strategy. Although there was a trend for reduced GFAP immunodensity in ChABC+GFs/trained group in comparison to the ChABC+GFs/untrained group, the difference between the two groups was not statistically significant. Interestingly, our examination also showed a significant attenuation in astrogliosis in ChABC+GFs/untrained group compared to the SCI vehicle/trained and SCI vehicle/untrained groups at the epicenter of the lesion (Fig. 2Q) which is in agreement with our previous results in a subacute SCI lesion after administration of ChABC+GFs [15]. Here, we did not observe any difference in lesional and peri-lesional astrogliosis between the two trained and untrained SCI vehicle groups as the result of treadmill motor exercise alone. Although, the differences between ChABC+GFs trained and untrained groups did not reach the significant level, the positive effects only obtained with the 3 combined treatments in the peri-lesional area suggest a potential moderate synergy. However, ChABC and GFs treatment seemed to be the key to induce the main effects.

Next, we studied how treatment with ChABC, GFs and training affect chronic inflammation assessed by the presence of macrophages/microglia within the lesional and peri-lesional regions (Fig. 3A–P, images depict representative sections at the epicenter and 1 mm rostral and caudal). Our neuroanatomical data at all the above-mentioned distances showed a significantly reduced macrophages/microglia in the chronic SCI lesion in the ChABC+GFs/trained group compared to the vehicle/untrained group and at the epicenter compared to the vehicle/trained group (Fig. 3R, *$p<0.05$, two-way ANOVA, Holm-Sidak *post hoc*). However, there was no significant difference between ChABC+GFs/trained and ChABC+GFs/untrained groups. Interestingly, rats in the ChABC+GFs/untrained group also showed less density of macrophages/microglia compared to the vehicle/untrained group that was significantly different at the epicenter and 1 mm rostral peri-lesional area, showing the effect of ChABC and GFs treatments on the reduction of inflammation process (Fig. 3Q, *$p<0.05$). This is also in agreement with our previous study that showed the positive effects of ChABC alone and in combination with GFs in attenuating lesional recruitment of macrophages/microglia in subacute SCI [15]. In the present chronic study, the significant reduction in macrophages/microglia at 2 mm rostral and 1 and 2 mm caudal to the epicenter only in ChABC+GFs/trained group suggests moderate synergistic effects of training with ChABC+GFs treatments.

ChABC, growth factors and daily training synergistically promote collateral sprouting of the corticospinal tract and serotonergic fibers after SCI

To assess whether our combined strategy would enhance neuroplasticity in the injured spinal cord, we studied the sprouting of two major descending pathways to the spinal cord: the corticospinal tract (CST) and serotonergic pathway. For studying the CST, we used anterograde BDA tracing to label the CST and its collateral fibers in the spinal cord (Fig. 4A–L). Of note, as we have shown previously, in our protocol to induce clip compressive SCI, the CST is disrupted by the injury and its axons caudal to the injury epicenter undergoes degeneration [11]. Moreover, CST axons proximal to the impact of injury are subject to axonal die-back and therefore are absent in rostral distances closer to the epicenter [11,35]. Accordingly, we examined the density of BDA labeling at starting at 5 mm distance rostral to the injury epicenter where the main CST is partially preserved following clip compression SCI [11]. To correct for inter-animal variation in the BDA labeling efficiency, we normalized the intensity of the BDA labeled collaterals in the gray matter to the intensity of BDA labeled main CST in the same section. Analysis of the dorsal and intermediate gray matter regions (boxed area depicted in Fig. 4A–L), at 5, 9 and 11 mm rostral points, revealed a significant increase in the density of BDA-labeled collaterals of the CST axons in the ChABC+GFs/trained group when compared to all other SCI experimental groups at 9 mm and to Vehicle/trained and untrained groups at 5 mm distances rostral to the lesion (Fig. 4M, *$p<0.05$, two-way ANOVA, Holm-Sidak *post hoc*). While the ChABC and GFs treatments together also demonstrated a non-significant trend toward a positive effect on promoting collateral sprouting of the CST in its target region at 5 mm rostral point, only the combination of these treatments with training was sufficient to significantly promote CST sprouting. Interestingly, in agreement with our previous reports with ChABC treatment, our combined strategy did not result in long distance axonal regeneration in the CST, as we did not detect any BDA traced CST fibers beyond the lesion [11].

We further examined the effects of ChABC+GFs/training on the plasticity of the descending serotonergic pathway that modulates neuronal activity and locomotion in the spinal cord [36–39]. In intact spinal cord, serotonergic fibers mainly terminate in the ventral and intermediate gray matter as well as lamina X and to lesser extent in the dorsal horn (Fig. 5A). As we reported previously, a sizable increase in serotonin immunoreactivity is seen in rostral white matter regions particularly in the lateral and dorsal

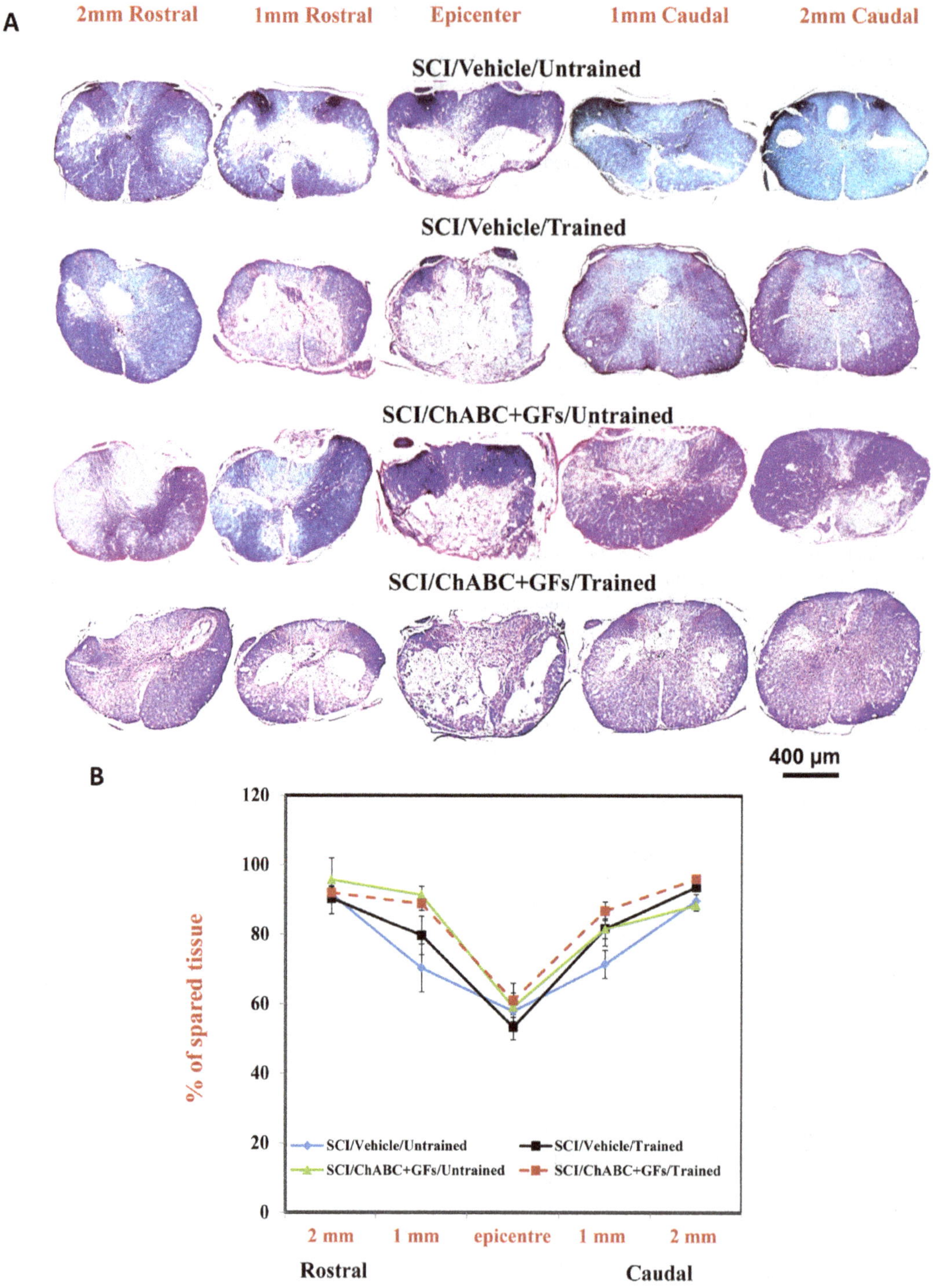

Figure 1. Morphometric analysis of the spinal cord lesion. (**A**) LFB/HE staining of cross sections of the injured spinal cord at various distances to the injury epicentre (both rostrally and caudally) is depicted for all experimental groups at seven weeks post-injury. The area of spared spinal cord tissue was traced and measured. (**B**) The percentage of spared tissue was calculated by normalizing the area of spared tissue to the total cross sectional area of the spinal cord. Although our quantitative analysis showed a positive trend in increasing tissue preservation in groups that received ChABC+GFs/Trained and ChABC+GFs/Untrained compared to Vehicle/Untrained counterpart in 1 mm rostral area, the difference was not statistically significant (Fig. 1B, Two-Way ANOVA, N = 3–6/group).

funiculi in our base-line SCI model (Fig. 5C) suggestive of spontaneous plasticity, increased expression of serotonin and/or accumulation of 5-HT in the serotonergic axons. Assessment of 5-HT immunodensity in multiple rostral and caudal distances to the injury epicenter (Fig. 5H) showed a significant increase in the density of serotonergic axons in ChABC+GFs/trained group (Fig. 5G) at all examined distances compared to both vehicle/untrained and vehicle/trained groups (Fig. 5C and E, $*p<0.05$). In addition, the 5-HT immunodensity was significantly increased in ChABC+GFs treated group with treadmill training relative to

Table 2. Percent of spared tissue.

Groups	2 mm rostral	1 mm rostral	Epicenter	1 mm caudal	2 mm caudal
SCI/Vehicle/Untrained	91.6±1.99	70.3±6.9	57.9±4.2	71.4±4	89.7±1.93
SCI/Vehicle/Trained	90.4±4.5	79.7±5.5	53.35±3.6	81.65±2.8	93.7±1
SCI/ChABC+GFs/Untrained	95.7±6.2	91.3±2.47	59.1±4.1	81.8±4.87	88.36±1.46
SCI/ChABC+GFs/Trained	91.9±1.95	88.8±1.91	61.03±4.8	86.8±2.65	95.91±0.6

Values are expressed as mean ± SEM.

the ChABC+GFs/untrained group (Fig. 5F, $*p<0.05$) at most distances excepted 1.5 mm rostral and caudal from the epicenter. On another hand, no difference was present between Vehicle/trained and Vehicle/untrained groups at all distances demonstrating a clear synergistic effect of the treadmill training with the pharmacological treatment toward an increase of 5-HT expression. Moreover, ChABC+GFs/untrained group showed a statistically significant elevation in 5-HT immunodensity at the epicenter as well as at 1.5 mm rostral and caudal points compared to both vehicle/untrained and vehicle/trained injured groups (Fig. 5H, $*p<0.05$). Serotonin density was also significantly higher at 3 mm rostral to the SCI epicenter in ChABC+GFs/untrained group compared to the vehicle/untrained counterpart. These findings collectively indicate that ChABC+GFs promote plasticity in serotonergic pathways and regular motor training enhances the magnitude of this response.

Recovery of kinematic parameters during treadmill locomotion

In accordance with our previous study on trained and untrained adult rats with a severe thoracic spinal cord clip compression [27], most of injured rats in the present study, regardless of treatment group, spontaneously recovered an impressive capability to generate efficient and coordinated hindlimb locomotor movements given the severity of the lesion. Consequently, the additional treadmill training provided during the 7-week recovery period failed to improve the locomotor parameters measured beyond this considerable spontaneous recovery at least at the end of experiment. In addition, none of the rats in the present study achieved full recovery in lateral balance during treadmill locomotion and only few animals recovered partial weight bearing (based on observations of the experimenters). Consequently, the trunk and/or tail of the rats were manually supported during treadmill training and/or kinematic recording sessions throughout the recovery period. The comparison of groups based on kinematic parameters indicated no significant effect of treadmill training throughout the recovery period. Consequently, to increase the statistical power and focus on the potential effects of ChABC + GFs treatment, the rats were then gathered in two groups: 1) ChABC + GFs treated and 2) vehicle treated animals. Figure 6 illustrates kinematic results of locomotor performance on treadmill from both groups before (*i.e.* baseline) and during the 7 weeks following SCI.

The data showed no significant difference between the two groups in the kinematics of locomotion on treadmill at later time-points. Overall, although weight support and lateral balance remained deficient, when the trunks of the rats were supported they were capable of producing a well-defined and coordinated spontaneous locomotor pattern on the treadmill. In fact, throughout the recovery period, the step cycle length and duration were similar to the baseline (no significant difference; Fig. 6A and B). Interestingly, when the tail and/or trunk support provided by the experimenters was removed, the performance of the rats decreased drastically, they fell on the ground and they were then no longer capable of following the treadmill belt. This observation suggests that after severe compressive SCI, the absence of external postural adjustment, such as during free overground locomotion, could mask the capability of the spinal cord to produce full locomotor pattern.

Although the step cycle length was near-normal at week 7 (Fig. 6A), the parts of the locomotor cycle in front and in back of the vertical projection of the hip was respectively lower ($p\leq0.001$; Fig. 6C left part) and higher ($p\leq0.001$; Fig. 6C right part). As we reported previously [27], these data demonstrate that the locomotor movements of the hindlimbs shifted backwards. Nevertheless, despite the postural support, the knee joint movement remained affected 7 weeks after SCI (see knee angle excursion in Fig. 6F) and its amplitude was half of the baseline value all along the recovery period ($p\leq0.001$; Fig. 6D). To maintain the amplitude of the whole locomotor pattern, the animals compensated by increasing the ankle amplitude in similar proportion than the decrease of the knee ($p\leq0.001$; Fig. 6E). The angular excursions of the hindlimbs joints (*i.e.* hip, knee, ankle and MTP) during locomotion were very similar between treated and untreated groups 7 weeks after SCI (Fig. 6F right panel). In addition, though the amplitude of knee and ankle changed (Fig. 6D and E) the global shape of angles joints excursion during locomotion returned close to normal at the end of the post-lesion period (Fig. 6F, right panel compared to the left).

The shape of hindlimb instant velocity during the swing phase was changed 7 weeks after SCI. Even if the acceleration and the peak of velocity in the first 20% of the swing were close to normal (comparison of the first 20% of the normalized swing phase duration between top and bottom panel in Fig. 6G), the injured rats decelerated shortly after (from about 30%; Fig. 6G bottom panel) while normal rats maintained the maximum speed until about 45% of the swing (Fig. 6G top panel). These findings suggest that although the injured rats were capable of reaching the highest velocity of a normal swing phase (*i.e.* about 0.9 $m.s^{-1}$); they lost the ability to maintain this speed. In normal rats, the rebound of velocity in the last 20% of the swing corresponds to the final ankle extension just before the foot landing (Fig. 6G top panel). In injured rats, this rebound is lost 7 weeks after SCI (Fig. 6G bottom panel) due to the incapability of landing the foot far enough in front of the hip vertical projection as shown in the figure 6C.

Recovery of locomotor coordination

SCI rats in both ChABC + GFs and vehicle treated groups recovered the capability of generating locomotor pattern with the hindlimbs; however, they never recovered coupling between anterior and posterior paws while the coordination between both hindlimbs remained similar to the baseline (Figure 7). In normal

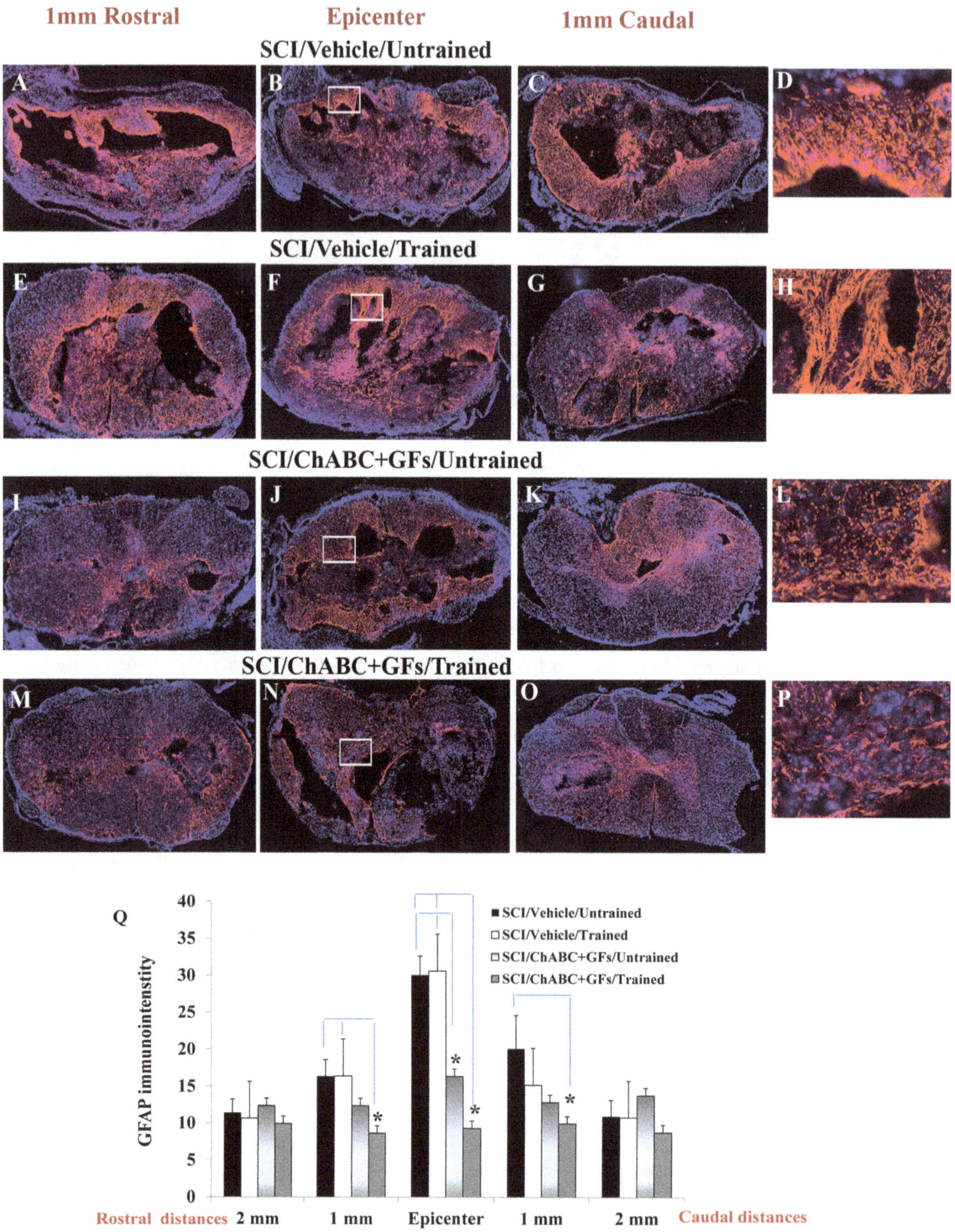

Figure 2. Effects of ChABC, GF and daily exercise on chronic astrogliosis after SCI. (**A–P**) Images show cross sections of the injured spinal cord immunostained for GFAP to mark astrocytes. Representative images from vehicle/untrained, vehicle/trained, ChABC+GFs/untrained and ChABC+GFs/trained injured rats are depicted at various rostral and caudal distances to the lesion epicenter. Confocal images show an overall reduction in the expression of GFAP particularly in the surrounding parenchymal region in ChABC+GFs/untrained and ChABC+GFs/trained groups relative to both Vehicle/Untrained and Vehicle/Trained groups. Images in D, H, L, and P depict magnified areas inside the boxed regions identified in B, F, J and N, respectively. (**Q**) Our quantitative analysis of GFAP immunointensity confirmed a significant reduction in astrogliosis in the ChABC+GFs/trained group at the SCI epicenter as well as 1 mm rostral and caudal in comparison to the Vehicle treated groups. ChABC+GFs/untrained group also demonstrated

a significant decrease in GFAP immunoreactivity at the epicenter compared to both vehicle treated groups (Two-way ANOVA, *$p<0.05$, n = 3–6/group). Although ChABC+GFs/trained group consistently showed less astrogliosis compared to the ChABC+GFs/untrained counterpart, our statistical analysis showed no significant differences between the two groups.

rats, the frequency of each of the four limbs is the same during locomotion and the anteroposterior coordination value remains very stable around 0.3 all along the treadmill locomotor session (Fig. 7A). After SCI, the coupling between anterior and posterior girdles was lost and unrecovered for all rats all along the post-injury period. This is demonstrated by the progressive drift of the cumulated coordination value during treadmill locomotor sequence at the end of the recovery period (Fig. 7B). In fact, this continuous drift was due to the de-synchronization of the fore- and hindlimbs frequencies after SCI suggesting the loss of neuronal coupling between corresponding CPGs. However, although some fluctuations around the baseline value (*i.e.* 0.5) were present during the post-SCI period, rats have recovered the coordination between both hindlimbs 7 weeks after SCI (Fig. 7C).

Distribution of walking rats and quality of the locomotor pattern

Data related to the distribution of rats capable to walk on treadmill at different time points show a trend of an earlier recovery in ChABC + GFs group for the three studied velocities 14, 20 and 26 $m.min^{-1}$ (Fig. 8). Two weeks after SCI, only rats from ChABC + GFs group were capable of walking on the treadmill at all velocities (14 $m.min^{-1}$: 21.73%; 20 $m.min^{-1}$: 13.04%; 26 $m.min^{-1}$: 4.34%; Fig. 8A1, B1 and C1). Three weeks after SCI, the distribution of walking rats was still greater in the treated group at 14 $m.min^{-1}$ (ChABC: 47.82%; Vehicle: 20%: Fig. 8A1) and 20 $m.min^{-1}$ (ChABC: 43.47%; Vehicle: 10%: Fig. 8B1) while only rats from treated group were capable to walk on treadmill at 26 $m.min^{-1}$ (26.08%; Fig. 8C1). Four weeks after SCI the distribution of rats capable of walking on treadmill was similar between groups for the less challenging speed (14 $m.min^{-1}$; Fig. 8A1). However, the proportion of walking rats 4 weeks post-lesion remained greater in ChABC + GFs treated group for the highest speeds, 20 $m.min^{-1}$ (ChABC + GFs: 69.56%; Vehicle: 50%; Fig. 8B1) and 26 $m.min^{-1}$ (ChABC + GFs: 65.21%; Vehicle: 40%; Fig. 8C1). In addition, the comparison of angular excursions of the hip, knee, ankle and MTP from representative rats 3 weeks after the lesion shows clearly that the gait of ChABC + GFs treated rats was more regular and consequently the locomotor patterns was more efficient at 14 and 20 $m.min^{-1}$ (Fig. 8A3 and B3). In addition, at the same period, the ChABC + GFs treated rats still showed a very regular locomotor pattern at the highest and most challenging speed (Fig. 8C3). Four weeks following SCI, although the distribution of walking rats remained in favor of ChABC + GFs treated group at 20 and 26 $m.min^{-1}$ (Fig. 8B1 and C1), the organization of angular patterns became equivalent throughout the groups (Fig. 8B4 and C4).

Relationship between neuroanatomical parameters and kinematic performance

Since the kinematic data showed no significant effect of treatments on treadmill locomotor performances, the global regression analysis was performed by combining the data from all groups. This approach aimed to highlight the main relationships between behavioural outcomes and various neuroanatomical indices of spinal cord tract integrity at the end of experiment. Figure 9 depicts the significant relationships of kinematic parameters with the overall density of corticospinal tract (CST) fibers (BDA; Fig. 9A–D), serotonergic fibers (5-HT; Fig. 9E) and presence of macrophages/microglia cells (OX42; Fig. 9F) in the injured spinal cord. Our analyses showed that density of the CST fibers in the injured spinal cord was positively correlated with the variability of the foot position at the onset of the swing (*i.e.* foot lift; Fig. 9A). The feet lift occurring at the transition between stance and swing phases, and the length variability of both phases were also positively correlated with the presence of CST fibers (Fig. 9B–C). Consequently, the inconsistent foot lift position could explain the positive relationship between the presence of CST fibers and the variability of the whole step cycle length (Fig. 9D). Similarly, 5-HT expression in the SCI site was positively correlated with the variability of the foot velocity in the last part of the swing phase (*i.e.* hindlimb extension part named E1 subphase; Fig. 9E). Taken together, these results strongly suggest that the change in the gait variability measured over time in the present study represents a plasticity mechanism mediated at least in part by the corticospinal tract whereby there is an attempt to constantly adapt the step cycle compared to a more repetitive robot-like locomotor pattern mainly controlled by spinal circuits. Interestingly, the presence of OX42-positive macrophages/microglia, which is representative of the extent of inflammation, and the foot velocity in the first part of the swing phase (*i.e.* hindlimb flexion part named F subphase) were negatively interrelated at the end of experiment (Fig. 9F). These data suggest that the increase of inflammation in the spinal cord could be related to the decrease in movement velocity especially during swing phase.

Discussion

In the present study, we investigated the impact of combining daily motor training on treadmill with pharmacological treatment consisting of ChABC as well as growth factors (GFs), containing EGF, bFGF and PDGF-AA, on the structural plasticity of the spinal cord and the recovery of locomotion in rats with clip compression spinal lesion at T7. We report evidence of neuroanatomical spinal plasticity with the combined therapy and modest neurobehavioural effects as exhibited by a trend for an earlier (3–4 weeks after SCI) return of bilateral hindlimb locomotion after SCI in animals treated with ChABC + GFs. However, this combinatorial approach did not induce long-term functionally significant improvement of our specific kinematic parameters at the end of the 7-week recovery period.

Combinatorial treatment enhances neuroanatomical plasticity in the spinal cord

The use of ChABC and GFs therapy was based on our previous work that showed promising results when combined with neural precursor cell (NPCs) transplantation in promoting neuroplasticity and remyelination in chronic SCI [11]. ChABC and GFs therapy also enhanced endogenous oligodendrocyte replacement and attenuated astrocyte generation and pre-lesional glial scarring and inflammation when applied subacutely following SCI [15]. Our goal in the present study was to determine whether addition of a regular motor training regimen, as a clinically viable therapy, to the ChABC and GFs treatment would synergistically improve the recovery of locomotion after SCI by enhancing activity dependent plasticity in spinal circuitry. On day four after SCI, we delivered ChABC and GFs intrathecally for one week. This

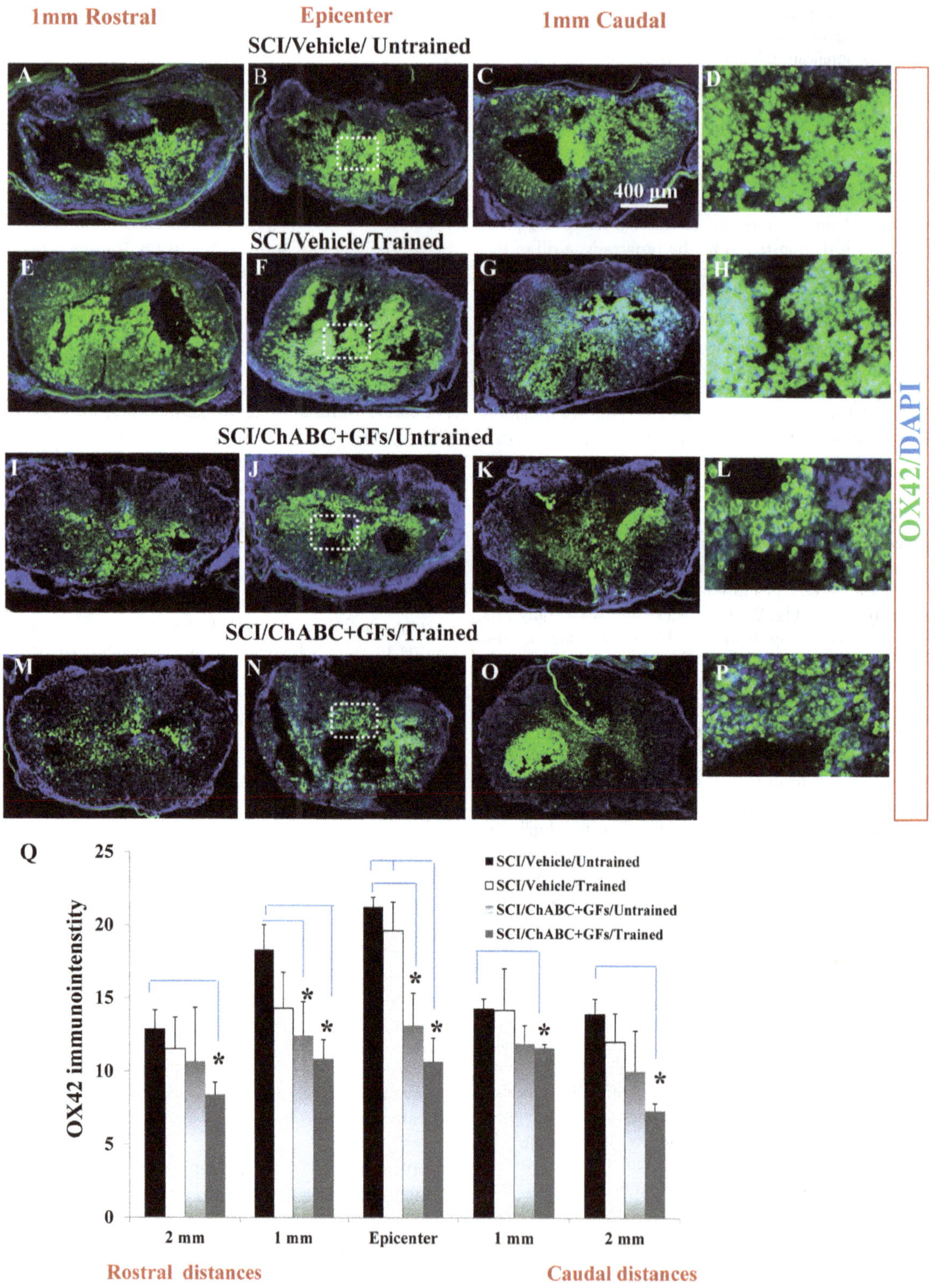

Figure 3. Effects of ChABC, GF and daily exercise on chronic presence of macrophages/microglia at the site of SCI lesion. (**A–P**) Confocal images showing the cross sections of the injured spinal cord immunostained for CD11b (OX42). Representative images from vehicle/untrained, vehicle/trained, ChABC+GFs/untrained and ChABC+GFs/trained injured rats are depicted at various rostral and caudal distances to the lesion epicenter. CD11b marks macrophages and microglia populations. Images in D, H, L, and P depict magnified areas inside the boxed regions identified in B, F, J and N, respectively. (**Q**) Our quantitative analysis of CD11b immunointensity showed reduced recruitment of macrophages/microglia in ChABC+GFs/trained group compared to the Vehicle/Untrained group at all distances and compared to the Vehicle/Trained group at the epicenter. Interestingly, ChABC+GFs/Untrained group also showed a significant reduction in CD11b immunoreactivity compared to the Vehicle/Untrained group at the injury epicenter (*$p<0.05$, Two way ANOVA, Holm-Sidak *post hoc*, N = 3–6/group).

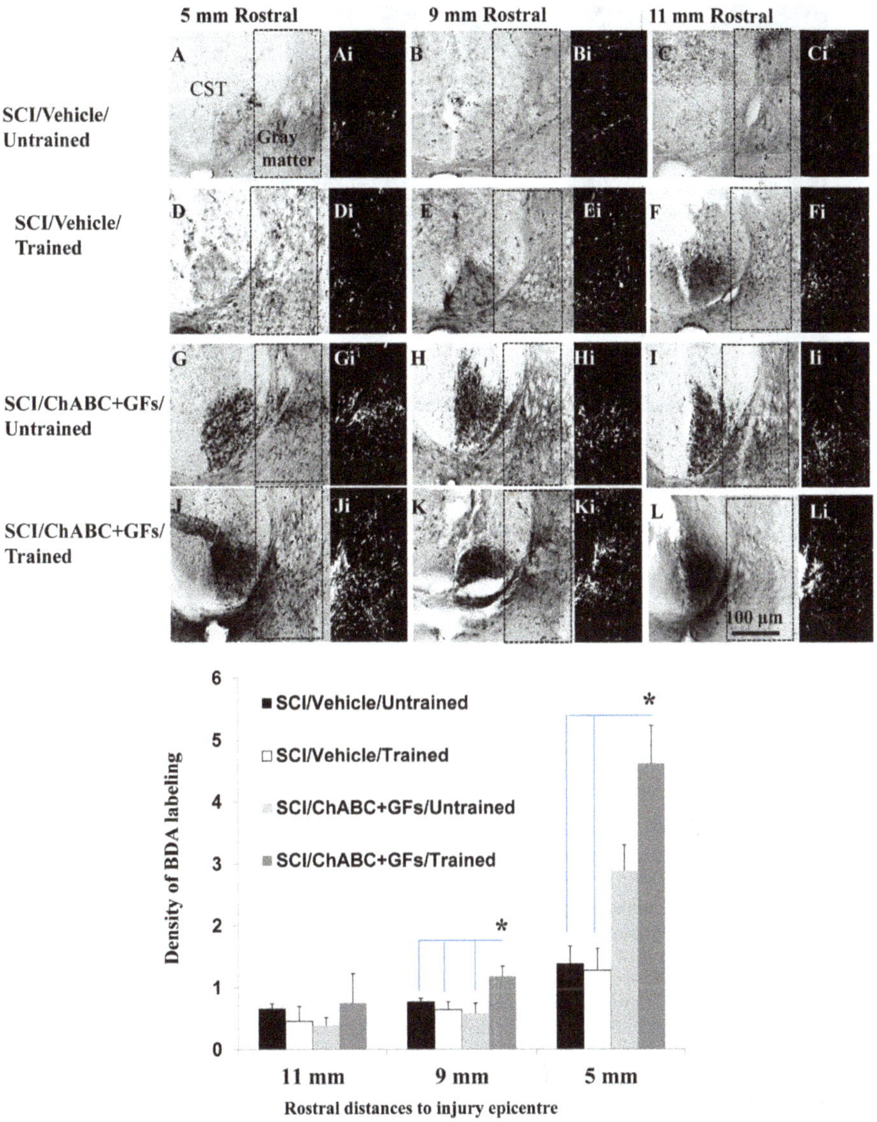

Figure 4. Synergistic effects of ChABC, GF and daily exercise enhance the collateral sprouting of the CST axons in the injured spinal cord. **(A–L)** Images of the BDA-labeled CST at 5, 9 and 11 mm rostral to the lesion are depicted in different experimental groups after unilateral injections of BDA into the sensorimotor cortex (Ai-Li). Inverted images were generated from the boxed region depicted in A–L for better visualization. BDA labeling was unilateral, so only contralateral CST is labeled. To correct for inter-animal variations in the BDA labeling efficiency, the intensity value of the BDA labeled collaterals in the gray matter were normalized to the intensity of BDA labeled fibers of the main CST. **(M)** Quantification of the areas depicted in Ai-Li at various distances revealed an increase in BDA density in the combined ChABC+GFs/trained treatment group compared to all other groups at 5 and 9 mm distances. Comparison of BDA-labeled collaterals among different injured groups also showed an increase in the density of BDA-labeled CST fibers in the ChABC+GFs/untrained group that was significantly higher than both vehicle treated groups at 5 mm rostral point to the SCI epicenter (*$p<0.05$, Two-way ANOVA, Holm-Sidak *post hoc*, N = 3–5).

delayed administration was specifically chosen for ChABC in SCI since: 1) CSPGs are highly upregulated and easily visualized within the spinal lesion at this time [15,40], 2) previous studies have shown the beneficial immunomodulatory effects of CSPGs in the acute phase of SCI [41], and 3) delayed therapies would facilitate a clinically relevant therapeutic time window of intervention for SCI. Our findings demonstrate that combining ChABC, GFs and daily exercise synergistically enhanced axonal plasticity in the descending CST and 5-HT spinal cord pathways. Additionally, the pharmacological treatment attenuated the evolution of astrocytic scar formation and chronic inflammation after SCI with a synergistic effect provided by treadmill training. These results are in general agreement with our previous studies in which we combined ChABC, GFs with NPC transplantation [11]. In fact, ChABC administration itself was sufficient to induce remarkable increase in collateral sprouting and/or preservation of the CST in rostral regions to the injury epicenter as well as sprouting of the serotonergic fibers within the lesional and peri-lesional areas [11]. Our neuroanatomical data here are also consistent with previous work by other groups indicating the overall positive impact of inhibiting CSPGs in improving injury microenvironment for repair and regeneration [16–18,22,42–45].

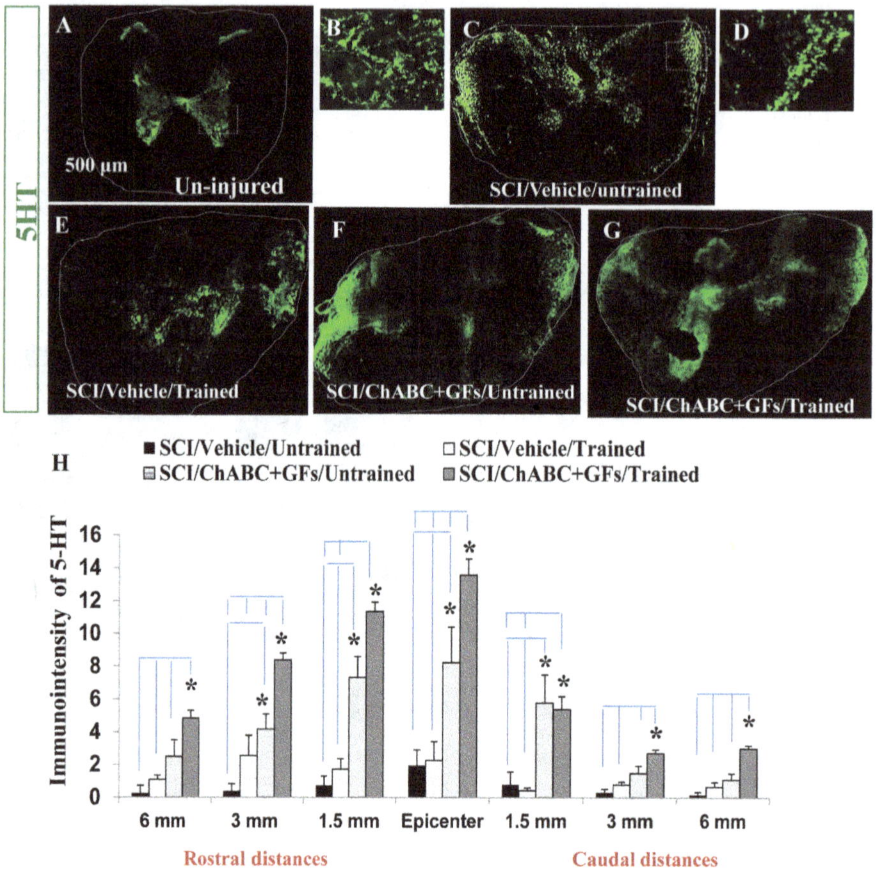

Figure 5. Combination of ChABC, GFs and training promotes plasticity of serotonergic fibers after SCI. (**A**) Transverse section of an uninjured spinal cord at mid-thoracic region demonstrates normal innervation pattern of serotonergic pathway (5-HT positive fibers) within the spinal cord. (**B**) Higher magnification of the boxed area in A shows the presence of serotonergic fibers in the gray matter areas representing of the signal that was quantified in our assessments. (C–G) At 7 weeks post-injury, 5-HT positive fibers in all experimental groups show significant changes in their localization (images shown for 1.5 mm rostral). In contrast to uninjured spinal cord, 5-HT immunoreactive fibers were sprouting in different regions of white matter in all injured groups. (**D**) Higher magnification of the boxed area in C shows the presence of serotonergic fibers in the white matter areas representing of the signal that was quantified in our assessments (H) Quantification of 5-HT immunointensity in the entire cross section of the spinal cord (traced areas in images) at various rostral and caudal distances revealed significantly increased level of 5-HT immunoreactivity in ChABC+ GFs/trained group compared to both vehicle treated group at all examined rostral and caudal distances (*$p<0.05$, Two-way ANOVA, Holm-Sidak *post hoc*, n = 3–6). Interestingly, at the epicenter and 1.5 mm rostral and caudal distances, the ChABC+GFs/untrained group also showed a significantly higher expression of 5-HT-immunoreactivity compared to the vehicle treated groups (*$p<0.05$, Two-way ANOVA, Holm-Sidak *post hoc*).

Absence of synergistic effects of treadmill training with ChABC and GF treatments on measurements of kinematic parameters at the end of the 7-week recovery period

Although the positive effects of ChABC administration on structural plasticity and regeneration in SCI has been established in the literature, its functional impact on specific motor patterns such as locomotion is still debated particularly in compressive/contusive models of SCI. To date, functional benefits of ChABC in SCI has been mainly achieved in partial transection models [12,13,16,18,19,22,44], and when ChABC was administered in more clinically-relevant models of SCI such as contusion and/or compression models as is the case in our study, its effects on functional recovery was minimal [11,43,46,47]. Recently, a study reported the transplantation of genetically modified Schwann cells to secrete endogenously D15A (neurotrophin mimicking the effects of NT-3 and BDNF) and ChABC in the injury site of rats with contusive SCI [21]. In agreement with our present and previous investigations [11], the data of this work showed a strong effect of the modified Schwann cells on the structural plasticity of the spinal cord (axonal regeneration, decrease of CSPGs, increase of myelination and 5-HT positive axons…) but a very moderate effect on the locomotor recovery (+0.5 improvement on the BBB scale compared to control group at the end of the experimental series lasting up to 14 weeks). Functional recovery with ChABC also seems to depend on the severity of SCI lesion. Caggiano and colleagues showed the positive effects of ChABC on hindlimb locomotor recovery only in rats with more severe compressive SCI [48]. Interestingly, in the same study, one experimental group with a moderate injury, comparable to the SCI severity in our present work, received no benefits on the recovery of locomotion from ChABC treatment [48].

Although, we show that rats in all experimental conditions had recovered the capability to generate fast, ample, coordinated and well-defined hindlimb locomotor movements on treadmill at the end of the 7 week recovery period and a trend of earlier return of locomotion in pharmacologically treated rats, our statistical analysis failed to detect any significant effects in treadmill trained animals (with or without pharmacological treatment). These results reinforce the conclusions of previous studies that showed

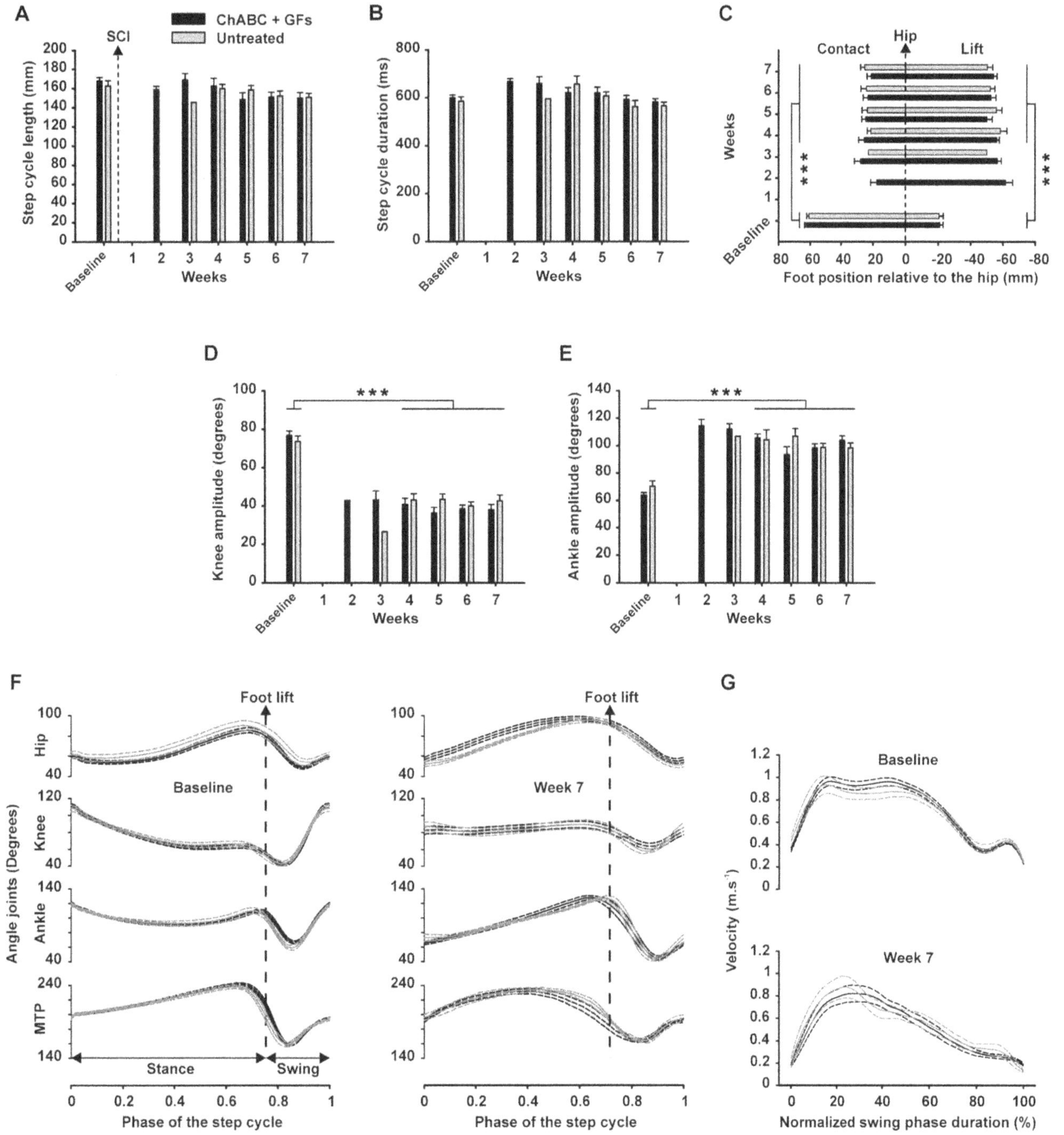

Figure 6. Kinematic analysis of locomotor patterns during the recovery period. Kinematic data were gathered in two groups (i.e. ChABC+ GFs and vehicle groups) and averaged before (baseline) and each week for 7 weeks after SCI. Because too few animals were capable to walk on treadmill during the three first weeks after SCI, statistical analysis were performed on baseline and week 4–7 only. (**A**) Mean length of the full step cycle (*i.e.* stance + swing phases) in millimeters is presented. (**B**) Mean duration of the full step cycle in milliseconds are shown. (**C**) Position of the foot contact (*i.e.* left part of the chart) and lift (*i.e.* right part) in millimeters relative to the vertical projection of the great trochanter are depicted (*i.e.* named hip in the chart and represented by the zero value). (**D**) Averaged amplitude of the knee joint in degrees and (**E**) averaged amplitude of ankle joint are presented. (**F**) Averaged angle excursions of the hip, knee, ankle and MTP, before (left panel) and 7 weeks after SCI (right panel) are shown. (**G**) Comparison of the averaged instant foot velocity (*i.e.* full lines) during swing phase before (top panel) and 7 weeks after SCI (bottom panel) for both groups, their respective SEM envelopes (*i.e.* dash line) are given. Symbol *** represent a significance threshold ≤0.001.

the absence of locomotor improvement in trained rats with incomplete SCI [27–29,49–51]. Interestingly, Caudle and colleagues report that when the hindlimbs of rats with mid thoracic contusion are immobilized on adapted wheelchair immediately after SCI, the overground locomotor performance of their hindlimbs decreases dramatically and then increases when the wheelchair is removed suggesting a substantial training effect of spontaneous locomotor movements [52]. Consequently, the

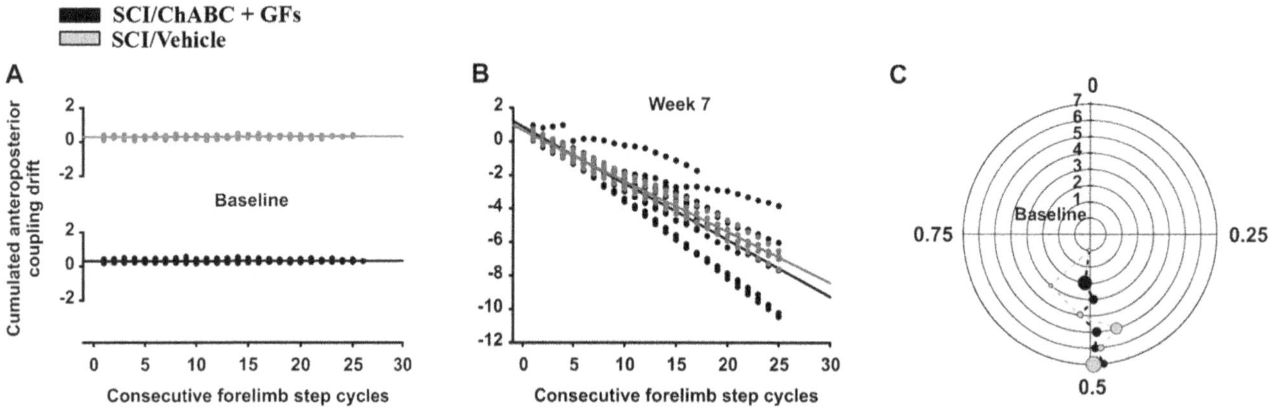

Figure 7. Limb coordination during locomotion. In **A** and **B**, coordination values plotted for each consecutive forelimb step cycle before and 7 weeks after SCI respectively. Usually the coordination measurement is expressed using polar coordinates. To simplify the representation of the coordination drift we converted these data to fit the Cartesian model by subtracting 1 to the polar values when two contacts of the forelimb with the treadmill belt occurred during one hindlimb step cycle (*i.e.* different stepping frequencies). This method renders an account of the intensity of the drift represented by the slope of the consecutive plots. (**C**) Hindlimbs coordination is expressed between 0 and 1 (*i.e.* theta) in a polar plot. The polar axis represents the delays from baseline (*i.e.* the innermost circle) to week 7 (*i.e.* the outermost) post-SCI. Circumference of the circles represent the normalized duration of right step cycle while the dots position on each circle represent the relative time position of the left foot contact averaged by group (see Alluin et al., 2011 for details). In addition, the size of each dot is proportional to the polar dispersion.

absence of treadmill training effect in the present study does not disclaim the beneficial effect of treadmill training after SCI but more likely represents the impact of continuous self-training of untrained SCI rats in their cage as previously suggested [26,27,49]. It is plausible that cage exercise in untrained and trained animals enhances their locomotor performance until a ceiling threshold is achieved beyond which any added treadmill training remains ineffective. In this context, it would be interesting in further experiment to challenge our combined strategy by increasing the severity of the spinal compression in order to lower the level of spontaneous recovery and reveal the potential benefits that might be concealed by the intrinsic locomotor capabilities. Further studies are required to elucidate the possibility that our combined therapy could improve functional recovery in a more severe compressive SCI with a lower degree of spontaneous locomotor recovery.

Other variables could also influence the outcomes of our training paradigm such as the duration and frequency of treadmill training and/or the optimal delay between SCI and the start of exercise training. An earlier study in spinal rats showed that the degree of locomotor recovery after SCI is correlated with the number of steps executed during each training session [53]. Therefore, it is plausible that the ten minutes duration of daily training in the present study might be insufficient to induce demonstrable activity-dependent functional improvement in clip compression SCI. Another variable is the impact of therapeutic time-window for initiating rehabilitation after SCI. In fact, studies by Smith and colleagues have shown the deleterious effect of swim training in acute phase of SCI on locomotor performance in rats with moderate contusive thoracic SCI [54]. The authors showed that starting training as early as 3 day after SCI could exert adverse effects on the recovery of locomotion by exacerbating the inflammatory response. Further studies are necessary to evaluate the impact of different variables in rehabilitation paradigms in SCI including time-window, frequency and duration of motor training.

Potential effects of combined ChABC and growth factors on fore-and hindlimbs coupling

Based on the absence of specific results induced by treadmill training, rats in the present study were consequently gathered into two experimental groups regardless of their training status: ChABC+GFs and vehicle treated groups. This was to focus on the effects of pharmacological treatments while increasing the statistical power of this new approach. Our kinematics analyses of ChABC+GFs and vehicle treated groups showed that injured rats generally regained plantar stepping with occasional weight bearing (not measured) and no evidence of forelimb-hindlimb coordination on treadmill (Fig. 7B). This recovery pattern corresponds to a BBB score of 9 to 10 which represents the baseline of our injury model as described previously [6,11]. However, although the anteroposterior coupling was globally disrupted in all animals of the present study, a subset of the ChABC+GFs treated group showed evidence of shorts bouts of coordinated frequency between forelimbs and hindlimbs (*i.e.* 3–5 consecutive step cycles) during their locomotor sequences 7 weeks after SCI (see few horizontal alignments of 3–5 consecutive black dots between 0–4, 5–8 and 15–20 forelimb step cycles in Fig. 7B). This transient period of coordination could be due to the perturbation of forelimb or hindlimb movements resulting in temporary forelimb-hindlimb synchronization. However, the fact that it was only evident in the ChABC+GFs group raises the potential benefits of the combined ChABC + GF treatment in establishing functional connections between upper and lower segments of the spinal cord.

It is noteworthy to mention that previous studies showing positive effects of ChABC on axonal regeneration and the potential functional connections used open field behavioural tasks to visually assess locomotion including coordination [11–13,19,22,44]. In the present study, we used precise measurement of coordination parameters using kinematics to assess fine locomotor improvements, which are normally unobservable or difficult to assess in open field evaluations. Given this, it is possible that moderate improvements in anteroposterior coupling may have occurred after ChABC treatment that had remained undetected in previous investigations. It is also possible that false positive anteroposterior coupling was observed on a short-term

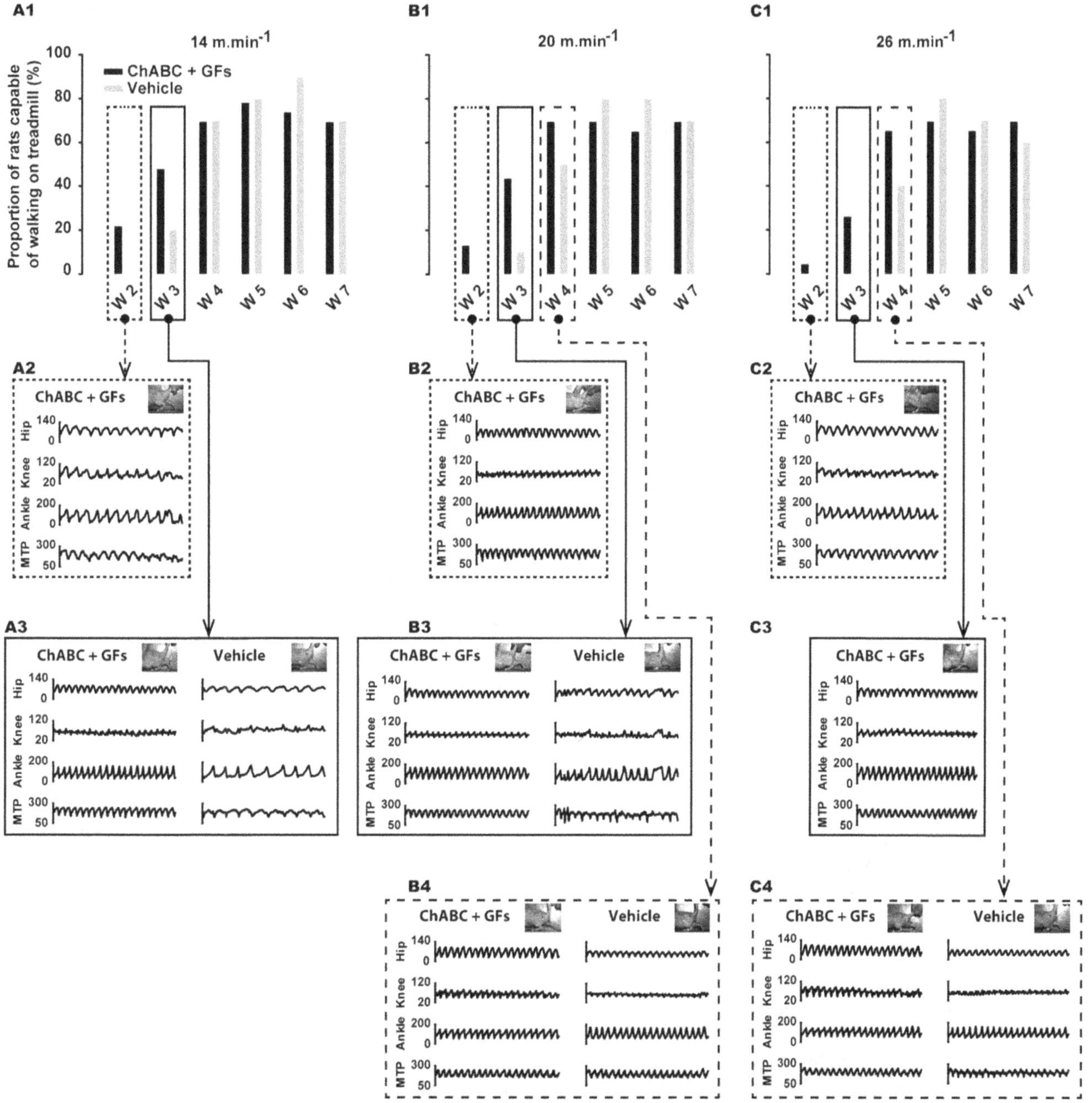

Figure 8. Frequency of rats that have recovered locomotion on treadmill at the three studied velocities and at the different time points throughout the recovery period. (**A1**, **B1** and **C1**), percent of rats capable of walking on treadmill at 14, 20 and 26 m.min^{-1} respectively, before and each week of the recovery period for ChABC+GFs and Vehicle groups. (**A2** and **A3**), raw angular excursions of hip, knee, ankle and MTP joints extracted from representative rats walking at 14 m.min^{-1} at week 2 and 3 respectively. (**B2**, **B3** and **B4**), raw angular excursions of hip, knee, ankle and MTP joints extracted from representative rats walking at 20 m.min^{-1} at week 2, 3 and 4 respectively. (**C2**, **C3** and **C4**), similar to B2, B3 and B4 for 26 m.min^{-1}. Data in A1, B1 and C1 are expressed in percentage of the group while the other panels below show angular data expressed in degrees.

scale. Nonetheless, in the present study, transient occurrences of anteroposterior coupling detected in ChABC+GFs treated group did not reach statistical significance. Future studies involving detailed analysis of interlimb coordination in a greater number of animals are essential to clarify the potential effect of ChABC+GFs treatment on forelimb-hindlimb coupling during locomotion in rat compressive SCI.

Some evidence of early locomotor recovery induced by the ChABC and GF treatments

Interestingly, our data on the percentage of rats capable of walking on treadmill at different time points after SCI, revealed not only a trend for an earlier recovery of locomotion in ChABC + GFs treated group, but also the improvement of stepping regularity and quality at early stages after SCI as demonstrated by comparison of raw angular excursions from representative rats

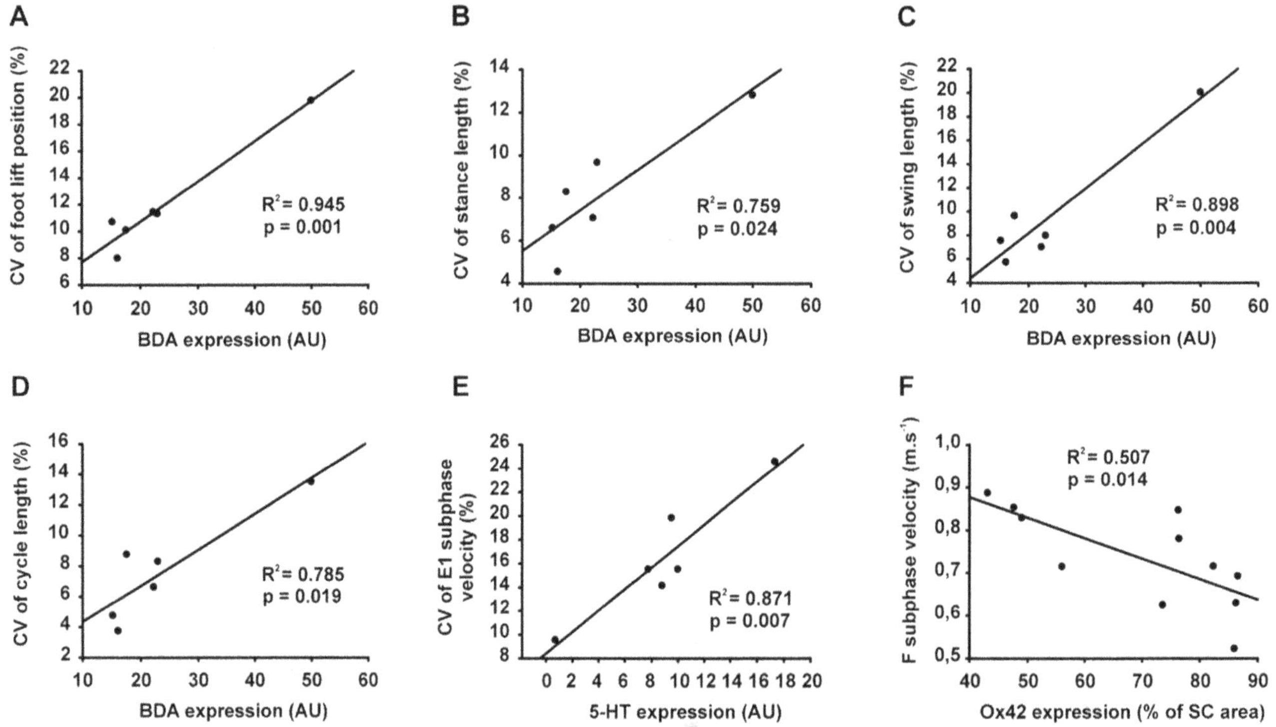

Figure 9. Relationships between behavior and neuroanatomical parameters. Given the absence of significant difference between groups for the behavioral features, available data from all rats were plotted together regardless of the groups. Given that the tissue preparation was different from one labelling protocol to the other, some animals were blindly selected in each group for each different procedure. In addition, among these selected animals not all have recovered the locomotion 7 weeks after SCI (as shown in Fig. 9 A1, B1 and C1). Taken together, this double restriction explains the limited number of plotted data in the present figure. (**A**) Global expression of BDA labeling from the spinal cord section studied was plotted against the coefficient of variation (CV) of the foot position at the onset of the swing phase. (**B**) Graph depicts overall BDA expression against the CV of stance phase length. (**C**) Overall BDA expression against the CV of swing phase length is shown. (**D**) Overall BDA expression against the CV of the step cycle length is depicted. (**E**) Graph shows overall 5-HT expression plotted against the CV of E1 subphase (*i.e.* 2nd part of the swing phase: extension of the hindlimb before foot contact) velocity. (**F**) Overall Ox42 expression is shown against averaged velocity of the F subphase (*i.e.* 1st part of the swing phase: initial flexion of the hindlimb following the foot lift). BDA and 5-HT quantifications are expressed in arbitrary unit (AU), CV is expressed in percentage of the mean and Ox42 labeling is expressed in percentage of the total spinal cord (SC) area. The coefficient of determination (R^2) and statistical significance (p) are given on each panel.

in both groups in Figure 8. Although these data did not reach statistical significance using our experimental design, the persistent trends at several consecutive time points and velocities suggest a possible effect of combined pharmacological treatment on the spinal cellular mechanisms early after the lesion. Immediately after SCI, influx of the inflammatory cells as well as the spinal shock occurs that targets the motoneurons below the lesion resulting in immediate loss of hindlimb movements and reflexes. This initial spinal shock is then followed by a gradual recovery of reflexes and, depending of the severity of lesion, regain of some motor functions. In the present study, we show a significant decrease in the presence of OX42 (CD11b) expressing macrophages/microglia in ChABC+GFs treated rats compared to vehicle counterparts (Fig. 3) suggesting the immunomodulatory effects of ChABC+GFs treatment on the injury induced-inflammatory response. Decrease in the inflammatory response in ChABC+GFs treated group may suggest a reduced period of spinal shock in these animals that could result in an earlier return of locomotor function observed in some of these animals. Here also, further investigations are needed to delineate the modulatory roles of these treatments on the recruitment of inflammatory cells as well as the impact of neuroinflammation inhibition on the time course of locomotor recovery after SCI.

Greater gait variability after SCI as a sign of greater supraspinal influence?

The correlation between the quantitative histological assessments and variability in the kinematic readouts is of interest. Such variability could be interpreted to mean that the step cycles are simply variable in nature or that the neuroplasticity induced by our treatment is aberrant and disrupting but it could also mean that the variability in the kinematic parameters reflect greater adaptability of these readouts. For instance, in a robotic locomotor performance in which the variability is dictated by the immediate environment only, such an automatic rhythmic behavior could be considered at the end of a spectrum where locomotion is principally defined by the operation of a spinal circuitry. However, it is considered that after partial SCI there are descending fibers re-innervating the spinal cord in an attempt to impose correcting inputs to the spinal cord. This might lead to a seemingly disorganized pattern but a pattern towards optimizing the motor performance despite the spinal lesion. We presume that the greater variability of the locomotor pattern may represent an attempt at a much more long-term functional recovery of the spinal cord. For instance, we can surmise that some degree of incoordination between the fore- and hindlimbs, as observed in the present study, might require adaptive corrections leading to a more apparent variability in the hindlimb step cycles. Our previous work in cats involved in a dual spinal lesion paradigm indicates that kinematic parameters of complete spinal cats are less variable than of hemisected cats suggesting that remnant descending pathways play a role in attempting to regulate the step cycle [55]. Similarly, in the present rat experiments, it could be postulated that as more supraspinal inputs reach the spinal cord through plastic mechanisms, the more variable step cycles may be represent as an attempt to continuously adapt the step cycles to the supraspinal inputs.

On the other hand, the recovery of hindlimb locomotion after partial spinal lesions depends also on intrinsic changes within the spinal cord itself. Indeed, several experiments in cats have shown that, after a thoracic hemisection, the spinal cord below the spinal lesion is durably changed since, after a further complete spinal section, the spinal cord can immediately express hindlimb locomotion whereas it usually takes 2–3 weeks of training to achieve such level of performance [56–59]. That such changes do occur in the spinal cord itself has consequences on the overall locomotor behavior of the animal since remnant inputs will encounter a more excitable spinal cord that has been changed by the previous lesion. In the present study, the large spinal lesion produced by the compression also leaves a great deal of autonomy to the spinal cord below the crush. It is therefore likely that such intrinsic spinal mechanisms also take place and those changes in intrinsic circuitry and neuroanatomical plasticity occurring below the lesion are part of the mechanisms leading to a seemingly faster optimal recovery of the hindlimb locomotor behavior [27].

Limitations and stringency of our behavioral assessment

Here, we assessed locomotor parameters on a treadmill but not as such changes in posture, in reflex transmission or in autonomic functions and it could be that some of the neuroanatomical changes seen reflect modifications of these parameters. Furthermore, changes in neuroanatomy and function may not be necessarily synergistic as seen here and in previous studies in which combined treatment of anti-Nogo-A antibody and training showed different beneficial effects but not synergistic [60]. Moreover, all parameters of improvement at a given time point may not reflect all the underlying processes that might be controlled by intrinsic neural mechanisms as well as environmental mechanisms such as provided by locomotor training. Thus, locomotor recovery after SCI can be defined from several points of views and with different degree of precision. Precise kinematic analyses such as employed here may be a double-edge sword. They provide an objective measurement of some specific parameters (step length for instance) but may fail to provide a complete global depiction of locomotion since not all kinematic parameters can be considered all the time at various speeds and epochs after SCI. Furthermore, the continuous scrolling of the belt during treadmill locomotion may provide afferent feedbacks from the hindlimbs, stimulating the locomotor system to generate locomotor movements and probably change the balance between spinal and supraspinal contributions to the control of locomotion decreasing the role of the supraspinal control while increasing that of the spinal circuitry.

Conclusions

Our findings demonstrate the beneficial effects of combined ChABC, growth factors and locomotor training on enhancing structural plasticity of the injured cord and despite an impressive spontaneous locomotor recovery observed in our model; we report modest neurobehavioral improvement in treated animals. However, the lack of significant kinematic evidence of sustained functional improvement beyond the spontaneous recovery, at least using our stringent video-based field-by-field analysis, suggests that additional approaches such as cell therapies and/or more appropriate locomotor training may be needed to optimize this therapeutic strategy.

Author Contributions

Conceived and designed the experiments: OA SKA MGF SR. Performed the experiments: OA SKA MKG HDM. Analyzed the data: OA SKA MKG HDM. Contributed to the writing of the manuscript: OA SKA SR MGF.

References

1. Sekhon LH, Fehlings MG (2001) Epidemiology, demographics, and pathophysiology of acute spinal cord injury. Spine 26: S2–12.
2. Tator CH (1998) Biology of Neurological Recovery and Functional Restoration after Spinal Cord Injury. Neurosurgery 42: 696–708.
3. van Hedel HJ, Dietz V (2010) Rehabilitation of locomotion after spinal cord injury. Restor Neurol Neurosci 28: 123–134.
4. Wilson JR, Grossman RG, Frankowski RF, Kiss A, Davis AM, et al. (2012) A clinical prediction model for long-term functional outcome after traumatic spinal cord injury based on acute clinical and imaging factors. J Neurotrauma 29: 2263–2271.
5. Fawcett JW, Curt A, Steeves JD, Coleman WP, Tuszynski MH, et al. (2007) Guidelines for the conduct of clinical trials for spinal cord injury as developed by the ICCP panel: spontaneous recovery after spinal cord injury and statistical power needed for therapeutic clinical trials. Spinal Cord 45: 190–205.
6. Karimi-Abdolrezaee S, Eftekharpour E, Wang J, Morshead C, Fehlings M (2006) Delayed Transplantation of Adult Neural Stem Cells Promotes Remyelination and functional recovery after Spinal Cord Injury. The Journal of Neuroscience, March 29, 26(13): 3377–3389.
7. Fouad K, Dietz V, Schwab ME (2001) Improving axonal growth and functional recovery after experimental spinal cord injury by neutralizing myelin associated inhibitors. Brain Res Brain Res Rev 36: 204–212.
8. Keirstead HS, Nistor G, Bernal G, Totoiu M, Cloutier F, et al. (2005) Human embryonic stem cell-derived oligodendrocyte progenitor cell transplants remyelinate and restore locomotion after spinal cord injury. J Neurosci 25: 4694–4705.
9. Lu P, Wang Y, Graham L, McHale K, Gao M, et al. (2012) Long-distance growth and connectivity of neural stem cells after severe spinal cord injury. Cell 150: 1264–1273.
10. Lu P, Blesch A, Graham L, Wang Y, Samara R, et al. (2012) Motor axonal regeneration after partial and complete spinal cord transection. J Neurosci 32: 8208–8218.
11. Karimi-Abdolrezaee S, Eftekharpour E, Wang J, Schut D, Fehlings MG (2010) Synergistic effects of transplanted adult neural stem/progenitor cells, chondroitinase, and growth factors promote functional repair and plasticity of the chronically injured spinal cord. J Neurosci 30: 1657–1676.
12. Bradbury EJ, Moon LD, Popat RJ, King VR, Bennett GS, et al. (2002) Chondroitinase ABC promotes functional recovery after spinal cord injury. Nature 416: 636–640.
13. Garcia-Alias G, Petrosyan HA, Schnell L, Horner PJ, Bowers WJ, et al. (2011) Chondroitinase ABC combined with neurotrophin NT-3 secretion and NR2D expression promotes axonal plasticity and functional recovery in rats with lateral hemisection of the spinal cord. J Neurosci 31: 17788–17799.
14. Fouad K, Schnell L, Bunge MB, Schwab ME, Liebscher T, et al. (2005) Combining Schwann cell bridges and olfactory-ensheathing glia grafts with chondroitinase promotes locomotor recovery after complete transection of the spinal cord. J Neurosci 25: 1169–1178.
15. Karimi-Abdolrezaee S, Schut D, Wang J, Fehlings MG (2012) Chondroitinase and growth factors enhance activation and oligodendrocyte differentiation of endogenous neural precursor cells after spinal cord injury. PLoS One 7: e37589.
16. Wang D, Ichiyama RM, Zhao R, Andrews MR, Fawcett JW (2011) Chondroitinase combined with rehabilitation promotes recovery of forelimb function in rats with chronic spinal cord injury. J Neurosci 31: 9332–9344.
17. Massey JM, Hubscher CH, Wagoner MR, Decker JA, Amps J, et al. (2006) Chondroitinase ABC digestion of the perineuronal net promotes functional collateral sprouting in the cuneate nucleus after cervical spinal cord injury. J Neurosci 26: 4406–4414.
18. Tom VJ, Kadakia R, Santi L, Houle JD (2009) Administration of chondroitinase ABC rostral or caudal to a spinal cord injury site promotes anatomical but not functional plasticity. J Neurotrauma 26: 2323–2333.
19. Lee H, McKeon RJ, Bellamkonda RV (2010) Sustained delivery of thermostabilized chABC enhances axonal sprouting and functional recovery after spinal cord injury. Proc Natl Acad Sci U S A 107: 3340–3345.

20. Garcia-Alias G, Barkhuysen S, Buckle M, Fawcett JW (2009) Chondroitinase ABC treatment opens a window of opportunity for task-specific rehabilitation. Nat Neurosci 12: 1145–1151.
21. Kanno H, Pressman Y, Moody A, Berg R, Muir EM, et al. (2014) Combination of engineered Schwann cell grafts to secrete neurotrophin and chondroitinase promotes axonal regeneration and locomotion after spinal cord injury. J Neurosci 34: 1838–1855.
22. Alilain WJ, Horn KP, Hu H, Dick TE, Silver J (2011) Functional regeneration of respiratory pathways after spinal cord injury. Nature 475: 196–200.
23. Carter LM, McMahon SB, Bradbury EJ (2011) Delayed treatment with chondroitinase ABC reverses chronic atrophy of rubrospinal neurons following spinal cord injury. Exp Neurol 228: 149–156.
24. Barritt AW, Davies M, Marchand F, Hartley R, Grist J, et al. (2006) Chondroitinase ABC promotes sprouting of intact and injured spinal systems after spinal cord injury. J Neurosci 26: 10856–10867.
25. Bukhari N, Torres L, Robinson JK, Tsirka SE (2011) Axonal regrowth after spinal cord injury via chondroitinase and the tissue plasminogen activator (tPA)/plasmin system. J Neurosci 31: 14931–14943.
26. Jakeman LB, Hoschouer EL, Basso DM (2011) Injured mice at the gym: review, results and considerations for combining chondroitinase and locomotor exercise to enhance recovery after spinal cord injury. Brain Res Bull 84: 317–326.
27. Alluin O, Karimi-Abdolrezaee S, Delivet-Mongrain H, Leblond H, Fehlings MG, et al. (2011) Kinematic study of locomotor recovery after spinal cord clip compression injury in rats. J Neurotrauma 28: 1963–1981.
28. Fouad K, Metz GA, Merkler D, Dietz V, Schwab ME (2000) Treadmill training in incomplete spinal cord injured rats. Behav Brain Res 115: 107–113.
29. Hutchinson KJ, Gomez-Pinilla F, Crowe MJ, Ying Z, Basso DM (2004) Three exercise paradigms differentially improve sensory recovery after spinal cord contusion in rats. Brain 127: 1403–1414.
30. Gauthier MK, Kosciuczyk K, Tapley L, Karimi-Abdolrezaee S (2013) Dysregulation of the neuregulin-1-ErbB network modulates endogenous oligodendrocyte differentiation and preservation after spinal cord injury. Eur J Neurosci.
31. Karimi-Abdolrezaee S, Eftekharpour E, Fehlings MG (2004) Temporal and spatial patterns of Kv1.1 and Kv1.2 protein and gene expression in spinal cord white matter after acute and chronic spinal cord injury in rats: implications for axonal pathophysiology after neurotrauma. Eur J Neurosci 19: 577–589.
32. Fehlings MG, Tator CH (1995) The relationships among the severity of spinal cord injury, residual neurological function, axon counts, and counts of retrogradely labeled neurons after experimental spinal cord injury. Exp Neurol 132: 220–228.
33. Eftekharpour E, Karimi-Abdolrezaee S, Wang J, Morshead C, Fehlings M (2007) Myelination of Congenitally Dysmyelinated Spinal Cord Axons by Adult Neural Precursor Cells Results in Formation of Nodes of Ranvier and Improved Axonal Conduction. The Journal of Neuroscience 27: 3416–3428.
34. Karimi-Abdolrezaee S, Schreyer DJ (2002) Retrograde repression of growth-associated protein-43 mRNA expression in rat cortical neurons. J Neurosci 22: 1816–1822.
35. Seif GI, Nomura H, Tator CH (2007) Retrograde axonal degeneration "dieback" in the corticospinal tract after transection injury of the rat spinal cord: a confocal microscopy study. J Neurotrauma 24: 1513–1528.
36. Ciranna L (2006) Serotonin as a Modulator of Glutamate- and GABA-Mediated Neurotransmission: Implications in Physiological Functions and in Pathology. Curr Neuropharmacol 4: 101–114.
37. Jordan LM, Liu J, Hedlund PB, Akay T, Pearson KG (2008) Descending command systems for the initiation of locomotion in mammals. Brain Res Rev 57: 183–191.
38. Schmidt BJ, Jordan LM (2000) The role of serotonin in reflex modulation and locomotor rhythm production in the mammalian spinal cord. Brain Res Bull 53: 689–710.
39. Husch A, Van Patten GN, Hong DN, Scaperotti MM, Cramer N, et al. (2012) Spinal cord injury induces serotonin supersensitivity without increasing intrinsic excitability of mouse V2a interneurons. J Neurosci 32: 13145–13154.
40. Gris P, Tighe A, Levin D, Sharma R, Brown A (2007) Transcriptional regulation of scar gene expression in primary astrocytes. Glia 55: 1145–1155.
41. Rolls A, Shechter R, London A, Segev Y, Jacob-Hirsch J, et al. (2008) Two faces of chondroitin sulfate proteoglycan in spinal cord repair: a role in microglia/macrophage activation. PLoS Med 5: e171.
42. Busch SA, Horn KP, Silver DJ, Silver J (2009) Overcoming macrophage-mediated axonal dieback following CNS injury. J Neurosci 29: 9967–9976.
43. Novotna I, Slovinska L, Vanicky I, Cizek M, Radonak J, et al. (2011) IT delivery of ChABC modulates NG2 and promotes GAP-43 axonal regrowth after spinal cord injury. Cell Mol Neurobiol 31: 1129–1139.
44. Starkey ML, Bartus K, Barritt AW, Bradbury EJ (2012) Chondroitinase ABC promotes compensatory sprouting of the intact corticospinal tract and recovery of forelimb function following unilateral pyramidotomy in adult mice. Eur J Neurosci 36: 3665–3678.
45. Fouad K, Pearse DD, Tetzlaff W, Vavrek R (2009) Transplantation and repair: combined cell implantation and chondroitinase delivery prevents deterioration of bladder function in rats with complete spinal cord injury. Spinal Cord 47: 727–732.
46. Mountney A, Zahner MR, Sturgill ER, Riley CJ, Aston JW, et al. (2013) Sialidase, chondroitinase ABC, and combination therapy after spinal cord contusion injury. J Neurotrauma 30: 181–190.
47. Yang YG, Jiang DM, Quan ZX, Ou YS (2009) Insulin with chondroitinase ABC treats the rat model of acute spinal cord injury. J Int Med Res 37: 1097–1107.
48. Caggiano AO, Zimber MP, Ganguly A, Blight AR, Gruskin EA (2005) Chondroitinase ABCI improves locomotion and bladder function following contusion injury of the rat spinal cord. J Neurotrauma 22: 226–239.
49. Heng C, de Leon RD (2009) Treadmill training enhances the recovery of normal stepping patterns in spinal cord contused rats. Exp Neurol 216: 139–147.
50. Ichiyama R, Potuzak M, Balak M, Kalderon N, Edgerton VR (2009) Enhanced motor function by training in spinal cord contused rats following radiation therapy. PLoS One 4: e6862.
51. Kuerzi J, Brown EH, Shum-Siu A, Siu A, Burke D, et al. (2010) Task-specificity vs. ceiling effect: step-training in shallow water after spinal cord injury. Exp Neurol 224: 178–187.
52. Caudle KL, Brown EH, Shum-Siu A, Burke DA, Magnuson TS, et al. (2011) Hindlimb immobilization in a wheelchair alters functional recovery following contusive spinal cord injury in the adult rat. Neurorehabil Neural Repair 25: 729–739.
53. Cha J, Heng C, Reinkensmeyer DJ, Roy RR, Edgerton VR, et al. (2007) Locomotor ability in spinal rats is dependent on the amount of activity imposed on the hindlimbs during treadmill training. J Neurotrauma 24: 1000–1012.
54. Smith RR, Brown EH, Shum-Siu A, Whelan A, Burke DA, et al. (2009) Swim training initiated acutely after spinal cord injury is ineffective and induces extravasation in and around the epicenter. J Neurotrauma 26: 1017–1027.
55. Barriere G, Frigon A, Leblond H, Provencher J, Rossignol S (2010) Dual spinal lesion paradigm in the cat: evolution of the kinematic locomotor pattern. J Neurophysiol 104: 1119–1133.
56. Barriere G, Leblond H, Provencher J, Rossignol S (2008) Prominent role of the spinal central pattern generator in the recovery of locomotion after partial spinal cord injuries. J Neurosci 28: 3976–3987.
57. Martinez M, Delivet-Mongrain H, Leblond H, Rossignol S (2012) Effect of locomotor training in completely spinalized cats previously submitted to a spinal hemisection. J Neurosci 32: 10961–10970.
58. Martinez M, Delivet-Mongrain H, Rossignol S (2013) Treadmill training promotes spinal changes leading to locomotor recovery after partial spinal cord injury in cats. J Neurophysiol 109: 2909–2922.
59. Rossignol SS, B.J.; Jordan,L.M (2014) Spinal plasticity underlying the recovery of locomotion after injury. In: Selzer MEC, S.; Cohen,L.G.; Kwakkel,G.; Miller,R.H., editor. Textbook of Neural Repair and Rehabilitation. Cambridge: Cambridge University Press.
60. Maier IC, Ichiyama RM, Courtine G, Schnell L, Lavrov I, et al. (2009) Differential effects of anti-Nogo-A antibody treatment and treadmill training in rats with incomplete spinal cord injury. Brain 132: 1426–1440.

12

Pooled Analysis of Non-Union, Re-Operation, Infection, and Approach Related Complications after Anterior Odontoid Screw Fixation

Nai-Feng Tian[1]*, Xu-Qi Hu[1], Li-Jun Wu[2], Xin-Lei Wu[2], Yao-Sen Wu[3], Xiao-Lei Zhang[1,4], Xiang-Yang Wang[1], Yong-Long Chi[1], Fang-Min Mao[1]*

1 Department of Orthopaedic Surgery, Second Affiliated Hospital of Wenzhou Medical University, Wenzhou, Zhejiang, China, **2** Institute of Digitized Medicine, Wenzhou Medical University, Wenzhou, Zhejiang, China, **3** Department of Orthopaedics, Second Affiliated Hospital, School of Medicine, Zhejiang University, Hangzhou, Zhejiang, China, **4** Center for Stem Cells and Tissue Engineering, School of Medicine, Zhejiang University, Hangzhou, Zhejiang, China

Abstract

Background: Anterior odontoid screw fixation (AOSF) has been one of the most popular treatments for odontoid fractures. However, the true efficacy of AOSF remains unclear. In this study, we aimed to provide the pooled rates of non-union, reoperation, infection, and approach related complications after AOSF for odontoid fractures.

Methods: We searched studies that discussed complications after AOSF for type II or type III odontoid fractures. A proportion meta-analysis was done and potential sources of heterogeneity were explored by meta-regression analysis.

Results: Of 972 references initially identified, 63 were eligible for inclusion. 54 studies provided data regarding non-union. The pooled non-union rate was 10% (95% CI: 7%–3%). 48 citations provided re-operation information with a pooled proportion of 5% (95% CI: 3%–7%). Infection was described in 20 studies with an overall rate of 0.2% (95% CI: 0%–1.2%). The main approach related complication is postoperative dysphagia with a pooled rate of 10% (95% CI: 4%–17%). Proportions for the other approach related complications such as postoperative hoarseness (1.2%, 95% CI: 0%–3.7%), esophageal/retropharyngeal injury (0%, 95% CI: 0%–1.1%), wound hematomas (0.2%, 95% CI: 0%–1.8%), and spinal cord injury (0%, 95% CI: 0%–0.2%) were very low. Significant heterogeneities were detected when we combined the rates of non-union, re-operation, and dysphagia. Multivariate meta-regression analysis showed that old age was significantly predictive of non-union. Subgroup comparisons showed significant higher non-union rates in age ≥70 than that in age ≤40 and in age 40 to <50. Meta-regression analysis did not reveal any examined variables influencing the re-operation rate. Meta-regression analysis showed age had a significant effect on the dysphagia rate.

Conclusions/Significances: This study summarized the rates of non-union, reoperation, infection, and approach related complications after AOSF for odontoid factures. Elderly patients were more likely to experience non-union and dysphagia.

Editor: Mohammed Shamji, Toronto Western Hospital, Canada

Funding: This work is supported by grants of National Natural Science Foundation of China (No. 81372014) and Natural Science Foundation of Zhejiang Province for Distinguished Young Scholars (No. LR12H06001). The funders had no role in study design, data collection and analysis, decision to publish, or preparation of the manuscript.

Competing Interests: The authors have declared that no competing interests exist.

* Email: tiannaifeng@163.com (NFT); spinemao@163.com (FMM)

Introduction

Odontoid fractures account for 10%–15% of all cervical spine fractures [1]. Despite of the frequency of odontoid fractures, its management remains controversial and ranges from conservative treatment to surgical intervention [2–7]. Conservative treatment consists of skull traction, cervical collar, brace, and halo vest. However, such methods are unpopular for unstable odontoid fractures (type II and shallow type III based on the classification of Anderson and D'lonzo [8]) because of the high non-union rate [2,3]. Moreover, they are often poorly tolerated in the elderly and in the multiply injured patients [6]. Posterior C1–C2 fusion has been advocated as it significantly increases the fusion rate [9,10]. Nevertheless, this technique is associated with extensive surgical exposure, autogenous bone harvest, and compromise of the cervical movement [2–6]. Anterior odontoid screw fixation (AOSF) has been one of the surgical treatments for unstable odontoid fractures since it was independently introduced by Bohler and Nakanishi [11,12]. This technique seems an ideal treatment as it preserves C1–C2 movement and obviates bone graft harvest.

To date, many clinical studies have evaluated the effectiveness of AOSF for odontoid fractures [12–77]. Nevertheless, clinicians may be confused about the true efficacy of this technique because of the wide variability of these reports. Previous reviews were mostly narrative or were investigations that did not weight the results of the single studies according to the number of participants [2,4–6]. Therefore, it is important to combine the results from different studies for clinical reference. In this study, we aimed to provide pooled rates of non-union, re-operation, infection, and approach related complications after surgical treatment of unstable odontoid fractures using AOSF. Furthermore, we tried to explore potential factors that affected these outcomes.

Materials and Methods

Search strategy and inclusion criteria

A computerized systematic search was conducted up to August 2013 using MEDLINE database. We screened all fields by the term "odontoid fracture" or "odontoid screw" or "odontoid fixation". Articles were limited to those published in English. We also searched the reference lists and relevant journals by hand. This meta-analysis was performed in accordance with the preferred reporting items for systematic reviews and meta-analyses (PRISMA) guidelines (when appropriate) (Checklist S1).

We included studies which were carried out on humans. The studies that discussed fusion results, and/or re-operations, and/or infections, and/or approach related complications after odontoid screw fixation for type II or type III odontoid fractures were selected. We also required a minimum sample size of five to ensure quality and comparability of data. Biomechanical studies, cadaveric studies, animal studies, case report, duplications, and review articles were excluded. Clinical studies with inadequate information or incomplete data were also excluded. We carefully reviewed the department/institute of each potential eligible study to screen whether there were any papers from the same surgical team. For papers that had overlapping patients determined through the overlapping research time, we only included the paper with the largest sample size for analysis.

Data extraction

Two investigators reviewed all identified articles to determine if an individual study was eligible for inclusion. Data from each study was extracted using a standardized form. Disagreements on eligibility and data between reviewers were resolved by consensus with the third reviewer. Studies were categorized into levels of evidence according to those published in the Journal of Bone and Joint Surgery (American) [78].

Data extracted consisted of study year, country, level of evidence, patients' mean age, sex proportion, mean follow-up duration, classification of the odontoid fracture, number of patients, number of non-unions, number of re-operations, number of infections, and number of approach related complications. Fusion status should be assessed according to radiological (static or dynamic) and/or computed tomography (CT) examinations. Because the fusion criteria might be different among the included studies, we used a universal definition of fusion for data extraction. Criteria for fusion success included formation of trabecular and cortex bony bridges through the fracture site, absence of sclerotic borders adjacent to the fracture site, and absence of movement of the fracture site confirmed on radiographs and/or CT scan. Radiolucent cleft, clear fracture line, fibrous union, or any movement at the fracture site were considered as non-union. Re-operation represented secondary surgical intervention for any reason after odontoid screw fixation. Infections indicated only those located at the surgical site including both superficial and deep ones. We extracted data on five types of approach related complications including postoperative dysphagia, postoperative hoarseness, esophageal /retropharyngeal injury, wound hematomas, and spinal cord injury. In this meta-analysis, data regarding the study characteristics and the outcomes of interest were extracted based on the average value of each study. For studies with overlapping patients, only the one with the largest sample size was entered into meta-analysis.

Statistical analysis

Meta-analyses were performed to pool the rates of non-union, re-operation, infection, and approach related complications. A Freeman-Tukey Double arcsine transformation was implemented to calculate the overall proportion. A test of heterogeneity was carried out, and cut-off p value of 0.1 was established as a threshold of homogeneity. Pooled estimates and 95% confidence intervals (CIs) were summarized by forest plots. Fixed-effect models were applied unless statistical heterogeneity was significant, in which case random-effect models were used. We further investigated potential sources of heterogeneity by arranging groups of studies according to relevant characteristics (year of publication, level of evidence, patients' mean age, sex, follow-up duration, fracture type, and study sample size) and by meta-regression analysis. Factors were examined both individually and in multiple-variable models. To avoid model instability, only factors that showed significant effects individually were enrolled into a multiple regression model. Publication bias was assessed using Egger test. All analyses were done in the statistical software R 3.0.1.

Results

In the initial screening, 972 potential studies were selected according to the search strategy. Hand-searching resulted in 12 additional papers. After reviewing titles and abstracts, 814 papers were found to be unrelated to the current topic. Of the remaining 170 papers, the full texts were read and 104 publications which did not meet eligibility criteria were excluded. Further three papers [71,73,76] were excluded due to potential overlapping patients. Consequently, sixty three papers met all inclusion criteria and were selected (Figure 1) [12–70,72,74,75,77]. Based on the level of evidence, there were 1 level II, 17 level III, and 45 level IV studies. The mean age ranged from 35 to 85.4 years. We divided the studies into five age subgroups (age ≤40, age 40 to <50, age 50 to <60, age 60 to <70, and age ≥70). The male to female ratio was 1.74. The follow-up duration ranged from 1.5 months to 9 years. 88.9% of the injuries were type II dens fractures according to Anderson and D'Alonzo's classification [8]. The characteristics of selected studies were summarized in Table S1 and Table S2.

54 studies [12–20,22–29,31–51,53–60,62,63,65–70] that reported fusion results were pooled. Six studies [21,52,61,72,74,75] were excluded from data synthesizing because of potential patients overlapping. Imaging methods used for fusion assessment included radiograph (static and/or dynamic) and CT scan. Radiograph was used in fifty two studies. CT scan was used in twenty six papers. Twenty five studies used both methods. In selected studies, a total of 1425 patients were evaluated. The non-union rates ranged from 0% to 62%. The pooled estimate for all studies was 10% (95% CI: 7%–13%). However, the estimate was associated with substantial heterogeneity ($p<0.001$) (Figure 2). We observed that the pooled non-union rate based on CT scan (12%, 95% CI: 7%–17%) was higher than that based on only X-rays (8%, 95% CI: 4%–13%). Nevertheless, the difference was statistically insignificant ($p=0.234$) after univariate meta-regression analysis. Therefore, we combine both image modalities into one database. Univariate meta-regression analysis showed that old age ($p=0.002$), less than one year follow-up ($p=0.017$), and publication after 2000 ($p=0.012$) were significantly predictive of non-union. The non-union rate increased with age, as estimates in the five age groups were 7%, 6%, 11%, 15%, and 25%, respectively (Figure 3). Subgroup comparisons showed that the non-union rate in age ≥

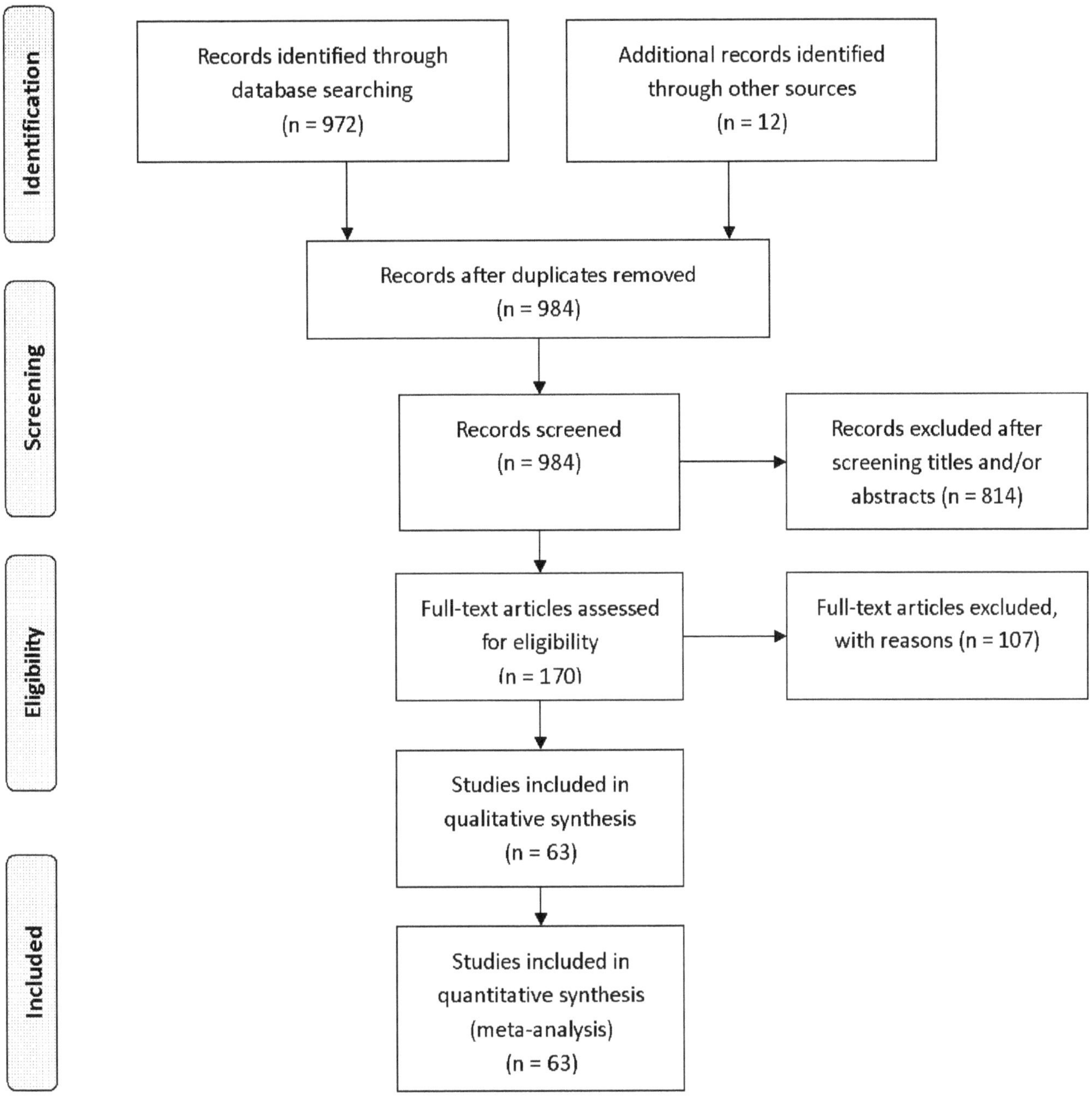

Figure 1. Selection of relevant publications, reasons for exclusion.

70 was significant higher than that in age ≤40 ($p = 0.015$) and in age 40 to <50 ($p = 0.015$). After multivariate meta-regression analysis, only age ($p = 0.016$) remained significant. No significant publication bias was detected ($p = 0.699$).

48 citations [12,14,15,17–20,22–24,26–31,33–35,38–56,58–60,62–67,69] provided re-operation information following odontoid screw fixation. Reasons for re-operation included screw loosening/pullout/cut-out/mal-position, fracture re-dislocation, unstable non-union, hematoma, and so on. The re-operation rates ranged from 0% to 24%. The random-effect pooled proportion was 5% (95% CI: 3%–7%) with pronounced heterogeneity ($p = 0.029$) (Figure 4). Meta-regression analysis revealed that none of the examined variables (year of publication, age, gender, follow-up duration, fracture type, or sample size) significantly influenced the re-operation rate. Egger test for publication bias showed no significant evidence for bias ($p = 0.343$).

Surgical site infection was assessed in 20 studies [15,19,21,22,24,31,33,34,41,45,47,49,50,60–62,66,67,69,70] with 563 surgeries. The reported infection rate was low, with estimates varied from 0% to 6%. The overall infection rate of all included studies was 0.2% (95% CI: 0%–1.2%) (Figure 5). As there was no substantial significant heterogeneity, further meta-regression analysis was not carried out. There was no significant publication bias ($p = 0.549$).

The main approach related complication was postoperative dysphagia. The pooled rate was 10% (95% CI: 4%–17%) with statistically significant heterogeneity (Figure 6). Meta-regression

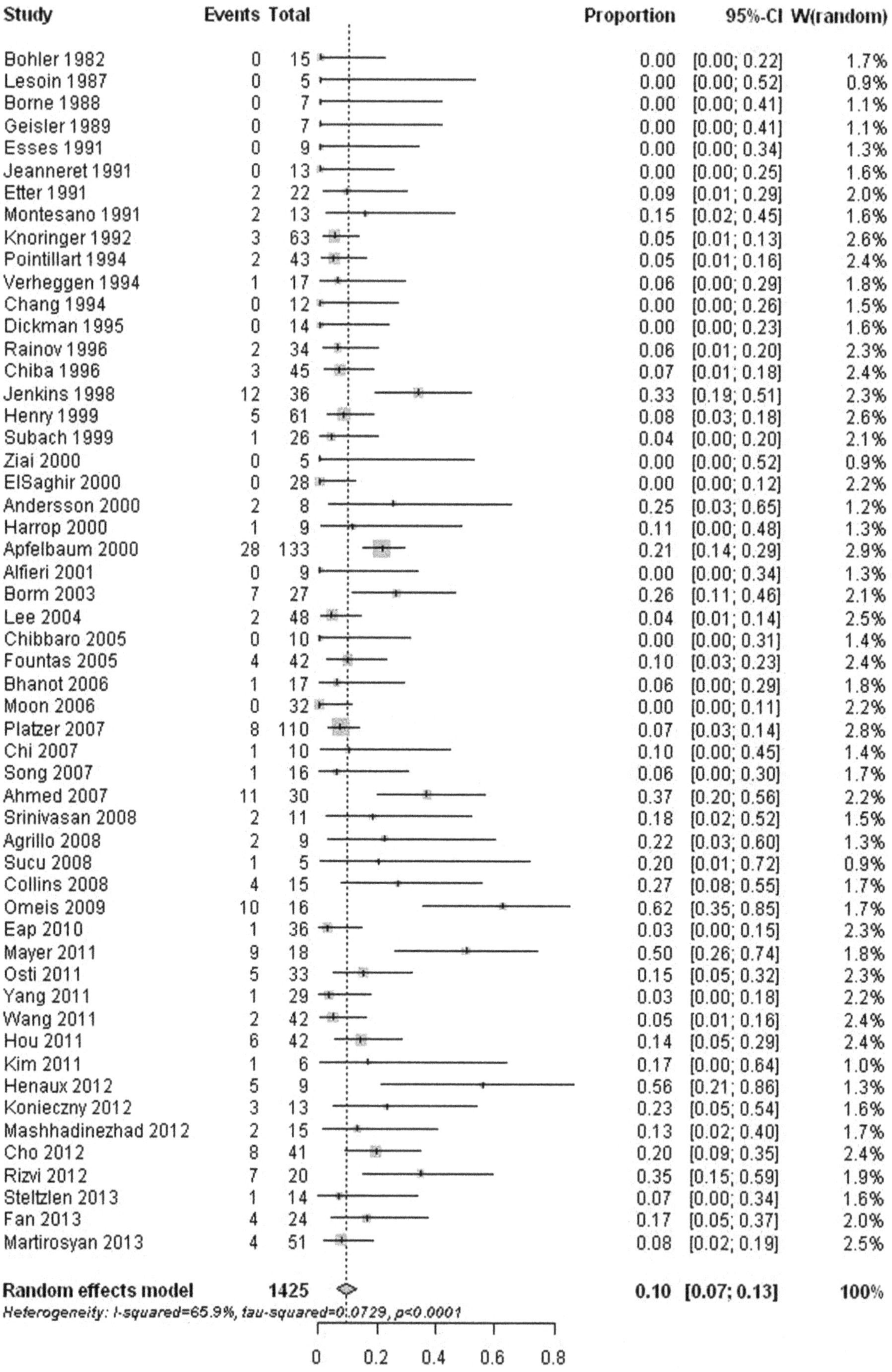
Study Events Total Proportion 95%-CI W(random)
Bohler 1982 0 15 0.00 [0.00; 0.22] 1.7%
Lesoin 1987 0 5 0.00 [0.00; 0.52] 0.9%
Borne 1988 0 7 0.00 [0.00; 0.41] 1.1%
Geisler 1989 0 7 0.00 [0.00; 0.41] 1.1%
Esses 1991 0 9 0.00 [0.00; 0.34] 1.3%
Jeanneret 1991 0 13 0.00 [0.00; 0.25] 1.6%
Etter 1991 2 22 0.09 [0.01; 0.29] 2.0%
Montesano 1991 2 13 0.15 [0.02; 0.45] 1.6%
Knoringer 1992 3 63 0.05 [0.01; 0.13] 2.6%
Pointillart 1994 2 43 0.05 [0.01; 0.16] 2.4%
Verheggen 1994 1 17 0.06 [0.00; 0.29] 1.8%
Chang 1994 0 12 0.00 [0.00; 0.26] 1.5%
Dickman 1995 0 14 0.00 [0.00; 0.23] 1.6%
Rainov 1996 2 34 0.06 [0.01; 0.20] 2.3%
Chiba 1996 3 45 0.07 [0.01; 0.18] 2.4%
Jenkins 1998 12 36 0.33 [0.19; 0.51] 2.3%
Henry 1999 5 61 0.08 [0.03; 0.18] 2.6%
Subach 1999 1 26 0.04 [0.00; 0.20] 2.1%
Ziai 2000 0 5 0.00 [0.00; 0.52] 0.9%
ElSaghir 2000 0 28 0.00 [0.00; 0.12] 2.2%
Andersson 2000 2 8 0.25 [0.03; 0.65] 1.2%
Harrop 2000 1 9 0.11 [0.00; 0.48] 1.3%
Apfelbaum 2000 28 133 0.21 [0.14; 0.29] 2.9%
Alfieri 2001 0 9 0.00 [0.00; 0.34] 1.3%
Borm 2003 7 27 0.26 [0.11; 0.46] 2.1%
Lee 2004 2 48 0.04 [0.01; 0.14] 2.5%
Chibbaro 2005 0 10 0.00 [0.00; 0.31] 1.4%
Fountas 2005 4 42 0.10 [0.03; 0.23] 2.4%
Bhanot 2006 1 17 0.06 [0.00; 0.29] 1.8%
Moon 2006 0 32 0.00 [0.00; 0.11] 2.2%
Platzer 2007 8 110 0.07 [0.03; 0.14] 2.8%
Chi 2007 1 10 0.10 [0.00; 0.45] 1.4%
Song 2007 1 16 0.06 [0.00; 0.30] 1.7%
Ahmed 2007 11 30 0.37 [0.20; 0.56] 2.2%
Srinivasan 2008 2 11 0.18 [0.02; 0.52] 1.5%
Agrillo 2008 2 9 0.22 [0.03; 0.60] 1.3%
Sucu 2008 1 5 0.20 [0.01; 0.72] 0.9%
Collins 2008 4 15 0.27 [0.08; 0.55] 1.7%
Omeis 2009 10 16 0.62 [0.35; 0.85] 1.7%
Eap 2010 1 36 0.03 [0.00; 0.15] 2.3%
Mayer 2011 9 18 0.50 [0.26; 0.74] 1.8%
Osti 2011 5 33 0.15 [0.05; 0.32] 2.3%
Yang 2011 1 29 0.03 [0.00; 0.18] 2.2%
Wang 2011 2 42 0.05 [0.01; 0.16] 2.4%
Hou 2011 6 42 0.14 [0.05; 0.29] 2.4%
Kim 2011 1 6 0.17 [0.00; 0.64] 1.0%
Henaux 2012 5 9 0.56 [0.21; 0.86] 1.3%
Konieczny 2012 3 13 0.23 [0.05; 0.54] 1.6%
Mashhadinezhad 2012 2 15 0.13 [0.02; 0.40] 1.7%
Cho 2012 8 41 0.20 [0.09; 0.35] 2.4%
Rizvi 2012 7 20 0.35 [0.15; 0.59] 1.9%
Steltzlen 2013 1 14 0.07 [0.00; 0.34] 1.6%
Fan 2013 4 24 0.17 [0.05; 0.37] 2.0%
Martirosyan 2013 4 51 0.08 [0.02; 0.19] 2.5%
Random effects model 1425 0.10 [0.07; 0.13] 100%
Heterogeneity: I-squared=65.9%, tau-squared=0.0729, p<0.0001
0 0.2 0.4 0.6 0.8

Figure 2. Forest plots showing the non-union rates (boxes) with 95% confidence of intervals (CIs; bars).

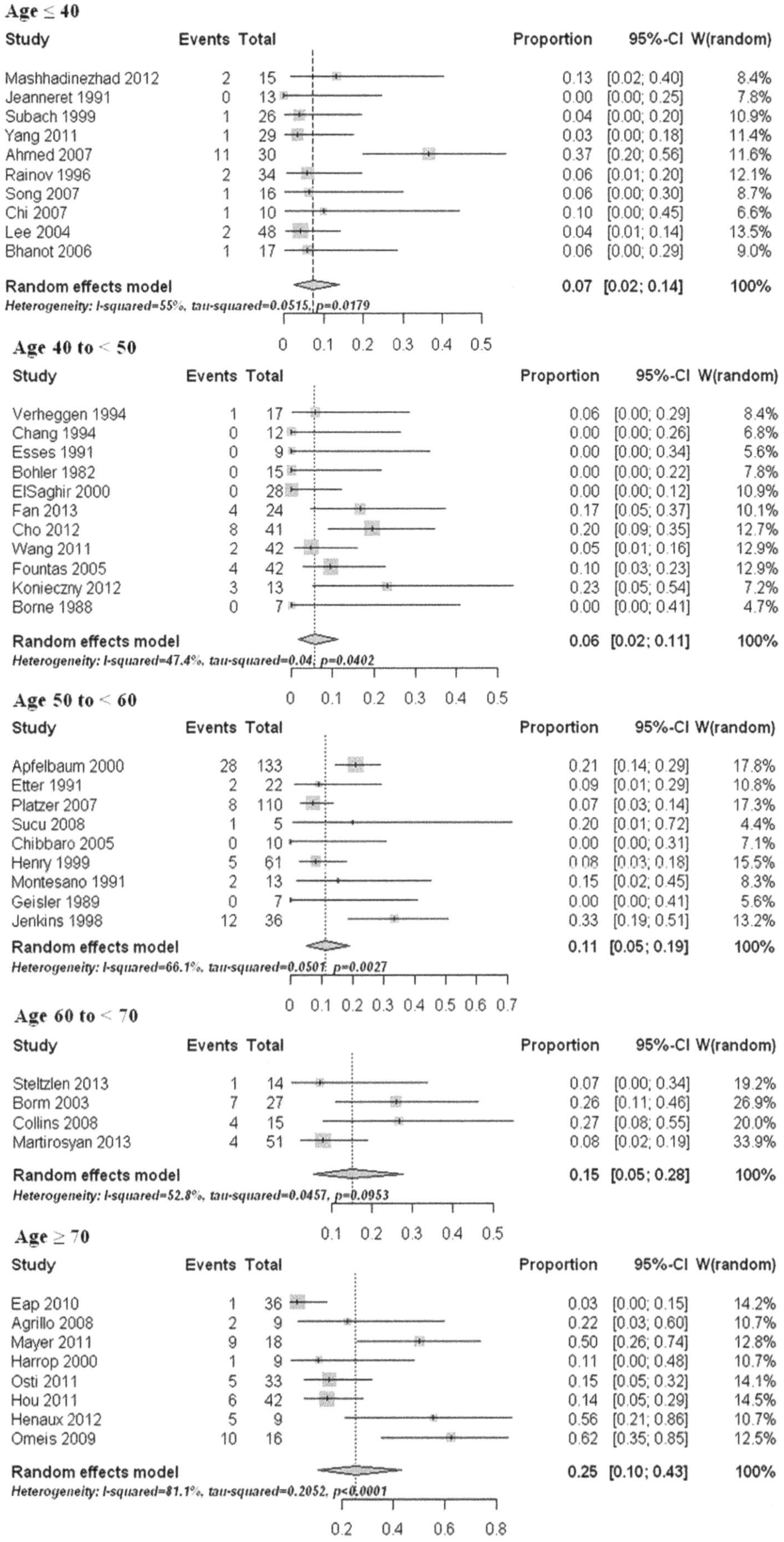
Age ≤ 40
Study Events Total Proportion 95%-CI W(random)
Mashhadinezhad 2012 2 15 0.13 [0.02; 0.40] 8.4%
Jeanneret 1991 0 13 0.00 [0.00; 0.25] 7.8%
Subach 1999 1 26 0.04 [0.00; 0.20] 10.9%
Yang 2011 1 29 0.03 [0.00; 0.18] 11.4%
Ahmed 2007 11 30 0.37 [0.20; 0.56] 11.6%
Rainov 1996 2 34 0.06 [0.01; 0.20] 12.1%
Song 2007 1 16 0.06 [0.00; 0.30] 8.7%
Chi 2007 1 10 0.10 [0.00; 0.45] 6.6%
Lee 2004 2 48 0.04 [0.01; 0.14] 13.5%
Bhanot 2006 1 17 0.06 [0.00; 0.29] 9.0%
Random effects model 0.07 [0.02; 0.14] 100%
Heterogeneity: I-squared=55%, tau-squared=0.0515, p=0.0179
0 0.1 0.2 0.3 0.4 0.5
Age 40 to < 50
Study Events Total Proportion 95%-CI W(random)
Verheggen 1994 1 17 0.06 [0.00; 0.29] 8.4%
Chang 1994 0 12 0.00 [0.00; 0.26] 6.8%
Esses 1991 0 9 0.00 [0.00; 0.34] 5.6%
Bohler 1982 0 15 0.00 [0.00; 0.22] 7.8%
ElSaghir 2000 0 28 0.00 [0.00; 0.12] 10.9%
Fan 2013 4 24 0.17 [0.05; 0.37] 10.1%
Cho 2012 8 41 0.20 [0.09; 0.35] 12.7%
Wang 2011 2 42 0.05 [0.01; 0.16] 12.9%
Fountas 2005 4 42 0.10 [0.03; 0.23] 12.9%
Konieczny 2012 3 13 0.23 [0.05; 0.54] 7.2%
Borne 1988 0 7 0.00 [0.00; 0.41] 4.7%
Random effects model 0.06 [0.02; 0.11] 100%
Heterogeneity: I-squared=47.4%, tau-squared=0.04, p=0.0402
0 0.1 0.2 0.3 0.4 0.5
Age 50 to < 60
Study Events Total Proportion 95%-CI W(random)
Apfelbaum 2000 28 133 0.21 [0.14; 0.29] 17.8%
Etter 1991 2 22 0.09 [0.01; 0.29] 10.8%
Platzer 2007 8 110 0.07 [0.03; 0.14] 17.3%
Sucu 2008 1 5 0.20 [0.01; 0.72] 4.4%
Chibbaro 2005 0 10 0.00 [0.00; 0.31] 7.1%
Henry 1999 5 61 0.08 [0.03; 0.18] 15.5%
Montesano 1991 2 13 0.15 [0.02; 0.45] 8.3%
Geisler 1989 0 7 0.00 [0.00; 0.41] 5.6%
Jenkins 1998 12 36 0.33 [0.19; 0.51] 13.2%
Random effects model 0.11 [0.05; 0.19] 100%
Heterogeneity: I-squared=66.1%, tau-squared=0.0501, p=0.0027
0 0.1 0.2 0.3 0.4 0.5 0.6 0.7
Age 60 to < 70
Study Events Total Proportion 95%-CI W(random)
Steltzlen 2013 1 14 0.07 [0.00; 0.34] 19.2%
Borm 2003 7 27 0.26 [0.11; 0.46] 26.9%
Collins 2008 4 15 0.27 [0.08; 0.55] 20.0%
Martirosyan 2013 4 51 0.08 [0.02; 0.19] 33.9%
Random effects model 0.15 [0.05; 0.28] 100%
Heterogeneity: I-squared=52.8%, tau-squared=0.0457, p=0.0953
0.1 0.2 0.3 0.4 0.5
Age ≥ 70
Study Events Total Proportion 95%-CI W(random)
Eap 2010 1 36 0.03 [0.00; 0.15] 14.2%
Agrillo 2008 2 9 0.22 [0.03; 0.60] 10.7%
Mayer 2011 9 18 0.50 [0.26; 0.74] 12.8%
Harrop 2000 1 9 0.11 [0.00; 0.48] 10.7%
Osti 2011 5 33 0.15 [0.05; 0.32] 14.1%
Hou 2011 6 42 0.14 [0.05; 0.29] 14.5%
Henaux 2012 5 9 0.56 [0.21; 0.86] 10.7%
Omeis 2009 10 16 0.62 [0.35; 0.85] 12.5%
Random effects model 0.25 [0.10; 0.43] 100%
Heterogeneity: I-squared=81.1%, tau-squared=0.2052, p<0.0001
0.2 0.4 0.6 0.8

Figure 3. Forest plots showing the non-union rates (boxes) with 95% confidence of intervals (CIs; bars) in different age groups.

Study	Events	Total	Proportion	95%-CI	W(random)
Bohler 1982	1	15	0.07	[0.00; 0.32]	1.5%
Borne 1988	0	7	0.00	[0.00; 0.41]	0.8%
Geisler 1989	0	7	0.00	[0.00; 0.41]	0.8%
Jeanneret 1991	0	13	0.00	[0.00; 0.25]	1.3%
Etter 1991	3	22	0.14	[0.03; 0.35]	2.0%
Montesano 1991	3	13	0.23	[0.05; 0.54]	1.3%
Knoringer 1992	4	63	0.06	[0.02; 0.15]	3.8%
Verheggen 1994	2	17	0.12	[0.01; 0.36]	1.6%
Pointillart 1994	1	43	0.02	[0.00; 0.12]	3.1%
Chang 1994	0	12	0.00	[0.00; 0.26]	1.2%
Rainov 1996	3	34	0.09	[0.02; 0.24]	2.7%
Chiba 1996	1	45	0.02	[0.00; 0.12]	3.2%
Jenkins 1998	3	36	0.08	[0.02; 0.22]	2.8%
Morandi 1999	0	17	0.00	[0.00; 0.20]	1.6%
Henry 1999	2	61	0.03	[0.00; 0.11]	3.8%
Subach 1999	2	26	0.08	[0.01; 0.25]	2.2%
ElSaghir 2000	4	28	0.14	[0.04; 0.33]	2.4%
Apfelbaum 2000	10	133	0.08	[0.04; 0.13]	5.2%
Harrop 2000	1	9	0.11	[0.00; 0.48]	1.0%
Borm 2003	4	27	0.15	[0.04; 0.34]	2.3%
Lee 2004	4	48	0.08	[0.02; 0.20]	3.3%
Fountas 2005	1	42	0.02	[0.00; 0.13]	3.1%
Chibbaro 2005	0	10	0.00	[0.00; 0.31]	1.1%
Moon 2006	0	32	0.00	[0.00; 0.11]	2.6%
Bhanot 2006	1	17	0.06	[0.00; 0.29]	1.6%
Platzer 2007	8	110	0.07	[0.03; 0.14]	4.9%
Ahmed 2007	1	30	0.03	[0.00; 0.17]	2.5%
Chi 2007	0	10	0.00	[0.00; 0.31]	1.1%
Song 2007	1	16	0.06	[0.00; 0.30]	1.6%
Collins 2008	3	15	0.20	[0.04; 0.48]	1.5%
Srinivasan 2008	0	11	0.00	[0.00; 0.28]	1.2%
Sucu 2008	0	5	0.00	[0.00; 0.52]	0.6%
Agrillo 2008	1	9	0.11	[0.00; 0.48]	1.0%
Koller 2009	1	11	0.09	[0.00; 0.41]	1.2%
Omeis 2009	1	16	0.06	[0.00; 0.30]	1.6%
Eap 2010	1	36	0.03	[0.00; 0.15]	2.8%
Osti 2011	8	33	0.24	[0.11; 0.42]	2.6%
Yang 2011	0	29	0.00	[0.00; 0.12]	2.4%
Hou 2011	1	42	0.02	[0.00; 0.13]	3.1%
Kim 2011	1	6	0.17	[0.00; 0.64]	0.7%
Wang 2011	0	42	0.00	[0.00; 0.08]	3.1%
Cho 2012	5	41	0.12	[0.04; 0.26]	3.0%
Henaux 2012	0	9	0.00	[0.00; 0.34]	1.0%
Mashhadinezhad 2012	2	15	0.13	[0.02; 0.40]	1.5%
Kantelhardt 2012	1	6	0.17	[0.00; 0.64]	0.7%
Rizvi 2012	7	40	0.18	[0.07; 0.33]	3.0%
Konieczny 2012	3	13	0.23	[0.05; 0.54]	1.3%
Steltzlen 2013	2	14	0.14	[0.02; 0.43]	1.4%
Random effects model		**1336**	**0.05**	**[0.03; 0.07]**	**100%**

Heterogeneity: I-squared=29.8%, tau-squared=0.0152, p=0.0294

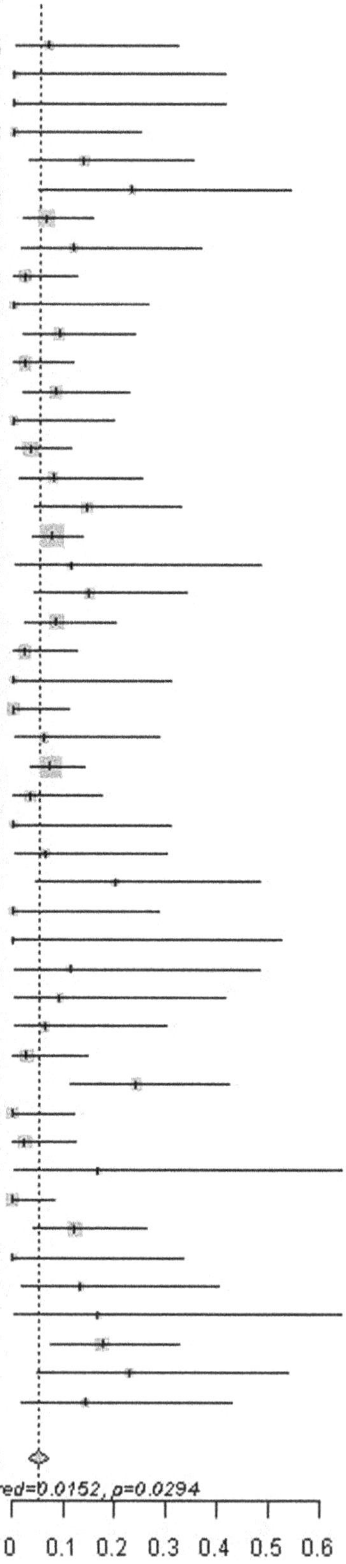

Figure 4. Forest plots showing the re-operation rates (boxes) with 95% confidence of intervals (CIs; bars).

analysis revealed that age had a significant effect on the estimate ($p<0.0001$). Subgroup comparisons indicated that the two old age groups (age 60 to <70 yrs and age ≥70 yrs) had significant higher dysphagia rates than those in the other three age groups (age ≤40, age 40 to <50, and age 50 to <60) ($p<0.05$). Pooled proportions for the other approach related complications like postoperative

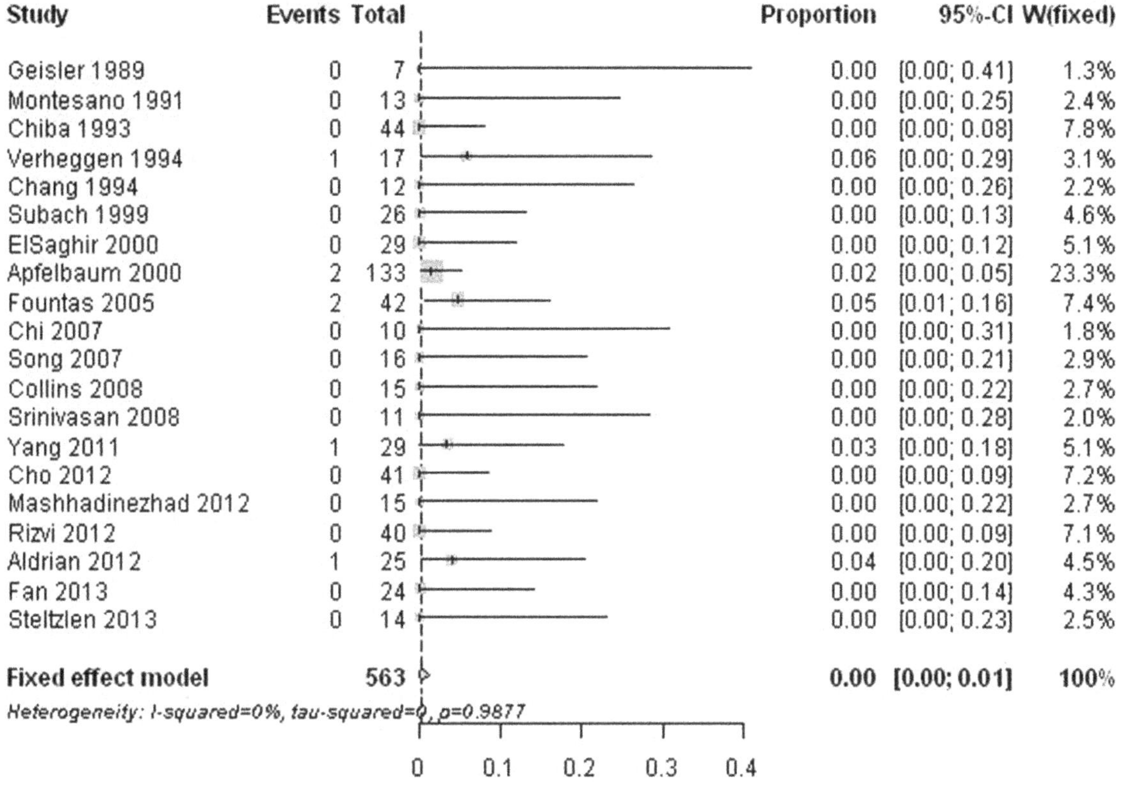
Study Events Total Proportion 95%-CI W(fixed)
Geisler 1989 0 7 0.00 [0.00; 0.41] 1.3%
Montesano 1991 0 13 0.00 [0.00; 0.25] 2.4%
Chiba 1993 0 44 0.00 [0.00; 0.08] 7.8%
Verheggen 1994 1 17 0.06 [0.00; 0.29] 3.1%
Chang 1994 0 12 0.00 [0.00; 0.26] 2.2%
Subach 1999 0 26 0.00 [0.00; 0.13] 4.6%
ElSaghir 2000 0 29 0.00 [0.00; 0.12] 5.1%
Apfelbaum 2000 2 133 0.02 [0.00; 0.05] 23.3%
Fountas 2005 2 42 0.05 [0.01; 0.16] 7.4%
Chi 2007 0 10 0.00 [0.00; 0.31] 1.8%
Song 2007 0 16 0.00 [0.00; 0.21] 2.9%
Collins 2008 0 15 0.00 [0.00; 0.22] 2.7%
Srinivasan 2008 0 11 0.00 [0.00; 0.28] 2.0%
Yang 2011 1 29 0.03 [0.00; 0.18] 5.1%
Cho 2012 0 41 0.00 [0.00; 0.09] 7.2%
Mashhadinezhad 2012 0 15 0.00 [0.00; 0.22] 2.7%
Rizvi 2012 0 40 0.00 [0.00; 0.09] 7.1%
Aldrian 2012 1 25 0.04 [0.00; 0.20] 4.5%
Fan 2013 0 24 0.00 [0.00; 0.14] 4.3%
Steltzlen 2013 0 14 0.00 [0.00; 0.23] 2.5%
Fixed effect model 563 0.00 [0.00; 0.01] 100%
Heterogeneity: I-squared=0%, tau-squared=0, p=0.9877
0 0.1 0.2 0.3 0.4

Figure 5. Forest plots showing the infection rates (boxes) with 95% confidence of intervals (CIs; bars).

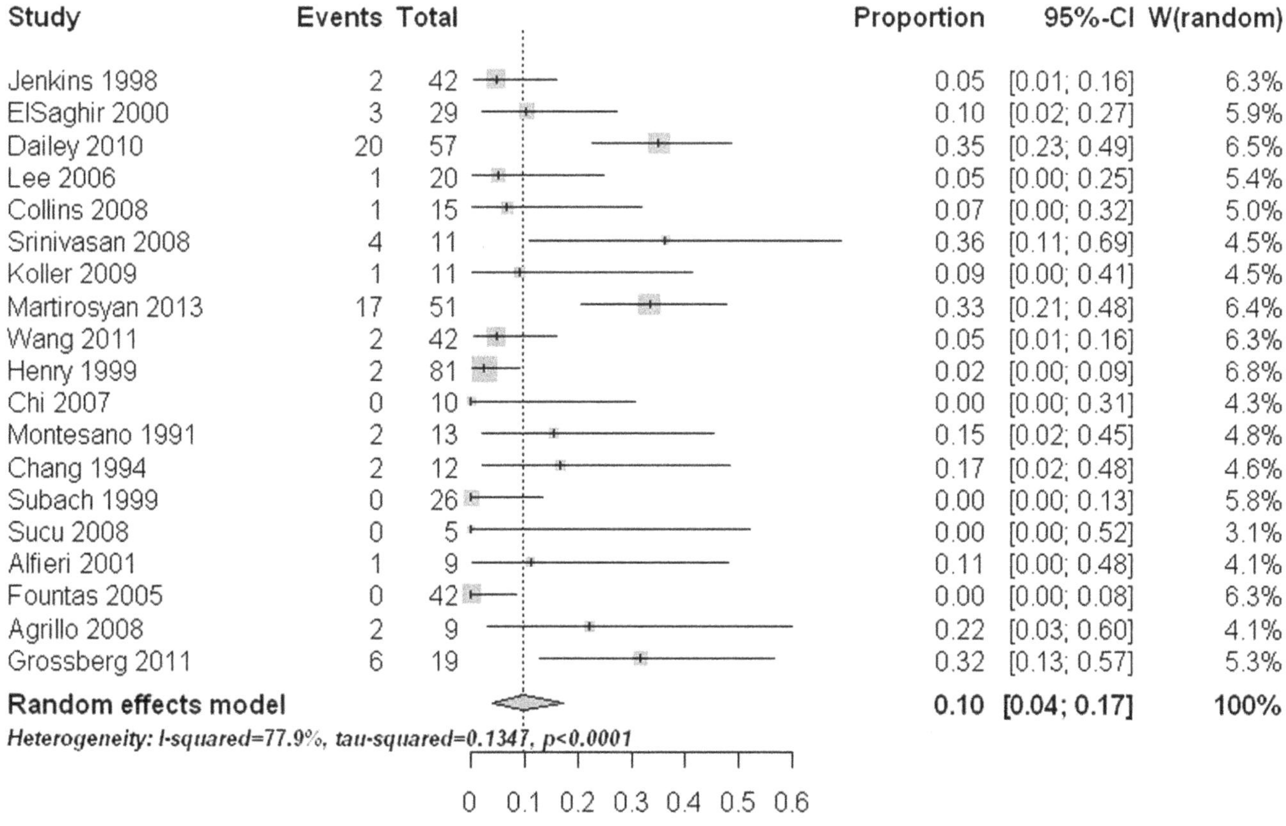
Study Events Total Proportion 95%-CI W(random)
Jenkins 1998 2 42 0.05 [0.01; 0.16] 6.3%
ElSaghir 2000 3 29 0.10 [0.02; 0.27] 5.9%
Dailey 2010 20 57 0.35 [0.23; 0.49] 6.5%
Lee 2006 1 20 0.05 [0.00; 0.25] 5.4%
Collins 2008 1 15 0.07 [0.00; 0.32] 5.0%
Srinivasan 2008 4 11 0.36 [0.11; 0.69] 4.5%
Koller 2009 1 11 0.09 [0.00; 0.41] 4.5%
Martirosyan 2013 17 51 0.33 [0.21; 0.48] 6.4%
Wang 2011 2 42 0.05 [0.01; 0.16] 6.3%
Henry 1999 2 81 0.02 [0.00; 0.09] 6.8%
Chi 2007 0 10 0.00 [0.00; 0.31] 4.3%
Montesano 1991 2 13 0.15 [0.02; 0.45] 4.8%
Chang 1994 2 12 0.17 [0.02; 0.48] 4.6%
Subach 1999 0 26 0.00 [0.00; 0.13] 5.8%
Sucu 2008 0 5 0.00 [0.00; 0.52] 3.1%
Alfieri 2001 1 9 0.11 [0.00; 0.48] 4.1%
Fountas 2005 0 42 0.00 [0.00; 0.08] 6.3%
Agrillo 2008 2 9 0.22 [0.03; 0.60] 4.1%
Grossberg 2011 6 19 0.32 [0.13; 0.57] 5.3%
Random effects model 0.10 [0.04; 0.17] 100%
Heterogeneity: I-squared=77.9%, tau-squared=0.1347, p<0.0001
0 0.1 0.2 0.3 0.4 0.5 0.6

Figure 6. Forest plots showing the rates of dysphagia (boxes) with 95% confidence of intervals (CIs; bars).

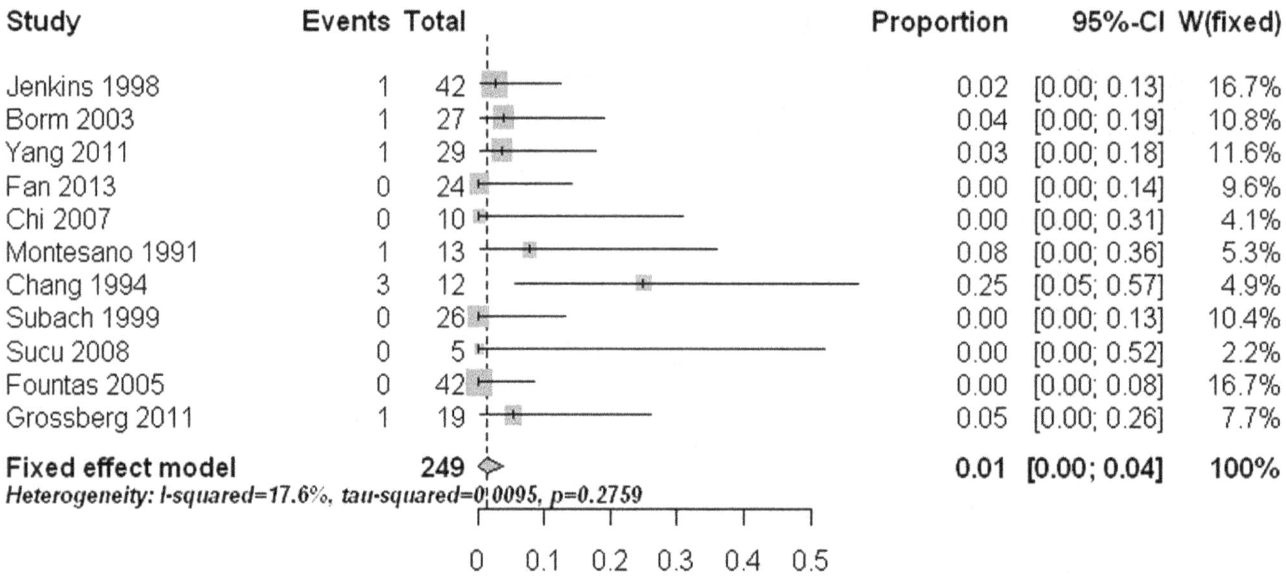
Study
Events Total
Proportion
95%-CI W(fixed)
Jenkins 1998 1 42 0.02 [0.00; 0.13] 16.7%
Borm 2003 1 27 0.04 [0.00; 0.19] 10.8%
Yang 2011 1 29 0.03 [0.00; 0.18] 11.6%
Fan 2013 0 24 0.00 [0.00; 0.14] 9.6%
Chi 2007 0 10 0.00 [0.00; 0.31] 4.1%
Montesano 1991 1 13 0.08 [0.00; 0.36] 5.3%
Chang 1994 3 12 0.25 [0.05; 0.57] 4.9%
Subach 1999 0 26 0.00 [0.00; 0.13] 10.4%
Sucu 2008 0 5 0.00 [0.00; 0.52] 2.2%
Fountas 2005 0 42 0.00 [0.00; 0.08] 16.7%
Grossberg 2011 1 19 0.05 [0.00; 0.26] 7.7%
Fixed effect model 249 0.01 [0.00; 0.04] 100%
Heterogeneity: I-squared=17.6%, tau-squared=0.0095, p=0.2759
0 0.1 0.2 0.3 0.4 0.5

Figure 7. Forest plots showing the rates of hoarseness (boxes) with 95% confidence of intervals (CIs; bars).

hoarseness (1.2%, 95% CI: 0%–3.7%) (Figure 7), esophageal / retropharyngeal injury (0%, 95% CI: 0%–1.1%) (Figure 8), wound hematomas (0.2%, 95% CI: 0%–1.8%) (Figure 9), and spinal cord injury (0%, 95% CI: 0%–0.2%) (Figure 10) were very low. No significant publication bias was detected (p>0.1)

Discussion

We conducted this study to provide a better understanding of the frequency of non-union, infection, re-operation, and approach related complications after anterior screw fixation for type II and type III odontoid fractures. Non-union can be one of the most important outcomes, because it may lead to spinal cord injury due to atlantoaxial instability. Pooled analysis from our study showed that the non-union rate after AOSF was 10%. It seemed that the fusion rate of AOSF (90%) was better than that of the conservative treatment (60%–80%) [3], and was comparable to that of the posterior fixation (89%–100%) [5]. Therefore, AOSF might be a good choice for type II and type III odontoid fractures in selected patients. This study revealed that the re-operation rate was 5% after AOSF. The reasons for re-operation included non-union, screw failure, fracture re-dislocation, and occasionally hematoma. Since non-union accounted for fifty percent of the cases undergoing re-operation, obtaining bony fusion becomes the first priority in AOSF. Not all of the non-unions underwent second surgical interventions, because some of them (fibrous unions) were radiologically stable. For these cases, long term follow up was still essential. The infection rate in surgical site was very low with only seven cases identified during our review [24,33,41,60,61]. The pooled estimate was 0.2% without significant heterogeneity among the studies. All infection cases were superficial and were resolved without sequelae.

Our study revealed that age had a significant impact on the non-union rate. The non-union rate in patients younger than 50

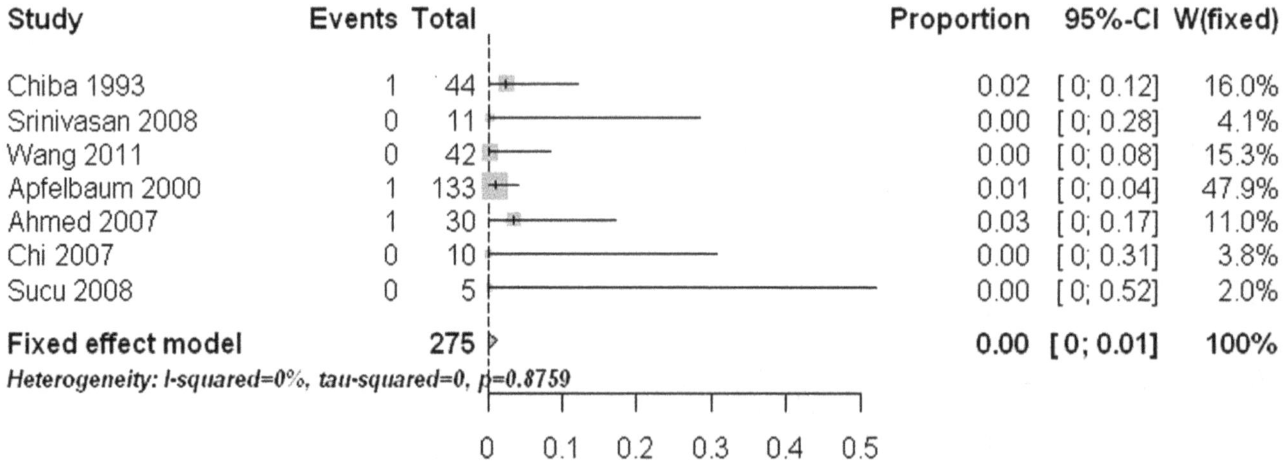
Study
Events Total
Proportion
95%-CI W(fixed)
Chiba 1993 1 44 0.02 [0; 0.12] 16.0%
Srinivasan 2008 0 11 0.00 [0; 0.28] 4.1%
Wang 2011 0 42 0.00 [0; 0.08] 15.3%
Apfelbaum 2000 1 133 0.01 [0; 0.04] 47.9%
Ahmed 2007 1 30 0.03 [0; 0.17] 11.0%
Chi 2007 0 10 0.00 [0; 0.31] 3.8%
Sucu 2008 0 5 0.00 [0; 0.52] 2.0%
Fixed effect model 275 0.00 [0; 0.01] 100%
Heterogeneity: I-squared=0%, tau-squared=0, p=0.8759
0 0.1 0.2 0.3 0.4 0.5

Figure 8. Forest plots showing the rates of esophageal /retropharyngeal injury (boxes) with 95% confidence of intervals (CIs; bars).

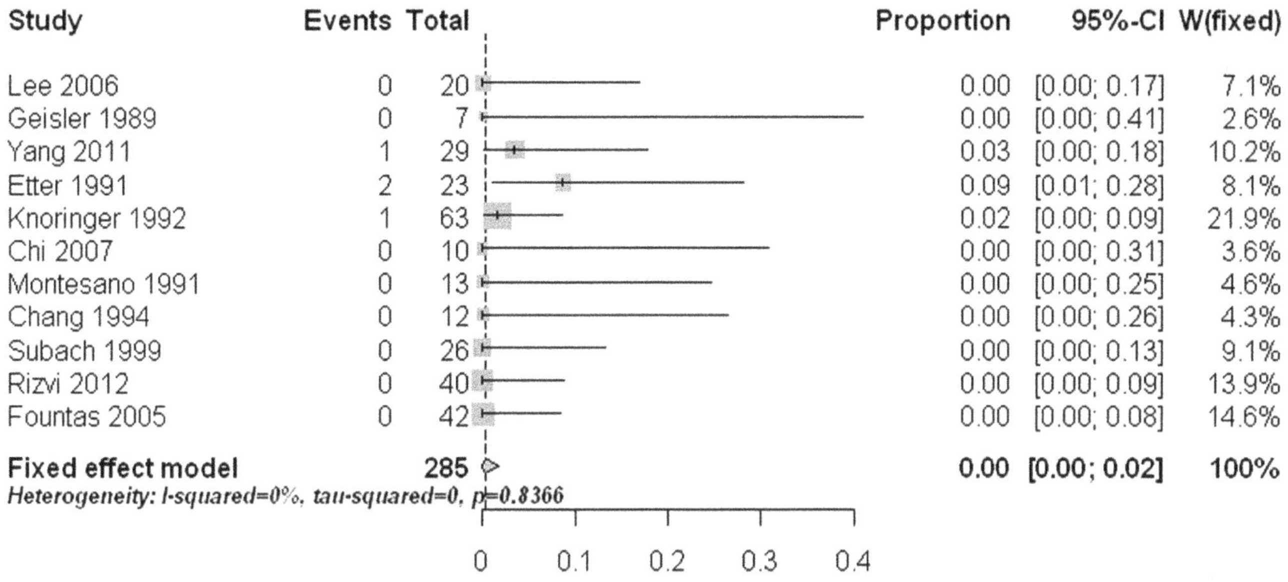
Study Events Total Proportion 95%-CI W(fixed)
Lee 2006 0 20 0.00 [0.00; 0.17] 7.1%
Geisler 1989 0 7 0.00 [0.00; 0.41] 2.6%
Yang 2011 1 29 0.03 [0.00; 0.18] 10.2%
Etter 1991 2 23 0.09 [0.01; 0.28] 8.1%
Knoringer 1992 1 63 0.02 [0.00; 0.09] 21.9%
Chi 2007 0 10 0.00 [0.00; 0.31] 3.6%
Montesano 1991 0 13 0.00 [0.00; 0.25] 4.6%
Chang 1994 0 12 0.00 [0.00; 0.26] 4.3%
Subach 1999 0 26 0.00 [0.00; 0.13] 9.1%
Rizvi 2012 0 40 0.00 [0.00; 0.09] 13.9%
Fountas 2005 0 42 0.00 [0.00; 0.08] 14.6%
Fixed effect model 285 0.00 [0.00; 0.02] 100%
Heterogeneity: I-squared=0%, tau-squared=0, p=0.8366
0 0.1 0.2 0.3 0.4

Figure 9. Forest plots showing the rates of wound hematomas (boxes) with 95% confidence of intervals (CIs; bars).

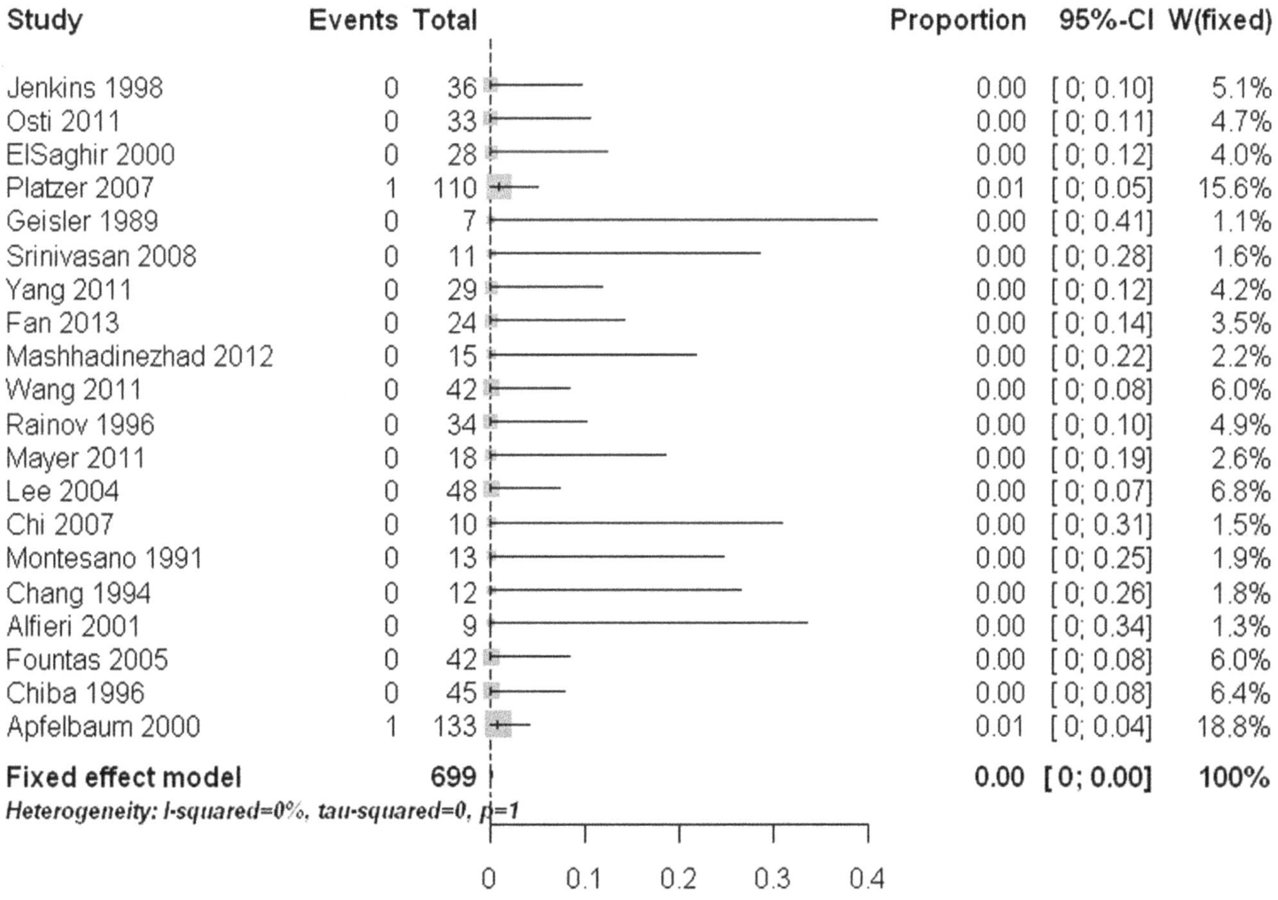
Study Events Total Proportion 95%-CI W(fixed)
Jenkins 1998 0 36 0.00 [0; 0.10] 5.1%
Osti 2011 0 33 0.00 [0; 0.11] 4.7%
ElSaghir 2000 0 28 0.00 [0; 0.12] 4.0%
Platzer 2007 1 110 0.01 [0; 0.05] 15.6%
Geisler 1989 0 7 0.00 [0; 0.41] 1.1%
Srinivasan 2008 0 11 0.00 [0; 0.28] 1.6%
Yang 2011 0 29 0.00 [0; 0.12] 4.2%
Fan 2013 0 24 0.00 [0; 0.14] 3.5%
Mashhadinezhad 2012 0 15 0.00 [0; 0.22] 2.2%
Wang 2011 0 42 0.00 [0; 0.08] 6.0%
Rainov 1996 0 34 0.00 [0; 0.10] 4.9%
Mayer 2011 0 18 0.00 [0; 0.19] 2.6%
Lee 2004 0 48 0.00 [0; 0.07] 6.8%
Chi 2007 0 10 0.00 [0; 0.31] 1.5%
Montesano 1991 0 13 0.00 [0; 0.25] 1.9%
Chang 1994 0 12 0.00 [0; 0.26] 1.8%
Alfieri 2001 0 9 0.00 [0; 0.34] 1.3%
Fountas 2005 0 42 0.00 [0; 0.08] 6.0%
Chiba 1996 0 45 0.00 [0; 0.08] 6.4%
Apfelbaum 2000 1 133 0.01 [0; 0.04] 18.8%
Fixed effect model 699 0.00 [0; 0.00] 100%
Heterogeneity: I-squared=0%, tau-squared=0, p=1
0 0.1 0.2 0.3 0.4

Figure 10. Forest plots showing the rates of spinal cord injury (boxes) with 95% confidence of intervals (CIs; bars).

years was 6%. Therefore, AOSF seems to be a good choice for young patients. Although the non-union rate reached 11% to 25% in patients aged 50 years or older, this rate was still acceptable as the non-union rate of conservative treatment for the elderly patients was very high (60% in Nourbakhsh' review [3], and 56%–72% in Huybregts' review [7]). Subgroup comparisons showed that age ≥70 had a significant higher non-union rate than the young had. Our findings were consistent with those reported by Platzer et al [46]. They observed that patients older than 65 years had a significantly higher non-union rate of 12% compared with that of 4% in younger individuals [46]. However, two other observational studies reported that age was not associated with fusion failure [38,62]. It was generally agreed that old patients had a higher chance to experience osteoporosis and diminished bone quality which might have an important effect on the fusion outcome. As none of the studies directly assessed osteoporosis of surgical patients, the bone quality information in different age groups was not clear. This could be one reason to explain the controversial results from different studies. Therefore, it is important for further studies to clarify the relationships among age, osteoporosis, and fusion outcomes after AOSF. Since elderly patients were more likely to experience non-unions, measures should be adopted to enhance the bony fusion in this population. Dailey et al [75] retrospectively analyzed the efficacy of AOSF in a group of patients with age over 70. They observed a significantly higher stabilization rate of 96% in patients when 2 screws were placed, compared with that of 56% in patients with only one screw used. However, in another group of relatively young patients, the difference became statistically insignificant [28]. Younger patients have better bone quality which could provide more stability at the surgical site. Thus, placing one screw may be sufficient. Nevertheless, the elderly patients might benefit from an additional screw which added rotational stability in the osteopenic bone [75].

Postoperative dysphagia was the main approach related complication after AOSF with pooled estimate of 10%, followed by postoperative hoarseness (1.2%). Esophageal /retropharyngeal injury, wound hematomas, and spinal cord injury were rare approach related complications. Noteworthy was that age also had a significant effect on postoperative dysphagia rate. Dysphagia is a known complication of anterior cervical spine surgery. A recent systematic review showed that female gender, advanced age, multilevel surgery, longer operating time and severe pre-operative neck pain may increase the risk of postoperative dysphagia after cervical spine surgery [79]. During our review, there was no study directly comparing the dysphagia rates among different age groups. Through this meta-analysis, we observed that age ≥60 had a significant higher dysphagia rate than the age <60 had. The possible reason for this fact was that the elderly patient's esophagus was less tolerant to retraction due to fibrosis [75]. Considering the relatively high dysphagia rate in the elderly after AOSF, strategies, such as using of perioperative methylprednisolone, monitoring of endotracheal tube cuff pressure, and preoperative tracheal/ esophageal traction exercise, may be employed to reduce the risk of this complication [79].

There are some limitations existing in this study. First, this meta-analysis only focused on the rates of non-union, re-operation, infection, and approach related complications. We did not pool other outcomes like functional results and patient satisfactory outcome because they were not always reported or were reported in various forms. Even the outcomes we combined were not always available. Second, during the extraction of fusion data, we found the fusion status was assessed using different imaging modalities and non-union was defined according to different standards. Thus, pooling of relevant data might lead to bias even though we had predefined unified criteria for non-union. Third, extensive and significant heterogeneities were detected when we combined the rates of non-union, re-operation, and dysphagia. We had explored the heterogeneity through meta-regression analysis according to several study characteristics, but we only found age had a significant effect on the non-union and dysphagia rate. After subgroup analysis, we still observed heterogeneity in each age group, which meant there were potential other factors influencing the two outcomes. For re-operation, we failed to find potential factors which could explain the heterogeneity. The factors we analyzed represented the average value of each study, which could limit the exploration of the heterogeneity. Moreover, the heterogeneity might also be ascribed to various factors, such as other patient characteristics, fracture subtypes, and surgical techniques used. Lastly, the level of evidence of our analysis is low as none of the enrolled studies were randomized controlled trials. Despite these weaknesses, our study obtains some clinical significance since we pooled estimates based on a relatively large sample. This study provides a quantitative description of the frequencies of non-union, re-operation, infection, and approach related complications after AOSF for odontoid fractures. These data can be helpful in making informed surgical decisions. Further studies may be necessary to pool the functional outcomes of using this technique and to determine the factors affecting the efficacy.

Supporting Information

Table S1 Characteristics of the studies included for analyzing non-union, re-operation, and infection.

Table S2 Characteristics of the studies included for analyzing approach related complications.

Checklist S1 PRISMA Checklist.

Author Contributions

Conceived and designed the experiments: NFT FMM. Performed the experiments: NFT XQH LJW XLW. Analyzed the data: NFT XQH YSW XLZ YLC. Contributed reagents/materials/analysis tools: XYW FMM. Wrote the paper: NFT FMM.

References

1. Husby J, Sorensen KH (1974) Fracture of the odontoid process of the axis. Acta Orthop Scand 45: 182–192.
2. Maak TG, Grauer JN (2006) The contemporary treatment of odontoid injuries. Spine (Phila Pa 1976) 31: S53–60; discussion S61.
3. Nourbakhsh A, Shi R, Vannemreddy P, Nanda A (2009) Operative versus nonoperative management of acute odontoid Type II fractures: a meta-analysis. J Neurosurg Spine 11: 651–658.
4. Harrop JS, Hart R, Anderson PA (2010) Optimal treatment for odontoid fractures in the elderly. Spine (Phila Pa 1976) 35: S219–227.
5. Patel AA, Lindsey R, Bessey JT, Chapman J, Rampersaud R (2010) Surgical treatment of unstable type II odontoid fractures in skeletally mature individuals. Spine (Phila Pa 1976) 35: S209–218.
6. Pal D, Sell P, Grevitt M (2011) Type II odontoid fractures in the elderly: an evidence-based narrative review of management. Eur Spine J 20: 195–204.
7. Huybregts JG, Jacobs WC, Vleggeert-Lankamp CL (2013) The optimal treatment of type II and III odontoid fractures in the elderly: a systematic review. Eur Spine J 22: 1–13.
8. Anderson LD, D'Alonzo RT (1974) Fractures of the odontoid process of the axis. J Bone Joint Surg Am 56: 1663–1674.

9. Brooks AL, Jenkins EB (1978) Atlanto-axial arthrodesis by the wedge compression method. J Bone Joint Surg Am 60: 279–284.
10. Grob D, Jeanneret B, Aebi M, Markwalder TM (1991) Atlanto-axial fusion with transarticular screw fixation. J Bone Joint Surg Br 73: 972–976.
11. Nakanishi T, Sasaki T, Tokita N, Hirabayashi K (1982) Internal fixation for the odontoid fracture. Orthop Trans 6: 176.
12. Bohler J (1982) Anterior stabilization for acute fractures and non-unions of the dens. J Bone Joint Surg Am 64: 18–27.
13. Lesoin F, Autricque A, Franz K, Villette L, Jomin M (1987) Transcervical approach and screw fixation for upper cervical spine pathology. Surg Neurol 27: 459–465.
14. Borne GM, Bedou GL, Pinaudeau M, Cristino G, Hussein A (1988) Odontoid process fracture osteosynthesis with a direct screw fixation technique in nine consecutive cases. J Neurosurg 68: 223–226.
15. Geisler FH, Cheng C, Poka A, Brumback RJ (1989) Anterior screw fixation of posteriorly displaced type II odontoid fractures. Neurosurgery 25: 30–37; discussion 37–38.
16. Esses SI, Bednar DA (1991) Screw fixation of odontoid fractures and nonunions. Spine (Phila Pa 1976) 16: S483–485.
17. Etter C, Coscia M, Jaberg H, Aebi M (1991) Direct anterior fixation of dens fractures with a cannulated screw system. Spine (Phila Pa 1976) 16: S25–32.
18. Jeanneret B, Vernet O, Frei S, Magerl F (1991) Atlantoaxial mobility after screw fixation of the odontoid: a computed tomographic study. J Spinal Disord 4: 203–211.
19. Montesano PX, Anderson PA, Schlehr F, Thalgott JS, Lowrey G (1991) Odontoid fractures treated by anterior odontoid screw fixation. Spine (Phila Pa 1976) 16: S33–37.
20. Knöringer P (1992) Internal fixation of dens fractures by double-threaded screws. Orthopedics and Traumatology: 231–245
21. Chiba K, Fujimura Y, Toyama Y, Takahata T, Nakanishi T, et al. (1993) Anterior screw fixation for odontoid fracture: clinical results in 45 cases. Eur Spine J 2: 76–81.
22. Chang KW, Liu YW, Cheng PG, Chang L, Suen KL, et al. (1994) One Herbert double-threaded compression screw fixation of displaced type II odontoid fractures. J Spinal Disord 7: 62–69.
23. Pointillart V, Orta AL, Freitas J, Vital JM, Senegas J (1994) Odontoid fractures. Review of 150 cases and practical application for treatment. Eur Spine J 3: 282–285.
24. Verheggen R, Jansen J (1994) Fractures of the odontoid process: analysis of the functional results after surgery. Eur Spine J 3: 146–150.
25. Dickman CA, Foley KT, Sonntag VK, Smith MM (1995) Cannulated screws for odontoid screw fixation and atlantoaxial transarticular screw fixation. Technical note. J Neurosurg 83: 1095–1100.
26. Chiba K, Fujimura Y, Toyama Y, Fujii E, Nakanishi T, et al. (1996) Treatment protocol for fractures of the odontoid process. J Spinal Disord 9: 267–276.
27. Rainov NG, Heidecke V, Burkert W (1996) Direct anterior fixation of odontoid fractures with a hollow spreading screw system. Acta Neurochir (Wien) 138: 146–153.
28. Jenkins JD, Coric D, Branch CL Jr (1998) A clinical comparison of one- and two-screw odontoid fixation. J Neurosurg 89: 366–370.
29. Henry AD, Bohly J, Grosse A (1999) Fixation of odontoid fractures by an anterior screw. J Bone Joint Surg Br 81: 472–477.
30. Morandi X, Hanna A, Hamlat A, Brassier G (1999) Anterior screw fixation of odontoid fractures. Surg Neurol 51: 236–240.
31. Subach BR, Morone MA, Haid RW Jr, McLaughlin MR, Rodts GR, et al. (1999) Management of acute odontoid fractures with single-screw anterior fixation. Neurosurgery 45: 812–819; discussion 819–820.
32. Andersson S, Rodrigues M, Olerud C (2000) Odontoid fractures: high complication rate associated with anterior screw fixation in the elderly. Eur Spine J 9: 56–59.
33. Apfelbaum RI, Lonser RR, Veres R, Casey A (2000) Direct anterior screw fixation for recent and remote odontoid fractures. J Neurosurg 93: 227–236.
34. ElSaghir H, Bohm H (2000) Anderson type II fracture of the odontoid process: results of anterior screw fixation. J Spinal Disord 13: 527–530; discussion 531.
35. Harrop JS, Przybylski GJ, Vaccaro AR, Yalamanchili K (2000) Efficacy of anterior odontoid screw fixation in elderly patients with Type II odontoid fractures. Neurosurg Focus 8: e6.
36. Ziai WC, Hurlbert RJ (2000) A six year review of odontoid fractures: the emerging role of surgical intervention. Can J Neurol Sci 27: 297–301.
37. Alfieri A (2001) Single-screw fixation for acute Type II odontoid fracture. J Neurosurg Sci 45: 15–18.
38. Borm W, Kast E, Richter HP, Mohr K (2003) Anterior screw fixation in type II odontoid fractures: is there a difference in outcome between age groups? Neurosurgery 52: 1089–1092; discussion 1092–1084.
39. Lee SC, Chen JF, Lee ST (2004) Management of acute odontoid fractures with single anterior screw fixation. J Clin Neurosci 11: 890–895.
40. Chibbaro S, Benvenuti L, Carnesecchi S, Marsella M, Serino D, et al. (2005) The use of virtual fluoroscopy in managing acute type II odontoid fracture with anterior single-screw fixation. A safe, effective, elegant and fast form of treatment. Acta Neurochir (Wien) 147: 735–739; discussion 739.
41. Fountas KN, Machinis TG, Kapsalaki EZ, Dimopoulos VG, Feltes CH, et al. (2005) Surgical treatment of acute type II and rostral type III odontoid fractures managed by anterior screw fixation. South Med J 98: 896–901.
42. Bhanot A, Sawhney G, Kaushal R, Aggarwal AK, Bahadur R (2006) Management of odontoid fractures with anterior screw fixation. J Surg Orthop Adv 15: 38–42.
43. Moon MS, Moon JL, Sun DH, Moon YW (2006) Treatment of dens fracture in adults: A report of thirty-two cases. Bull Hosp Jt Dis 63: 108–112.
44. Ahmed N, Loutfy M, Shershera W, Sleem A (2007) Fixation of Type II Odontoid Fractures with Anterior Single Screw. EJNS 22 137–146
45. Chi YL, Wang XY, Xu HZ, Lin Y, Huang QS, et al. (2007) Management of odontoid fractures with percutaneous anterior odontoid screw fixation. Eur Spine J 16: 1157–1164.
46. Platzer P, Thalhammer G, Ostermann R, Wieland T, Vecsei V, et al. (2007) Anterior screw fixation of odontoid fractures comparing younger and elderly patients. Spine (Phila Pa 1976) 32: 1714–1720.
47. Song KJ, Lee KB, Kim KN (2007) Treatment of odontoid fractures with single anterior screw fixation. J Clin Neurosci 14: 824–830.
48. Agrillo A, Russo N, Marotta N, Delfini R (2008) Treatment of remote type ii axis fractures in the elderly: feasibility of anterior odontoid screw fixation. Neurosurgery 63: 1145–1150; discussion 1150–1141.
49. Collins I, Min WK (2008) Anterior screw fixation of type II odontoid fractures in the elderly. J Trauma 65: 1083–1087.
50. Srinivasan U, Dhillon C, Mahesha K, Kumar P (2008) Anterior single lag screw fixation in type II Dens fracture—indian experience. Indian Journal of Neurotrauma 5: 87–91
51. Sucu HK, Akkol I, Minoglu M, Gelal F (2008) Percutaneous anterior odontoid screw fixation. Minim Invasive Neurosurg 51: 106–108.
52. Koller H, Acosta F, Forstner R, Zenner J, Resch H, et al. (2009) C2-fractures: part II. A morphometrical analysis of computerized atlantoaxial motion, anatomical alignment and related clinical outcomes. Eur Spine J 18: 1135–1153.
53. Omeis I, Duggal N, Rubano J, Cerabona F, Abrahams J, et al. (2009) Surgical treatment of C2 fractures in the elderly: a multicenter retrospective analysis. J Spinal Disord Tech 22: 91–95.
54. Eap C, Barresi L, Ohl X, Saddiki R, Mensa C, et al. (2010) Odontoid fractures anterior screw fixation: a continuous series of 36 cases. Orthop Traumatol Surg Res 96: 748–752.
55. Hou Y, Yuan W, Wang X (2011) Clinical evaluation of anterior screw fixation for elderly patients with type II odontoid fractures. J Spinal Disord Tech 24: E75–81.
56. Kim SK, Shin JJ, Kim TH, Shin HS, Hwang YS, et al. (2011) Clinical outcomes of halo-vest immobilization and surgical fusion of odontoid fractures. J Korean Neurosurg Soc 50: 17–22.
57. Mayer M, Zenner J, Auffarth A, Atzwanger J, Romeder F, et al. (2011) Efficacy of anterior odontoid screw fixation in the elderly patient: a CT-based biometrical analysis of odontoid fractures. Eur Spine J 20: 1441–1449.
58. Osti M, Philipp H, Meusburger B, Benedetto KP (2011) Analysis of failure following anterior screw fixation of Type II odontoid fractures in geriatric patients. Eur Spine J 20: 1915–1920.
59. Wang J, Zhou Y, Zhang ZF, Li CQ, Zheng WJ, et al. (2011) Comparison of percutaneous and open anterior screw fixation in the treatment of type II and rostral type III odontoid fractures. Spine (Phila Pa 1976) 36: 1459–1463.
60. Yang YL, Fu BS, Li RW, Smith PN, Mu WD, et al. (2011) Anterior single screw fixation of odontoid fracture with intraoperative Iso-C 3-dimensional imaging. Eur Spine J 20: 1899–1907.
61. Aldrian S, Erhart J, Schuster R, Wernhart S, Domaszewski F, et al. (2012) Surgical vs nonoperative treatment of Hadley type IIA odontoid fractures. Neurosurgery 70: 676–682; discussion 682–673.
62. Cho DC, Sung JK (2012) Analysis of risk factors associated with fusion failure after anterior odontoid screw fixation. Spine (Phila Pa 1976) 37: 30–34.
63. Henaux PL, Cueff F, Diabira S, Riffaud L, Hamlat A, et al. (2012) Anterior screw fixation of type IIB odontoid fractures in octogenarians. Eur Spine J 21: 335–339.
64. Kantelhardt SR, Keric N, Giese A (2012) Management of C2 fractures using Iso-C(3D) guidance: a single institution's experience. Acta Neurochir (Wien) 154: 1781–1787.
65. Konieczny MR, Gstrein A, Muller EJ (2012) Treatment algorithm for dens fractures: non-halo immobilization, anterior screw fixation, or posterior transarticular C1–C2 fixation. J Bone Joint Surg Am 94: e144(141–146).
66. Mashhadinezhad H, Samini F, Mashhadinezhad A, Birjandinejad A (2012) Clinical results of surgical management in type II odontoid fracture: a preliminary report. Turk Neurosurg 22: 583–587.
67. Rizvi SA, Fredo HL, Lied B, Nakstad PH, Ronning P, et al. (2012) Surgical management of acute odontoid fractures: surgery-related complications and long-term outcomes in a consecutive series of 97 patients. J Trauma Acute Care Surg 72: 682–690.
68. Martirosyan NL, Kalb S, Cavalcanti DD, Lochhead RA, Uschold TD, et al. (2013) Comparative Analysis of Isocentric 3-dimensional C-arm Fluoroscopy and Biplanar Fluoroscopy for Anterior Screw Fixation in Odontoid Fractures. J Spinal Disord Tech 26: 189–193.
69. Steltzlen C, Lazennec JY, Catonne Y, Rousseau MA (2013) Unstable odontoid fracture: Surgical strategy in a 22-case series, and literature review. Orthop Traumatol Surg Res. Epub ahead of print.
70. Fan K, Liao J, Niu C, Chen L, Chen W, et al. (2013) Anterior single-screw fixation in 24 patients with Type II odontoid fractures. Formosa n Journal of Musculosk eletal Disorde rs 4 26–31

71. Fujii E, Kobayashi K, Hirabayashi K (1988) Treatment in fractures of the odontoid process. Spine (Phila Pa 1976) 13: 604–609.
72. Berlemann U, Schwarzenbach O (1997) Dens fractures in the elderly. Results of anterior screw fixation in 19 elderly patients. Acta Orthop Scand 68: 319–324.
73. Fountas KN, Kapsalaki EZ, Karampelas I, Feltes CH, Dimopoulos VG, et al. (2005) Results of long-term follow-up in patients undergoing anterior screw fixation for type II and rostral type III odontoid fractures. Spine (Phila Pa 1976) 30: 661–669.
74. Lee SH, Sung JK (2006) Anterior odontoid fixation using a 4.5-mm Herbert screw: The first report of 20 consecutive cases with odontoid fracture. Surg Neurol 66: 361–366; discussion 366.
75. Dailey AT, Hart D, Finn MA, Schmidt MH, Apfelbaum RI (2010) Anterior fixation of odontoid fractures in an elderly population. J Neurosurg Spine 12: 1–8.
76. Cho DC, Sung JK (2011) Is All Anterior Oblique Fracture Orientation Really a Contraindication to Anterior Screw Fixation of Type II and Rostral Shallow Type III Odontoid Fractures? J Korean Neurosurg Soc 49: 345–350.
77. Grossberg J, Spader H, Belknap T, Oyelese A (2011) The use of the Mayfield Frame facilitates trajectory in anterior odontoid screw fixation. 27th annual meeting of the AANS/CNS section on disorder of the spine and peripheral nerves.
78. Wright JG, Swiontkowski MF, Heckman JD (2003) Introducing levels of evidence to the journal. J Bone Joint Surg Am 85-A: 1–3.
79. Cho SK, Lu Y, Lee DH (2013) Dysphagia following anterior cervical spinal surgery: a systematic review. Bone Joint J 95-B: 868–873

13

Age-Dependent Transcriptome and Proteome Following Transection of Neonatal Spinal Cord of *Monodelphis domestica*

Norman R. Saunders[1]*, Natassya M. Noor[1], Katarzyna M. Dziegielewska[1], Benjamin J. Wheaton[1], Shane A. Liddelow[1,2], David L. Steer[3], C. Joakim Ek[4], Mark D. Habgood[1], Matthew J. Wakefield[5,6], Helen Lindsay[5,7], Jessie Truettner[8], Robert D. Miller[9], A. Ian Smith[3], W. Dalton Dietrich[8]

1 Department of Pharmacology & Therapeutics, The University of Melbourne, Victoria, Australia, **2** Department of Neurobiology, Stanford University, Stanford, California, United States of America, **3** Department of Biochemistry and Molecular Biology, Monash University, Clayton, Victoria, Australia, **4** Department of Neuroscience and Physiology, University of Gothenburg, Gothenburg, Sweden, **5** Walter & Eliza Hall Institute of Medical Research, Victoria, Australia, **6** Department of Genetics, The University of Melbourne, Victoria, Australia, **7** Institute of Molecular Life Sciences, University of Zurich, Zurich, Switzerland, **8** The Miami Project to Cure Paralysis, University of Miami, Miller School of Medicine, Miami, Florida, United States of America, **9** Center for Evolutionary & Theoretical Immunology, Department of Biology, University of New Mexico, Albuquerque, New Mexico, United States of America

Abstract

This study describes a combined transcriptome and proteome analysis of *Monodelphis domestica* response to spinal cord injury at two different postnatal ages. Previously we showed that complete transection at postnatal day 7 (P7) is followed by profuse axon growth across the lesion with near-normal locomotion and swimming when adult. In contrast, at P28 there is no axon growth across the lesion, the animals exhibit weight-bearing locomotion, but cannot use hind limbs when swimming. Here we examined changes in gene and protein expression in the segment of spinal cord rostral to the lesion at 24 h after transection at P7 and at P28. Following injury at P7 only forty genes changed (all increased expression); most were immune/inflammatory genes. Following injury at P28 many more genes changed their expression and the magnitude of change for some genes was strikingly greater. Again many were associated with the immune/inflammation response. In functional groups known to be inhibitory to regeneration in adult cords the expression changes were generally muted, in some cases opposite to that required to account for neurite inhibition. For example myelin basic protein expression was reduced following injury at P28 both at the gene and protein levels. Only four genes from families with extracellular matrix functions thought to influence neurite outgrowth in adult injured cords showed substantial changes in expression following injury at P28: Olfactomedin 4 (*Olfm4*, 480 fold compared to controls), matrix metallopeptidase (*Mmp1*, 104 fold), papilin (*Papln*, 152 fold) and integrin α4 (*Itga4*, 57 fold). These data provide a resource for investigation of *a priori* hypotheses in future studies of mechanisms of spinal cord regeneration in immature animals compared to lack of regeneration at more mature stages.

Editor: Michelle L. Baker, CSIRO, Australia

Funding: This project was supported by the Victoria Neurotrauma Initiative. The funders had no role in study design, data collection and analysis, decision to publish, or preparation of the manuscript.

Competing Interests: The authors have declared that no competing interests exist.

* E-mail: n.saunders@unimelb.edu.au

Introduction

The studies of Aguayo and colleagues in the 1980s [1,2], which repeated an old experiment of Tello [3] using implants and bridges of sciatic nerve to promote regeneration of the central nervous system (CNS) resulted in a concentrated effort to understand the mechanisms underlying the failure of the adult mammalian spinal cord to exhibit regenerative recovery following injury. Since then several such inhibitory mechanisms have been described including myelin inhibitory factors [4,5] and proteoglycans [6–8]. So far no effective therapy has emerged and disappointingly, attempts to replicate apparently promising animal studies have been mostly unsuccessful (e.g., [9–13]). One reason for this may simply be that the responses of the injured CNS are so complex that a repair strategy based on modifying only one aspect of this process is unlikely to be successful. A strong indication of the complexity of the response of the spinal cord to injury came first from the microarray study by Aimone and colleagues [14]. Similarly complex findings following brain injury have been reported [15]. Verhaagen et al. [16] provided an overview of 25 gene expression profiling studies (over the period of 2001 to 2009, see [16]) of spinal cord injury in rodents. The sites examined were at or around the lesion, which were mainly a contusion in the thoracic spinal cord. The studies used microarrays (generally Affymetrix) to investigate gene expression over a wide range of post injury times (30 min to 90 days). One of these studies involved embryonic spinal cord, which was uninjured but compared to adult injured spinal cord [17]. To date, only one RNA-Seq dataset of injured spinal cord has been published [18] although additional information may perhaps be gleaned from an RNA-Seq study that examined the effects of transplanted progenitor/stem cells following spinal cord injury [19].

Verhaagen et al. [16] reported that the observed changes in gene expression across this large number of studies were "remarkably consistent" and summarized the results under 8 functional categories that showed changed expression. Genes in some of these groups were generally upregulated: immediate early genes, proinflammatory genes, phagocytosis & induction of the complement system, neuronal genes (some implicated in neurite outgrowth or synaptic plasticity). Other groups showed a mixture of up- and downregulation: genes related to apoptosis, angiogenesis. Some showed predominantly downregulation: genes encoding neurotransmitter synthesis and other aspects of synaptic function, ion channels. Surprisingly, no mention was made of genes that generate various extracellular matrix factors such as proteoglycans, as this family of proteins has been implicated in several studies to be involved in the failure of neurite outgrowth following injury (see [20]).

In contrast to the lack of functional recovery from severe spinal cord injury in adult mammals, immature animals show a significant degree of recovery. This has been demonstrated in two species of marsupial opossum, where substantial growth of axons across a lesion was observed. Some of these axons were shown to be regenerating and some were growing as a part of normal development [21–23]. This response to injury appears to be age dependent [23–25] providing an opportunity to compare gene regulation in a mammalian species at a stage of development when regeneration and axon growth occurs and one when it does not [25,26]. To undertake a similar study in rodents would require *in utero* transection of the spinal cord at around E15 (permissive stage, [27]) and at a stage that was non-permissive but with bodyweight bearing locomotion (probably E19–20).

Some preliminary studies in developing spinal cord have been carried out using human microarrays [28], mouse microarrays [24] and tammar wallaby microarrays [29] as well as different forms of polymerase chain reaction methods [24,30]. These showed that there is indeed substantial age-dependent gene regulation in the response of the spinal cord to injury [24,28–30]. The most comprehensive study of these responses was that by Mladinic et al., [29] using a combination of microarray (tammar wallaby, a marsupial species) and qRT-PCR for specific genes of interest. These authors divided the genes identified into categories relating to whether changes in expression (up- or downregulation) might be expected to be contributing to successful growth of axons across a lesion made at P8, but not at P13. However, these studies used *in vitro* preparations of isolated *Monodelphis* spinal cord at 25°C, which may have had an influence on some aspects of the response to injury (see General Discussion).

With the recent sequencing of the opossum genome [31] and the advent of high throughput RNA sequencing (RNA-Seq) it is now possible to examine overall gene expression changes in response to injury in this species. In the present study we investigated both the transcriptome and the proteome in the segment of cord rostral to the site of injury following a complete spinal cord transection in opossums at an age when axonal growth across a lesion and substantially normal locomotor development occur (postnatal day 7, P7) and compared this with an older age when no axon growth can be seen, but nevertheless a demonstrable body weight-bearing locomotion is present (P28, [25]). A study of changes in the spinal cord proteome caudal to the site of injury following spinal cord transection in *Monodelphis* at these two ages has been previously published [32].

Materials and Methods

Animals used

Monodelphis domestica were obtained from a colony based at the University of Melbourne Medical Sciences Animal House Facility, Melbourne, Australia. Procedures were performed according to National Health and Medical Research Council guidelines, with the approval of the University of Melbourne Animal Ethics Committee (Ethics #0707108). Pups of both sexes were used. Day of birth was designated as postnatal day zero, P0 (see [25,26]).

The pups were assigned to two age groups and spinal cord injuries (SCIs) were performed at either P7 or P28. At P7, whole litters (6–7 pups) were operated on. Separate litters of pups were kept as controls as there is no consistent way to mark these very young animals without increasing the risk of cannibalisation by the mother [22]. Injuries at P28 were usually made on half the pups in a litter, since at P28 their ears can be marked. The remaining pups from these litters were anaesthetised but remained uninjured and were used as controls. For RNA-Seq and proteomic analyses experimental and control pups were collected at 24 h (+24 h) post surgery. For morphological studies, animals were collected as unoperated controls and at 0 h and 24 h post injury in both age groups. The total number of animals used in the transcriptomic study was: P8 control ($n = 24$), P7+24 h ($n = 24$), P29 control ($n = 12$), P28+24 h ($n = 12$). These were obtained from several separate litters. In the proteomic study the number of animals and weights of tissues used are shown in Table 1. For the morphological studies at least 3 pups at each age were used, usually from different litters [32,33].

Spinal cord transection

At P7, *Monodelphis* pups are still attached to the mothers' teats [34]. The female adult *Monodelphis* were anaesthetized with 2–3% isofluorane; the same anaesthetic was administered to the P7 pups via a small facemask during the surgical procedure. Pups at P28 are no longer attached to the mother and were separately anaesthetized with isofluorane throughout the surgical procedure [25].

Complete spinal cord transection was performed at thoracic level 10 (T10) using sharp sterilized fine scissors. Skin was closed using surgical grade glue (Vetbond, 3 M, St. Paul, MN, USA). Animals were returned to their cages and allowed to recover for 24 hours (+24 h) post injury. At the end of the experimental period, control and injured animals were terminally anaesthetized with an overdose of isofluorane and spinal cords were dissected out.

The cords were separated into two segments, the upper (rostral to the injury) and lower (caudal to the injury) divided at T10 (site of transection), or corresponding segments from control animal spinal cords. Samples were stored at −80°C until used. Rostral segments of the cords were used in the present study. For morphological studies spinal cords were dissected out, fixed in Bouin's fixative and paraffin embedded as described previously [32,33].

RNA extraction

Samples of rostral cord were homogenized using Qiashredder columns (Qiagen, Valencia, CA, USA) and total RNA was extracted using the RNeasy Plus Mini Kit (Qiagen) according to standard supplier protocol. Total RNA samples were quantified using a NanoDrop ND-100 UV-VIS spectrophotometer (Thermo Scientific, Wilmington, DE, USA) and quality checked on an RNA chip using and Agilent 2100 Bioanalyzer (Agilent, Santa Clara,

Table 1. Number, tissue weight and protein concentration of spinal cord tissue used for proteomic analysis in this study.

Age group	Number of cords	Tissue weight (mg)	Total protein concentration (μg/μl)
P7+24 h transected	11	37.7	4.7
P8 control	11	27.8	5.14
P28+24 h transected	4	66.5	6.97
P29 control	4	87	8.74

Samples rostral to the site of injury (T10) were used in proteomic analysis for control and transected spinal cords of *Monodelphis domestica* at P7 or P28. Note that individual cords were pooled from more than one litter.

CA, USA). Only samples with an RNA Integrity Number close to 9 were kept for further sequencing experiments.

RNA sequencing

RNA sequencing was performed at the Australian Genome Research Facility (Melbourne, Australia). A cDNA library was prepared from 10 μg of total RNA from pools of two individuals using the RNA-Seq Sample Preparation Kit (Illumina, San Diego, CA, USA) according to the standard manufacturer protocol. Quality of the library was verified using a DNA 1000 chip using the Agilent 2100 Bioanalyzer (Agilent) and quantified by fluorimetry. The library was subjected to 100 bp single end read cycles of sequencing on an Illumina Genome Analyzer IIx (Illumina) as per manufacturer protocol. Cluster generation was performed on a c-Bot (Illumina) with a single read cluster generation kit. Sequencing was performed using a 36-cycle sequencing kit v4. In total 16 separate sequencing lanes were run on the platform. Two separate runs were conducted from separately collected samples, which were: rostral spinal cords from P8 control, P7+24 h injury, P29 controls and P28+24 h injury.

Statistical analysis of RNA-Seq data

Gene expression level analysis. Short reads were trimmed to remove ambiguous bases from the start and segments with low quality scores from the end. Trimmed reads were mapped with Bowtie2 version 2.0.4 [35] to the Ensembl *Monodelphis domestica* genome, release 69 [36]. The number of reads mapped to nuclear genes was determined with HTSeq [37], using the default "union" counting option.

An average of 4.6 M mapped reads were obtained per sample. Raw data are available at: Gene Expression Omnibus (http://www.ncbi.nlm.nih.gov/geo/) under accession code GSE54805. Differential expression between the adult and embryonic samples was detected using an exact test in the Bioconductor [38] 6dger package version 2.6.12 [39]. Genes considered to be significantly differentially expressed were those with a *p*-value of less than 0.05 after false discovery rate correction. Changes in expression were considered significant where there was a fold change greater than 2.00 and an adjusted *p*-value of less than 0.05. Gene targets with fold changes less than 2.00 were considered unchanged. Genes that showed changes according to the above criteria are shown Table S1 (P7+24 h) and Table S2 (P28+24 h).

Gene ontology level analysis. Gene Ontology (GO) analysis was completed using GOSeq software [40]. Differentially expressed genes were split into up- and down-regulated groups and a separate GOSeq enrichment test was applied for each set. A final Benjamini-Hochberg correction was applied to adjust for multiple tests.

Illumina RNA sequencing data have been deposited with the Gene Expression Omnibus http://www.ncbi.nlm.nih.gov/geo/) under accession code GSE54805.

Proteomics

Methods for the 2-dimensional separation of proteins, selection of protein bands and mass spectrometry have been published previously [32] but are described here in full.

Sample preparation for proteomic analysis. Spinal cord segments rostral to the site of injury performed at P7 or P28 were collected 24 hours after transection (P7+24 h or P28+24 h) together with corresponding segments from age-matched controls. Tissue was pooled from several pups (n = 4–20) in order to obtain a total of a minimum of 30 mg (wet tissue weight) per sample (Table 1). Pooled tissue samples were homogenized 1:10 w/v in homogenization buffer containing 0.32 mM sucrose, 25 mM Tris, 1 mM MgCl2, pH 7. This was done by passing the samples through 20 Gauge (G), 21 G, 25 G and 27 G needles until the suspension offered no more resistance. Samples were centrifuged at 2000×*g* for 2 minutes at 4°C and supernatants retained for further analysis. Total protein concentration was estimated using the Bradford Assay [40] with a protein standard (Sigma-Aldrich, St Louis, MO, USA) to ensure the consistency of the extraction process as all samples were normalized weight to volume. The same volume for all samples was used throughout the study (Table 1).

The clean-up step. Contaminants were removed from 50 μl aliquots of each sample using the 2-dimensional (2D) clean-up kit (GE Healthcare Bio-Sciences Corp., Piscataway, NJ, USA) as detailed in the Manufacturer's Protocol (Procedure B). Fifty μl aliquots of each sample were used for the clean-up. Samples were centrifuged for 10 minutes at 8000×*g* and wash buffer was removed without disturbing the pellet. Acetone present in the wash buffer was evaporated before moving to the next step. Six clean-up samples were prepared for each age group,

Off-gel Fractionator. An Off-gel Fractionator 3100 (Agilent Technologies, Santa Clara, CA, USA) was used in accordance with the Manufacturer's Protocol. Immobilized pH gradient (IPG) strips (12 cm, pH 3–10, Linear, Agilent Technologies, Santa Clara, CA, USA) were used for this separation. A total of 150 μl from cleaned-up sample (see above) was rehydrated (as specified by Manufacturer's Protocol) and prepared for each lane together with IPG strips (also rehydrated with the Off-gel buffer prior to sample loading). Each sample was run in duplicate on two separate IEF lanes. The fractionator was set to run under the default Manufacturer's settings until the current was reduced to zero. Samples from each well were collected and the Bradford assay [40] was performed on each sample. Variation in protein concentrations between the duplicates was within ±10%. For further analysis duplicates of each sample fraction were combined and all

Off-gel fractions were used. Aliquots (25 μl) from each fraction were subjected to a further clean-up step as described above. Again, duplicates were prepared for each sample. In the final step, the wash buffer was carefully decanted without disturbing the pellet before pellets were dried at 37.5°C in a heat block for 10 minutes to fully evaporate any wash buffer residue.

Lithium dodecyl sulfate –polyacrylamide gel electrophoresis (LDS-PAGE). The obtained dried pellet was re-suspended in 5 μl LDS sample buffer (Invitrogen, Carlsbad, CA, USA) [23], 2 μl reducing agent (Invitrogen, Carlsbad, CA, USA) and 13 μl deionized water. The mixture was heated in a 37.5°C heat block for 10 minutes. Pre-cast 4–12% NuPage Bis-Tris 10 well Mini Gels (Invitrogen, Carlsbad, CA, USA) were used with 2-(N-morpholino) ethanesulfonic acid (MES)-SDS running buffer (Invitrogen, Carlsbad, CA, USA) diluted 1:20. Samples from each fraction from injured and control animals were loaded as duplicates. One lane of each gel contained a molecular weight standard (NovexH Sharp pre-stained standard, Invitrogen, Carlsbad, CA, USA). Gels were run at 200 V constant voltage for approximately 35 minutes.

Silver Staining and Densitometric Gel Analysis. Separated protein bands were visualised using silver stain. Gels were stained for 10–15 min (Silver Stain Plus Kit, Bio-Rad Laboratories, Hercules, CA, USA) according to the Manufacturer's Protocol. Silver stained gels were scanned on a flatbed scanner (Agfa Duoscan, Mortsel, Belgium) and analysed using 1D gel analysis software, GeneTools V4.01.02 (Syngene, Synoptics Ltd, Cambridge, England). The number of bands visible in each lane was counted and consistency between duplicates in each lane was checked. Protein profiles from injured spinal cord samples were compared to those from controls for each fraction. Differences in band intensity, staining pattern or molecular weight changes were recorded. A relative change threshold of ±0.5 compared to control (set as 1) was accepted to identify proteins that changed their expression following spinal injury. This threshold was set after evaluation of technical variability of the methods employed [32,41]. As is usually the case for such proteomic studies it was not possible to make a sufficient number of biological replicates for a statistical analysis to be applied. The results are therefore presented as an increase or decrease compared to controls.

Mass Spectrometry

Tryptic digestion. Each protein band of interest was individually and manually excised from gels and de-stained in 50 mM ammonium bicarbonate with 50% acetonitrile. Obtained gel pieces were washed and dehydrated in 50 mM ammonium bicarbonate and acetonitrile in alternating wash steps until completely dehydrated. Once dehydrated, gel pieces were subsequently rehydrated in 0.5 μg trypsin (Promega corp., Madison, WI, USA) and 20 mM ammonium bicarbonate solution for in-gel digestion by incubating at 37°C overnight and sonicated (Health Sonics, Livermore CA, USA) for 10 minutes prior to analysis.

LC-MS/MS. Tryptic digests were analysed by LC-MS/MS using the HCT ULTRA ion trap mass spectrometer (Bruker Daltonics, Bremen, Germany) coupled online with nanoflow HPLC (Ultimate 3000, Thermo Scientific, Breman, germany). Samples injected onto a pepmap100, 75 μm id, 100 Å pore size, reversed phase nano column with 95% buffer A (0.1% Formic acid) at a flow rate of 300 nl/minute. The peptides were eluted over a 30-minute gradient to 70% B (80% Acetonitrile 0.1% formic acid). The eluant is nebulised and ionised using the Bruker ESI electrospray source via the nanoflow ESI sprayer with a capillary voltage of 4000 V, dry gas at 200°C and flow rate of 5.0l/minute and nebuliser gas at 6psi. Peptides are selected for MSMS analysis in autoMSn mode with smart parameter settings selected with a target mass of 900 m/z and active exclusion released after 1 minute. Data obtained from LC-MS/MS were searched against a custom database downloaded from the National Center for Biotechnology Information (NCBI) ftp site and Swiss-Prot databases using the MASCOT search engine (version 2.1, Matrix Science Inc., London, UK) with all taxonomy selected.

Identified proteins were categorized by relevance to spinal cord injury, obtained from search of relevant literature published in PubMed (http://www.ncbi.nlm.nih.gov/pubmed).

Morphology and Immunohistochemistry

Bouin's-fixed, paraffin embedded spinal cords from P8, P7+24 h, P29 and P28+24 h animals (n = 3–4) were obtained from previous studies [32,33] with some additional material collected specifically for this project. All sections were cut in either coronal or sagittal plane at 5 μm thickness. Ten consecutive sections were placed on each glass slide. Routine hematoxylin and eosin (H&E) staining was performed on every 10th slide for general morphology. Immunocytochemistry using the PAP (peroxidase-anti-peroxidase) detection method [32,42] was applied to map the cellular distribution of individual proteins. Briefly, sections were dewaxed in histolene (Fronine, Australia) followed by rehydration in ethanol of decreasing concentration and final wash in phosphate buffered saline with 0.2% Tween20 (PBS/Tween). After blocking non-specific binding sites with Peroxidase and Protein Blockers (DAKO) sections were incubated with primary antibodies (rabbit anti- human IL-1β, Endogen, USA). This was followed by consecutive incubations with appropriate secondary antibodies (swine anti rabbit, DAKO, 1:200 dilution and rabbit PAP, Sigma, 1:200 dilution) and developed with DAKO DAB+ detection kit. Finally the stained sections were dehydrated through graded alcohol and histolene and mounted with Ultramount (Fronine, Australia). Control sections did not contain the primary antibody and these always appeared blank.

The presence of myelin was detected in paraffin sections by the histological stain Luxol Fast Blue as described in detail previously [25].

Results and Discussion

General Morphology of the injury site of *Monodelphis* spinal cord injured at P7 or P28

The morphological appearance of the spinal cord of *Monodelphis* after injury is illustrated in H&E stained sections in Fig. 1. Note the completeness of the transections at P7 and P28 (Fig. 1A&B) and the obvious bleeding into the wound site in the P28 spinal cord (Fig. 1B). It was noticeable that at the time of injury bleeding was more prominent in the P28 spinal cords than at P7. It is likely that bleeding occurred in some of the P7 injured cords collected for RNA-Seq analysis, but the P28 cords were probably more contaminated, which may account for the presence of upregulated blood-related genes at P28 but not P7 following injury (see below). Note also that the gap between the rostral and caudal ends of the transected spinal cord at 24 h post injury was much greater in the P28 (Fig. 1D) cord compared to the P7 cord (Fig. 1C). A similar difference between P7 and P14 transected cords was reported previously [24]. This difference was attributed to greater arching of the back in the P14 *Monodelphis*. The even larger gap in transected spinal cords of older opossum may contribute to the lack of neurite growth across the site of injury in P28 pups. Nevertheless at both ages 24 h after injury the cut ends of the

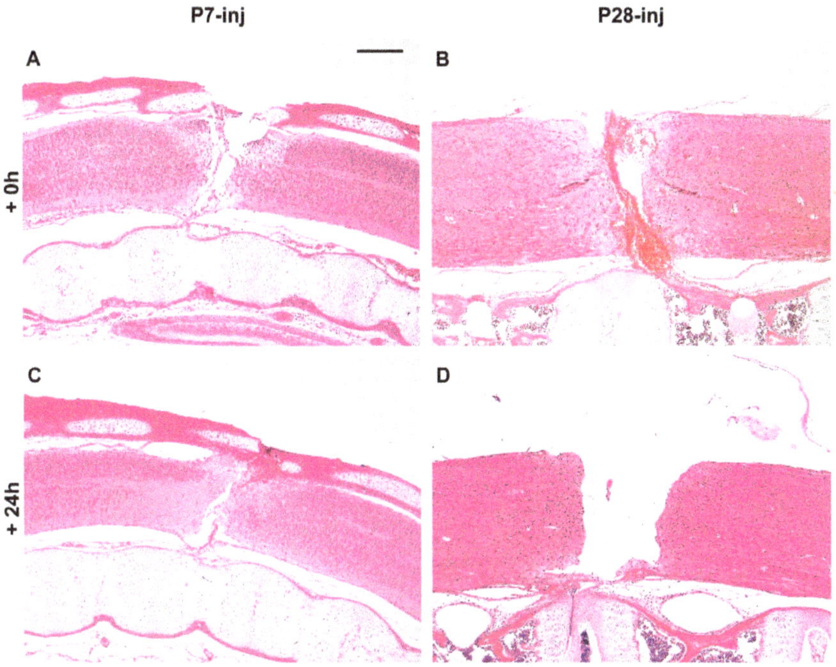

Figure 1. ***Monodelphis domestica*** **spinal cords injured at P7 or P28.** Longitudinal sections (hematoxylin & eosin staining) of spinal cords injured at P7 or P28 shown immediately after complete spinal transection at T10 (A, B) or 24 hours later (C, D). Note obvious bleeding into the injury site at P28 (B), which was more pronounced than at P7 (A) One day after transection (+24 h) the gap between severed ends of the cord was larger in P28 injured animals (D) than in P7 injured animals (C). Rostral end is to the left, caudal to the right, dorsal is uppermost. Scale bar is 500 μm.

spinal cord were clearly sealed without showing much cellular damage in the surrounding spinal cord tissue.

Transcriptomic analysis of postnatal *Monodelphis* spinal cord following transection

The gene expression responses to injury have been examined in the segment of spinal cord rostral to a complete spinal transection (T10) at two postnatal ages: P7 when substantial axon growth occurs across the lesion site and P28 when no such axon growth occurs [25]. Gene expression patterns were investigated using high throughput RNA-Seq analysis at 24 h after injury. Genes were assigned to functional categories based on published information on function, taking account of studies of gene expression changes in injured adult spinal cord (e.g., [16,17,20,43]) as well as those we deduce might have effects on neurite outgrowth at P7 and P28, 24 h after spinal cord transection (Fig. 2 and Tables S2 and S3). Only a single assignment was made for each gene (Tables 2–4, S5), although many appear to have multiple functions.

Changes in gene ontology

There was a striking difference in the number of genes that changed their expression level at the two ages; many more were changed at P28 than at P7 following injury and the magnitude of many gene expression changes at P28 was much greater (Fig. 2). In addition at P7 no genes were downregulated (>-2 fold) in response to injury in contrast to many at P28. It is also striking that at P7 almost all of the genes affected were immune/inflammatory related. Only four genes identified in the P7 injury group were categorized in the other functional groups.

Twenty-four hours following injury at P28 about half as many genes were upregulated as were downregulated and the largest category upregulated was also immune/inflammatory while the largest category of downregulated genes was enzymes & metabolism. However, nearly all categories identified in the P28 injury group contained genes that were both up- and downregulated. These gene expression changes following injury at the two ages are summarized in Fig. 2.

Gene expression in postnatal *Monodelphis* spinal cord 24 h following transection at P7

At P7+24 h only 40 genes showed a significant expression change of ≥2 fold (Fig. 3 and Table S1); all of these were upregulated, none was downregulated. The gene descriptions and details of the statistical analysis are shown in Table S1 and illustrated in Fig. 3. Thirty-six of these genes were in the immune/inflammatory group (Table S1); the highest expressed of these were interleukin 1β, which was 54 fold higher than uninjured control spinal cord and a *novel* gene (C-C motif chemokine similar to *Ccl8* and *Ccl13*) which was 33 fold higher than uninjured control spinal cord. The four non immune-related genes upregulated at this age (green in Fig. 3) were the metalloproteinase inhibitor *Timp* (3.2 fold), one novel gene related to cell proliferation and apoptosis (similar to *Samd9/Samd9l* sterile alpha motif domain 9), which was upregulated 4 fold, the syntaxin binding protein *Stxbp2* was upregulated 2.7 fold and a novel gene similar to MT3 Metallothionein 3, upregulated 2 fold. It has been shown before that in adult spinal cord injury, one of the main functional groups of genes to show regulatory changes soon after injury is the inflammatory group (e.g., [16]). The finding that almost all of the gene expression changes identified at 24 h after spinal cord injury at P7 were immune/inflammatory genes with only single members of other gene families shown to have marked expression changes, suggests that the overwhelming inflammatory response at this age may reflect a general response to injury. It does itself appear to affect the outgrowth of neurites, which has previously been shown to be profuse at this age [21,22]. The absence of an immune/

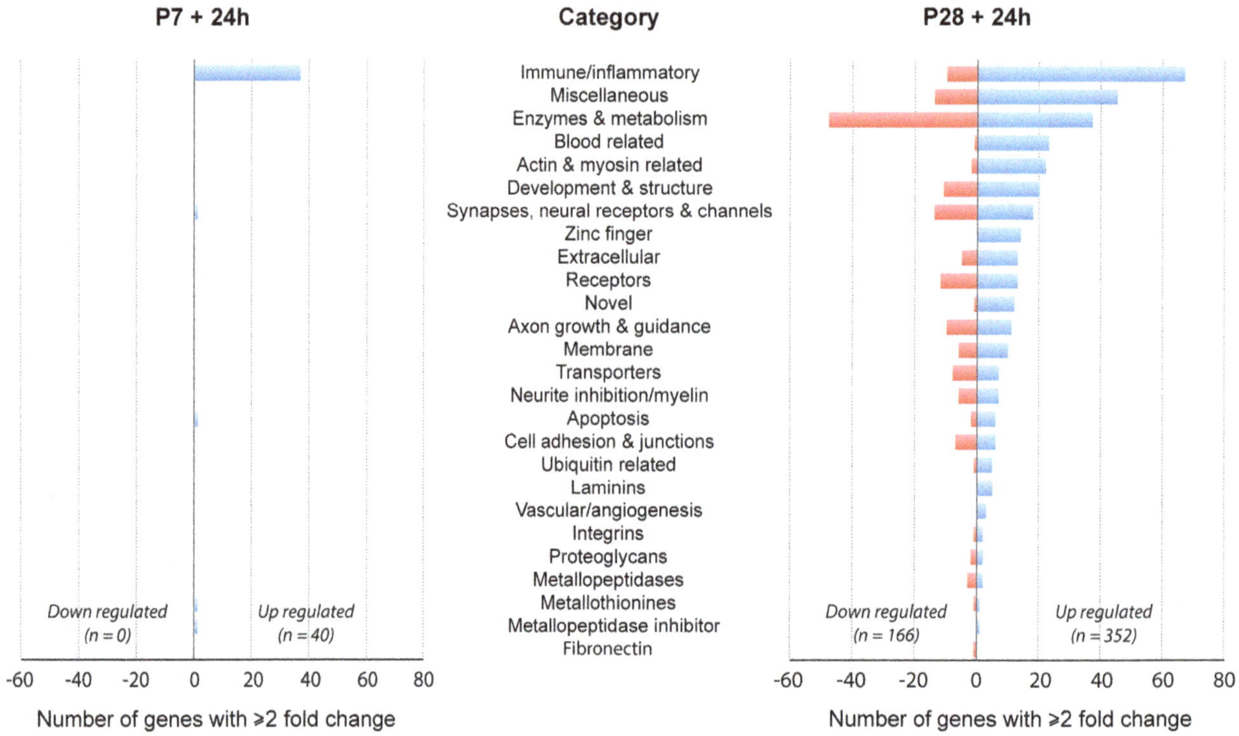

Figure 2. Changes in gene expression in spinal cord 24 h following transection at P7 or P28 in *Monodelphis domestica*. Numbers of genes in each functional category that showed ±≥2 fold change compared to uninjured aged matched controls. Note dominance of immune/inflammatory genes particularly at P7. Also note that at P28 many more genes showed expression changes (both up and down). See Tables S1 and S2 for gene descriptions, fold change and p values.

inflammatory response to injury in isolated postnatal *Monodelphis* spinal cord [28,29] supports this conclusion; this is discussed further below. Given the successful growth of axons across the lesion site at this age it would appear that the injury does little to interfere with the process, because most of the known genes associated with axon growth or inhibition were unaffected.

The immature state of the immune system at the end of the first week of postnatal life in *Monodelphis* may help to explain the complexity of immune/inflammatory genes upregulated at this time, compared with P28 (see below). That the majority of immune/inflammatory genes are upregulated is consistent with responses that are generally associated with non-specific or innate cell types, and with the early stage of development at P7/P8. At the end of the first week of postnatal life in the opossum, the αβ T cell receptor (*Tcr*) is present, although the thymus itself is still relatively immature [44]. T cells expressing the *γδTcr*, a lineage that has been implicated in playing a role in wound healing, are first detectable at P8 [44,45]. The ontogeny of antibody producing B cells is similarly at an early transitional point. Cells committed to the B cell lineage are found in prenatal embryos and within the first 24 postnatal hours B cells that have rearranged their heavy chain antibody genes are detected [46]. But the first wave of light chain gene rearrangements necessary for developing mature B cells is not detected until P7 at the earliest. T and B cells at this stage are fairly limited in their diversity, most likely consistent with low numbers of cells. Given the immature state of the adaptive side of the immune system it may not be surprising that components of the innate immune system such as complement components *C1q* and *Factor B* are upregulated.

Upregulated transcripts such as those encoding Sialic acid-binding immunoglobulin-type lectins (*Siglecs*) and *Vsig4* have been implicated in inhibitory regulation of inflammation and adaptive immune responses through regulation of B and T cells. *Siglecs* are involved in the cell adhesion and phagocytosis, among other things, and are expressed on a variety of immune system cells including macrophages. They have been implicated in binding pathogen associated molecular patterns (*Pamps*), transmitting inhibitory signals and participating in B cell tolerance (reviewed in [47]). Likewise, *Vsig4* is a receptor for the complement component 3 fragments, *C3b* and *iC3b* and has been implicated in being a negative regulator of T cells [48]. We were only able to obtain antibody cross-reactivity for one of the protein products of the large number of genes that showed upregulation (Il-1β). Its distribution in P7 and P28 spinal cord 24 h after injury is illustrated in Fig. 4 (for description see below).

Only two genes at P7 that might be expected to be related to a neural response to injury were upregulated >2 fold (Table S1). These were metallopepetidase inhibitor 1 (*Timp1*, 3.2 fold) and syntaxin binding protein 2 (*Sxbp2*, 2.7 fold). As these were also similarly upregulated following injury at P28 (Fig. 5) it seems unlikely that they account for successful neurite outgrowth at P7, which was lacking at P28.

Gene expression in postnatal *Monodelphis* spinal cord 24 h following transection at P28, including comparison with injury at P7

Examination of the whole gene list shows that at P28+24 h there were 332 genes that increased their expression by 2 fold or more (Table S2); 149 genes reduced their expression by 2 fold or more. This contrasts with the response at P7 when no genes were found to be downregulated (Fig. 2 and Fig. 3, Table S1). For comparison of the response at 24 h after injury, all 40 genes that

Table 2. Change in expression of neurite inhibitory and axon growth/guidance genes 24 h following spinal cord injury at P28.

SYMBOL	GENE DESCRIPTION	FOLD
NEURITE INHIBITION/MYELIN		
Efna4	ephrin-A4	5.0
Arhgap6	Rho GTPase activating protein 6	3.1
Gmip	GEM interacting protein encodes a member of the ARHGAP family of Rho/Rac/Cdc42-like GTPase activating proteins.	3.0
Novel	similar to SMPD3 sphingomyelin phosphodiesterase	2.4
Novel	similar to OPHN1 oligophrenin 1,encodes Rho-GTPase-activating protein	2.3
Mpz	myelin protein zero	1.8
Rtn4	Nogo, myelin inhibitory factor	1.2
Mog	myelin oligodendrocyte glycoprotein	−1.7
Mag	myelin associated glycoprotein	−1.8
Arhgef10	Rho guanine nucleotide exchange factor (GEF) 10	−2.0
Arhgap35	Rho GTPase activating protein 35	−2.1
Mbp	myelin basic protein	−2.2
Plp1	proteolipid protein 1	−2.4
AXON GROWTH & GUIDANCE		
Hhipl2	HHIP-like 2, hedgehog interacting protein-like 2	6.5
Sgsm3	small G protein signaling modulator 3	4.5
Slit3	slit homolog 3 (Drosophila) interacts with Robo; axon repellent	4.0
Novel	similar to DNAH7 dynein, axonemal, heavy chain	3.1
Robo3	roundabout, axon guidance receptor, homolog 3 (Drosophila)	3.0
Mical1	microtubule assoc monoxygenase, calponin & LIM domain containing 1	2.3
Serpinf1	serpin peptidase inhib, clade F α-2 antiplasmin, pigment epithelium factor)	2.3
Tgfb3	transforming growth factor, β 3, regulator of ECMs and integrins	2.2
Ntn5	netrin 5	2.1
Tcerg1l	transcription elongation regulator 1-like	2.0
Elmo3	engulfment and cell motility 3	2.0
Cntn2	contactin 2 (axonal) [Source:HGNC Symbol;Acc:2172]	−2.0
Sema4f	sema domain, immunoglobulin domain (Ig), transmembrane domain (TM)	−2.0
Astn1	astrotactin 1, neuronal adhesion molecule required for glial-guided migration of young postmitotic neuroblasts, previously described in developing brain	−2.1
Olig2	oligodendrocyte lineage transcrip factor 2, enhances myelination after SCI	−2.1
Pak7	p21 protein (Cdc42/Rac)-activated kinase 7	−2.3
Plekhb1	pleckstrin homology domain containing, family B (evectins) member 1	−2.4
Sema5a	sema domain, seven thrombospondin repeats (type 1 and type 1-like), transmembrane domain TMand short cytoplasmic domain, (semaphorin) 5A	−2.4
Sema3e	sema domain, immunoglobulin domain (Ig), short basic domain, secreted	−2.5
Pak2	p21 protein (Cdc42/Rac)-activated kinase 2	−2.9
Gas7	growth arrest-specific 7, neurite outgrowth in some cultured neurons	−7.7

Change in expression of neurite inhibitory and axon growth/guidance genes in rostral spinal cord 24 h following spinal cord injury at P28. Note that most of the myelin inhibitory factor genes have not changed their expression in response to injury (fold <2).

showed a change in expression at P7+24 h (Table S1) are compared with the top 40 genes that increased in expression at P28+24 h (from Table S2 as shown in Fig. 5). It is noteworthy that several genes upregulated following injury at both ages showed a much greater change at P28+24 h than even the top gene at P7+ 24 h (Fig. 5 and Cf Tables S1 and S2). Genes that changed expression 24 h following spinal transection at P28 are listed by functional category in Table S3 and are next considered.

Immune-inflammatory genes. Seventy-four genes were classified as immune-inflammatory at P28 (Fig. 2 and Table S3); of these 66 were upregulated and the remaining 8 were downregulated. Twenty-three of the immune/inflammatory genes upregulated following injury at P28 were also upregulated following injury at P7 (Fig. 5) however, only 2 were upregulated substantially more than following injury at P7 (a novel C-C motif chemokine similar to *Ccl8* and *Ccl13*, 322 compared to 33.4 fold and C type lectin/mannose receptor similar to *Mrc1*, 9.3 compared to 3.6 fold); the others were either upregulated to a similar extent or only marginally more than at P7 (Fig. 5).

The difference in the response between P7 and P28 is in the complexity. The much greater P28 response in immune/ inflammatory genes may be a reflection of the state of

Table 3. Change in expression of extracellular matrix factor genes in 24 h following spinal cord injury at P28.

SYMBOL	GENE DESCRIPTION	FOLD
EXTRACELLULAR MATRIX		
Olfm4	olfactomedin 4, also OlfD, hOlfD, ECM glycoprotein that facilitates cell adhesion.	480
Mgp	matrix Gla protein	5.1
Col21a1	collagen, type XXI, alpha 1	4.8
Novel	similar to AMY cluster collagen COL25A1	4.3
Col24a1	collagen, type XXIV, alpha 1	3.5
Lox	lysyl oxidase	3.4
Ecm1	extracellular matrix protein 1	3.2
Pxdn	peroxidasin homolog (Drosophila)	2.9
Col7a1	collagen, type VII, alpha 1	2.9
Sod3	superoxide dismutase 3, extracellular	2.6
Srrm4	serine/arginine repetitive matrix 4	2.4
Fbn3	fibrillin 3	2.3
Col27a1	collagen, type XXVII, alpha 1	2.0
Col15a1	collagen, type XV, alpha 1	−2.0
Dag1	dystroglycan 1 (dystrophin-associated glycoprotein 1)	−2.0
Emilin2	elastin microfibril interfacer 2	−2.1
Nfasc	neurofascin, L1 family immunoglobulin cell adhesion molecule with multiple IGcam and fibronectin domains: neurite outgrowth, neurite fasciculation	−2.2
Nid2	nidogen 2 (osteonidogen) binds collagens I and IV and laminin	−2.2
FIBRONECTIN		
Elfn2	extracellular leucine-rich repeat and fibronectin type III domain containing 2	−2.9
METALLOPEPTIDASES		
Adam11	ADAM metallopeptidase domain 11	3.0
Adamts10	ADAM metallopeptidase with thrombospondin type 1 motif, 10	2.5
Ermp1	endoplasmic reticulum metallopeptidase 1	−2.0
Adam17	ADAM metallopeptidase domain 17	−2.1
Cndp1	carnosine dipeptidase 1 (metallopeptidase M20 family)	−2.2
METALLOPEPTIDASE INHIBITOR		
Timp1	TIMP metallopeptidase inhibitor 1	4.4
METALLOTHIONINES		
Mmp1	matrix metallopeptidase 1 (interstitial collagenase)	104
Mmp15	matrix metallopeptidase 15 (membrane-inserted)	−2.4
PROTEOGLYCANS		
Papln	papilin, proteoglycan-like sulfated glycoprotein	152
Bcan	brevican	2.1
Novel	similar to HS2ST1 heparan sulfate 2-O-sulfotransferase 1	−2.6
Extl1	exostoses (multiple)-like 1	−3.0
LAMININS		
Lamc3	lamin gamma 3	4.8
Lamb2	lamini beta 2	2.6
Lamc2	laminin gamma 2	2.4
Lamc1	laminin gamma 1	2.2
Lama4	laminin alpha 4	2.0
INTEGRINS		
Itgb1bp2	integrin beta 1 binding protein (melusin) 2	6.2
Itga2b	integrin, alpha 2b (platelet glycoprotein IIb of IIb/IIIa complex, antigen CD41)	6.1
Itga4	integrin, alpha 4 (antigen CD49D, alpha 4 subunit of VLA-4 receptor)	−57

Change in expression of extracellular matrix (ECM) factor genes 24 h following spinal cord injury at P28, subdivided into ECM, metallopeptidases, inhibitors, proteoglycans, laminins and integrins.

development of the immune system. By P28 the opossum immune system is fully mature in cellular composition [46,49]. There were 44 additional immune/inflammatory genes upregulated after injury at P28 and 9 that were downregulated (Table S3); none of these showed detectable expression changes at P7. The distribution of Il-1β immunostaining in P28 spinal cord 24 h after injury is illustrated in Fig. 4. In P7 injured cords no immunoreactivity for the cytokine could be detected in the cord but was clearly visible in the connective tissue and forming bone surrounding the spinal cord, confirming cross-species cross-reactivity (Fig. 4A). In contrast in P28 injured cords Il-1β immunoreactivity was detected in several cells of monocytic appearance mostly in close proximity to the central canal (Fig. 4B&C). These cells were present in spinal segments both rostral (Fig. 4B&C) and caudal to the site of the injury. They were not visible in control cords nor were they present in P7 injured tissue.

Blood-related. At P28, 24 h after injury 25 genes in this functional group were upregulated between 2 fold (von Willebrand factor precursor) and 99 fold (novel, haptoglobin-related protein; see Table S5). Only 2 genes in this category were upregulated following injury at P7: a *novel* gene (Similar to Gp6 glycoprotein VI (platelet)) was upregulated 7.8 fold compared to 2.3 fold at P28 and *Trem3* (triggering receptor expressed on myeloid cells 2) which was upregulated 12.4 fold at P7 but was unchanged at P28. One gene in this group was downregulated at P28: *Thbs2* (-4 fold). The observation that bleeding following operation on the cords at P28 was greater than at P7 (Fig. 1) perhaps accounts for the presence of some of the much greater number of genes with changed regulation at P28 (see Fig. 2).

Neurite inhibitory, growth/guidance and extracellular matrix genes. Studies of spinal cord injury in adult animals have shown upregulation of genes with protein products that inhibit neurite outgrowth following axonal injury by a variety of mechanisms. Many of these have been targets for therapies aimed at improving function following spinal cord injury. The main groups are:

(i) Those associated with myelin and the ephrin genes (e.g., [20,50–52]).
(ii) Extracellular matrix genes, including metallopeptidases and proteoglycans [20].
(iii) RhoA activation by myelin associated inhibitors and chondroitin sulphate proteoglycans [43].
(iv) Genes involved in axon growth and guidance [53].

Only *Timp1* (tissue inhibitor of metalloproteinase) in this category was found to change expression following injury at P7 (3.2 fold, Table S1). Genes that increased or decreased their expression in this category at P28 are listed in Table 2.

Many inhibitory factors converge on Rho, an intracellular GTPase. These include myelin-derived inhibitory factors, semaphorins, chondroitin sulphate proteoglycans (CPSGs), ephrins, netrins and repulsive guidance molecules (RGMs; see [43]). Neither *Rho* nor its downstream effector Rho kinase (*Rock*) changed expression by 24 h after spinal cord injury at P28. Four Rho family members were identified that change expression level after injury at P28. Amongst other Rho family members, two were upregulated 3 fold (*Arhgap6, Gmip*) and 2 were downregulated 2 fold (*Arhgef10, Arhgap35*) see Table 2. Thus even if any of the numerous upstream neurite inhibitory factors changed expression after injury, it seems unlikely they would be effective in influencing neurite outgrowth. In fact, very few were found to change expression. Following injury at P28, none of the seven myelin-associated genes identified was upregulated. Five did not change expression (*Rtn4* also known as *Nogo, Mpz, Mag, Mog, Ngr*) and only two were marginally downregulated (*Mbp, Plp1*). These findings are consistent with the morphological observation that myelination is not complete at this stage of spinal cord development (Fig. 6).

Luxol Fast Blue stain for myelin demonstrated that the process of myelination in the thoracic region of *Monodelphis* spinal cord does not begin until about 3 weeks of age. There was no myelin staining at P8 (Fig. 6A). By P28 the distinctive myelin staining was apparent; however, the thickness of the myelinated white matter was still smaller than in the adult (compare Fig. 6B with Fig. 6A in [25]). From preliminary studies we have established that myelination is relatively rapid after P28 and by P35 the staining pattern of the thoracic cord is very similar to that in the adult (unpublished observations).

Of seven ephrin and nine ephrin receptor genes identified, only Ephrin-A4 (*Eph4a*) was upregulated (5 fold). *Eph4A* -/- mutant mice have been suggested to show greater axon growth after spinal cord injury [54] but others have not confirmed this [55]. Even if *Eph4A* is involved in inhibition of axon growth the lack of change in *Rho/Rock* expression suggests it would not have contributed in the present experiments. Equally, myelin inhibition is unlikely to have contributed to the failure of axons to grow across a lesion made at P28.

Twenty-one genes associated with axon growth and guidance during spinal cord development were identified as having changed expression levels following injury at P28 (Table 2). Eight were downregulated 2 to 3 fold and could therefore have possibly contributed to the lack of axon growth. The others were upregulated (Table 2) including *Hhipl2* (hedgehog interacting protein-like- 2, 6.5 fold) and *Sgsm3* (small G protein signalling modulator 3) and are thus unlikely to have contributed to lack of axon growth at P28. Amongst six netrin genes identified, only *Ntn5* was marginally upregulated (2.1 fold) and amongst seven CSPGs only one was marginally upregulated (Brevican, *Bcan*, 2 fold). Neither of the repulsive guidance molecules, *Rgma, Rgmb*, changed expression following injury.

Thirty-nine genes with extracellular matrix products, including fibronectin, metallopeptidases, metallothionines, laminins, integrins and proteoglycans showed changed expression following injury at P28 (Table 3). Of these, twenty-six were upregulated 2 to 480 fold and thirteen were downregulated (2 to 3 fold) except for *Itga4* which showed expression levels 57 fold less than controls). The most strikingly upregulated were olfactomedin 4 (*Olfm4*, 480 fold), papilin, proteoglycan-like sulfated glycoprotein (*Papln* 152 fold, see below) and matrix metallopepetidase 1 (*Mmp1*, 104 fold). *Olfm4* is a member of the 4-member olfactomedin family. Originally identified as the human granulocyte colony-stimulating factor stimulated clone-1 (hGC-1; [56]), *Olfm4* has been suggested to be specifically expressed in gut and pancreas [57] in contrast to *Olfm1*, which was reported to be specifically expressed in brain [58]. It is an extracellular matrix glycoprotein that facilitates cell adhesion by binding to cadherin and lectins [57], although it is not clear if this is its function in the spinal cord. *Olfm4* has been implicated in suppressing inflammation. Mice deficient in *Olfm4* have a stronger anti-bacterial response including enhanced inflammation to *Helicobacter pylori* [59]. However, it may be that its function in the extracellular matrix of the spinal cord may be more relevant to the present study.

Using western blotting and immunocytochemistry MMP1 has been found to be increased 24 h following spinal cord injury in rats, [60] and in human postmortem studies using immunocytochemistry [61]. Its gene expression does not appear to have been studied. The protein has been localized in macrophages and

Table 4. Change in expression of channel, synapse, neural receptor, actin, myosin and related genes 24 h following spinal cord injury at P28.

SYMBOL	GENE DESCRIPTION	FOLD
SYNAPSES, NEURAL RECEPTORS & CHANNELS		
Gpr26	G protein-coupled receptor 26	6.6
Trpc7	transient receptor potential cation channel, subfamily C, member 7	4.6
Hcrt	hypocretin (orexin) neuropeptide precursor	3.8
Novel	Similar to UNC80 unc-80 homolog (C. elegans)	3.7
Sytl1	synaptotagmin-like 1	3.0
Fchsd1	FCH and double SH3 domains 1	3.0
Adora2a	adenosine A2a receptor	3.0
Fam40b	family with sequence similarity 40, member B, correct symbol STRIP2	3.0
Clcn2	chloride channel, voltage-sensitive 2	2.6
Bzrap1	benzodiazapine receptor (peripheral) associated protein 1	2.6
Mast1	microtubule associated serine/threonine kinase 1	2.4
Trpt1	tRNA phosphotransferase 1	2.4
Stxbp2	syntaxin binding protein 2	2.3
Mcoln1	mucolipin 1	2.3
C10orf10	chromosome 10 open reading frame 10	2.3
Ano8	anoctamin 8	2.1
Cacnb3	calcium channel, voltage-dependent, beta 3 subunit	2.1
Adrbk2	adrenergic, beta, receptor kinase 2	2.0
Camkk1	calcium/calmodulin-dependent protein kinase 1α, modulation of neuron survival	2.0
Syt2	synaptotagmin II	−1.8
Trpc4ap	transient receptor potential cation channel, subfamily C, member 4 assoc prot	−2.1
Gprc5b	G protein-coupled receptor, family C, group 5, member B	−2.1
Ncs1	neuronal calcium sensor 1	−2.1
Kif1b	kinesin family member 1B	−2.2
Gab1	GRB2-associated binding protein 1	−2.2
Kcnj10	potassium inwardly-rectifying channel, subfamily J, member 10	−2.3
Shroom2	shroom family member 2	−2.5
Syn3	synapsin III	−2.5
Gpr17	G protein-coupled receptor 17	−2.6
Gabrb1	gamma-aminobutyric acid (GABA) A receptor, beta 1	−2.9
Gpr75	probable G-protein coupled receptor 75	−2.9
Kcnj12	potassium inwardly-rectifying channel, subfamily J, member 12	−5.8
Novel	similar to CLCNKA/CLCNKB chloride channel	−27
ACTIN, MYOSIN & RELATED		
Trdn	triadin	206
Myl1	myosin, light chain 1, alkali; skeletal, fast	139
Mylpf	myosin light chain, phosphorylatable, fast skeletal muscle	22
MYH4	myosin, heavy chain 4, skeletal muscle	18
Acta1	actin, alpha 1, skeletal muscle	8.6
Mybpc3	myosin binding protein C, cardiac	4.8
Parvg	parvin, gamma	4.7
Novel	LOC100015891 Similar to Myosin heavy chain	4.6
Pgam2	phosphoglycerate mutase 2 (muscle)	4.3
Myof	myoferlin	4.2
Nexn	nexilin (F actin binding protein)	4.0
Myo19	myosin XIX	3.7
Tpm2	tropomyosin 2 (beta) member of the actin filament binding protein family	3.1
Miox	myo-inositol oxygenase	2.9

Table 4. Cont.

SYMBOL	GENE DESCRIPTION	FOLD
Speg	SPEG complex locus	2.8
Novel	similar to actinin alpha, F-actin cross-linking protein	2.8
Tagln	transgelin 22 kDa actin-binding protein	2.7
Ryr3	ryanodine receptor 3 brain ryanodine receptor-calcium release channel	2.7
Ttll9	tubulin tyrosine ligase-like family, member 9	2.6
Neb	nebulin	2.6
Myo1f	myosin IF	2.6
Novel	LOC100014836 similar to ACTA1 actin, alpha 1, skeletal muscle	2.2
Popdc3	popeye domain containing 3	−2.2
Kif13b	kinesin family member 13B	−2.3

Change in expression of channel, synapse, neural receptor, actin, myosin and related genes 24 h following spinal cord injury at P28. Note that myosin and actin genes are important structural and functional components of synapses.

astrocytes in the human study [61] but also in neurons in the rat study [60]. MMPs are a family of peptidases that degrade extracellular matrix proteins. Early increased expression of for example *Mmp-9* is thought to have deleterious effects whereas the later upregulation of MMP-2 may be beneficial as part of the repair process [62]. The role of MMP-1 following spinal cord injury is unknown but given its early and substantial upregulation in P28 *Monodelphis* spinal cord following injury described here, it may be contributing to the lack of neurite outgrowth at this age.

Proteoglycans, particularly chondroitin sulphate proteoglycans (CSPGs) are known to be upregulated following injury to adult spinal cord and are thought to be a major component of neurite inhibition following injury [20]. These proteoglycans were not found to be upregulated in the current study (see above). However, a novel gene similar to papilin, *Papln* proteoglycan-like sulfated glycoprotein was upregulated 152 fold; this gene has not previously been identified in spinal cord but perhaps it also has neurite inhibitory properties as in the case of CSPGs. Several collagens have been identified in the post injury scar that restricts neurite outgrowth following spinal cord injury in the adult [20]. In the present study three collagen genes were upregulated (Table 3) and may have contributed to the lack of neurite outgrowth at P28, as collagen is an important component of the glial scar [20]; one was marginally downregulated (-2 fold). It seems unlikely that the rather modest changes in expression of metalloproteinase genes, some of which increased and others decreased (Table 3), would

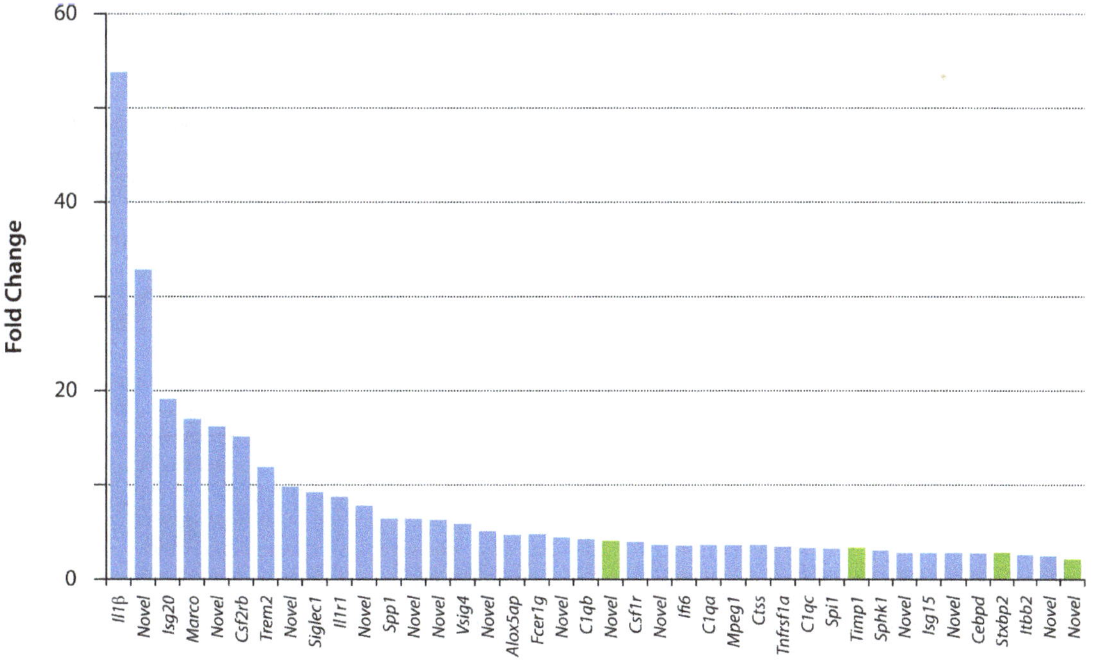

Figure 3. Changes in gene expression 24 h following spinal transection at P7. Only 40 genes changed their expression levels by ≥2 fold. All were upregulated. See Table S1 for gene descriptions and statistics. There were 12 "novel" genes; search of GO categories showed that these have immune/inflammatory properties. Note that only four of the genes in this figure (green bars) are not in the immune/inflammatory category (blue bars).

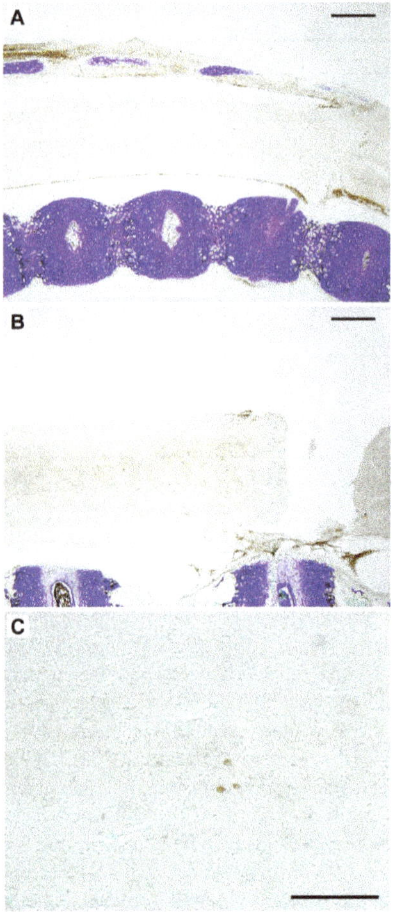

Figure 4. Interleukin-1β in *Monodelphis* spinal cord 24 hours after a complete transection at P7 or P28. In the segment of the cord rostral to the site of injury Il-1β was detected using cross-reacting antibodies to the human cytokine. Note strong immunopositive signal in the tissue surrounding the cords at P7-injured (A) and P28 (B) but lack of significant staining within the spinal tissue especially at P7 (A). One day following injury at P28 a few immunopositive cells with the general morphology of monocytes were detected, especially in segments of the cord more rostral to the injury (C). Scale bars A, B = 500 μm, C = 100 μm.

have contributed to the lack of neurite outgrowth at P28. Of 13 laminins, 5 were upregulated 2.0–4.8 fold (Table 3).

Integrins are an important receptor family promoting axon growth during development and regeneration following injury to peripheral nerves. They interact with the extracellular matrix factors described above (e.g. collagen, laminin, tenascin, vitronectin). Integrins are cell surface proteins. They bind to molecules in the extracellular matrix and transduce extrinsic cues that regulate the cytoskeleton leading to modulation of axon growth (for references see [63]). In contrast to their activity in developing nervous system and peripheral nerve regeneration, there appears to be little change in integrin expression following injury to the adult central nervous system [63]. Integrins are also present on the surface of leukocytes; for example, antibodies to integrin α4vβ1 reduced neutrophil and monocyte/macrophage influx into adult spinal cord following injury [64]. In the present study there was a substantial reduction (57 fold) in expression of *Itga4* (integrin α4) following injury at P28. Lane et al. [24] reported a small infiltration of granulocytes at 24 h following spinal cord transection in *Monodelphis* at P7. At P14 the infiltration was 2–3 times larger but was delayed compared to P7 injuries. This may explain why we do not see many granulocytes 24 hours after injury in the P28 spinal cords. However, we observe some monocytic cells as illustrated in Fig. 4. Only two other integrins (*Itgibp2, Itga2b*) showed a change in expression, increasing about 6 fold in both cases. However, these integrins have not previously been identified in spinal cord so their possible role in lack of neurite outgrowth is unclear.

Rho signaling proteins regulate the dynamics of cytoskeleton and cell motility [65]. Rho appears to be the common target of the main mechanisms that limit neurite outgrowth following spinal cord injury: myelin inhibitors, CSPGs, and guidance inhibitors [43]. Given the rather small and opposing changes in expression of Rho family genes and of many of the genes that target Rho following injury in adult spinal cords (see above) it seems unlikely that Rhos and inhibitory factors that target them contribute to the lack of axon growth following injury at P28. However, many of the axons passing through the site of injury have their cell bodies of origin in the brainstem, where changes in Rho genes might be expected to be manifest. Changes in brainstem gene expression will be the subject of a separate report (Saunders *et al.*, in preparation) but preliminary examination of the RNA-Seq data suggests that here too changes in expression of Rho-related genes following spinal cord injury are also marginal.

Cell adhesion and intercellular junctions. There were twelve genes in this functional category (S3). Only four were upregulated (2.2. to 3 fold). The other seven decreased their expression (-2 to -3 fold). Most of these genes have not previously been identified in spinal cord. *Pdch1* appears to play a role in spinal cord development in the mouse [66] and *Pdch18* in chick and zebrafish developing spinal cord [67,68]. *Gjc2* encodes the gap junction protein connexin-47; a mutation of this gene has been associated with hypomyelination [69]. Of all the genes identified in this group only *Icam-1* has been found to change expression in injured adult spinal cord. Thus its expression has been found to increase following spinal cord injury in rats; endothelial cell upregulation of *Icam1* was suggested to increase adhesion and extravasation of leukocytes 1–2 days following injury [70]. The possible importance of ICAM-1 in the response to injury is indicated by the report that intravenous injection of ICAM-1 monoclonal antibody 30 min after spinal cord injury in rats reduced motor disturbance and enhanced recovery [71].

Channels, synapses and neural receptors. In previous studies of adult spinal cord it has been reported that some ion channel genes, including those for sodium, potassium and calcium are downregulated shortly after injury [16]. In the present study four channel genes were downregulated (Table 4), including one potassium channel (*Kcnj12*, -5.8 fold) and one chloride channel (a novel gene, similar to *Clcnka/Clcnkb* chloride channel) that was markedly downregulated (27 fold). In addition three channel genes were upregulated (*Trpc7, Clcn2, Cacnb3*, Table 4).

In reviewing a large number of microarray studies of adult rodent spinal cord Verhaagen *et al.* [16] also reported genes encoding enzymes involved in neurotransmitter synthesis and genes encoding proteins involved in synaptic vesicle transport and docking as well as expression of glutamate receptors, which were generally downregulated following spinal cord injury. In our dataset in this category, there were five genes that were upregulated (2 to 3 fold) and six that were downregulated (2.1 to 2.9 fold) see Table 4. Myosin and actin are important for normal structure and function of neural synapses [72–74]. Genes related to these protein products have been listed separately in Table 4. Twenty-three were identified with significant changes in expression; all but one (*Popdc*, -2.2 fold) was upregulated. Of those

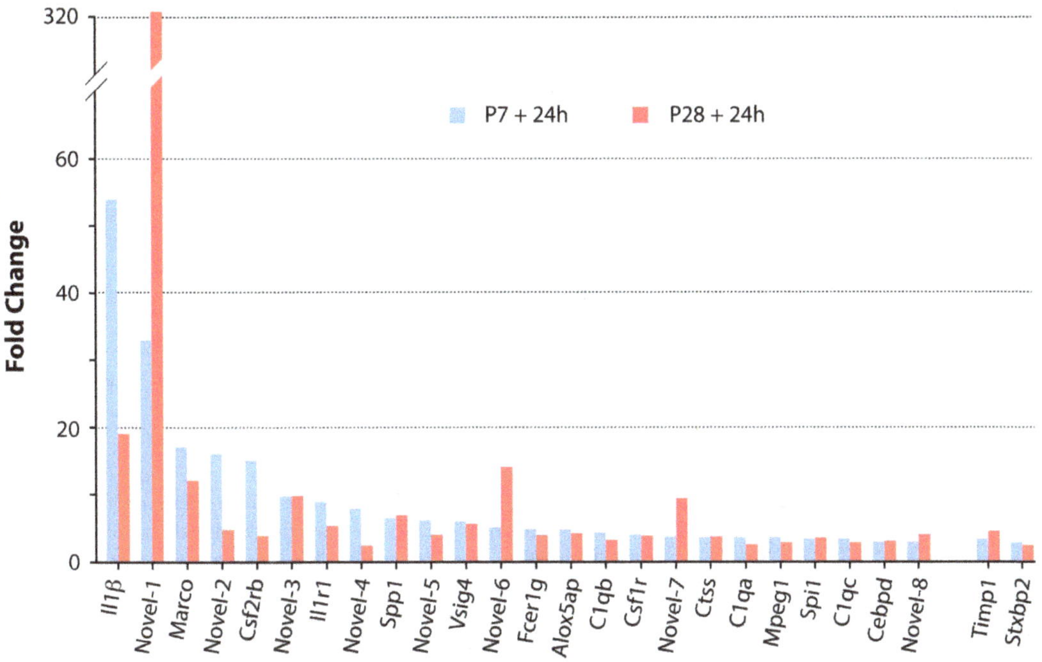

Figure 5. Comparison of expression levels of the twenty-six genes that changed expression in spinal cord 24 h following transection at both P7 and P28. All but two of these genes (Timp1 and Stxbp2) were in the immune/inflammatory category. The magnitude of the expression changes was generally similar at the two ages, but more genes (six: IL1β, MARCO, novel-2, CSF2RB, IL1-R1, novel-4) showed greater upregulation at P7 than at P28 (three: novel-1, novel-6, novel-7). A search of Ensembl, NCBI "Gene" and GO categories showed that all of these novel genes are involved in immune/inflammatory functions (see Tables S1 and S2).

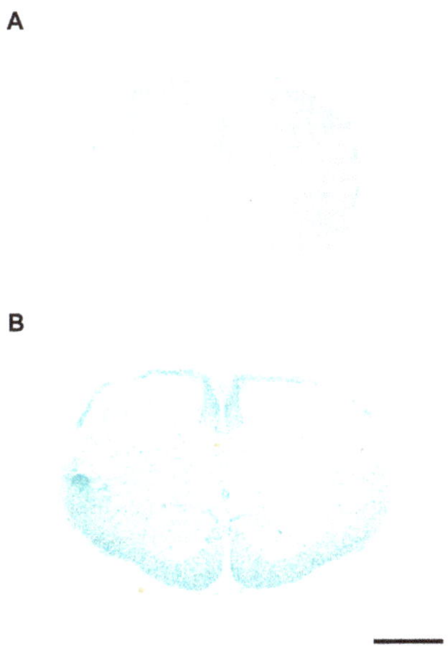

Figure 6. Myelin staining in the developing spinal cord of *Monodelphis domestica*. Transverse sections through thoracic spinal cord of P8 (A) and P29 (B) spinal cord stained with Luxol fast blue (LFB). There was no LFB stained myelin at P8 (A) but relatively well- developed myelin was present at P28 (B). However even at P28 the myelination is only beginning to appear (first detected between P21 and P28) and does not reach adult levels until several weeks later (not illustrated). Dorsal is uppermost. Scale bar is 500 μm.

upregulated, some increased their expression very substantially: *Triadin* (206 fold), *Myl1* (139 fold), *Mylpf* (22 fold) and a *novel* gene *LOC100027326*, myosin-4-like (18 fold). Triadin was first discovered as an important intrinsic membrane glycoprotein in the sarcoplasmic reticulum of skeletal muscle [75]. Although initially thought to be exclusive to skeletal muscle, according to Dulhunty *et al.*, [76] it has been found in a range of tissues. However, it does not seem to have been identified previously in spinal cord, but there is one report of Triadin 2 (the cardiac isoform) in mouse brain [77] together with the intracellular calcium channel proteins ryanodine receptors (RyR) 1 and 3. *Ryr3* was upregulated in the present study (Table 4). Ryanodine receptors and Triadin are essential components of sarcoplasmic Ca^{2+} transduction in skeletal muscle [76]. Their presence in spinal cord suggests that they may have a role in Ca^{2+} storage and release there too. *Myl1* and the *novel* gene (*myosin-4-like*) have not been identified in spinal cord previously. *Mylpf* a gene involved in muscle contraction has been found to be downregulated in the spinal cord in response to acrylamide [78]. These genes and those listed in Table 4 show changes in expression following injury that is presumably related to changes in synaptic function at later stages after the injury. They may reflect some of the changes in gene expression and neural circuits in opossum spinal cord caudal to the injury site following injury at P28 [26]. These may be important for the weight bearing locomotion displayed by these animals when adult, in spite of the lack of axonal growth across the lesion (25). However, it seems unlikely that these changes in synapse-related genes are contributing to this lack of axon growth following injury at P28.

Apoptosis and ubiquitin. Only one apoptosis-related gene was upregulated at P7 following injury: a *novel* gene, related to *Samd9*. In contrast, five genes with products that are involved in apoptosis were upregulated 3 to 6 fold in the P28 injured cords:

Dnajb13 (*Hsp40* homologue), three *novel* genes and *Plac8* (Table S3). *Faim2*, a gene for Fas apoptotic inhibitory molecule was downregulated (−2.3 fold) as was the apoptosis-associated tyrosine kinase *Aatk* (Table S3). This suggests a degree of apoptotic activity that was not present following injury at P7. Lane *et al.* [24] reported a large increase in pyknotic cells 3 h after spinal cord transection in P7 and P14 *Monodelphis*. This returned to control levels by 24 h, which may account for the limited expression changes in apoptotic-related genes at P7 and P28 in the present study conducted 24 hours after injury (Tables S1, S2 and S3).

Four ubiquitin-related genes increased expression (4.0 to 7.6 fold, Table S3). Only one was downregulated (a novel gene similar to *Ubr3*, -2 fold). These genes, *Wsb1, Cul7, Cul9* and *Ubr3* are all genes for different E3 ubiquitin ligases that ubiquitinate various target proteins, signaling them for protein degradation. WSB1 is a hedgehog inducible ubiquitin ligase socs-box-containing WD-40 protein. Currently, there is no evidence for this process following spinal cord injury; however, it is an E3 ubiquitin ligase for thyroid hormone-activating type 2 iodothyronine deiodinase [79], which is a HIPK2-interacting protein [80]. The cullin family of genes codes for *cullin E3 ligase* scaffold protein, which interacts with *Rbx1.* In this study, we identified two cullin family members with >2 fold change, *Cul7* and *Cul9.* CUL7 has only been shown to bind with FBXW8 [81]. However, there is some evidence that this protein heterodimerizes with CUL1, facilitating polyubiquitination of target proteins [81]. The specific function of CUL7 in the spinal cord is otherwise unknown; however, CUL1 [82] and CUL3 [83] have been shown to be important during embryonic development through interaction with cyclin E. *Cul7* knockout-mice also show neonatal lethality [84]. CUL9, previously known as PARC on the other hand has been shown to bind and promote p53-dependent apoptosis [85]. The last of the E3 protein ligase genes identified is *Ubr3*, ubiquitin protein ligase E3 component n-recognin 3. This gene codes for a ligase that specifically targets the N-terminal residues for degradation [86]. Although its role has not been previously described in spinal cord injury, this ligase has been shown to play a role in olfactory and tactile sensory systems [86].

Vascular/angiogenesis and transporters. Three genes with vascular/angiogenic properties were upregulated 2.5 to 3.8 fold (Table S3). Of fifteen transporter genes seven were upregulated (3 to 12 fold) and eight were downregulated (−2 to −5 fold). Only two have previously been identified in spinal cord (*Sclc18a3*, vesicular acetylcholine transporter and *Atp2a1*, both downregulated). There was only one efflux transporter gene (*Abcc5, Mrp5*, upregulated 4.5 fold). Most of the influx transporters were ion carriers, some upregulated, others downregulated. Of two monocarboxylic transporters one (*Slc16a4*) was upregulated (8 fold) and one (*Slc16a1*) downregulated (−2 fold). The highest change in expression was that of the vitamin C transporter *Slc23a3* (12 fold). It seems unlikely that any of these changes are directly related to the lack of axon growth following injury at P28.

Development and structure. Thirty-one genes were classified as development and structure related genes (Table S3). Of these, twenty were upregulated, 2.1 to 21 fold and eleven were downregulated, (−2 to −11 fold). Several of these genes have important roles in neural development. For example *Fuz*, which was upregulated 21 fold, is a planar polarity gene, mutations of which are associated with neural tube defects [87]. *Hoxb1* (12 fold) and *Hoxb3* (2.4 fold) are transcription factors involved in patterning of the caudal central nervous system [88,89]. *Hoxd4* (2.4 fold) does not appear to have been identified previously in spinal cord but *Hoxd10* has been implicated in determining motor neuron numbers and spinal nerve trajectories in lumbar spinal cord of mice [90]. There were two insulin growth factor-like genes, one upregulated (*Igf2bp2*, 2.5 fold) and one downregulated (*Igfbpl1*, −11 fold); there was also one IGF-like receptor (*Igflr1*, 5.2 fold). None of these have previously been identified in spinal cord. Only five of the remaining genes have been identified previously in spinal cord (*Tube1, Notch3, Rhou, Sort1, Vim*). Of these, tubulin protein has been reported in spinal cord injury, where it was upregulated 2.7 fold [91] compared with a 4.5 fold in gene expression, and vimentin (*Vim*) was upregulated [92]. Given that many of these genes are of unclear function in normal or injured spinal cord it cannot be concluded whether they contribute to the lack of neurite outgrowth following injury at P28, although this seems unlikely.

Proteomic analysis in postnatal *Monodelphis* spinal cord following transection

The changes in proteomic expression have been examined in the segment of the cord rostral to the lesion compared to age-matched controls. Proteins identified from gel bands that showed changes in the density were classified under the same functional categories as those used in the RNA-Seq analysis (see above).

Protein expression in postnatal *Monodelphis* spinal cord 24 h following transection at P7

Compared to P8 age-matched controls, in cords injured at P7 and analysed 24 h later there were only four proteins with increased band intensity (upregulated). Almost all of the rest of the proteins identified at this age (twenty-six) showed reduced band intensity (downregulated); one protein was identified with both an increased and a decreased density that depended on the fraction in which the protein was separated (Tables S4 and S6). The identity of these proteins and their classification into functional categories are shown in Table S4. Four of the functional groups: Neurite Inhibition, Guidance & Extracellular; Apoptosis & Ubiquitin; Synapses, Neural Receptors & Channels and Development & Structure are illustrated in Fig. 7.

Neurite inhibition, guidance and extracellular proteins. One neurite inhibitory protein, myelin basic protein, was upregulated, whereas a protein that interacts with the myelin inhibitory protein, NOGO (Ubiquinol-cytochrome c reductase core protein II, see [93]) was downregulated. Three tubulin proteins were also downregulated (Fig. 7A and Table S4).

Apoptosis and ubiquitin-related. All six of the proteins in this group were downregulated. Three were ubiquitin-related, two were peroxiredoxins with an antioxidant protective role [94] and one was an immunoproteasome protein, which also is involved in processing of class 1 MHC peptides (http://www.ncbi.nlm.nih.gov/gene/5689). This is illustrated in Fig. 7B (data in Table S4).

Synapses, neural receptors and channels. Six of the seven proteins in this group were down regulated. Their functions appear to relate to intracellular structure, motility and transport. The one protein that was upregulated was a vesicle transport and fusion protein (valosin).

All of the proteins assigned to the development and structure and the metabolic-associated protein groups were downregulated; two stress response genes changed in opposite directions (Fig. 7C and Table S4).

Development and structure

Four proteins in this group (glial fibrillary acidic protein, transgelin-2, peptidylprolyl isomerase A-like and phosphatidylethanolamine-binding protein 1) were downregulated. None was upregulated (Fig. 7D and Table S4).

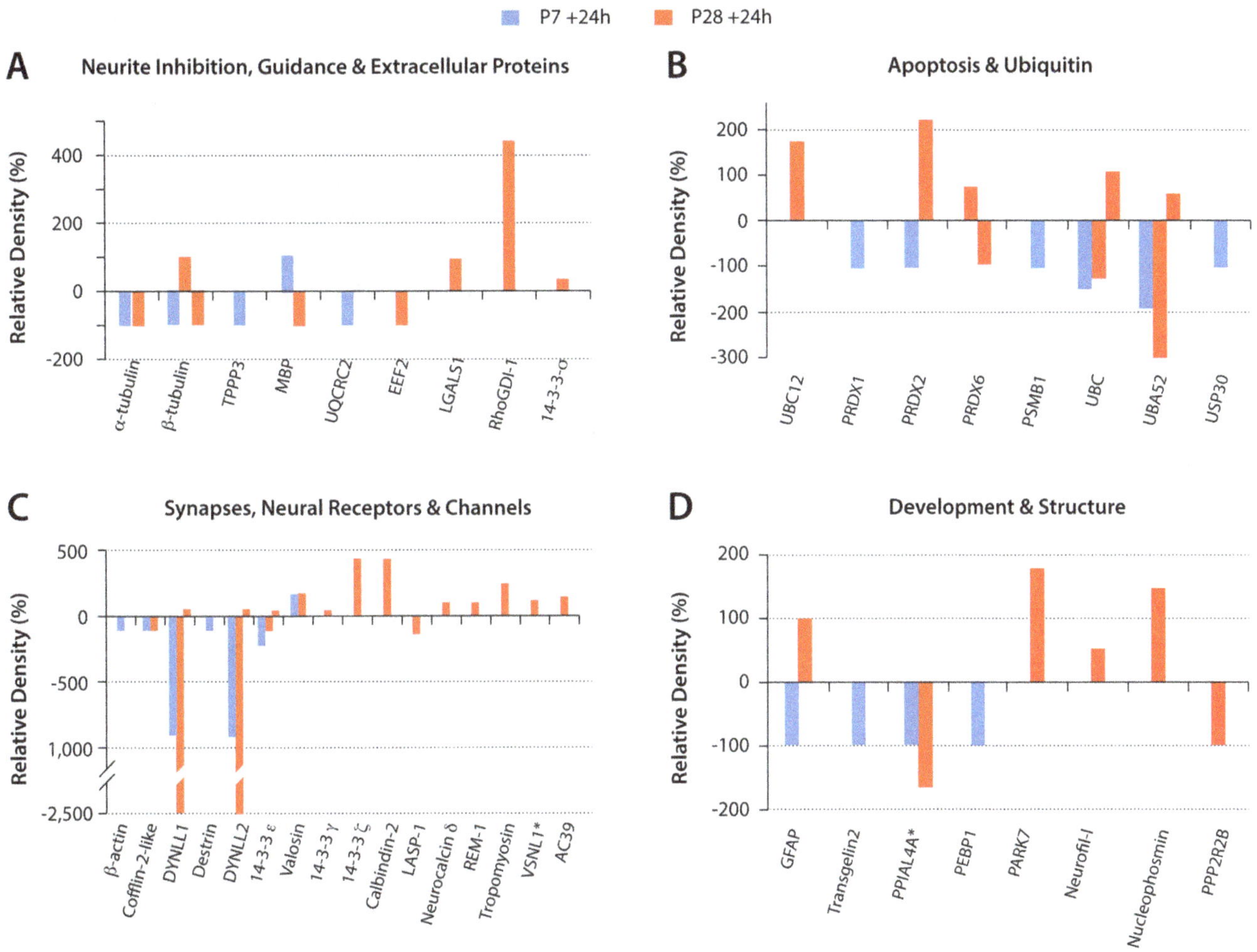

Figure 7. Proteins by functional groups with changed expression levels after spinal transection at P7 or P28. Estimates of protein expression levels from densitometry measurements. Values are expressed as % change from control values (100%). y axis: Relative Density (%). Proteins grouped by functions as listed in Tables S4 and S5. Abbreviations: TPPP3-Brain specific protein; UQCRC2-Ubiquinol-cytochrome c reductase core protein II; EEF2-Elongation factor 2 isoform 1; LGALS1-galactin1; MBP–Myelin basic protein; PRDX1-peroxiredoxin1; PRDX2–peroxiredoxin 2; PRDX6–peroxiredoxin 6; PSMB1-Proteasome subunit β type 1; UBC–Ubiquitin C; UBA52-Ubiquitin A-52; USP30-Ubiquitin specific peptidase 30 phosphoglycerate kinase; BC12-NEDD8-conjugating enzyme UBC12; DYNLL1- Cytoplasmic dynein light chain 1; DYNLL2-Dynein light chain LC8 type 2; VSLN1-Visinin like-1; AC39-AC39/physophilin; GFAP–glial fibrillary acidic protein; TAGLN2-transgelin 2; PPIAL4A - Peptidylprolyl isomerase A-like PEBP1 - Phosphatidylethanolamine-binding protein 1; PARK7 - Parkinson protein 7; Neurofil-L – Neurofilament-L subunit; PPP2R2B - Protein phosphatase 2 regulatory subunit B. Two proteins, VSNL1 and PPIAL4A (marked with *) are mean values as their expression levels changes were detected in more than one fraction (see Table S4 and S5 for individual changes). Note also that a few of the proteins listed showed both up- and downregulation but only in P28 injury group.

Blood-related proteins. Two hemoglobin proteins, hemoglobin-α and hemoglobin subunit β-M showed changes in band density; hemoglobin-α was increased in Off gel fraction 12 and reduced in fraction 9 (Table S4), hemoglobin subunit β-M was increased. Neither of these proteins has been identified previously in spinal cord. It is possible that their presence was due to blood contamination in the injured cords (see Fig. 1).

Protein expression in postnatal *Monodelphis* spinal cord 24 h following transection at P28

Following injury at P28 (P28+24 h) compared to P29 controls twenty eight protein bands were identified with increased intensity, fourteen protein bands with reduced intensity and thirteen that showed both increased or decreased intensity depending on the Off-gel fraction in which they were present (Fig. 8, Table S6) most likely reflecting changes in post-translational modifications [31]. The variability in the proteome following injury at P28 is in contrast to the response to injury at P7 when almost all of the proteins identified were downregulated (Fig. 7).

Immune-inflammatory proteins. In contrast to the very large number of genes in this functional category that changed their regulation at P28 following injury, only three proteins were identified here (Table S5). One was *Anxa2* (annexin a2), which showed decreased expression, although the expression of its gene was unchanged. Annexin2 is involved in recruitment and activation of immune cells [95]. A protein that is likely to have immune related functions was also identified (immunoglobulin lambda-like polypeptide 5-like) and found to be upregulated (Table S5). However, its actual function appears to be unknown. A third protein was Melanocortin 1 Receptor, which is said to have anti-inflammatory and immunomodulatory effects [96]. The discrepancy between the large number of identified genes and

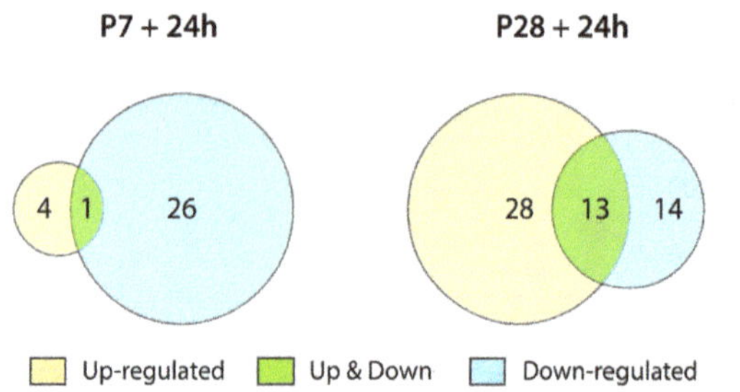

Up	Down	Up & Down	Up	Down	Up & Down
13%	84%	3%	51%	25%	24%

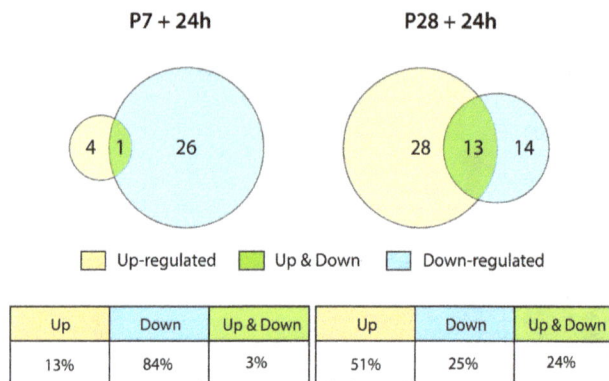

Figure 8. Summary of numbers of proteins that changed expression levels 24 h following spinal transection at P7 or P28. All but five of the proteins identified at P7 as showing a change in expression after injury were downregulated. At P28 half of the proteins were upregulated.

small number of proteins is most likely to be due to the sensitivity of detection methods: proteomic analysis is not likely to detect molecules within relatively low concentration range as is the case for most cytokines. It is also possible that some of the genes detected by RNA-Seq. analysis were not yet translated into their protein products within the time frame used in this study (24 hours).

Neurite inhibition and guidance proteins. Unlike results following injury at P7, at P28 myelin basic protein was downregulated (Fig. 7A). On the other hand Rho GTPase activating protein, through which many of the neurite inhibitory factors act (see above) was increased. Two other proteins that have been suggested to influence neurite outgrowth (Elongation Factor 2 Isoform 1 [97] and Lectin, galactoside-binding, soluble 1 (Galectin 1) [98,99]) changed in opposite directions (Fig. 7A, Table S5). Galectin-1 has also been described in neutrophils at the site of a spinal cord injury made 24 h earlier and in macrophages/ microglia at 3 days post injury [100]. This increase in Galectin-1 protein was not accompanied by a change in transcript expression (Table S6).

Apoptosis and ubiquitin. Five of the eight proteins in this category were upregulated in contrast to P7 injured spinal cord when the proteins in this group were all downregulated (Fig. 7B). However, there were three proteins in this group, which were identified as a band in a different fraction that showed decreased density (periredoxin-6, ubiquitin c and ubiquitin A52, Fig. 7B, Table S5). Detailed studies of the apoptotic activity in *Monodelphis* spinal cord after injury have not been conducted, mostly due to the lack of cross-reactivity of commercially available antibodies commonly used as markers for this process.

Synapses, receptors and channels. There were twelve proteins in this category, including three members of 14-3-3 proteins (ε, γ, ξ) that were upregulated. These are involved in tyrosine 3-monooxygenase/tryptophan 5-monooxygenase activation signal transduction. Seven proteins involved in synaptic structure and function were upregulated, but only two (Cofilin and LIM & SH3 protein) were downregulated (Fig. 7C, Table S5). It seems unlikely that these proteins would play a role in the lack of neurite outgrowth following injury at P28, but they may indicate an early aspect of synaptic reorganisation in the injured spinal cord.

Development and structure. There were eight proteins identified as changing their expression in this category, including glial fibrillary acidic protein (GFAP). All but two (PPIAL4A, PPP2R2B) were upregulated (Fig. 7D, Table S5). However two of the upregulated proteins also appeared as bands in other fractions that indicated downregulation. These changes may be a reflection of developmental reorganization of spinal cord tissue rather than involvement in blocking neurite outgrowth at P28.

Stress response proteins. Five proteins with changed expression were identified in this category (Table S5). Two were upregulated (heat shock proteins HSP84b and HSP90B1), two were downregulated (glucose regulated heat shock protein 70kDa, protein 5; novel heat shock protein) and one (heat shock protein 90) was both increased or decreased depending on the fraction. Heat shock proteins are highly expressed cellular proteins in all species examined so far [101]. Stressors of various kinds generally result in an increase in the levels of these proteins e.g., HSP70 and HSP90 [101]. Several authors have reported this effect early after spinal cord injury in adult animals [102,103]. However, down-regulation of some heat shock proteins by various drug treatments has been reported in spinal cord injury (see [104] for references). It has therefore been suggested that both up- and down-regulatory changes in heat shock proteins may have neuroprotective effects, reflecting a complex role in protective responses to injury [104].

Blood-related proteins. As observed following P7 injury two hemoglobins showed a change in regulation. However, following injury at P28 hemoglobin α was decreased whereas at P7 different fractions showed either a decrease or/and an increase (Cf Tables S4 and S5). For hemoglobin β, the changes were the opposite; that is at P7 this protein was increased but at P28 different fractions showed opposite changes. In addition to these two hemoglobins, two other proteins showed an increase following injury at P28: the plasma carrier protein albumin and NADPH-flavin reductase, which is involved in heme metabolism. As suggested for P7 it may be that these blood-related proteins originate from blood contamination of the spinal cord as a consequence of the injury (see Fig. 1).

Comparison of gene and protein expression

Based on the proteins identified, we searched for corresponding genes or family of genes associated with these proteins. Table S6 shows the matches of proteins and genes identified from RNA-Seq analysis that were up- or downregulated (proteins ±0.5 band density, genes ±2 fold change). A few proteins did not have IDs that corresponded to a gene in our RNA-Seq dataset. This may be due to incompleteness of the annotation of the opossum genome. Most of the genes corresponding to up- or downregulated proteins that we identified as changing their expression following injury at either P7 or P28 did not show changes in the RNA-Seq analysis. In only two cases did both gene and protein changed both at P28. (i) Hemoglobin beta M was identified in three different fractions. In two of these the protein was upregulated and in the third it was decreased. The corresponding gene is a *novel* opossum gene (LOC100019389) that was upregulated 2.2 fold. (ii) A second upregulated gene (*Blvrd*) corresponded to an upregulated protein (NADPH-flavin reductase) that is involved in heme metabolism. The protein products of these genes may perhaps be explained by blood contamination in the injured spinal cord. However, this would not explain the presence of these genes. Erythrocytes are no longer nucleated in opossums after birth and hemoglobin transcripts have been identified in cerebral endothelial cells of neonatal mice [105], which may thus explain the changes in gene expression found in the present study.

There are several reasons why there were so many more genes that showed changes in expression that was the case for the proteins. The main one is likely to be that the protein extraction method used was favorable for soluble cytoplasmic proteins, whereas many of the products of genes identified are associated with cell membranes and intracellular structures such as microtubules and actin filaments. It is also possible that the increased expression of some of the genes had not yet resulted in increased protein synthesis within the 24 h period following injury. In addition, as mentioned earlier, the sensitivity of the two methods is very different and many proteins whose genes showed changes are not present in cord tissue in concentrations high enough to be detected by silver staining of separated bands. In addition we have identified previously that some of the observed changes in the bands intensity are due to post translational modifications rather than changes in corresponding gene expression [32,33].

General Discussion

The most striking observation from this study is the large number of genes and proteins that change their level of expression within 24h after spinal cord injury in the neonatal opossum. The number of these changes was much greater following injury at P28 compared to P7, particularly when considering transcriptome changes. At P7 there were no genes that showed significant decrease (i.e., ≥−2 fold) in expression. In contrast most of (84%) of the proteins that changed expression at P28 were downregulated. This could in part be due to tissue loss following injury, thus reducing the amount of protein-containing tissue sampled but is also likely to be a reflection of the timing of these experiments: early tissue loss is followed by a later adaptation of the cellular response, as reflected by transcriptome changes detected.

The comparatively muted response to injury at P7 may indicate that the injury was introduced at an age when substantial spinal cord growth occurs as part of normal development and that this was little impaired by the trauma. Whereas by P28, when many of the spinal cord tracts are established, the response is more "adult-like" in the inability of the injured spinal cord to display a regenerative response [25]. By far the largest category of genes to respond to injury was the immune/inflammatory group. There were twenty-four genes that changed expression after injury at both ages, all increasing their expression. Nineteen changed to a similar extent at both ages (< two times difference between the ages). More genes in this category showed a larger increase in expression at P7 than at P28; only three novel genes at P28 showed substantially higher increases (322, 14 and 9.3 fold) in expression than at P7 (Fig. 5).

In vivo compared to *in vitro* opossum spinal cord injury experiments

Several previous studies have assessed the importance of the developmental stage and the consequences of spinal cord injury on patterns of gene expression in the opossum [28–30]. In these investigations, changes in specific families of genes associated with axonal growth as well as inhibitory molecules were emphasized. In contrast, more extensive changes in gene expression were documented in the present study. There are several possibilities for these differences that relate to the experimental design of the studies. At a technical level the coverage of RNA Sequencing is potentially much greater than that of a microarray chip. In papers in which an isolated spinal cord preparation was used [29,30] the tissues were bathed in a room temperature solution (24–25°C; [28]) during and after the spinal cord injury. Mild levels of hypothermia are known to be neuroprotective after brain and spinal cord injury and may alter specific secondary injury mechanisms including alterations in gene expression [106–109]. Thus, the hypothermic conditions that were used in the isolated opossum spinal cord preparation may have influenced some injury-induced gene expression changes compared to *in vivo* spinal cord injury preparations conducted at normal body temperature (31–34°C in the opossum [110]). In addition, because these opossum studies used an isolated spinal cord preparation, the involvement of acute systemic responses to spinal cord injury would also be expected to differ in comparison to *in vivo* injury conditions, due to the lack of blood circulation. Thus the well-described inflammatory response to spinal cord injury involving infiltration of different types of immune cells after experimental and clinical neurotrauma [111–113] would not occur in the absence of a circulation. These injury-modeling conditions may therefore help explain some differences in patterns of gene expression between the *in vitro* versus *in vivo* spinal cord injury studies. The relative contributions of lower temperature and absence of immune cell infiltration are hard to judge. The lower temperature of the *in vitro* preparations does not appear to have suppressed other aspects of the response to injury compared to the absence of an immune/inflammatory response. Since there was a lack of neurite growth across the lesion both at P13 *in vitro* and P28 *in vivo* it seems unlikely that the large number of additional immune/inflammatory genes that changed their expression at P28 compared to P7 *in vivo* was a major factor in this lack of neurite outgrowth. Also it is apparent from the Supplementary data in Mladinic *et al.*, [29] that only a few immune genes were detected and they changed little in response to injury at either age. This would suggest that the lack of a circulation in the *in vitro* preparations might have been the main factor in the absence of much of an inflammatory response in these isolated preparations. In addition, it is clear from studies of injured adult spinal cord that changes in expression of immune and inflammatory genes and proteins are mainly of significance in relation to secondary injury that follows the primary injury with a time course that has been variously estimated to be days to weeks (see [114,115]).

To what extent may the observed changes in gene and protein expression account for the lack of neurite outgrowth at P28 following injury?

Twenty-nine of thirty-four genes suggested to influence neurite growth (Table 2) only changed their expression to a limited extent in the range +3 to −3 fold change, with equal numbers up- and downregulated. In addition, key inhibitory genes either did not change their expression (*Nogo, Mag, Mog*) or were downregulated (*Mbp, Plp1*), rather than upregulated. Thus it seems unlikely that the explanation for the lack of neurite outgrowth is accounted for by inhibitory activity of the protein products of these genes. There were similar numbers of opposing changes in protein expression for this functional group after injury at P28 (Fig. 7, Table S5) and myelin basic protein was downregulated as was its gene. Most extracellular matrix genes (Table 3) also showed relatively small and opposing changes in expression, but there were some notable exceptions. Three genes showed very large increases in expression: olfactomedin 4 (480 fold), *Mmp1* (104 fold) and *Papln* (*papilin*, proteoglycan-like sulfated glycoprotein, 152 fold). One gene in this category showed a marked decrease in expression: integrin α4 (−57 fold). Overall, there were some thirty-four genes that increased their expression by >10 fold following injury at P28 and only four that showed reduced expression of >10 fold. Of the upregulated genes almost half were in the immune and blood-related functional categories, which for reasons outlined above were probably not contributing to the lack of neurite outgrowth. Only three of the substantially upregulated genes (*Olfm4, Mmp-1, Papln*) and one markedly downregulated gene (*Itga4*) are in a functional category (see Table 5) in which there is evidence for effects on neurite outgrowth. Proteoglycans generally seem to have inhibitory effects on neurite outgrowth [20]. *Mmp-1* has been reported to be increased by one day after injury in adult spinal cord, but MMPs as a group appear to have rather complex effects following spinal cord injury, some deleterious and others beneficial [116,117]. It is not known what the function of olfactomedin-4 may be in spinal cord injury, but it binds to cadherins and lectins [57]. Olfactomedin-1 promotes neurite outgrowth by binding to the Nogo A receptor complex (NgR1) and inhibiting the growth cone collapse induced by myelin inhibitors [118]. Several integrins (α6, α7, α9 and β1) have been implicated in promoting axon growth during development and in the response of the peripheral nervous system to injury [63]. Integrin α4β1 is expressed by leukocytes that invade spinal cord tissue following injury [64]. However, it has also been described as having a role in regenerating growth cones following injury to sensory neurons where it provides a signaling pathway for re-expression of fibronectin (for references see [119]). Thus its downregulation could be contributing to the lack of neurite outgrowth in P28 injured spinal cord, particularly if combined with inhibitory effects of MMP1 and papilin.

An additional possibility is that changes in the growth potential of brainstem neurons with axons that project to the spinal cord may be reduced by P28 in opossums. This is an aspect of the failure of neural regeneration in injured adult spinal cord that has been little studied. However, its importance is suggested by the experiments of Kobayashi et al. [120] who showed that infusion of BDNF and NT-4/5 prevented atrophy of rat rubrospinal axons after cervical axotomy. This treatment evoked upregulation of a number of regeneration-associated genes, which they considered correlated with an increased regenerative capacity of axotomized rubrospinal neurons.

Comparing proteome results from segments of spinal cord rostral and caudal to the transection

The present study reports on the changes in gene and protein expression in the segment of spinal cord rostral to the site of transection of the spinal cord. These changes would be expected to affect centrally projecting neurites from sensory neurons, should they regenerate following injury. There is only limited information about changes in gene expression in the segment of cord caudal to the site of injury in postnatal opossums [24]. That study used a combination of a mouse microarray of genes encoding cytokines and chemokines with some qPCR validation, as discussed above. However, we have previously published a proteomic analysis of the spinal cord segment caudal to the injury in the same animals that have been used in the present study for the segments of cord rostral to the lesion [32].

There were ten proteins in the P7 injured spinal cords that were common to the two segments of cord (Table 6). All but two of these had bands that were decreased in density compared to the controls. Cofilin and peptidylprolyl isomerase A-like proteins were reduced in the rostral spinal cord and increased in the caudal segment. In the P28 injured spinal cord there were fourteen proteins that were common to both segments of cord (Table 7). All but four of the proteins had bands that changed in the same direction in both cord segments, but several of these proteins had bands that increased or decreased in different fractions. As observed at P7, cofilin and peptidylprolyl isomerase a-like decreased in the rostral segment but increased in the caudal segment. Annexin-A2 decreased in the rostral cord but increased in the caudal segment. Tropomyosin on the other hand increased in the rostral segment but decreased caudally. There were more proteins that were identified as changing their regulation only in one segment or the other. These are listed in Tables S7A & S7B for P7+24 h and Tables S7C & S7D for P28+24 h. As we discussed in detail previously [32] some of the observed changes in identified proteins were more likely to be due to post-translational modifications than changes in the expression of their coding genes.

Limitations of the Study

This study was restricted to the changes in gene and protein expression that could be identified 24 h after injury at P7 or at P28 in the cord segment rostral to the transection (T10). Further changes in gene and protein expression may well occur at later times following injury as suggested by studies in injured adult spinal cord [16,103].

This study was initiated early in the adoption of RNA-Seq and involved a small number of samples. Although technical variability is low, a large degree of biological variability was observed, consistent with level of manipulation required in the experimental preparation of samples. This variability is likely to have reduced the number of genes observed to be statistically significantly differentially expressed. This reduced power necessitated the simplification of the analytical design to exclude direct modeling of interaction between development and injury.

In presenting the data we have concentrated on functional categories that previous work in the injured adult spinal cord suggested to be important for the characteristic failure of neurites to grow following injury to the adult spinal cord. This is something that has been known since the time of Ramon y Cajal [121]. Our description has tended to emphasize the genes that showed the largest changes in expression, many of which had not previously been implicated in the failure of neurite outgrowth following spinal cord injury. Since little is known about the functions of some of these genes (e.g., olfactomedin 480 fold; triadin 206 fold and several novel opossum genes, see Table S3) their role in failure of neurite outgrowth is speculative, as was considered in the General Discussion above.

An alternative possibility is that relatively small changes in expression of a large number of key genes may account for the lack of neurite outgrowth. This has been considered in the General Discussion, above.

An important limitation on providing an overall functional view of the large number of expression changes in both genes and proteins is that we were unsuccessful in attempts at pathway analysis, with identified pathways consisting of small number of genes with only one differentially expressed member. We hypothesize that this was primarily because of limitations in the functional annotation of the opossum genome. We also eschewed the use of heat maps for presenting our data in favour of a numerical approach of presenting data in graphs and tables. The visual approach of heat maps puts undue emphasis on expression differences by using colour coding which, although eye catching, may give a misleading impression of the statistical validity of differences in gene expression.

The number of antibodies available that cross react with opossum material is very limited. At this stage it is therefore not possible to define in which cell populations these genes and their protein products are expressed. In future studies it is planned to localize some of the key genes using *in situ* hybridisation.

It may be considered by some that the lack of overlap between the genes we have identified in RNA-Seq analysis and the protein gene products identified in the proteomic part of the study may indicate a fault in the experimental design. There are several reasons for this lack of overlap. The most obvious one is the difference in the sensitivity of the two methods as detection of the

Table 5. Genes that changed most in expression (±≥10 FOLD) 24 h following spinal cord injury at P28.

SYMBOL	GENE DESCRIPTION	FOLD
MOST UPREGULATED GENES		
IMMUNE & INFLAMMATORY		
Novel	C-C motif chemokine similar to CCL8 and CCL13	322
Dok3	docking protein 3	266
Novel	C-C motif chemokine similar to CCL2, CCL7, CCL8, CCL11 and CCL13	197
Pstpip1	proline-serine-threonine phosphatase interacting protein 1	167
Lrrc33	leucine rich repeat containing 33 Official name NRROS	160
Novel	similar to TARM1 T cell-interacting, activating receptor on myeloid cells 1	22
Il1b	interleukin 1, β	20
Vav1	VAV1 guanine nucleotide exchange factor	17
Osmr	oncostatin M receptor	14
Lgals4	lectin, galactoside-binding, soluble, 4	14
Amh	anti-Mullerian hormone	12
Marco	macrophage receptor with collagenous structure	12
Igsf22	immunoglobulin superfamily, member 22	12
Novel	LOC100020928 C-C motif chemokine similar to CCL3 and CCL4	10
BLOOD-RELATED		
Novel	similar to HPR, haptoglobin-related protein	99
Novel	similar to TARM1 T cell-interacting, activating receptor on myeloid cells 1	22
EXTRACELLULAR MATRIX		
Olfm4	olfactomedin 4, ECM glycoprotein that facilitates cell adhesion.	480
METALLOTHIONINE		
Mmp1	matrix metallopeptidase 1 (interstitial collagenase)	104
PROTEOGLYCAN		
Papln	papilin, proteoglycan-like sulfated glycoprotein	152
ACTIN, MYOSIN & RELATED		
Trdn	triadin	206
Myl1	myosin, light chain 1, alkali; skeletal, fast	139
Mylpf	myosin light chain, phosphorylatable, fast skeletal muscle	22
Myh4	myosin, heavy chain 4, skeletal muscle	18
TRANSPORTERS		
Slc23a3	solute carrier family 23, sodium-dependent vitamin C transporter 3	12
DEVELOPMENT & STRUCTURE		
fuz	fuzzy homolog (Drosophila) cell polarity, ciliogenesis & cell movement.	21
hoxb1	homeobox B1, transcription factor role in morphogenesis	12
des	desmin	12
MEMBRANE		
Novel	novel protein with potential transmembrane domains	254
Novel	novel protein with potential transmembrane domains	241
Tmem106a	transmembrane protein 106A	157
ENZYMES & METABOLISM		
Pstpip1	proline-serine-threonine phosphatase interacting protein 1	167
Novel	similar to ATP13A5 ATPase type 13A5	23
MISCELLANEOUS		
Ttc40	tetratricopeptide repeat domain 40	89
ZINC FINGER		
Novel	similar to ZC3H13 zinc finger CCCH-type containing 13	352
MOST DOWN REGULATED GENES		
Itga4	integrin, α 4 (antigen CD49D, alpha 4 subunit of VLA-4 receptor)	−57
Novel	similar to CLCNKA/CLCNKB chloride channel	−27

Table 5. Cont.

SYMBOL	GENE DESCRIPTION	FOLD
Igfbpl1	insulin-like growth factor binding protein-like 1	−11
Gxylt2	glucoside xylosyltransferase 2	−16

doi:10.1371/journal.pone.0099080.t005

protein by even silver staining is several orders of magnitude less than that for RNA. The second main difference is the timing of the extraction protocol—many genes are transcribed much earlier than the translation of their products. Our study was performed at one time point only (24 h post injury). The third, and most biologically relevant possibility is that proteomic analysis identifies not only changes in the concentration levels of individual proteins but also in their post-translational modifications. This would be difficult to detect at the transcriptome level. That this may be the case has been suggested in our earlier proteomic study in which RT-qPCR was used to examine the expression levels of the genes of some of the proteins identified as changing following injury. Many of the identified proteins showed changes in their isoelectric mobility but not in their gene expression [32]. This is important because it indicates that analysis of the transcriptome alone may in fact not provide a comprehensive overall picture of changes occurring in the whole tissue in response to injury.

Despite these limitations the unique nature of these data provide a valuable resource for the investigation of the *a priori* hypotheses of mechanisms of spinal cord regeneration and as a foundation for future studies.

Conclusions

Morphological repair and functional recovery following spinal cord injury requires a complex but coordinated set of cellular responses; they are particularly complicated because they involve sites close to the injury (local) as well as distant locations such as neuronal cells bodies of axotomised axons. The very large number of genes that changed their expression level significantly following injury, particularly in the more mature spinal cord at P28, is very striking. It reinforces microarray studies of injured adult spinal cord that also show expression changes in a large number of genes [16] indicating just how complicated the response of the spinal cord to injury is. It seems unlikely that the preoccupation of most studies of trying to identify a single gene or protein will provide a therapy for patients with spinal cord injuries, unless key upstream regulatory genes and their proteins can be identified.

In the present study we report on the changes detected in transcript and protein expression that follow complete spinal cord transection at two different ages (P7 and P28) in postnatal *Monodelphis domestica.* P7 pups were chosen because at this age the animals show substantial axon growth across the lesion. This axon growth is partly regenerative from injured axons and partly due to axon growth that occurs as continued postnatal development of the spinal cord [21]. When these animals reach adulthood their locomotor behavior is essentially normal [25]. P28 animals were chosen for comparison because following a similar complete transection there is no axon growth across the lesion although the animals, when adult, exhibit weight-bearing locomotion [25]. The present study was designed to see whether short-term changes in gene and protein expression that occur after a complete spinal transection at T10 might account for these differences in axon growth and subsequent behaviour. Although some immune/inflammatory genes were highly upregulated (Table S3), comparison of the results presented in this study together with previously published work on *Monodelphis* spinal cord *in vitro* suggests that immunological/inflammatory genes may not be involved in the differential response to primary injury we observe at the two ages. However, as we discuss above, they are more likely to be important in the secondary phase of the process.

From the analysis of known functional groups of genes and proteins presented here we conclude that there appear to be at

Table 6. Proteins that changed level 24 h following spinal cord injury at P7 in *Monodelphis* in segments rostral and caudal to site of transection.

Protein	Rostral SC	Caudal SC
14-3-3	↓	↑↓
cofilin	↓	↑
destrin	↓	↓
Hemoglobin α	↑↓	↓
Hemoglobin subunit β M	↑	↑↓
Peptidylprolyl isomerase a-like	↓	↑
Pyruvate dehydrogenase	↓	↓
Tubulin α	↓	↓
Tubulin β	↓	↓
ubiquitin	↓	↓

↑increased band density, ↓ decreased band density. Some proteins showed an increase or decrease in different fractions (↑↓).

Table 7. Proteins that changed level 24 h following spinal cord injury at P28.in *Monodelphis* in segments rostral and caudal to site of transection.

Protein	Rostral SC	Caudal SC
14-3-3 protein	↑	↑↓
albumin	↑	↑↓
Alpha enolase	□	↑↓
Annexin-a2	↓	↑
ATP synthase subunit β, mitochondrial	↑	↑↓
cofilin	↓	↑
GFAP	↑	↑
Glyceraldehyde 3 phosphate dehydrogenase	↑↓	↑↓
Hemoglobin subunit β M	↑↓	↑↓
Neurofilament L subunit	↑	↓
Peptidylprolyl isomerase A-like	↓	↑
Tropomyosin	↑	↓
Tubulin α	↑↓	↑↓
ubiquitin	↑↓	↑

↑increased band density, ↓ decreased band density. Some proteins showed an increase or decrease in different fractions (↑↓).

least three not mutually exclusive general mechanisms that may be involved in the age-related response to injury and in particular the lack of neurite outgrowth following injury at P28:

(i) Changes in expression of genes and proteins that are known to be involved in axon guidance and inhibition (Table 2). However, these were not significant at P7 and at P28 they were relatively small and many were in opposing directions. One example is two of the key *Rho* activating genes (*Arhgap6*, 3.1 fold; *Arhgef10*, −2.1 fold) that are central to control of many of the downstream neurite inhibitory factors. In addition, almost all of the myelin-associated genes and their proteins were either unchanged or downregulated (Tables 2 and 6) which perhaps makes this explanation less likely.

(ii) Down regulation of essential neurotrophic genes in brain stem neurons with axonal projections to the spinal cord. This will be the subject of a separate study (Saunders et al., in preparation).

(iii) Major changes in expression of a few genes at P28 that produce extracellular matrix proteins (Table 3). Most of these have not previously been described in studies of adult spinal cord injury, but they are members of gene families that have been implicated. These seem to be plausible candidates to explain the failure of neurite growth following injury that will be worthy of further study.

This study provides a large database of changes in expression of genes and proteins at 24 h after spinal cord injury at two ages in postnatal *Monodelphis*. We have provided a detailed analysis based on functional groups thought to be important in the response of the spinal cord to injury. There were several novel genes that showed strikingly large changes in expression following injury at P28. Their identity and function will need to be determined before their roles in the response to injury can be considered.

Supporting Information

Table S1 Data used for analysis of gene expression changes 24 h following spinal cord transection at P7. Gene symbols, description and ENSEMBL ID shown. Log2FC = Log_2 fold change. These values were derived by comparing expression at P7+24 h with P8 control. See Methods for details of statistical analysis used. Updated 13 May 2013.

Table S2 Data used for analysis of gene expression changes 24 h following spinal cord transection at P28. Gene symbols, description and ENSEMBL ID shown. Log2FC = Log_2 fold change. These values were derived by comparing expression at P28+24 h with P29 control. See Methods for details of statistical analysis used. Updated 13 May 2014.

Table S3 Gene expression P28+24 h following spinal cord transection. Genes categorized by function with their ID and description included. FC = Fold Change compared to P29 controls. Updated 13 May 2014.

Table S4 Proteins that changed expression level 24 h following spinal cord injury at P7 in *Monodelphis domestica*. Arrows indicate direction of change in gel band density (upregulation ↑or downregulation ↓). Relative change is densitometry value of gel band at P7+24 h compared to P8 control. Gene name symbol or provisional ID in genome and protein function are included.

Table S5 Proteins that changed expression level 24 h following spinal cord injury at P28 in *Monodelphis domestica*. Arrows indicate direction of change in gel band density (upregulation ↑ or downregulation ↓). Relative change is densitometry value of gel band at P28+24 h compared to P29 control. Gene name, symbol or provisional ID in genome and protein function are included.

Table S6 Proteomic results of identified proteins in different fractions and bands compared with expression of their respective genes in the transcriptome. ***Column A*** shows fraction in which protein was identified, ***Column B*** shows band in gel in which protein was identified. Note that some proteins were identified in more than one fraction or band. ***Column C*** is ENSEMBL protein ID, where known. ***Column D*** is protein name. ***Column E*** and ***F*** show whether protein band density was increased ≥0.5 compared to age-matched controls 24 h following spinal cord injury at P7 or P28. ***Column G*** shows corresponding gene symbol or name. ***Column H*** shows ENSEMBL gene ID. ***Column I*** and ***J*** show gene expression level 24 h following injury at P7 or P28. Note the relative lack of correlation between identified changes in the transcriptome and the proteome. Updated 13 May 2014

Table S7 A. Proteins that were identified as changing expression level in the spinal cord *rostral* but not caudal to the site of transection 24 h after injury at P7. ↑ increased band density, ↓ decreased band density. Some proteins showed an increase or decrease in different fractions (↑↓). **B. Proteins that were identified as changing in expression level in the spinal cord *caudal* but not rostral to the site of transection 24 h after injury at P7.** ↑ increased band density, ↓ decreased band density. Some proteins showed an increase or decrease in different fractions (↑↓). **C.** *Monodelphis* spinal cord. Proteins that were identified in the spinal cord *rostral* but not caudal to the site of transection 24 h after injury at P28. ↑ increased band density, ↓ decreased band density. Some proteins showed an increase or decrease in different fractions (↑↓). **D:** *Monodelphis* spinal cord. Proteins that were identified in the spinal cord *caudal* but not rostral to the site of transection 24 h after injury at P28. ↑ increased band density, ↓ decreased band density. Some proteins showed an increase or decrease in different fractions (↑↓).

Author Contributions

Conceived and designed the experiments: NRS NMN KMD BJW SAL DLS CJE MDH MW HL JT RDM AIS WDD. Performed the experiments: NRS NMN KMD BJW SAL DLS CJE MDH MW HL JT RDM AIS WDD. Analyzed the data: NRS NMN KMD BJW SAL DLS CJE MDH MW HL JT RDM AIS WDD. Contributed reagents/materials/analysis tools: NRS NMN KMD BJW SAL DLS CJE MDH MW HL JT RDM AIS WDD. Wrote the paper: NRS NMN KMD BJW SAL DLS CJE MDH MW HL JT RDM AIS WDD.

References

1. Aguayo AJ, David S, Bray GM (1981) Influences of the glial environment on the elongation of axons after injury: transplantation studies in adult rodents. The Journal of experimental biology 95: 231–240.
2. David S, Aguayo AJ (1981) Axonal elongation into peripheral nervous system "bridges" after central nervous system injury in adult rats. Science 214: 931–933.
3. Tello F (1911) La influencia del neurotropismo en la regeneracion de los centros nerviosos. Trab Laborator Invest Biol University Madrid 9: 123–159.
4. Akbik F, Cafferty WB, Strittmatter SM (2011) Myelin associated inhibitors: A link between injury-induced and experience-dependent plasticity. Experimental neurology.
5. Buchli AD, Schwab ME (2005) Inhibition of Nogo: a key strategy to increase regeneration, plasticity and functional recovery of the lesioned central nervous system. Annals of medicine 37: 556–567.
6. Bradbury EJ, Carter LM (2011) Manipulating the glial scar: chondroitinase ABC as a therapy for spinal cord injury. Brain research bulletin 84: 306–316.
7. Fawcett JW (2006) Overcoming inhibition in the damaged spinal cord. Journal of neurotrauma 23: 371–383.
8. Galtrey CM, Fawcett JW (2007) The role of chondroitin sulfate proteoglycans in regeneration and plasticity in the central nervous system. Brain research reviews 54: 1–18.
9. Hurtado A, Marcillo A, Frydel B, Bunge MB, Bramlett HM, et al. (2012) Anti-CD11d monoclonal antibody treatment for rat spinal cord compression injury. Experimental neurology 233: 606–611.
10. Pinzon A, Marcillo A, Pabon D, Bramlett HM, Bunge MB, et al. (2008) A re-assessment of erythropoietin as a neuroprotective agent following rat spinal cord compression or contusion injury. Experimental neurology 213: 129–136.
11. Pinzon A, Marcillo A, Quintana A, Stamler S, Bunge MB, et al. (2008) A re-assessment of minocycline as a neuroprotective agent in a rat spinal cord contusion model. Brain research 1243: 146–151.
12. Sharp KG, Flanagan LA, Yee KM, Steward O (2012) A re-assessment of a combinatorial treatment involving Schwann cell transplants and elevation of cyclic AMP on recovery of motor function following thoracic spinal cord injury in rats. Experimental neurology 233: 625–644.
13. Steward O, Sharp K, Yee KM, Hofstadter M (2008) A re-assessment of the effects of a Nogo-66 receptor antagonist on regenerative growth of axons and locomotor recovery after spinal cord injury in mice. Experimental neurology 209: 446–468.
14. Aimone JB, Leasure JL, Perreau VM, Thallmair M (2004) Spatial and temporal gene expression profiling of the contused rat spinal cord. Experimental neurology 189: 204–221.
15. Crack PJ, Gould J, Bye N, Ross S, Ali U, et al. (2009) The genomic profile of the cerebral cortex after closed head injury in mice: effects of minocycline. Journal of neural transmission 116: 1–12.
16. Verhaagen J, Van Kesteren RE, Bossers KA, Macgillavry HD, Mason MR, et al. (2012) Molecular target discovery for neural repair in the functional genomics era. Handbook of clinical neurology 109: 595–616.
17. Gris P, Murphy S, Jacob JE, Atkinson I, Brown A (2003) Differential gene expression profiles in embryonic, adult-injured and adult-uninjured rat spinal cords. Molecular and cellular neurosciences 24: 555–567.
18. Chen K, Deng S, Lu H, Zheng Y, Yang G, et al. (2013) RNA-seq characterization of spinal cord injury transcriptome in acute/subacute phases: a resource for understanding the pathology at the systems level. PloS one 8: e72567.
19. Kumamaru H, Ohkawa Y, Saiwai H, Yamada H, Kubota K, et al. (2012) Direct isolation and RNA-seq reveal environment-dependent properties of engrafted neural stem/progenitor cells. Nature communications 3: 1140.
20. Fawcett JW, Schwab ME, Montani L, Brazda N, Muller HW (2012) Defeating inhibition of regeneration by scar and myelin components. Handbook of clinical neurology 109: 503–522.
21. Fry EJ, Stolp HB, Lane MA, Dziegielewska KM, Saunders NR (2003) Regeneration of supraspinal axons after complete transection of the thoracic spinal cord in neonatal opossums (Monodelphis domestica). J Comp Neurol 466: 422–444.
22. Saunders NR, Kitchener P, Knott GW, Nicholls JG, Potter A, et al. (1998) Development of walking, swimming and neuronal connections after complete spinal cord transection in the neonatal opossum, Monodelphis domestica. J Neurosci 18: 339–355.
23. Wang XM, Terman JR, Martin GF (1998) Regeneration of supraspinal axons after transection of the thoracic spinal cord in the developing opossum, Didelphis virginiana. J Comp Neurol 398: 83–97.
24. Lane MA, Truettner JS, Brunschwig JP, Gomez A, Bunge MB, et al. (2007) Age-related differences in the local cellular and molecular responses to injury in developing spinal cord of the opossum, Monodelphis domestica. Eur J Neurosci 25: 1725–1742.
25. Wheaton BJ, Callaway JK, Ek CJ, Dziegielewska KM, Saunders NR (2011) Spontaneous development of full weight-supported stepping after complete spinal cord transection in the neonatal opossum, Monodelphis domestica. PloS one 6: e26826.
26. Wheaton BJ, Noor NM, Whish SC, Truettner JS, Dietrich WD, et al. (2013) Weight-bearing locomotion in the developing opossum, Monodelphis domestica following spinal transection: remodeling of neuronal circuits caudal to lesion. PloS one 8: e71181.
27. Saunders NR, Balkwill P, Knott G, Habgood MD, Mollgard K, et al. (1992) Growth of axons through a lesion in the intact CNS of fetal rat maintained in long-term culture. Proc Biol Sci 250: 171–180.
28. Farlow DN, Vansant G, Cameron AA, Chang J, Khoh-Reiter S, et al. (2000) Gene expression monitoring for gene discovery in models of peripheral and central nervous system differentiation, regeneration, and trauma. Journal of cellular biochemistry 80: 171–180.
29. Mladinic M, Lefevre C, Del Bel E, Nicholls J, Digby M (2010) Developmental changes of gene expression after spinal cord injury in neonatal opossums. Brain research 1363: 20–39.
30. Mladinic M, Wintzer M, Del Bel E, Casseler C, Lazarevic D, et al. (2005) Differential expression of genes at stages when regeneration can and cannot

occur after injury to immature mammalian spinal cord. Cellular and molecular neurobiology 25: 407–426.
31. Mikkelsen TS, Wakefield MJ, Aken B, Amemiya CT, Chang JL, et al. (2007) Genome of the marsupial Monodelphis domestica reveals innovation in non-coding sequences. Nature 447: 167–177.
32. Noor NM, Steer DL, Wheaton BJ, Ek CJ, Truettner JS, et al. (2011) Age-dependent changes in the proteome following complete spinal cord transection in a postnatal South American opossum (Monodelphis domestica). PloS one 6: e27465.
33. Noor NM, Mollgard K, Wheaton BJ, Steer DL, Truettner JS, et al. (2013) Expression and cellular distribution of ubiquitin in response to injury in the developing spinal cord of Monodelphis domestica. PloS one 8: e62120.
34. Saunders NR, Adam E, Reader M, Mollgard K (1989) Monodelphis domestica (grey short-tailed opossum): an accessible model for studies of early neocortical development. Anat Embryol (Berl) 180: 227–236.
35. Langmead B, Salzberg SL (2012) Fast gapped-read alignment with Bowtie 2. Nature methods 9: 357–359.
36. Flicek P, Amode MR, Barrell D, Beal K, Brent S, et al. (2011) Ensembl 2011. Nucleic acids research 39: D800–806.
37. Anders A (2011) HTSeq: Analysing high-throughput sequencing data with Python. Available: http://www.huber.embl.de/users/anders/HTSeq. Accessed 2014, May 14.
38. Gentleman RC, Carey VJ, Bates DM, Bolstad B, Dettling M, et al. (2004) Bioconductor: open software development for computational biology and bioinformatics. Genome biology 5: R80.
39. McCarthy DJ, Chen Y, Smyth GK (2012) Differential expression analysis of multifactor RNA-Seq experiments with respect to biological variation. Nucleic acids research 40: 4288–4297.
40. Young MD, Wakefield MJ, Smyth GK, Oshlack A (2010) Gene ontology analysis for RNA-seq: accounting for selection bias. Genome biology 11: R14.
41. Gerner C, Frohwein U, Gotzmann J, Bayer E, Gelbmann D, et al. (2000) The Fas-induced apoptosis analyzed by high throughput proteome analysis. The Journal of biological chemistry 275: 39018–39026.
42. Dziegielewska KM, Daikuhara Y, Ohnishi T, Waite MP, Ek J, et al. (2000) Fetuin in the developing neocortex of the rat: distribution and origin. J Comp Neurol 423: 373–388.
43. McKerracher L, Ferraro GB, Fournier AE (2012) Rho signaling and axon regeneration. International review of neurobiology 105: 117–140.
44. Parra ZE, Baker ML, Lopez AM, Trujillo J, Volpe JM, et al. (2009) TCR mu recombination and transcription relative to the conventional TCR during postnatal development in opossums. Journal of immunology 182: 154–163.
45. Jameson J, Ugarte K, Chen N, Yachi P, Fuchs E, et al. (2002) A role for skin gammadelta T cells in wound repair. Science 296: 747–749.
46. Wang X, Sharp AR, Miller RD (2012) Early postnatal B cell ontogeny and antibody repertoire maturation in the opossum, Monodelphis domestica. PloS one 7: e45931.
47. Pillai S, Netravali IA, Cariappa A, Mattoo H (2012) Siglecs and immune regulation. Annual review of immunology 30: 357–392.
48. Vogt L, Schmitz N, Kurrer MO, Bauer M, Hinton HI, et al. (2006) VSIG4, a B7 family-related protein, is a negative regulator of T cell activation. The Journal of clinical investigation 116: 2817–2826.
49. Miller RD (2010) Those other mammals: the immunoglobulins and T cell receptors of marsupials and monotremes. Seminars in immunology 22: 3–9.
50. Duffy P, Wang X, Siegel CS, Tu N, Henkemeyer M, et al. (2012) Myelin-derived ephrinB3 restricts axonal regeneration and recovery after adult CNS injury. Proceedings of the National Academy of Sciences of the United States of America 109: 5063–5068.
51. Pernet V, Schwab ME (2012) The role of Nogo-A in axonal plasticity, regrowth and repair. Cell and tissue research 349: 97–104.
52. Goldshmit Y, Spanevello MD, Tajouri S, Li L, Rogers F, et al. (2011) EphA4 blockers promote axonal regeneration and functional recovery following spinal cord injury in mice. PloS one 6: e24636.
53. Hollis ER II, Zou Y (2012) Expression of the Wnt signaling system in central nervous system axon guidance and regeneration. Frontiers in molecular neuroscience 5: 5.
54. Goldshmit Y, Galea MP, Wise G, Bartlett PF, Turnley AM (2004) Axonal regeneration and lack of astrocytic gliosis in EphA4-deficient mice. J Neurosci 24: 10064–10073.
55. Cruz-Orengo L, Figueroa JD, Torrado A, Puig A, Whittemore SR, et al. (2007) Reduction of EphA4 receptor expression after spinal cord injury does not induce axonal regeneration or return of tcMMEP response. Neurosci Lett 418: 49–54.
56. Zhang J, Liu WL, Tang DC, Chen L, Wang M, et al. (2002) Identification and characterization of a novel member of olfactomedin-related protein family, hGC-1, expressed during myeloid lineage development. Gene 283: 83–93.
57. Liu W, Chen L, Zhu J, Rodgers GP (2006) The glycoprotein hGC-1 binds to cadherin and lectins. Experimental cell research 312: 1785–1797.
58. Kulkarni NH, Karavanich CA, Atchley WR, Anholt RR (2000) Characterization and differential expression of a human gene family of olfactomedin-related proteins. Genetical research 76: 41–50.
59. Liu W, Yan M, Liu Y, Wang R, Li C, et al. (2010) Olfactomedin 4 down-regulates innate immunity against Helicobacter pylori infection. Proceedings of the National Academy of Sciences of the United States of America 107: 11056–11061.
60. Xu J, Kim GM, Ahmed SH, Yan P, Xu XM, et al. (2001) Glucocorticoid receptor-mediated suppression of activator protein-1 activation and matrix metalloproteinase expression after spinal cord injury. The Journal of neuroscience: the official journal of the Society for Neuroscience 21: 92–97.
61. Buss A, Pech K, Kakulas BA, Martin D, Schoenen J, et al. (2007) Matrix metalloproteinases and their inhibitors in human traumatic spinal cord injury. BMC neurology 7: 17.
62. Zhang H, Adwanikar H, Werb Z, Noble-Haeusslein LJ (2010) Matrix metalloproteinases and neurotrauma: evolving roles in injury and reparative processes. The Neuroscientist: a review journal bringing neurobiology, neurology and psychiatry 16: 156–170.
63. Eva R, Andrews MR, Franssen EH, Fawcett JW (2012) Intrinsic mechanisms regulating axon regeneration: an integrin perspective. International review of neurobiology 106: 75–104.
64. Fleming JC, Bao F, Chen Y, Hamilton EF, Relton JK, et al. (2008) Alpha4beta1 integrin blockade after spinal cord injury decreases damage and improves neurological function. Experimental neurology 214: 147–159.
65. Hall A, Lalli G (2010) Rho and Ras GTPases in axon growth, guidance, and branching. Cold Spring Harbor perspectives in biology 2: a001818.
66. Redies C, Heyder J, Kohoutek T, Staes K, Van Roy F (2008) Expression of protocadherin-1 (Pcdh1) during mouse development. Developmental dynamics: an official publication of the American Association of Anatomists 237: 2496–2505.
67. Kubota F, Murakami T, Tajika Y, Yorifuji H (2008) Expression of protocadherin 18 in the CNS and pharyngeal arches of zebrafish embryos. The International journal of developmental biology 52: 397–405.
68. Lin J, Wang C, Redies C (2012) Expression of delta-protocadherins in the spinal cord of the chicken embryo. The Journal of comparative neurology 520: 1509–1531.
69. Biancheri R, Rosano C, Denegri L, Lamantea E, Pinto F, et al. (2013) Expanded spectrum of Pelizaeus-Merzbacher-like disease: literature revision and description of a novel GJC2 mutation in an unusually severe form. European journal of human genetics: EJHG 21: 34–39.
70. Isaksson J, Farooque M, Holtz A, Hillered L, Olsson Y (1999) Expression of ICAM-1 and CD11b after experimental spinal cord injury in rats. Journal of neurotrauma 16: 165–173.
71. Hamada Y, Ikata T, Katoh S, Nakauchi K, Niwa M, et al. (1996) Involvement of an intercellular adhesion molecule 1-dependent pathway in the pathogenesis of secondary changes after spinal cord injury in rats. Journal of neurochemistry 66: 1525–1531.
72. Hirokawa N, Niwa S, Tanaka Y (2010) Molecular motors in neurons: transport mechanisms and roles in brain function, development, and disease. Neuron 68: 610–638.
73. van den Berg R, Hoogenraad CC (2012) Molecular motors in cargo trafficking and synapse assembly. Advances in experimental medicine and biology 970: 173–196.
74. Kneussel M, Wagner W (2013) Myosin motors at neuronal synapses: drivers of membrane transport and actin dynamics. Nature reviews Neuroscience 14: 233–247.
75. Knudson CM, Stang KK, Moomaw CR, Slaughter CA, Campbell KP (1993) Primary structure and topological analysis of a skeletal muscle-specific junctional sarcoplasmic reticulum glycoprotein (triadin). The Journal of biological chemistry 268: 12646–12654.
76. Dulhunty A, Wei L, Beard N (2009) Junctin - the quiet achiever. The Journal of physiology 587: 3135–3137.
77. Li C, Dong S, Wang H, Hu Y (2011) Microarray analysis of gene expression changes in the brains of NR2B-induced memory-enhanced mice. Neuroscience 197: 121–131.
78. Seale SM, Feng Q, Agarwal AK, El-Alfy AT (2012) Neurobehavioral and transcriptional effects of acrylamide in juvenile rats. Pharmacology, biochemistry, and behavior 101: 77–84.
79. Dentice M, Bandyopadhyay A, Gereben B, Callebaut I, Christoffolete MA, et al. (2005) The Hedgehog-inducible ubiquitin ligase subunit WSB-1 modulates thyroid hormone activation and PTHrP secretion in the developing growth plate. Nature cell biology 7: 698–705.
80. Choi DW, Seo YM, Kim EA, Sung KS, Ahn JW, et al. (2008) Ubiquitination and degradation of homeodomain-interacting protein kinase 2 by WD40 repeat/SOCS box protein WSB-1. The Journal of biological chemistry 283: 4682–4689.
81. Ponyeam W, Hagen T (2012) Characterization of the Cullin7 E3 ubiquitin ligase—heterodimerization of cullin substrate receptors as a novel mechanism to regulate cullin E3 ligase activity. Cellular signalling 24: 290–295.
82. Dealy MJ, Nguyen KV, Lo J, Gstaiger M, Krek W, et al. (1999) Loss of Cul1 results in early embryonic lethality and dysregulation of cyclin E. Nature genetics 23: 245–248.
83. Singer JD, Gurian-West M, Clurman B, Roberts JM (1999) Cullin-3 targets cyclin E for ubiquitination and controls S phase in mammalian cells. Genes & development 13: 2375–2387.
84. Arai T, Kasper JS, Skaar JR, Ali SH, Takahashi C, et al. (2003) Targeted disruption of p185/Cul7 gene results in abnormal vascular morphogenesis. Proceedings of the National Academy of Sciences of the United States of America 100: 9855–9860.

85. Pei XH, Bai F, Li Z, Smith MD, Whitewolf G, et al. (2011) Cytoplasmic CUL9/PARC ubiquitin ligase is a tumor suppressor and promotes p53-dependent apoptosis. Cancer research 71: 2969–2977.
86. Tasaki T, Sohr R, Xia Z, Hellweg R, Hortnagl H, et al. (2007) Biochemical and genetic studies of UBR3, a ubiquitin ligase with a function in olfactory and other sensory systems. The Journal of biological chemistry 282: 18510–18520.
87. Seo JH, Zilber Y, Babayeva S, Liu J, Kyriakopoulos P, et al. (2011) Mutations in the planar cell polarity gene, Fuzzy, are associated with neural tube defects in humans. Human molecular genetics 20: 4324–4333.
88. Jungbluth S, Bell E, Lumsden A (1999) Specification of distinct motor neuron identities by the singular activities of individual Hox genes. Development 126: 2751–2758.
89. Yau TO, Kwan CT, Jakt LM, Stallwood N, Cordes S, et al. (2002) Auto/cross-regulation of Hoxb3 expression in posterior hindbrain and spinal cord. Developmental biology 252: 287–300.
90. Lin AW, Carpenter EM (2003) Hoxa10 and Hoxd10 coordinately regulate lumbar motor neuron patterning. Journal of neurobiology 56: 328–337.
91. Afjehi-Sadat L, Brejnikow M, Kang SU, Vishwanath V, Walder N, et al. (2010) Differential protein levels and post-translational modifications in spinal cord injury of the rat. Journal of proteome research 9: 1591–1597.
92. Xiao L, Ma ZL, Li X, Lin QX, Que HP, et al. (2005) cDNA microarray analysis of spinal cord injury and regeneration related genes in rat. Sheng li xue bao: [Acta physiologica Sinica] 57: 705–713.
93. Hu WH, Hausmann ON, Yan MS, Walters WM, Wong PK, et al. (2002) Identification and characterization of a novel Nogo-interacting mitochondrial protein (NIMP). Journal of neurochemistry 81: 36–45.
94. Zhu H, Santo A, Li Y (2012) The antioxidant enzyme peroxiredoxin and its protective role in neurological disorders. Experimental biology and medicine 237: 143–149.
95. Swisher JF, Khatri U, Feldman GM (2007) Annexin A2 is a soluble mediator of macrophage activation. Journal of leukocyte biology 82: 1174–1184.
96. Catania A (2008) Neuroprotective actions of melanocortins: a therapeutic opportunity. Trends in neurosciences 31: 353–360.
97. Iketani M, Iizuka A, Sengoku K, Kurihara Y, Nakamura F, et al. (2013) Regulation of neurite outgrowth mediated by localized phosphorylation of protein translational factor eEF2 in growth cones. Developmental neurobiology 73: 230–246.
98. McGraw J, Oschipok LW, Liu J, Hiebert GW, Mak CF, et al. (2004) Galectin-1 expression correlates with the regenerative potential of rubrospinal and spinal motoneurons. Neuroscience 128: 713–719.
99. McGraw J, Gaudet AD, Oschipok LW, Kadoya T, Horie H, et al. (2005) Regulation of neuronal and glial galectin-1 expression by peripheral and central axotomy of rat primary afferent neurons. Experimental neurology 195: 103–114.
100. Kurihara D, Ueno M, Tanaka T, Yamashita T (2010) Expression of galectin-1 in immune cells and glial cells after spinal cord injury. Neuroscience research 66: 265–270.
101. Lindquist S, Craig EA (1988) The heat-shock proteins. Annual review of genetics 22: 631–677.
102. Chen A, McEwen ML, Sun S, Ravikumar R, Springer JE (2010) Proteomic and phosphoproteomic analyses of the soluble fraction following acute spinal cord contusion in rats. Journal of neurotrauma 27: 263–274.
103. Yan X, Liu J, Luo Z, Ding Q, Mao X, et al. (2010) Proteomic profiling of proteins in rat spinal cord induced by contusion injury. Neurochemistry international 56: 971–983.
104. Reddy SJ, La Marca F, Park P (2008) The role of heat shock proteins in spinal cord injury. Neurosurgical focus 25: E4.
105. Daneman R, Zhou L, Agalliu D, Cahoy JD, Kaushal A, et al. (2010) The mouse blood-brain barrier transcriptome: a new resource for understanding the development and function of brain endothelial cells. PloS one 5: e13741.
106. Chatzipanteli K, Yanagawa Y, Marcillo AE, Kraydieh S, Yezierski RP, et al. (2000) Posttraumatic hypothermia reduces polymorphonuclear leukocyte accumulation following spinal cord injury in rats. Journal of neurotrauma 17: 321–332.
107. Kinoshita K, Chatzipanteli i K, Vitarbo E, Truettner JS, Alonso OF, et al. (2002) Interleukin-1beta messenger ribonucleic acid and protein levels after fluid-percussion brain injury in rats: importance of injury severity and brain temperature. Neurosurgery 51: 195–203; discussion 203.
108. Truettner JS, Alonso OF, Bramlett HM, Dietrich WD (2011) Therapeutic hypothermia alters microRNA responses to traumatic brain injury in rats. Journal of cerebral blood flow and metabolism: official journal of the International Society of Cerebral Blood Flow and Metabolism 31: 1897–1907.
109. Truettner JS, Suzuki T, Dietrich WD (2005) The effect of therapeutic hypothermia on the expression of inflammatory response genes following moderate traumatic brain injury in the rat. Brain research Molecular brain research 138: 124–134.
110. Kraus DB, Fadem BH (1987) Reproduction, development and physiology of the gray short-tailed opossum (Monodelphis domestica). Lab Anim Sci 37: 478–482.
111. Alexander JK, Popovich PG (2009) Neuroinflammation in spinal cord injury: therapeutic targets for neuroprotection and regeneration. Progress in brain research 175: 125–137.
112. Bethea JR, Dietrich WD (2002) Targeting the host inflammatory response in traumatic spinal cord injury. Current opinion in neurology 15: 355–360.
113. Fleming JC, Norenberg MD, Ramsay DA, Dekaban GA, Marcillo AE, et al. (2006) The cellular inflammatory response in human spinal cords after injury. Brain: a journal of neurology 129: 3249–3269.
114. Ek CJ, Habgood MD, Callaway JK, Dennis R, Dziegielewska KM, et al. (2010) Spatio-temporal progression of grey and white matter damage following contusion injury in rat spinal cord. PLoS One 5: e12021.
115. Ek CJ, Habgood MD, Dennis R, Dziegielewska KM, Mallard C, et al. (2012) Pathological changes in the white matter after spinal contusion injury in the rat. PloS one 7: e43484.
116. Veeravalli KK, Dasari VR, Rao JS (2012) Regulation of proteases after spinal cord injury. Journal of neurotrauma 29: 2251–2262.
117. Veeravalli KK, Dasari VR, Tsung AJ, Dinh DH, Gujrati M, et al. (2009) Human umbilical cord blood stem cells upregulate matrix metalloproteinase-2 in rats after spinal cord injury. Neurobiology of disease 36: 200–212.
118. Nakaya N, Sultana A, Lee HS, Tomarev SI (2012) Olfactomedin 1 interacts with the Nogo A receptor complex to regulate axon growth. The Journal of biological chemistry 287: 37171–37184.
119. Gardiner NJ (2011) Integrins and the extracellular matrix: key mediators of development and regeneration of the sensory nervous system. Developmental neurobiology 71: 1054–1072.
120. Kobayashi NR, Fan DP, Giehl KM, Bedard AM, Wiegand SJ, et al. (1997) BDNF and NT-4/5 prevent atrophy of rat rubrospinal neurons after cervical axotomy, stimulate GAP-43 and Talpha1-tubulin mRNA expression, and promote axonal regeneration. The Journal of neuroscience: the official journal of the Society for Neuroscience 17: 9583–9595.
121. Ramon y Cajal S (1928) Degeneration and regeneration of the nervous system. May RM, translator; De Felipe J, Jones EG, editors: Oxford University Press.

The Effects of Controlled Release of Neurotrophin-3 from PCLA Scaffolds on the Survival and Neuronal Differentiation of Transplanted Neural Stem Cells in a Rat Spinal Cord Injury Model

Shuo Tang[1]⁹, Xiang Liao[2]⁹, Bo Shi[3], Yanzhen Qu[4], Zeyu Huang[1], Qiang Lin[5]*, Xiaodong Guo[4]*, Fuxing Pei[1]*

1 Department of Orthopaedics, West China Hospital, Sichuan University, Chengdu, China, **2** Department of Pain Medicine, Shenzhen Nanshan Hospital, Shenzhen, China, **3** Department of Orthopaedics, Mianyang Center Hospital, Mianyang, China, **4** Department of Orthopaedics, Union Hospital, Tongji Medical College, Huazhong University of Science and Technology, Wuhan, China, **5** Department of Orthopaedics, Guangdong hospital of traditional Chinese medicine, Guangzhou, China

Abstract

Neural stem cells (NSCs) have emerged as a potential source for cell replacement therapy following spinal cord injury (SCI). However, poor survival and low neuronal differentiation remain major obstacles to the use of NSCs. Biomaterials with neurotrophic factors are promising strategies for promoting the proliferation and differentiation of NSCs. Silk fibroin (SF) matrices were demonstrated to successfully deliver growth factors and preserve their potency. In this study, by incorporating NT-3 into a SF coating, we successfully developed NT-3-immobilized scaffolds (membranes and conduits). Sustained release of bioactive NT-3 from the conduits for up to 8 weeks was achieved. Cell viability was confirmed using live/dead staining after 14 days in culture. The efficacy of the immobilized NT-3 was confirmed by assessing NSC neuronal differentiation in vitro. NSC neuronal differentiation was 55.2±4.1% on the NT-3-immobilized membranes, which was significantly higher than that on the NT-3 free membrane. Furthermore, 8 weeks after the NSCs were seeded into conduits and implanted in rats with a transected SCI, the conduit+NT-3+NSCs group achieved higher NSC survival (75.8±15.1%) and neuronal differentiation (21.5±5.2%) compared with the conduit+NSCs group. The animals that received the conduit+NT-3+NSCs treatment also showed improved functional outcomes, as well as increased axonal regeneration. These results indicate the feasibility of fabricating NT-3-immobilized scaffolds using the adsorption of NT-3/SF coating method, as well as the potential of these scaffolds to induce SCI repair by promoting survival and neuronal differentiation of transplanted NSCs.

Editor: Wenhui Hu, Temple University School of Medicine, United States of America

Funding: This work was financially supported by the National Natural Science Foundation of China (NSFC, No. 81401787, 81371939 and 81000812), the International Science & Technology Cooperation Program of China (2013DFG32690), as well as the Science & Technology Bureau of Chengdu City-West China Hospital Joint Foundation (ZH13034). The funders had no role in study design, data collection and analysis, decision to publish, or preparation of the manuscript.

Competing Interests: The authors have declared that no competing interests exist.

* Email: qiang_linm@163.com (QL); xiaodongguo@hust.edu.cn (XDG); peifuxing@vip.163.com (FXP)

⁹ These authors contributed equally to this work.

Introduction

Trauma-induced spinal cord injuries (SCI) resulting in significant motor impairment or paralysis remain a critical public health concern with approximately 100,000 new cases each year [1]. SCI interrupts connections between the brain and the spinal cord, which transmit motor control and somatic sensory signals. Victims of SCI often suffer from severe neurological disabilities. However, effective treatment is currently limited because of the complexity of the pathophysiology of the injured spinal cord. SCI triggers a series of events, including systemic and local inflammatory responses, subsequent death of neuronal and glial cells, and formation of cavities and glial scars in the injury site [2].

Cell transplantation therapy provides a potential source of cells to repopulate the damaged spinal cord and aid in functional recovery by replacing damaged circuits, increasing plasticity, and promoting cell survival and regeneration of host axons [3]. Neural stem cells (NSCs) have the potential to proliferate, migrate, and differentiate into the three major cell types of the central nerve system, oligodendrocytes, astrocytes, and neurons, to replace lost cells or rescue dysfunctional cells [4,5]. However, poor cell survival and uncontrolled differentiation of transplanted NSCs are the current limitations of this approach [6]. Transplanted NSCs have a much greater tendency to astrocytically differentiate, and they rarely undergo neuronal differentiation. Neurons that have differentiated from transplanted NSCs can extend axons into the host spinal cord in both rostral and caudal directions over remarkably long distances, and connections with the host axons are then formed. The host axons can also regenerate into the sites of transplanted NSCs and promote host-to-graft connectivity [7]. The differentiation into oligodendrocytes can promote remyelination of regenerated axons [8]. However, the differentiation of transplanted NSCs into astrocytes may be problematic because reactive gliosis is believed to be an inhibitor of regeneration [9].

Therefore, increasing the rate of survival and differentiation of NSCs into neuronal cells is important.

Neurotrophins (NTs), such as nerve growth factor (NGF), brain-derived neurophic factor, and neurotrophin-3 (NT-3), are important in neuronal survival and differentiation [10,11]. Among these factors, NT-3 facilitates the differentiation of NSCs into neurons and supports the survival and maturation of neurons [12]. Combining NSC transplantation with NT-3 is considered a potentially useful approach for the treatment of SCI [13]. NSC transplantation and soluble NT therapies are limited by the poor survival of injected cells and the short half-life of injected NTs. The external pump/catheter system is used as a controlled release system for delivering drugs into the intrathecal space through a catheter. However, this method is prone to infection and has not been approved for long-term delivery in SCI patients in the USA [14]. To address these issues, tissue-engineered scaffolds have been developed for the treatment of SCI. Biodegradable scaffolds and NSC transplantation each have unique advantages as therapeutic strategies for SCI. Biodegradable scaffolds have many advantages as a delivery system, not only for sustained NT-3 delivery but also for the delivery of NSCs to the injured spinal cord [15]. Furthermore, scaffolds can also bridge the lesion with a 3D permissive environment, which can fill the tissue gap and concomitantly support axonal regeneration [16].

Thus, the incorporation of NT-3 within a biodegradable scaffold offers an opportunity to promote the survival and differentiation of NSCs. Most of the current approaches in incorporating growth factors in biomaterials include physically entrapping soluble growth factors into the scaffolds or covalently immobilizing growth factors onto synthetic polymer scaffolds [17]. By immobilizing growth factors within scaffolds, the growth factors are protected against cellular inactivation and digestion [18]. As a result, the immobilized growth factors can overcome the diffusional limitations of soluble factors, thereby allowing sustained activity. However, most of the covalent immobilization methods require the use of organic solvents or cross-linking agents, which may limit the biological activity of the growth factors. Furthermore, by using these methods, the immobilization of growth factors is not a simple task [19].

Silk fibroin (SF), a natural protein, has been recently found to be biocompatible, slowly biodegradable, and endowed with excellent mechanical properties and processability [20]. SF matrices can successfully deliver growth factors while preserving their potency [21]. Interestingly, SF in aqueous solution can precipitate due to β-sheet formation. SF adsorbs onto various substrates spontaneously and forms a layer, which eventually forms a robust and stable coating through mild all-aqueous processes [22]. Growth factors can be incorporated into the SF matrix during these processes. With the degradation of SF, growth factors can be released. In our previous study, Poly(ε-caprolactone)-block-poly(l-lactic acid-co-ε-caprolactone) (PCLA) scaffolds with precise hierarchical pore architectures were fabricated using injection molding combined with thermally induced phase separation [23]. In the present study, the PCLA scaffolds (membranes and conduits) were fabricated first, and then NT-3 was immobilized within the scaffolds by coating the scaffold with a solution of SF and NT-3. NSCs were cultured in vitro, and their differentiation into neural cells was measured after seeding on the NT-3-immobilized membranes. A rat spinal cord transection model was utilized to evaluate the efficacy of the NT-3 immobilized conduit with the adhered NSCs in vivo.

Materials and Methods

Ethics Statement

All experimental protocols were approved by the Ethics Committee in Sichuan University (protocol # 2013-C-206). The animals were maintained on a standard laboratory diet in plastic cages at ambient temperature, and allowed free mobilization in compliance with the requirements of the International Council on Laboratory Animal Science.

Scaffold fabrication and NT-3 immobilization

PCLA: [PCL27-b-P(LLA405- co-CL14) (PCLA); $Mn = 8.8\times10^4$, $PDI = 1.22$, $T = 171.2°C$, and $\Delta H = 39.3\,J/g$. PCLA was first dissolved in dioxane with a concentration of 60 mg/ml at 50°C, and the mold was chilled to the preset temperature of −40°C. The hot PCLA/dioxane solution was quickly injected into the cold mold using a syringe, as previously described [24]. The temperature of the system was maintained at −40°C for 2 h to induce the solid-liquid phase separation of the polymer solution. Then, the temperature of the cold trap was adjusted to −20°C, and the solvents were sublimated through a two-day lyophilizing process. Finally, the mold was removed, and the 2D scaffolds (membranes) and the 3D scaffolds (conduits) for in vitro and in vivo studies, respectively, were obtained. The prepared conduit had an inner diameter of 3.0 mm, a wall thickness of 0.5 mm and a length of 2.0 mm.

The SF aqueous solution was prepared as previously described [22]. Briefly, cocoons from *Bombyx mori* were boiled in ultra-purified water (UPW) containing 0.02 M Na_2CO_3, thoroughly rinsed with distilled water to extract the glue-like sericin proteins and wax, and then dissolved in 9 M LiBr at 55°C to obtain a 3% (w/v) aqueous SF solution. NT-3 (PeproTech, Rocky Hill, NJ, USA) was embedded by adding 20 μg of NT-3 to 1 ml of SF solution. The NT-3/SF solution was subsequently sterilized using a 0.22 μm filter (Millipore, Tullagreen, Ireland). The scaffolds were immersed in the NT-3/SF solution for 2 h at room temperature. Then, the scaffolds were freeze-dried overnight and subsequently treated with 90% (v/v) methanol in UPW for 15 min to induce formation of SF crystalline β-sheet structure. The scaffolds were stored in a desiccator and rinsed with sterile PBS three times before use.

Determination of kinetics of NT-3 release from NT-3 immobilized PCLA scaffold

Five conduits were separately immersed in 500 μl PBS (10 mM, pH 7.4) and kept in a gently shaking incubator (20 rpm) at 37°C for various time periods up to 8 weeks. The release of NT-3 was examined on day 1, with further measurements after 2, 3, 4, 5, 6, and 7 days. After that, continuous measurements were performed for 8 weeks at 1 week intervals. At each time interval, the supernatant was removed completely and replaced with fresh buffer. The amounts of NT-3 in the collected supernatants were measured using enzyme-linked immunosorbent assay (ELISA; Becton Dickinson, Franklin Lakes, NJ, USA) in accordance with the manufacturer's instructions. The absorbance was measured at 450 nm using a plate reader (Model 680; Bio-RAD, Hercules, CA, USA). The NT-3 concentration was determined by comparing the reading to the standard curve. The amounts of NT-3 in each conduit were calculated based on the cumulative amounts of bioactive NT-3 released in PBS and normalized by the mass of the conduit.

Isolation and culture of rat brain-derived NSCs

Primary NSCs were isolated from E14 Sprague-Dawley (SD) rats, expressing green fluorescent protein (GFP) for the in vivo study and non-GFP for the in vitro study. The transgenic SD rats expressing GFP were purchased from Cyagen Biotechnology Company Ltd. (Guangzhou, China). Whole hippocampi were dissected and dissociated in Hanks' balanced salt solution (HBSS). After centrifugation at 1000 rpm for 5 min, the supernatant containing cell debris was removed. The pelleted cells were resuspended in growth medium, which contained Neurobasal media (Gibco-Invitrogen, Carlsbad, CA, USA), B27 neural supplement (Gibco-Invitrogen), 2 mM L-glutamine (Sigma-Aldrich, St Louis, MO, USA), 1% penicillin-streptomycin (Sigma-Aldrich), 20 ng/ml epidermal growth factor (Gibco-Invitrogen), and 20 ng/ml bFGF (Gibco-Invitrogen). The cells were then plated onto 75 ml culture flasks, with fresh medium every 3 days. The cultured cells typically grew as suspending neurospheres and were passaged once a week. The expression of nestin, a marker of NSCs, was assessed by immunocytochemistry.

PCLA membrane studies

PCLA membrane were placed in 24-well plates and sterilized with 70% ethanol for 5 min, followed by washing three times with PBS solution prior to use. NSCs were spun down at 1500 rpm for 5 min, and the resultant pellet was re-suspended and dissociated in fresh growth media. The cell solution was then added so that each well contained 10 000 cells, and the final volume of media in the wells was 500 μl. After 24 h, the media was removed and replaced with differentiation media – Neurobasal media containing B27 supplement, L-glutamine, penicillin-streptomycin, and 1% fetal bovine serum (FBS). Half-volume media changes were performed every 48 h thereafter.

The viability of cells on the membranes was determined using a live/dead assay (Molecular Probes, Eugene, OR), in accordance with the manufacturer's protocol. Briefly, after 14 days of culture, the PCLA membranes were rinsed with 0.1 M PBS (pH 7.4) three times, followed by staining in 2 ml 0.1 M PBS containing 2 mM of calcein-AM and 4 mM ethidium homodimer (EthD-III) for 30 min at 37°C. The cells were washed again with PBS and then imaged using an Olympus fluorescent microscope. Live cells stained with calcein-AM showed a green color, and dead cells stained with EthD-III showed a red color. Cell viability was calculated by counting the percentage of calcein-AM-positive cells over the total number of cells from five randomly chosen fields of view per sample.

Differentiation was determined using immunocytochemistry staining following the standard protocol. The following primary antibodies were used for immunohistochemical analysis: rabbit anti-2',3'-cyclic nucleotide 3'-phosphodiesterase (CNPase, 1:100, Cell Signaling Technology, Beverly, MA), mouse anti-glial fibrillary acidic protein (GFAP; 1:500, Sigma, St. Louis, MO) for astrocytes, and rabbit anti-microtubule-associated protein 2 (MAP2; 1:500, Sigma, St. Louis, MO) for neurons. Briefly, the samples were fixed in 4% paraformaldehyde for 20 min at 4°C and then permeabilized with 0.3% Triton X-100 for 5 min. Non-specific binding was blocked with 10% goat serum and 1% bovine serum albumin (BSA) for 1 h at room temperature. The samples were subsequently incubated with the primary antibodies overnight at 4°C. After washing with PBS, the samples were incubated at room temperature for 2 h with secondary fluorescent antibodies: Alexa Fluor 488-conjugated goat anti-rabbit IgG or Alexa Fluor 594-conjugated goat anti-mouse IgG (1:500, Invitrogen, Carlsbad, CA, USA). The nuclei were stained with 4',6-diamidino-2-phenylindole (DAPI; Sigma-Aldrich, St Louis, MO, USA). The samples were viewed under an Olympus fluorescent microscope. Cell differentiation was calculated by counting the percentage of MAP2-, GFAP- and CNPase-positive cells from five randomly chosen fields of view per sample using ImageJ software (National Institutes of Health, Bethesda, MD).

Seeding of NSCs into PCLA conduits

Sterile conduits were incubated in complete media overnight, prior to cell seeding. Before seeding the NSCs into the conduits, the NSCs were digested into single cell suspension. The media inside the tubes were then replaced with 80 μl of cell suspension, which contained GFP-positive cells (passage 4) at a cell density of 4×10^6 cells per 80 μl. For the *in vivo* study, the conduits containing the neurosphere suspension were rotated manually every 15 min for 1 hour to achieve uniform cell seeding. These conduits were then transferred to new wells, which contained growth media, and incubated for 24 h prior to implantation into the transected spinal cords. Scanning electron microscopy (SEM, JSM-5800LV) (JEOL, Tokyo, Japan) was used to observe the cell morphology after 24 h of culture. The cell density inside the channels was not uniform and covered mainly the lower half of the channels due to gravity.

Animal surgery and post-operative care

All of the animal experiments were approved and performed according to the regulations of the Animal Ethical Committee of our university. Adult male rats (220–250 g, purchased from the Experimental Animals Center of Sichun University) were divided randomly into three groups. 1, conduit+NT-3+NSCs group ($n = 8$): the transected spinal cord was bridged by an NT-3 immobilized conduit with NSCs; 2, conduit+NSCs group ($n = 7$): the transected spinal cord was bridged by a conduit with NSCs; 3, conduit+NT-3 group ($n = 7$): the transected spinal cord was bridged by an NT-3 immobilized conduit without NSCs. Each rat was anesthetized with an intraperitoneal injection of sodium pentobarbital (50 mg/kg) before the operation. We performed all of the surgical procedures under a microscope and under sterile conditions. The backs of rats were shaved and aseptically prepared. After checking of the lowest lumbar level, a laminectomy was performed to expose the T8-10 spinal segments. The posterior aspect of the spinal cord was exposed and the dura was cut vertically using microforceps and microscissors. An angled microscissor was used to transect the spinal cord competely and the stumps were retracted, creating a 2.0-mm gap in the spinal cord of T9. To prevent unexpected reflex movements and bleeding, we applied two drops of 1% lidocaine with epinephrine onto the spinal cord. The conduit was grafted into the lesion site in a manner such that the cut ends of both spinal stumps were apposed to the NSCs-containing conduit. The exposed spinal cord with the implanted conduit was covered with muscles and fascia. The skin was repositioned and closed with sutures.

After surgery, the rats were injected with 5.0 ml saline subcutaneously and allowed to recuperate. Buprenorphine (0.03 mg/kg) was administered subcutaneously for 3 days to minimize pain. Enroflaxacin (2.5 mg/kg) was administered subcutaneously for 7 days for prophylactic treatment against postoperative infections. Bladders were manually expressed thrice daily for the duration of the experiment. Functional recovery was assessed weekly during the 8 week survival period using the Basso, Beattie, Bresnahan (BBB) open field locomotor scale [25]. BBB scoring was conducted by two observers blinded to the experimental groups. All of the animals were evaluated weekly for 8 weeks.

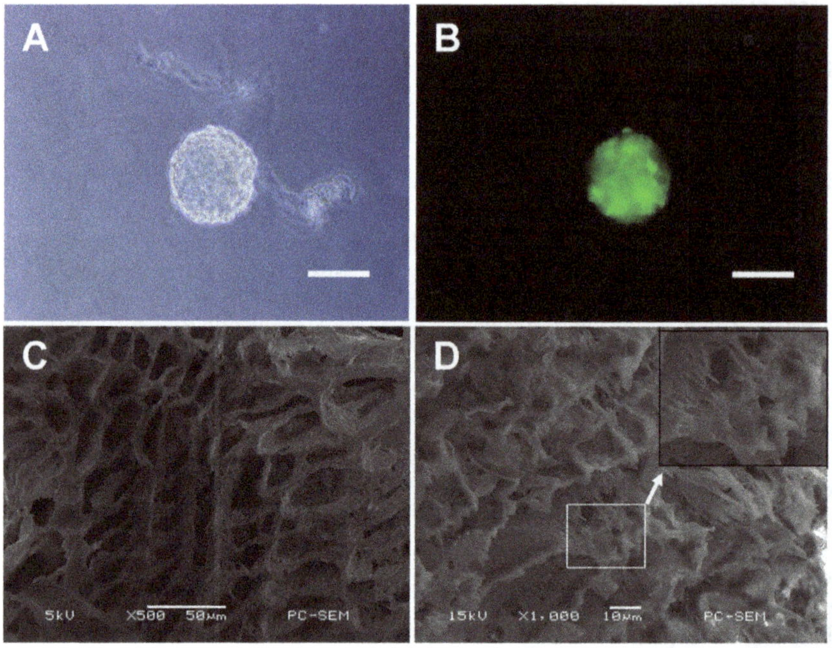

Figure 1. Neurosphere and PCLA scaffold. (A) A neurosphere visualized under a light microscope. (B) GFP-positive neurosphere visualized under a fluorescent microscope. (C) SEM images of the inner wall of the PCLA conduit without NSCs. (D) NSCs adhered to the inner wall of the PCLA conduit. The black box show representative cells from the white box at higher magnification to enhance visualization of cellular morphology under SEM. Scale bars = 100 μm in A–B, 50 μm in C, and 10 μm in D.

Tissue preparation and cell counts of GFP-positive cells

The animals were sacrificed via transcardial perfusion with 4% paraformaldehyde in 0.1 M PBS at 8 weeks after implantation. The spinal cords were carefully removed, postfixed in 4% paraformaldehyde for 5 h, and then transferred to 0.1 M PBS containing 30% sucrose at 4°C overnight. Afterwards, they were frozen and embedded in an optimal cutting temperature (OCT) compound (Sakura, Tokyo, Japan), and then cut into 15 μm sections on a freezing microtome for cell count and histological analysis.

To quantify cell survival, every tenth equidistant frozen section of the spinal cord was selected from each animal and counterstained with the nuclear dye DAPI. The samples were examined using a Zeiss LSM 710 laser scanning confocal microscope (LSCM; Zeiss, Oberkochen, Germany). A minimum of five random fields containing the GFP-positive transplanted NSCs were photographed over multiple tissue sections of each animal. Cell survival was calculated by manually counting GFP-positive cells associated with DAPI stained nuclei across the sample.

Histological analysis

In addition to the antibodies previously described, mouse anti-neurofilament 200 (NF200; 1:500, Sigma, St. Louis, MO) for axons was also used. The secondary antibodies were Alexa Fluor 594-conjugated goat anti-mouse or goat anti-rabbit IgG antibodies (1:500, Invitrogen, Carlsbad, CA, USA). The sections were washed with PBS and permeabilized with 0.3% Triton X-100 for 5 min. Non-specific binding was blocked using 10% goat serum and 1% BSA for 1 h at room temperature. After washing with PBS, the sections were incubated in primary antibody overnight at 4°C. Afterwards, sections were washed with 0.1 M PBS, and corresponding secondary antibodies was added for 1 h at 25°C. After another series of washes, the nuclei were stained with DAPI. Finally, the immunostained samples were mounted onto glass slides with mounting medium and viewed under the LSCM. In all the immunohistochemistry procedures, appropriate negative controls were used without the primary antibodies.

For histological analysis, every tenth equidistant frozen section of the spinal cord was selected from each animal. A minimum of five random fields containing the GFP-positive transplanted NSCs were photographed per sample. Phenotypic analysis of transplanted NSCs was calculated based on identification of GFP-positive cells associated with a DAPI stained nucleus and the immunohistological marker of interest. The number of NF200-positive axons in the conduits was also counted.

Statistical analysis

Analysis of variance (ANOVA) was used to test for the statistical significance, and the results were accepted when two-tailed $P < 0.05$. Tukey's post-test was performed to compare individual pairs of means if ANOVA $P<0.05$. The results are presented as mean ± standard deviation.

Results

Isolation and culture of NSCs

NSCs were isolated from the whole hippocampi of E14 SD rats. The NSCs aggregated as free-floating neurospheres (Fig. 1A), as observed under a phase contrast microscope after 5 days of culture. The formation of neurospheres is considered the gold standard for the identification of NSCs. Then, the NSCs were assessed using nestin, a marker for neural precursors. The immunocytochemistry results indicated that the neurospheres showed positive immunoreactivity to nestin, a known protein marker of NSCs (Fig. 1B). These data indicated that NSCs maintained their undifferentiated status in the defined medium. The NSCs grafted into the NT-3-immobilized PCLA conduits were shown in Fig. 1C and D.

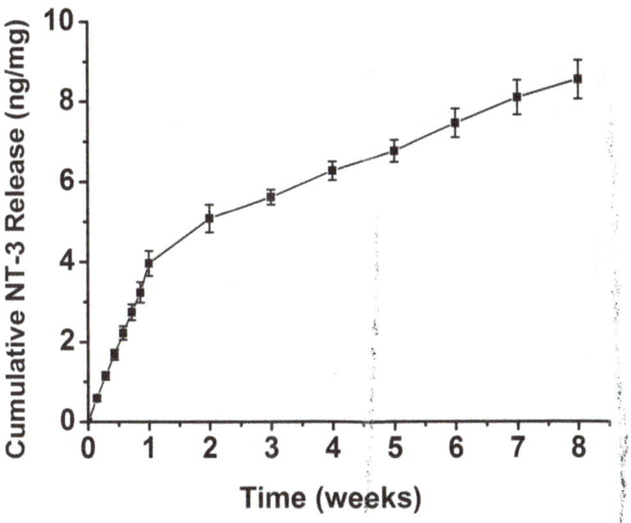

Figure 2. Cumulative release profile of bioactive NT-3 from NT-3-immobilized PCLA-SF conduits in vitro. n = 3.

Determination of kinetics of NT-3 release from NT-3 immobilized scaffolds

NT-3 was released from NT-3-immobilized conduits in vitro for at least 8 weeks (Fig. 2). The release profile was composed of two parts, an initial burst in the first week followed by a sustained release. After an initial burst release in the first week, the NT-3-immobilized conduits released NT-3 at a stable and constant rate in the following seven weeks. The cumulative amount of released NT-3 was 8.56 ng/mg.

Viability and differentiation of NSCs on NT-3-immobilized PCLA membranes

To determine the viability of the NSCs on the membranes, the seeded cells were cultured for 14 days, and then stained with calcein-AM and EthD-III. The cell viability on PCLA-SF-NT-3, PCLA-SF, and PCLA membranes were determined to be 94.52±3.37%, 87.12±2.63%, and 86.86±3.61%, respectively (Fig. 3A–D). The percentage of live cells was highest on PCLA-SF-NT-3 membranes. No significant difference in viability was found between the PCLA-SF and PCLA membranes.

To evaluate the differentiation of seeded NSCs on the NT-3-immobilized PCLA membranes, we stained the cells with MAP-2, GFAP, and CNPase (Fig. 4A–I). At day 14, the percentages of MAP-2-positive cells on PCLA, PCLA-SF, and PCLA-SF-NT-3 membranes were determined to be 18.6±2.2%, 25.3±3.2%, 55.2±4.1%, respectively. The percentages of GFAP-positive cells and CNPase-positive cells were the lowest in the PCLA-SF-NT-3 group, compared with the PCLA and PCLA-SF groups (Fig. 4J).

Long-term survival and differentiation of NSCs after SCI

The surgical procedures are shown in Fig. 5A and B. During the experiment, no rats exhibited wound complications. At explantation, no inflammatory signs or adverse tissue reactions were observed. General observation of both ends of the lesion site revealed reparative tissue completely filling the gap between the transected cord stumps 8 weeks after implantation (Fig. 5C).

At 8 weeks after implantation, NSC survival was observed in the conduit+NT-3+NSCs and conduit+NSCs groups. Fluorescent microscopy of frozen sections showed GFP-positive transplanted NSCs in the bridge tissue (Fig. 5D, E). The overall survival of the transplanted NSCs was quantified for each group. The conduit+NT-3+NSCs group exhibited an average GFP-positive cell density of 75.8±15.1%, whereas the conduit+NSCs group exhibited only

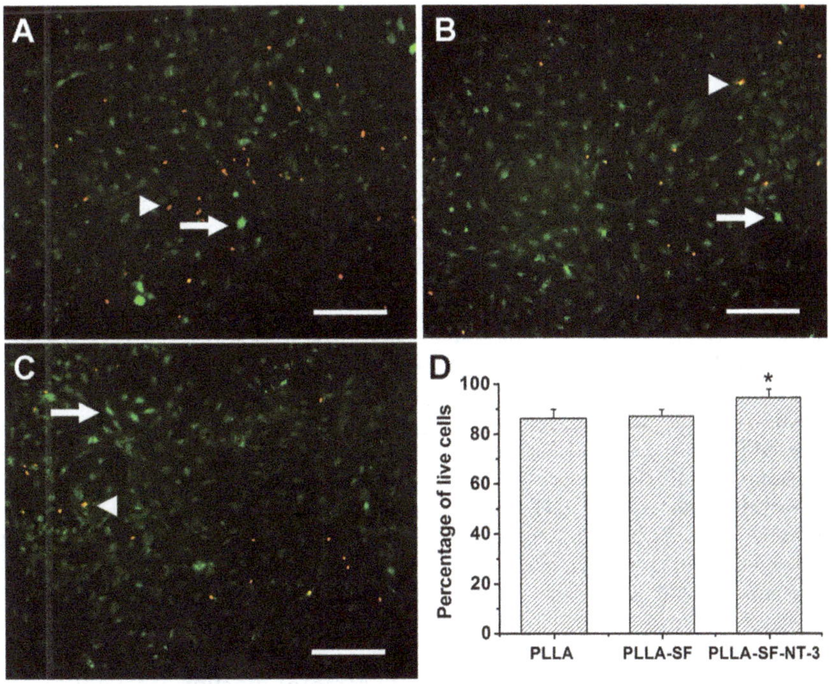

Figure 3. Fluorescent staining for cell viability of NSCs grown on PCLA (A), PCLA-SF (B), and PCLA-SF-NT-3 (C) membranes for 14 days. Living cells (white arrows) were in green and dead cells (white arrowheads) were in red. (D) The percentage of live cells. Scale bars = 100 μm; *$P<0.05$; n = 4.

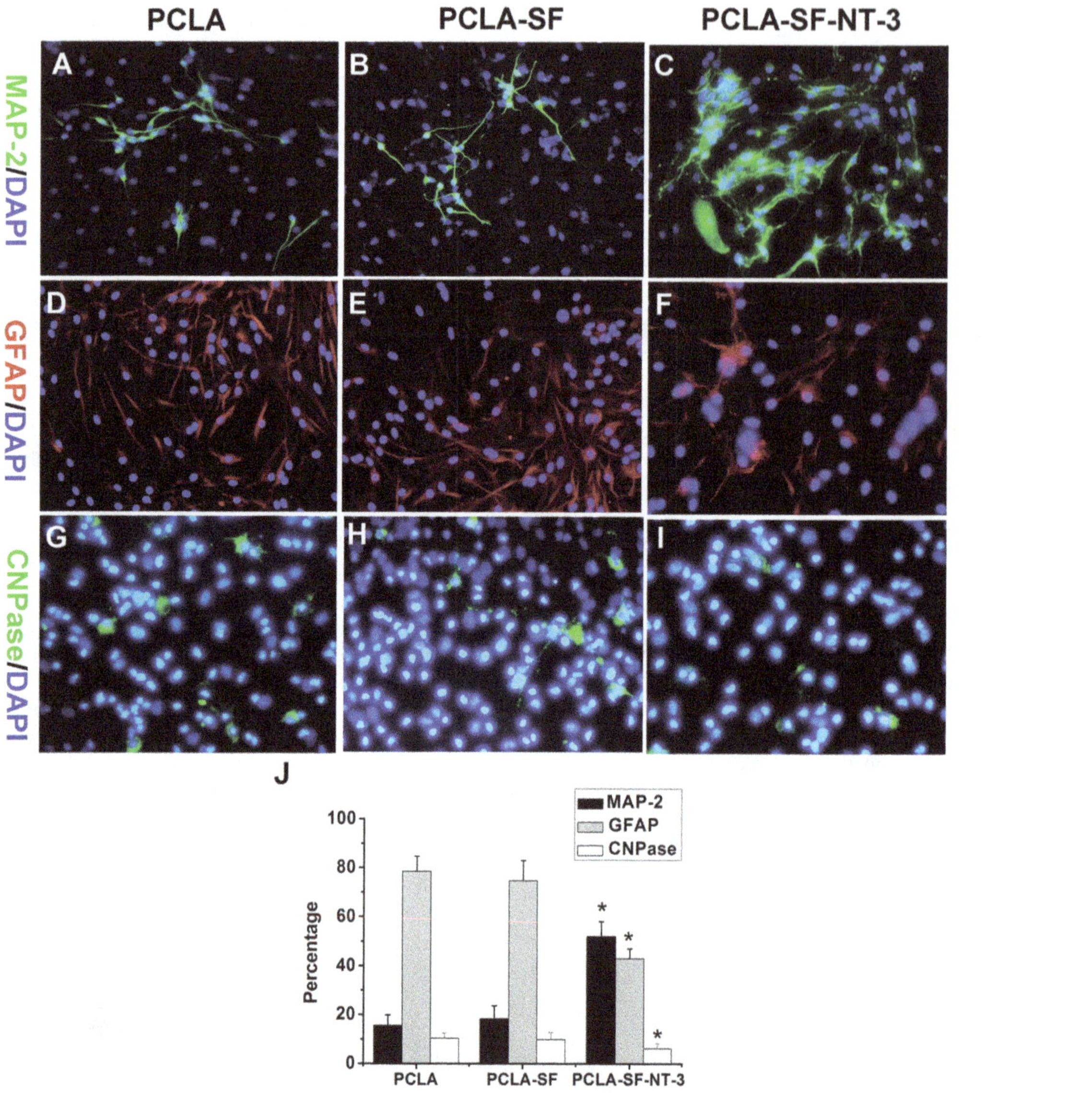

Figure 4. Differentiation of NSCs in vitro. (A–I) Cells cultured on PCLA (A, D, G), PCLA-SF (B, E, H), and PCLA-SF-NT-3 (C, F, I) membrane were immunostained with MAP-2 for neurons (A–C), GFPA for astrocytes (D–F), CNPase for oligodendrocytes (G–I). The nuclei were stained with DAPI. (J) Quantitative analysis of the NSC differentiation in vitro. Scale bars = 25 μm, $^*P<0.05$; n = 4.

32.3±10.2% GFP positive cell density (Fig. 5F). The conduit+NT-3+NSCs group showed significantly improved long-term survival of NSCs compared with the conduit+NSCs group.

NSC differentiation after 8 weeks was examined. Immunofluorescent images showed that GFP-positive cells co-localized with MAP-2 positive mature neurons, GFAP-positive astrocytes, or CNPase-positive oligodendrocytes of the conduit+NT-3+NSCs and conduit+NSCs groups (Fig. 6A–F). The results are summarized in Fig. 6G. MAP-2 staining for neurons showed that 21.5±5.2% neuronal differentiation of NSCs in the conduit+NT-3+NSCs group, which was higher than that in the conduit+NSCs group. In contrast, the percentages of GFAP-positive cells and CNPase-positive cells in the conduit+NT-3+NSCs group were lower, compared with the conduit+NSCs group.

Axon regeneration

Axon regeneration across the bridge was identified by NF200 staining at 8 weeks after implantation. Fluorescent microscopy showed that the regenerating axons were visible in the conduit+NT-3+NSCs group, whereas few regenerating axons were found in the conduit+NSCs group (Fig. 7A and B). The number of NF-200 positive axons in the NSCs contained conduit was determined to be 75.3±7.2 in the conduit+NT-3+NSCs group, and 48.3±6.2 in the conduit+NSCs group. The difference in the number of NF200-positive axons between the two groups was statistically significant (Fig. 7C).

Locomotor function recovery

Animals were monitored weekly for hindlimb function using the BBB open field locomotor scale. BBB scores were 0 when the spinal cord was completely transected. A time-dependent increase

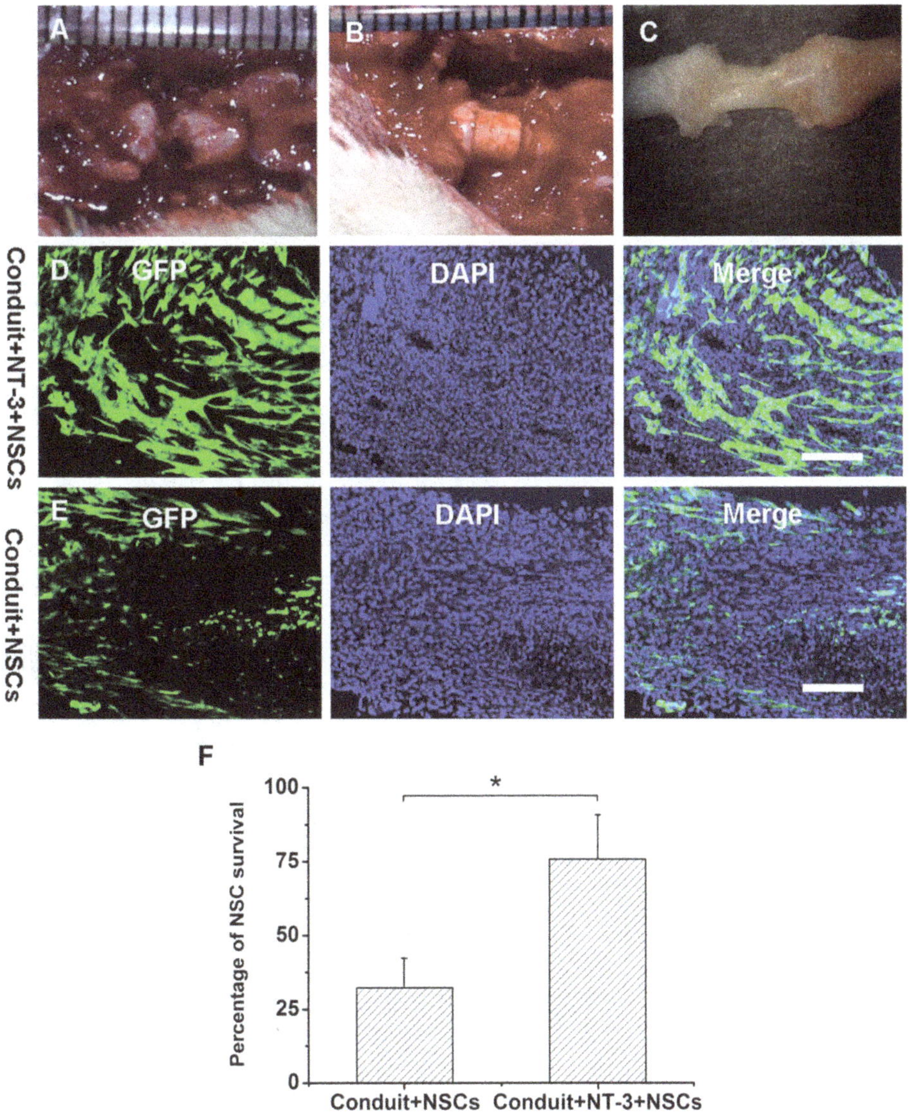

Figure 5. Conduit implantation after spinal cord transection facilitates tissue bridging and NSC survival. (A–B) Surgical procedure for implantation of conduits into completely transected rat spinal cords. (C) Gross appearance of spinal cords 8 weeks after implantation of the conduits. (D–E) Confocal fluorescent images of NSC survival in the conduit+NT-3+NSCs (D) and conduit+NSCs (E) groups 8 weeks after implantation. (F) Percentage of NSC survival for each group. Scale bar = 100 μm; $^{*}P<0.05$; n = 7.

in the BBB scores was displayed in the conduit+NT-3+NSCs, conduit+ NSCs, and conduit+NT-3 groups.

No significant difference was observed among the three groups until 3 weeks. However, at 4 weeks and thereafter, the conduit+ NT-3+NSCs group displayed significant behavioral improvement compared with the other two groups (Fig. 8).

Discussion

NSCs-based transplantation therapy is currently considered a potentially useful approach for SCI treatment [26]. A major challenge in NSCs-based transplantation therapy is to increase the rate of survival and neuronal differentiation of grafted NSCs. NT-3 is one of the best candidates in stimulating the survival and differentiation of NSCs. However, NT-3 has a short half-life and easily diffuses through tissue and cerebrospinal fluid. Moreover, maintaining a sufficient concentration of NT-3 at the injury site to elicit an effect is difficult [27]. In the present study, we utilized SF β-sheet formation to immobilize NT-3 within the PCLA scaffolds, in which the bioactivity of NT-3 can be maintained, and its release can be controlled for 8 weeks. We then investigated the effects of NT-3-immobilized scaffolds on the survival and neuronal differentiation of NSCs in vitro and in a rat spinal cord transection model. The results showed that the NT-3-immobilized scaffolds enhanced the survival and neuronal differentiation of NSCs in vitro and 8 weeks after implantation in rats. Functional recovery and regeneration of NF200-positive axons were also promoted.

Maintaining the integrity and activity of NT-3 is critical for effective NT-3 delivery. In this study, NT-3 ELISA kits were used to quantify the release of growth factors from the conduits. The release profiles showed that the release of bioactive NT-3 was sustained over 8 weeks. The sustained release is due to the proteolytic degradation of SF coating [28]. The rate of NT-3 release was highest in the first 7 d, and NT-3 release continued at a

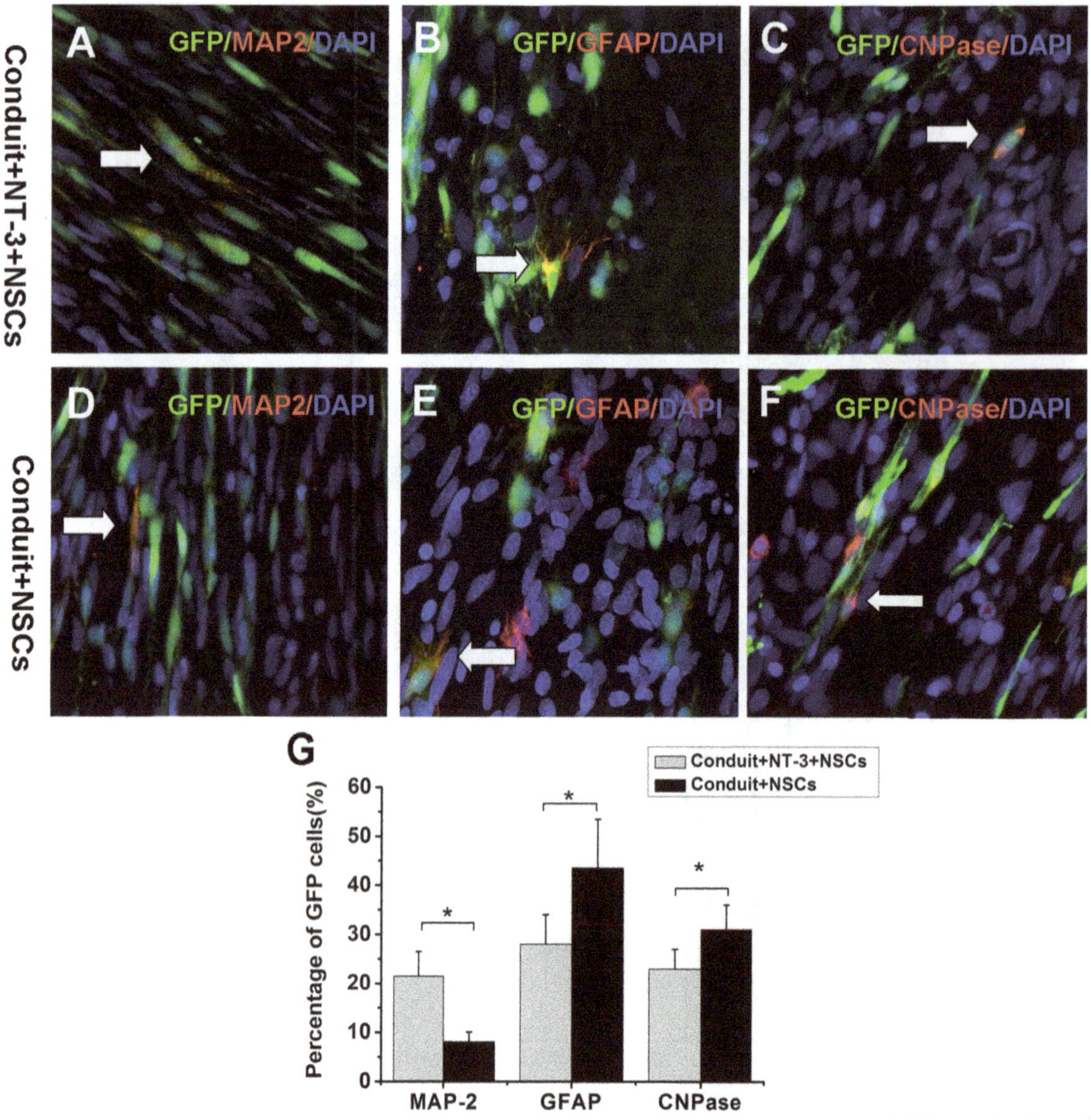

Figure 6. Differentiation profiles of NSCs in vivo. (A–F) Tissue samples were immunostained with MAP-2 for neurons (A, D), GFAP for astrocytes (B, E), and CNPase for oligodendrocytes (C, F) from the conduit+NT-3+NSCs (A–C) and conduit+NSCs groups (D–F). White arrows indicate the representative differentiated cells. (G) Quantification of NSC differentiation profile for each group. Scale bar = 20 μm. $^*P<0.05$; n = 7.

slower rate for up to 8 wks. This can be ascribed to the inactive of released NT-3 in PBS during the testing interval, and ELISA can only detect the intact NT-3. In the present study, a daily testing interval was initially set, and then the testing interval was changed to weekly.

Currently, the development of biomaterials for neural tissue regeneration and stem cell implantation is a prominent research focus in regenerative medicine. SF has been shown to have excellent biocompatibility both in vitro and in vivo, good mechanical properties, and a slow biodegradation rate [20]. The crystal structure of SF is composed of hydrophilic domains (silk I) and hydrophobic domains (silk II). Hydrophobic blocks make up the crystalline regions of SF due to their ability to form intermolecular β-sheets. Methanol treatement dehydrates and destabilizes the unstable silk I state of SF, leading to a switch to the silk II (predominant) conformation, which is more stable and characterized by an increase in β-sheet content [29]. Therefore, by treating the adsorbed SF/NT-3 molecules on the surface of the scaffolds with methanol, the NT-3 molecules are entrapped in the SF coating. In the present study, SF coating was used as NT-3 reservoir, which played an important role in stabilizing the bioactivity of NT-3. No obvious cytotoxicity of the biomaterials could be observed for the NSCs, due to the biocompatibility of the scaffold and the sustained release of NT-3. In our previous work, we also immobilized NGF within nanofibrous nerve conduits in a concentration gradient pattern by SF coating to guide the dorsal root ganglia (DRG) neurite outgrowth [23]. In sum, the NT-3-immobilized PCLA-SF scaffold is a promising NT-3 delivery system, which increases NSC survival.

SCI results in loss of both sensory and motor neuron function, even neuronal damage and death, as well as axonal demyelination. Despite the presence of endogenous NSC populations within the adult spinal cord, the extent of neuronal differentiation from these endogenous precursor cells, even after infusion of exogenous

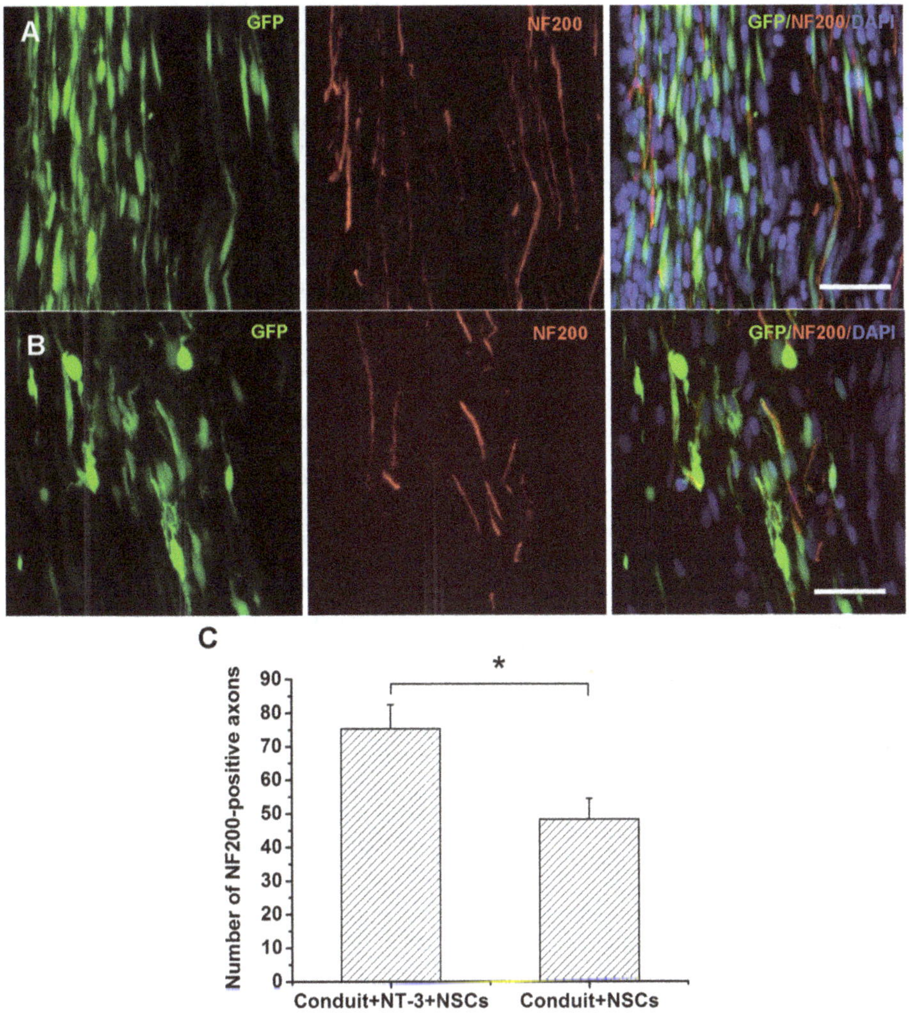

Figure 7. Axonal regeneration. NF200-positive axons were observed in the conduit+NT-3+NSCs (A) and conduit+NSCs (B) groups 8 weeks after implantation. (C) Histograms showing the number of NF200-positive axons for each group. Scale bar = 20 μm, *$P<0.05$; n = 7.

growth factors, is not sufficient to stimulate neuroplasticity, and rescue neuronal loss after SCI [30]. Thus, restoration of the neuron population by cell transplantation therapy is an attractive strategy in constructing a neural network after SCI. In the present study, enhanced survival and differentiation of transplanted NSCs in vitro and in vivo was achieved using the NT-3 delivery system. Each conduit was seeded with NSCs prior to implantation, and cell survival was assayed 8 weeks after implantation. The conduit+NT-3+NSCs group had a higher density of GFP-positive cells, compared with the conduit+NSCs group. Hence, the NT-3-immobilized scaffolds enhanced the survival of the NSCs not only in vitro but also in vivo.

On the NT-3-immobilized membranes, NSCs differentiated into neurons with a significantly high percentage in vitro. However, when the NT-3-immobilized scaffolds were implanted into the injured spinal cord, this differentiation percentage decreased in vivo, yet was still significantly higher than the control group. Despite this lower cell survival in vivo, the NT-3 group still had the highest effect in terms of NF200-positive axon regeneration and functional recovery. Therefore, although this differentiation percentage was lower in vivo than in vitro, the NT-3 delivery system is still meaningful.

Complete spinal cord transection is the most severe injury model and results in loss of hindlimb movement immediately after injury. In the present study, the conduit+NT-3+NSCs group showed a statistically significant improvement in hindlimb function, resulting in some movement of hindlimb joints. Immunohistochemistry showed that the NF200-positive axons were densest across the tissue bridge. Axon regeneration has been demonstrated in several SCI models [31,32]. We believe that this finding is important because these axons may provide a structural basis for re-establishment of a neuronal network for physiological signal transduction across the injury site. Lu et al. seeded NSCs derived from human fetal spinal cord in growth-factor-containing fibrin to derive neurons [7]. The graft-derived neurons were found to extend large numbers of axons into the host spinal cord in both rostral and caudal directions. These axons in the host spinal cord formed dense bouton-like terminals around the host dendrites and cell bodies. Synapse formation was identified by immunohistochemistry and electron microscopy, which supported the observed enhanced functional recovery [33]. In our study, the enhanced functional recovery in the conduit+NT-3+NSCs group can be ascribed to the relatively high amount of NF200-positive axons.

Remarkable progress in guiding neuronal differentiation has been achieved by priming NSCs to neuron-restricted progenitor

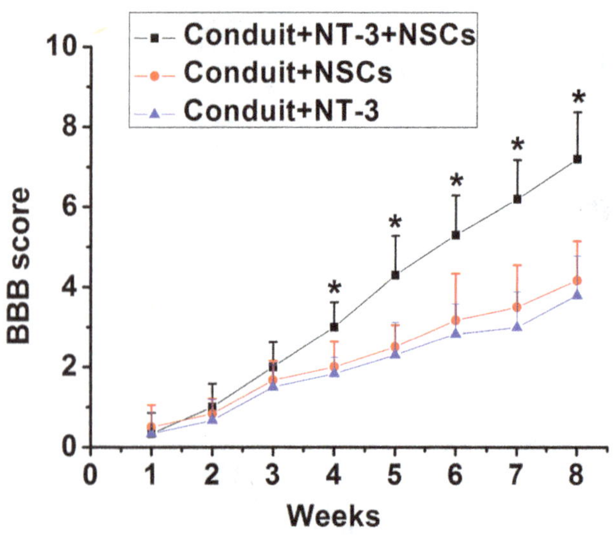

Figure 8. BBB locomotor scores were evaluated weekly for 8 weeks after SCI. At 4 weeks and thereafter, the conduit+NT-3+NSCs group displayed significant behavioral improvement compared with the other two groups. *$P<0.05$; $n=6$.

cells in vitro and addition of growth factors, including NTs, sonic hedgehog protein, and retinoid acid [34,35]. NTs, particularly NT-3, are considered to be the most promising strategy for future clinical application. NT-3 could not only facilitate the survival and proliferation of NSCs, but also induce the differentiation of NSCs into neurons. NT-3 acts via its corresponding receptor tyrosine kinases (TrkA, TrkB, and TrkC). NT-3 preferentially binds to TrkC, and then activates the Akt/MAP kinase signal pathway, which is involved in neurotransmitter regulation and neural peptide synthesis [36]. In several investigations, genetically modified NSCs were utilized to overexpress NT-3 to affect the survival and differentiation of surrounding cells. However, gene transduction is limited by various problems, including concerns about the safety and efficiency of gene transfection and the potential adverse effects of exogenous gene expression [37]. In contrast, PCLA-SF has several advantages for NT-3 delivery. First, SF adsorption and β-sheet formation is a simple method to immobilize growth factors. Multiple growth factors can also be immobilized simultaneously with SF coating, which synergistically improve functional recovery. Furthermore, drugs that eliminate the inhibitory environment or enhance the regenerative ability of axons could also be included. Second, the present NT-3 delivery system is safe. Both PCLA and SF are recommended scaffold materials because of their unique features, such as biocompatibility and biodegradability, for tissue engineering for the repair and regeneration of injured tissues [38,39].

Conclusions

By incorporating NT-3 into SF coating, we successfully developed an NT-3-immobilized PCLA scaffold as a delivery system. Seeding NSCs within these NT-3-immobilized PCLA scaffolds not only enhanced the survival of grafted cells but also promoted neuronal differentiation both in vitro and in a rat SCI model. At 8 weeks after implantation, the conduit+NT-3+NSCs group showed significant improvement in axon regeneration and functional recovery. Our results suggest that PCLA conduits immobilized with NT-3 have the potential for SCI repair by promoting survival and neuronal differentiation of transplanted NSCs. In addition, SF adsorption and coating are simple methods for immobilizing bioactive molecules. In the future, drugs that eliminate the inhibitory environment and enhance regeneration can be immobilized within the scaffolds for a synergistic effect.

Acknowledgments

The authors appreciate Jixiang Zhu (Department of Biomedical Engineering, Guangzhou Medical University, China) for his kind help in material fabrication.

Author Contributions

Conceived and designed the experiments: XG. Performed the experiments: ST XL ZH. Analyzed the data: BX YQ. Contributed reagents/materials/analysis tools: QL. Wrote the paper: FP.

References

1. Adams M, Cavanagh JF (2004) International Campaign for Cures of Spinal Cord Injury Paralysis (ICCP): another step forward for spinal cord injury research. Spinal Cord 42: 273–280.
2. Fleming JC, Norenberg MD, Ramsay DA, Dekaban GA, Marcillo AE, et al. (2006) The cellular inflammatory response in human spinal cords after injury. Brain 129: 3249–3269.
3. Johnson PJ, Tatara A, McCreedy DA, Shiu A, Sakiyama-Elbert SE (2010) Tissue-engineered fibrin scaffolds containing neural progenitors enhance functional recovery in a subacute model of SCI. Soft Matter 6: 5127–5137.
4. Kim H, Zahir T, Tator CH, Shoichet MS (2011) Effects of dibutyryl cyclic-AMP on survival and neuronal differentiation of neural stem/progenitor cells transplanted into spinal cord injured rats. PLoS One 6: e21744.
5. Yang Z, Duan H, Mo L, Qiao H, Li X (2010) The effect of the dosage of NT-3/chitosan carriers on the proliferation and differentiation of neural stem cells. Biomaterials 31: 4846–4854.
6. Abematsu M, Tsujimura K, Yamano M, Saito M, Kohno K, et al. (2010) Neurons derived from transplanted neural stem cells restore disrupted neuronal circuitry in a mouse model of spinal cord injury. J Clin Invest 120: 3255–3266.
7. Lu P, Wang Y, Graham L, McHale K, Gao M, et al. (2012) Long-distance growth and connectivity of neural stem cells after severe spinal cord injury. Cell 150: 1264–1273.
8. Guo X, Zahir T, Mothe A, Shoichet MS, Morshead CM, et al. (2012) The effect of growth factors and soluble Nogo-66 receptor protein on transplanted neural stem/progenitor survival and axonal regeneration after complete transection of rat spinal cord. Cell Transplant 21: 1177–1197.
9. Johnson PJ, Tatara A, Shiu A, Sakiyama-Elbert SE (2010) Controlled release of neurotrophin-3 and platelet-derived growth factor from fibrin scaffolds containing neural progenitor cells enhances survival and differentiation into neurons in a subacute model of SCI. Cell Transplant 19: 89–101.
10. Weishaupt N, Blesch A, Fouad K (2012) BDNF: the career of a multifaceted neurotrophin in spinal cord injury. Exp Neurol 238: 254–264.
11. Chao MV (2003) Neurotrophins and their receptors: a convergence point for many signalling pathways. Nat Rev Neurosci 4: 299–309.
12. Yang Z, Duan H, Mo L, Qiao H, Li X (2010) The effect of the dosage of NT-3/chitosan carriers on the proliferation and differentiation of neural stem cells. Biomaterials 31: 4846–4854.
13. Wang JM, Zeng YS, Wu JL, Li Y, Teng YD (2011) Cograft of neural stem cells and schwann cells overexpressing TrkC and neurotrophin-3 respectively after rat spinal cord transection. Biomaterials 32: 7454–7468.
14. Wang Y, Lapitsky Y, Kang CE, Shoichet MS (2009) Accelerated release of a sparingly soluble drug from an injectable hyaluronan-methylcellulose hydrogel. J Control Release 140: 218–223.
15. Krych AJ, Rooney GE, Chen B, Schermerhorn TC, Ameenuddin S, et al. (2009) Relationship between scaffold channel diameter and number of regenerating axons in the transected rat spinal cord. Acta Biomater 5: 2551–2559.
16. Straley KS, Foo CW, Heilshorn SC (2010) Biomaterial design strategies for the treatment of spinal cord injuries. J Neurotrauma 27: 1–19.
17. Tang S, Zhao J, Xu S, Li J, Teng Y, et al. (2012) Bone induction through controlled release of novel BMP-2-related peptide from PTMC(11)-F127-PTMC(11) hydrogels. Biomed Mater 7.
18. Chiu LL, Weisel RD, Li RK, Radisic M (2011) Defining conditions for covalent immobilization of angiogenic growth factors onto scaffolds for tissue engineering. J Tissue Eng Regen Med 5: 69–84.
19. Meade KA, White KJ, Pickford CE, Holley RJ, Marson A, et al. (2013) Immobilization of heparan sulfate on electrospun meshes to support embryonic stem cell culture and differentiation. J Biol Chem 288: 5530–5538.
20. Wenk E, Merkle HP, Meinel L (2011) Silk fibroin as a vehicle for drug delivery applications. J Control Release 150: 128–141.

21. Shchepelina O, Drachuk I, Gupta MK, Lin J, Tsukruk VV (2011) Silk-on-silk layer-by-layer microcapsules. Adv Mater 23: 4655–4660.
22. Uebersax L, Mattotti M, Papaloizos M, Merkle HP, Gander B, et al. (2007) Silk fibroin matrices for the controlled release of nerve growth factor (NGF). Biomaterials 28: 4449–4460.
23. Tang S, Zhu J, Xu Y, Xiang AP, Jiang MH, et al. (2013) The effects of gradients of nerve growth factor immobilized PCLA scaffolds on neurite outgrowth in vitro and peripheral nerve regeneration in rats. Biomaterials 34: 7086–7096.
24. He L, Zhang Y, Zeng C, Ngiam M, Liao S, et al. (2009) Manufacture of PLGA multiple-channel conduits with precise hierarchical pore architectures and in vitro/vivo evaluation for spinal cord injury. Tissue Eng Part C Methods 15: 243–255.
25. Basso DM, Beattie MS, Bresnahan JC (1995) A sensitive and reliable locomotor rating scale for open field testing in rats. J Neurotrauma 12: 1–21.
26. Yang Z, Duan H, Mo L, Qiao H, Li X (2010) The effect of the dosage of NT-3/ chitosan carriers on the proliferation and differentiation of neural stem cells. Biomaterials 31: 4846–4854.
27. Willerth SM, Rader A, Sakiyama-Elbert SE (2008) The effect of controlled growth factor delivery on embryonic stem cell differentiation inside fibrin scaffolds. Stem Cell Res 1: 205–218.
28. Lu Q, Wang X, Hu X, Cebe P, Omenetto F, et al. (2010) Stabilization and release of enzymes from silk films. Macromol Biosci 10: 359–368.
29. Taddei P, Monti P (2005) Vibrational infrared conformational studies of model peptides representing the semicrystalline domains of Bombyx mori silk fibroin. Biopolymers 78: 249–258.
30. Obermair FJ, Schroter A, Thallmair M (2008) Endogenous neural progenitor cells as therapeutic target after spinal cord injury. Physiology (Bethesda) 23: 296–304.
31. Steward O, Sharp K, Selvan G, Hadden A, Hofstadter M, et al. (2006) A re-assessment of the consequences of delayed transplantation of olfactory lamina propria following complete spinal cord transection in rats. Exp Neurol 198: 483–499.
32. Kim D, Adipudi V, Shibayama M, Giszter S, Tessler A, et al. (1999) Direct agonists for serotonin receptors enhance locomotor function in rats that received neural transplants after neonatal spinal transection. J Neurosci 19: 6213–6224.
33. Abematsu M, Tsujimura K, Yamano M, Saito M, Kohno K, et al. (2010) Neurons derived from transplanted neural stem cells restore disrupted neuronal circuitry in a mouse model of spinal cord injury. J Clin Invest 120: 3255–3266.
34. Lowry N, Goderie SK, Lederman P, Charniga C, Gooch MR, et al. (2012) The effect of long-term release of Shh from implanted biodegradable microspheres on recovery from spinal cord injury in mice. Biomaterials 33: 2892–2901.
35. Santos T, Ferreira R, Maia J, Agasse F, Xapelli S, et al. (2012) Polymeric nanoparticles to control the differentiation of neural stem cells in the subventricular zone of the brain. ACS Nano 6: 10463–10474.
36. Lim MS, Nam SH, Kim SJ, Kang SY, Lee YS, et al. (2007) Signaling pathways of the early differentiation of neural stem cells by neurotrophin-3. Biochem Biophys Res Commun 357: 903–909.
37. Lu HX, Hao ZM, Jiao Q, Xie WL, Zhang JF, et al. (2011) Neurotrophin-3 gene transduction of mouse neural stem cells promotes proliferation and neuronal differentiation in organotypic hippocampal slice cultures. Med Sci Monit 17: R305–R311.
38. Sandker MJ, Petit A, Redout EM, Siebelt M, Muller B, et al. (2013) In situ forming acyl-capped PCLA-PEG-PCLA triblock copolymer based hydrogels. Biomaterials 34: 8002–8011.
39. Wang X, Hu X, Daley A, Rabotyagova O, Cebe P, et al. (2007) Nanolayer biomaterial coatings of silk fibroin for controlled release. J Control Release 121: 190–199.

15

STAT3 Modulation to Enhance Motor Neuron Differentiation in Human Neural Stem Cells

Rajalaxmi Natarajan[1], Vinamrata Singal[1], Richard Benes[1], Junling Gao[1], Hoi Chan[1], Haijun Chen[2], Yongjia Yu[3], Jia Zhou[2], Ping Wu[1]*

1 Department of Neuroscience and Cell Biology, The University of Texas Medical Branch, Galveston, Texas, United States of America, **2** Department of Pharmacology & Toxicology, The University of Texas Medical Branch, Galveston, Texas, United States of America, **3** Department of Radiation Oncology, The University of Texas Medical Branch, Galveston, Texas, United States of America

Abstract

Spinal cord injury or amyotrophic lateral sclerosis damages spinal motor neurons and forms a glial scar, which prevents neural regeneration. Signal transducer and activator of transcription 3 (STAT3) plays a critical role in astrogliogenesis and scar formation, and thus a fine modulation of STAT3 signaling may help to control the excessive gliogenic environment and enhance neural repair. The objective of this study was to determine the effect of STAT3 inhibition on human neural stem cells (hNSCs). *In vitro* hNSCs primed with fibroblast growth factor 2 (FGF2) exhibited a lower level of phosphorylated STAT3 than cells primed by epidermal growth factor (EGF), which correlated with a higher number of motor neurons differentiated from FGF2-primed hNSCs. Treatment with STAT3 inhibitors, Stattic and Niclosamide, enhanced motor neuron differentiation only in FGF2-primed hNSCs, as shown by increased homeobox gene Hb9 mRNA levels as well as $HB9^+$ and microtubule-associated protein 2 $(MAP2)^+$ co-labeled cells. The increased motor neuron differentiation was accompanied by a decrease in the number of glial fibrillary acidic protein (GFAP)-positive astrocytes. Interestingly, Stattic and Niclosamide did not affect the level of STAT3 phosphorylation; rather, they perturbed the nuclear translocation of phosphorylated STAT3. In summary, we demonstrate that FGF2 is required for motor neuron differentiation from hNSCs and that inhibition of STAT3 further increases motor neuron differentiation at the expense of astrogliogenesis. Our study thus suggests a potential benefit of targeting the STAT3 pathway for neurotrauma or neurodegenerative diseases.

Editor: Wenhui Hu, Temple University School of Medicine, United States of America

Funding: This study is supported by John S. Dunn Research Foundation, TIRR Foundation Mission Connect, Gillson Longenbaugh Foundation, and Moody Foundation. The funders had no role in study design, data collection and analysis, decision to publish, or preparation of the manuscript.

Competing Interests: The authors have declared that no competing interests exist.

* Email: piwu@utmb.edu

Introduction

Acute spinal cord injury (SCI) and amyotrophic lateral sclerosis (ALS) are characterized by death of cholinergic motor neurons accompanied by reactive astrogliosis, *i.e.* hypertrophy and proliferation of astrocytes and alterations in their gene expression patterns. Typically, after spinal cord injury, initial motor neuron death is mediated by mechanical or physical forces. The massive death of residual neurons is due to secondary apoptotic, necrotic and excitotoxic processes, which initiate cascades of neuro-inflammatory responses by proinflammatory molecules, leading to reactivation and proliferation of nearby astrocytes. Similarly, prominent astrogliosis is a pathological hallmark of ALS in humans and animal models. For instance, transgenic rats carrying $SOD1^{G93A}$ mutation exhibited astrogliosis along with the loss of ventral motor neurons and astrocytic glutamate transporter [1,2]. Moreover, recent studies show that astrocytes derived from familial and sporadic ALS patients exhibit non-autonomous toxicity to motor neurons [3,4]. Thus, it is clear that increased astrogliosis resulting from acute spinal injury or chronic neurodegenerative conditions creates a highly gliogenic cellular environment, which is not conducive to the formation or long-term survival of motor neurons. Hence, in such patients, potential therapy should employ a two-pronged approach: 1) reduce the local gliogenic environment and 2) switch the environmental milieu such that it promotes/sustains neurogenesis.

In rodent models of SCI, levels of pro-inflammatory interleukin such as IL-6 peak acutely in the injured areas and lead to activation of the JAK1-STAT3 signaling pathway, which contributes to development of neuropathic pain [5,6]. Moreover, in previous work, conditional ablation of STAT3 increased motor deficits after spinal cord injury [7]. STAT3 signaling is also upregulated in certain neurodegenerative diseases. For instance, spinal cord microglia, reactive astrocytes and motor neuron nuclei of ALS patients showed increased levels of phosphorylated STAT3 [8]. ALS mouse models also exhibited persistent activation and nuclear translocation of phosphorylated STAT3 [9]. Together these studies support the hypothesis that after SCI, and perhaps in neurodegenerative conditions, activation of STAT3 signaling causes various undesirable outcomes. Hence, to promote neurogenesis in these tissues, it might be important to inhibit STAT3 activity. However, this hypothesis must be considered in the light of a growing body of literature suggesting that STAT3 is an injury-induced signaling mechanism critical for various aspects of nerve regeneration [7,10–13]. For instance, intrathecal administration of STAT3 inhibitors after nerve injury or spinal ligation reduced symptoms of neuropathic pain in rats [6,10]. Moreover, it is known that *in vitro* suppression of STAT3 [11] or its conditional deletion *in vivo* [12] induces neurogenesis and inhibits astrogliosis. Thus, it appears that the key to enhance neurogenesis and thereby, neural repair in SCI or ALS patients, would be to precisely regulate STAT3 pathway, such that it is inhibited at exactly the right time and to the right levels.

For stem cell researchers, replacing lost motor neurons in SCI or ALS patients by either transplantation of exogenous neural stem/progenitor cells or modulating endogenous adult stem cells to produce new motor neurons *in vivo* is a desirable but challenging goal. Previous studies from our laboratory have shown that the fate of human neural stem cells (hNSCs) can be modulated by precise amounts of certain growth factors in the surrounding environment [14,15]. For instance, human fetal brain-derived NSCs primed with basic fibroblast growth factor (FGF2), heparin and laminin (FHL) differentiated into cholinergic motor neurons [14,15], whereas epidermal growth factor (EGF), leukemia inhibitory factor (LIF) and laminin (ELL)-primed hNSCs generated glutamate and γ-aminobutyric acid (GABA) neuronal subtypes and showed minimal capability to form cholinergic motor neurons [15].

Thus, spinal damage from injury or degenerative disease causes loss of motor neurons, astrogliosis and a significant increase in STAT3, which increases astrocyte activation. In this study, we asked if pharmacological inhibition of STAT3 in the presence of FGF2 will enhance differentiation of hNSCs to motor neurons and reduce astrocytosis in an *in vitro* paradigm, more amenable to molecular analyses. Among the commercially available STAT3 inhibitors, we chose Stattic and Niclosamide because of their potency and relative specificity in inhibiting the STAT3 signaling pathway. Stattic has been shown to specifically inhibit STAT3 over STAT1, STAT5, c-Myc/Max, Jun/Jun and Lck in HepG2 cell lines [16]. Similarly, Niclosamide displays selectivity for STAT3 over STAT1, STAT5, JAK1, JAK2 and Src kinases [17]. Thus far, no studies have reported the effectiveness of these inhibitors in obtaining neurons from neural stem cells. This study shows that blocking STAT3 activity in FGF2-primed hNSCs increases expression of markers specific to motor neurons and decreases astrocyte markers, presumably by blocking nuclear transport of tyrosine-phosphorylated form of STAT3.

Methods/Materials

Human NSC Culture

Human fetal brain NSCs, the line K048 generously provided by C.N. Svendsen as we previously described [14], were cultured as free-floating "neurospheres" in 75-cm^2 flasks with growth medium containing DMEM (high glucose, L-glutamine)/Ham's F12 (3:1; Invitrogen/Gibco, Grand Island, NY), and supplemented with 15 mM HEPES (Sigma, St. Louis, MO), 1.5% D-glucose (Sigma), 67 IU/ml/67 μg/ml penicillin/streptomycin (Mediatech, Inc/CellGro, Manassas, VA), 25 μg/ml bovine insulin (Sigma), 100 μg/ml human transferrin (Sigma), 100 μM putrescine (Sigma), 20 nM progesterone (Sigma), 30 nM sodium selenite (Sigma), 20 ng/ml recombinant human EGF (Invitrogen), 20 ng/ml recombinant human FGF2 (R&D Systems, Minneapolis, MN), 5 μg/ml heparin (R&D Systems), 10 ng/ml recombinant human LIF (Millipore), and 2 mM L-glutamine (Sigma). Cells were passaged every 7 days. Cultured spheres were pelleted by centrifugation at 216×g for 10 min, resuspended in 0.025% trypsin (Sigma) plus 1.5% D-glucose dissolved in calcium- and magnesium-free Dulbecco's phosphate buffered saline (CMF-dPBS, CellGro), and incubated for 10 min at 37°C with periodic trituration. 250 U/ml DNAse was added to break down aggregated DNA in cases of excessive cell lysis. The reaction was stopped by using 1.2 mg/ml of trypsin inhibitor (Sigma) diluted in conditioned medium that was spared from the original cell culture. Cells were mechanically triturated with a 5-ml serological pipet till no visible clumps. Cells were quantified using trypan blue exclusion and hemacytometer counting. After passaging, 5×10^6 cells were seeded into a 75-cm^2 flask in 5 ml of conditioned and 10 ml of fresh medium and incubated at 37°C with 8.5% CO_2 to maintain pH 7.2–7.5. Prior to plating cells, new flasks were treated with conditioned medium (7 ml/75 cm^2) at 37°C for at least 1 hr, which helped to prevent initial adhesion of cells to the bottom of new culture flasks.

Priming, Inhibitor Treatment and Differentiation

Priming of hNSC was carried out in 25 cm^2 flasks (T25 flasks). These flasks were precoated with 2 mL of 0.1 mg/mL poly-D-lysine (Sigma) for one hour and then with 2 mL dPBS containing 1 μg/cm^2 laminin overnight. Approximately 2 million cells were plated per T25 flask, and primed with either FGF2/heparin/laminin (FHL) or EGF/LIF/laminin (ELL) medium, based on our previous experiments revealing the effects of different priming media on motor neuron differentiation [15]. The priming was carried out for either 1 day for Western blot analyses of protein phosphorylation or 4 days for mRNA measurement by RT-PCR and motor neuron differentiation by immunostaining (see below).

Specific inhibitors for STAT3, Stattic, Niclosamide or HJC0142, were applied to hNSCs during the priming period. After screening various compounds, we decided to use Stattic (Tocris Biosystems, Elsville, MO), Niclosamide (Tocris Biosystems) and HJC0142 (developed in house [18,19]). We tested Stattic with the following dosages for hNSC treatments: 0.5 μM, 2 μM after researching various dosages and utilizing the IC_{50}. We tested Niclosamide with the following dosages: 0.25 μM, 0.5 μM, 1 μM. Stattic was added every day during the 4-day priming period, whereas Niclosamide was administered once. After testing various concentrations, 0.5 μM HJC0149 was selected for further experiments.

Semiquantitative Reverse Transcription-Polymerase Chain Reaction (RT-PCR)

Cells were washed with PBS, and total RNA was extracted using Qiagen RNA Isolation Kit (Qiagen, Valencia, CA). Reverse transcription was performed using the High Capacity cDNA Reverse Transcription Kit (AB Applied Biosystems, Carlsbad, CA) according to the manufacturer's instructions. Twenty ng of cDNA was used in the following PCR reaction using empirically determined conditions to allow a quantitative analysis [15]. PCR amplification was performing using REDTaq DNA Polymerase (Sigma) with a program of 95°C for 5 minutes, 35 cycles of 94°C for 30 seconds, 65°C for 1 minute, 72°C for 1 minute, an extension of 72°C for 5 minutes for Hb9 amplification; a program of 95°C for 5 minutes, 23 cycles of 94°C for 30 seconds, 60°C for 30 seconds, 72°C for 90 seconds, and an extension of 72°C for 5 minutes was used for GAPDH amplification. The following reverse and forward primers were utilized: HB9: AGCT-GGGCCGGCACCTTCC and CCGCCGCCGCCCTTCTG-TTTCTC; GAPDH: TGAAGGTCGGAGTCAACGGA and GATGGCATGGACTGTGGTCAT. PCR products were visualized on an ethidium bromide-stained1.5% agarose gel and the bend intensities under UV light were captured and analyzed with a Chemi-Imager 4400 v5.5 with the Alpha-Ease software. The HB9 expression levels were normalized to that of GAPDH.

Western Blot Analysis

T25 flasks pre-coated with 0.01% poly-D-lysine/dPBS and 0.5 μg/cm^2 Laminin/dPBS for 1 hr at 37°C respectively were plated with ~2.2 million cells. The cells were primed with FHL or ELL along with various concentrations of STAT3 inhibitors, Stattic (0.5 μM, 2 μM) and Niclosamide (0.25 μM and 2 μM) for 24 hrs. The cells were washed with 4 ml dPBS and incubated with 150 μl of solution containing 1x cell lysis buffer (Cell Signaling Technology, Danvers, MA) and 1 mM PMSF (Sigma). The cells were scraped and the lysate rocked for 1 hr at 4°C. Subsequently, the lysate was centrifuged at 14,000×g at 4°C for 10 min and the supernatant was collected in a fresh microfuge tube. Lysates were either used fresh or stored at −80°C. Protein concentration was determined using Bio-Rad Protein Assay. Samples were warmed in a solution containing LDS sample buffer and NuPAGE reducing buffer at 75°C and 2 μg of protein was loaded per well. Proteins were separated using NuPAGE 4–12% bis-tris gel (Invitrogen) electrophoresis (110 V for 90 min) using the recommended running buffer. The proteins were transferred onto a nitrocellulose membrane by running at 120 V/2 h. The blots were blocked with 5% phosphoBLOCKER (for phosphoproteins) or with non-fat dry milk (for regular proteins) for 1 hr at room temperature. The blots were incubated overnight with the following primary antibodies (Cell Signaling Technology): rabbit anti-pSTAT Tyr-705 (1:1,000), rabbit anti-pSTAT3 Ser 727 (1:1,000), total rabbit anti-STAT3 (1:1,000) and mouse anti-GAPDH (1:1,000). The membranes were washed 3×10 min in TBST with vigorous shaking, followed by incubating with HRP-conjugated secondary antibodies: goat anti-rabbit (1:5,000) and sheep anti-mouse (1:2,000) for 1 hr at room temperature. The membranes were rinsed again as before, and incubated with ECL or ECL Plus reagents (for phosphoproteins, Amersham). The bend intensities were measured and analyzed with an Alpha Innotech Imager.

Immunofluorescence

Cells were primed on glass coverslips in 24-well plates (precoated as described in the priming section) with 0.12 million cells per well. We tested two dosages along with controls: 0.25 μm Niclosamide and 0.5 μm Stattic. Cells stayed in either FHL or ELL medium for 4 days (Stattic treatment was added every day at the same time) and were placed in 1X B27 medium for differentiation for 9 days. B27 medium was made from 50x B27 (Gibco/Invitrogen) and dPBS. After 9 days, cells were fixed in ice-cold 4% paraformaldehyde for 20 min and washed with PBS, and post-fixed with methanol, and then washed with TBS 3 times for 5 minutes each. Cells were permeabilized using 0.25% Triton-X and blocked using 5% Normal Goat Serum. Slides were incubated overnight with the primary antibodies against MAP2 (Chemicon, 1:500) and Hb9 (Santa Cruz Biotechnology, Santa Cruz, CA, 1:100) in a double labeling, GFAP (Chemicon, 1:1,000), pSTAT3-Tyr 705 (Cell signaling Technology, 1:100) or pSTAT3-Ser727 (Cell signaling Technology, 1:100). After three washes with TBS for 15 minutes each, cells were incubated in the following secondary antibodies depending on the type of primary antibody: Alexa 568 goat anti-mouse antibody (Invitrogen, 1:400) or Alexa 488 goat anti-rabbit antibody (Invitrogen, 1:400). Cells were counter-stained with DAPI to locate the nucleus, and then coverslips were mounted on microscope slides using Fluromount-G. Cells were visualized by using fluorescence or confocal microscope. At least 10 randomly-selected fields of cells were imaged per treatment condition for every experiment and each experiment was independently performed 3–4 times. Images for each fluorophore are achieved individually. The total cell number in each field is determined by DAPI staining. Cells with clear nuclear Hb9 staining were counted as Hb9$^+$. Cells that exhibited distinct neurite extensions with MAP2 labeling were counted as MAP2$^+$. The ratio of Hb9$^+$/MAP2$^+$ is calculated accordingly. The localization of active STAT3 is examined with anti-pSTAT3-Y705 antibody. The pY705 immunoreactivity was quantified by an NIS-Element software to determine the average ratio of pY705 immunoreactivity inside a DAPI-labeled nucleus over pY705 in the whole cell.

WST-1 Assay

Cells were primed and then incubated in 37°C at 8.5% CO_2 for 72 hours (approximately 0.03 million cells/well) in a 96-well plate in either FHL or ELL medium. After 72 hrs, cells were retrieved and approximately 10 μl of WST-1 reagent (Roche Applied Science, Indianapolis, IN) was added to each well. After approximately 2–3 hours (or after noticing a considerable color change) the plate was moved to the microplate reader, which provided an output spectrophotometric analysis at a wavelength of 450 nm.

Statistical/Data Analysis

All experiments were repeated at least three times. Results were analyzed with Prism software (GraphPad Software, San Diego, CA). Data are shown as mean±S.E.M and are compared with One-way ANOVA followed by post-hoc tests, or Student's *t*-test. A p value <0.05 is considered statistically significant.

Results

FGF2 Priming Reduces Tyrosine Phosphorylated STAT3 in hNSCs

Our previous studies showed that growth factors, EGF and FGF2, have opposite effects on specification of motor neurons from hNSCs, via differential actions on the PI3K/Akt/GSK3B pathway [20]. To determine if priming of hNSCs with FGF2 or EGF affects the activation of STAT3, we performed Western blot analysis using phospho-specific antibodies: tyrosine 705 (pSTAT3-Y705) or serine 727 (pSTAT3-S727). Lysates from neurospheres and hNSCs primed with either FGF2/Heparin/Laminin (FHL) or EGF/LIF/Laminin (ELL) for 24 hr were probed with antibodies against pSTAT3-Y705 or pSTAT3-Ser 727 (Fig. 1A). Densitometric analysis was performed to measure pSTAT3-Y705 or pSTAT3-S727 levels and the ratios of pSTAT3-Y705/total STAT3 or pSTAT3-S727/total STAT3 were graphically represented (Fig. 1A). We found that unprimed hNSCs grown as free-floating neurospheres (Fig. 1B) had considerable amounts of pSTAT3-Y705, pSTAT3-S727 and total STAT3 (Fig. 1A, sphere). As expected, a further 20% increase in the amount of pSTAT3-Y705 was observed upon EGF priming (Fig. 1A, ELL) while there was no change in the amounts of pSTAT3-S727 levels (Fig. 1A, ELL). Upon ELL priming, the cells attained the expected long, radiating morphology with limited migrating potential (Fig. 1C). On the other hand, priming with FGF2 (in the absence of EGF) consistently yielded a 50% reduction in the levels of pSTAT3-Y705 compared to unprimed neurospheres (Fig. 1A, FHL). This effect of FGF2 was specific to tyrosine phosphorylation because pSTAT3-S727 levels remained unchanged upon FGF2 priming (Fig. 1A, FHL). Moreover, as expected, FGF2-treated cells exhibited uniform sizes with more pyramidal morphology

(Fig. 1D). Thus, this indicates that stimulation with FGF2 specifically decreases tyrosine 705-, but not serine 727-, phosphorylation of STAT3. Moreover, it also shows that stimulation of hNSCs with EGF results in a moderate upregulation of tyrosine 705-, but not serine 727-, phosphorylation of STAT3. Thus, it appears that in hNSCs only tyrosine phosphorylation of STAT3 is responsive to growth factors.

STAT3 Inhibitors, Stattic and Niclosamide, Exhibit Dose-dependent Viability in Human Neural Stem Cells

To identify the optimal dosage of Stattic and Niclosamide that inhibit STAT3 activity but do not exhibit any morphological or cytotoxic effects, we performed morphological analysis and WST-1 viability assays in the presence of these inhibitors under EGF or FGF2 priming conditions. As previously

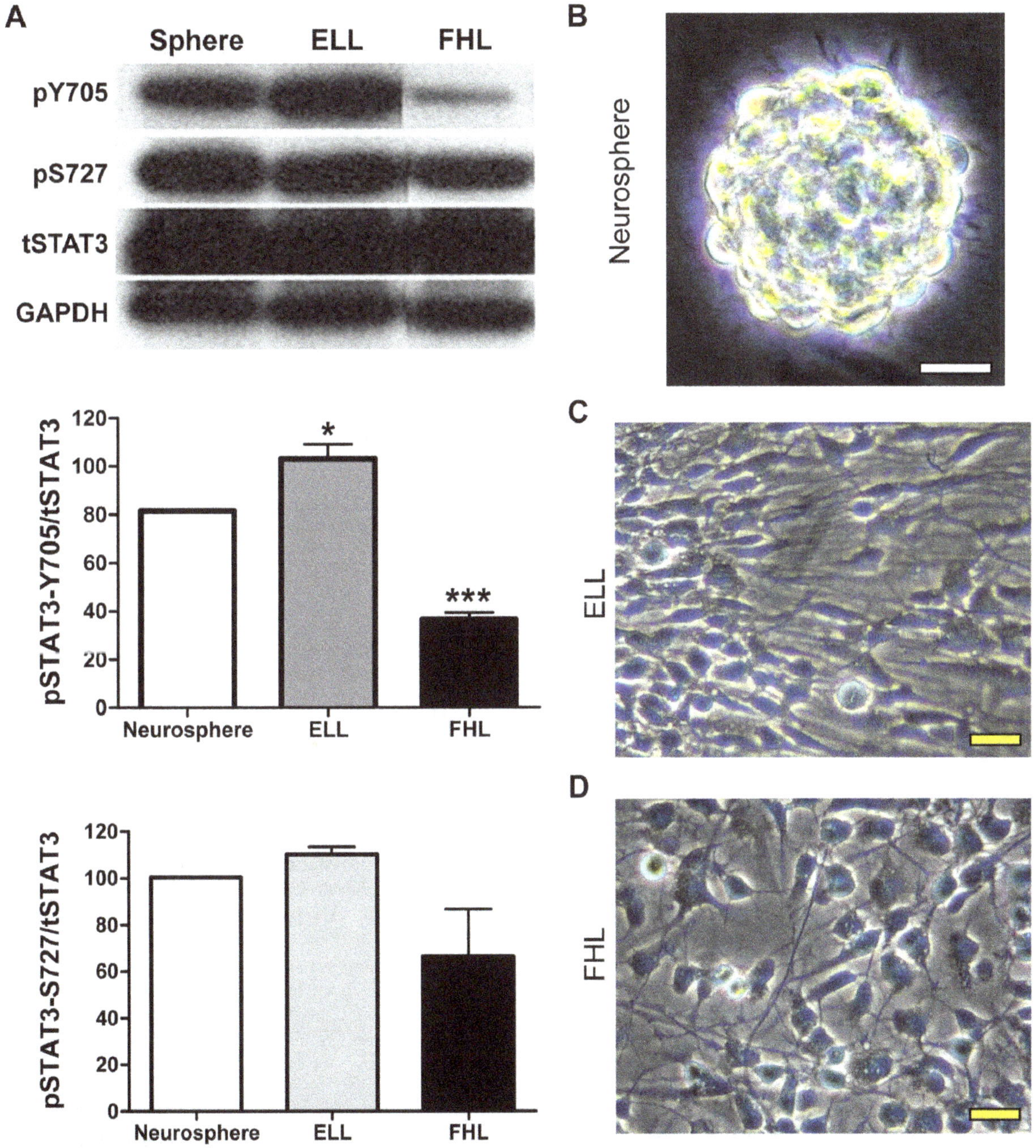

Figure 1. EGF and FGF2 have opposite effects on STAT3 phosphorylation in hNSCs. (**A**) Lysates from neurospheres as well as hNSCs primed with either EGF (ELL) or FGF2 (FHL) for 24 hrs were analyzed by immunoblotting using antibodies against phosphorylated STAT3-Tyr705 (pY705) or STAT3-Ser727 (pS727). The blots were stripped and re-probed for total STAT3 (tSTAT3) and GAPDH (loading control). Densitometric analysis was performed and ratios of phosphorylated STAT3 to total STAT3 (pSTAT3/tSTAT3) are graphically represented as Mean ± SEM (n = 3). $^*p < 0.05$ and $^{***}p < 0.001$ by One-way ANOVA with Tukey post-hoc test. pSTAT3-Y705 is increased in EGF-primed cells, but reduced in FGF2-primed cells when compared to unprimed neurospheres. pSTAT3-S727 levels, however, remain unchanged after either priming. Representative phase contrast images of primary culture hNSCs are shown as neurospheres (**B**), one day after ELL- (**C**) or FHL-priming (**D**). Scale bars, 20 µm. hNSCs: human neural stem cells; ELL: EGF plus LIF and laminin; FHL: FGF2 plus heparin and laminin.

reported, FHL-primed hNSCs had uniform cell size, shape and retained the ability to migrate (Fig. S1A) On the other hand, ELL-primed cells had diverse shapes, long radiating projections and limited migrating capacities (Fig. S1B, control). Upon treatment with various doses of Stattic, ELL- and FHL-primed hNSCs exhibited morphological features similar to their corresponding control cells (compare Fig. S1C to Fig. S1A and Fig. S1D to Fig. S1B). However, higher doses of Stattic resulted in cytotoxicity, under both ELL and FHL priming conditions (Fig. S1E, S1F). The WST-1 assay indicated that concentrations up to 2.5 μM Stattic did not affect cell viability whereas treatment with higher concentrations of Stattic led to the loss of cell viability in both ELL- and FHL-primed hNSCs (Fig. 2A). Similarly, cells treated with lower concentrations of Niclosamide and primed with ELL or FHL exhibited expected morphological features, well comparable to their corresponding controls (Compare Fig. S2A to Fig. S2C and Fig. S2B to Fig. S2D). However, both ELL- and FHL-primed hNSCs treated with higher concentrations of Niclosamide (2 μM and 5 μM) resembled FHL-treated cells more than ELL-treated controls (Fig. S2E and S2F). In addition, the WST-1 cell viability assay indicated that cells treated with 2 μM Niclosamide showed moderate cytotoxicity only in ELL-primed cells while higher doses (5 μM) of Niclosamide had significantly decreased viability when primed with either growth factor (Fig. 2B). Based on WST-1 cell viability and morphological analysis, sub-lethal doses of Stattic (0.5 or 2.5 μM) and Niclosamide (0.25 μM) were chosen for further studies.

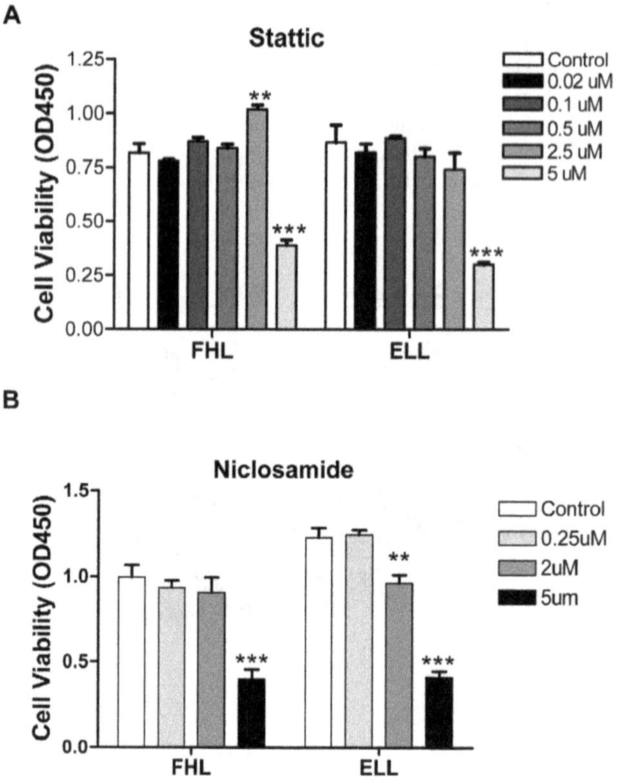

Figure 2. Stattic and Niclosamide exhibit dose-dependent effects on hNSCs. Cell viability is determined by WST-1 assay in FHL- or ELL-primed hNSCs treated with varying doses of Stattic and Niclosamide. (**A**) Low doses of Stattic (up to 2.5 μM) did not affect viability in either FHL or ELL conditions. Higher concentrations of Stattic, such as 5 μM, are toxic to cells. (**B**) Low doses of Niclosamide reduced the number of viable cells in ELL-primed group whereas higher concentrations of Niclosamide (5 μM) were toxic to both FHL- and ELL-primed cells. Data are presented as mean ± SEM (n = 6), ***$p<0.0001$; **$p<0.01$ by One-way ANOVA with Tukey post-hoc tests. hNSCs: human neural stem cells; ELL: EGF plus LIF and laminin; FHL: FGF2 plus heparin and laminin.

STAT3 Inhibition Increased Motor Neuron Differentiation in hNSCs

To test if STAT3 inhibition affects motor neuron specification of hNSCs, we analyzed mRNA and protein expression levels of Hb9, a known marker of motor neurons. To compare Hb9 mRNA levels upon STAT3 inhibition, cells primed with either ELL or FHL were treated with various sub-lethal concentrations of either Stattic or Niclosamide for 24 hrs followed by RT-PCR analysis. We observed a consistently significant increase in Hb9 mRNA levels in FHL-primed cells with increasing concentrations of Stattic (Fig. 3A). Treatment with 0.5 μM Stattic resulted in roughly double the Hb9/GAPDH ratio compared to untreated FHL controls (Fig. 3A). However, further increase in Stattic concentrations did not increase Hb9 mRNA yield, indicating that this concentration of Stattic provides the level of STAT3 that results in optimal expression of Hb9 mRNA. Similarly, we observed a dose-dependent increase in Hb9 mRNA levels upon Niclosamide treatment and found that FHL-primed cells treated with 0.25 μM Niclosamide had significantly increased the Hb9/GAPDH ratio compared to FHL-primed untreated cells (Fig. 3B). On the other hand, treatment with Stattic (0.5uM) or Niclosamide (0.25 uM) in ELL-primed cells did not result in any significant increase in Hb9/GAPDH ratio (Fig. 3C). This indicates that precise control of STAT3 levels along with FGF2 leads to optimal Hb9 mRNA expression. Moreover, as reported previously, the ratio of Hb9/GAPDH in FHL-primed control cells is usually at least 2-fold higher than the ratio of Hb9/GAPDH in ELL-primed control cells (Fig. 3A–B Control vs Fig. 3C Control). To confirm that the increase in Hb9 mRNA levels in FHL-primed hNSC treated with optimal doses of Stattic or Niclosamide was accompanied by a corresponding increase in Hb9 protein levels, immunofluorescent analysis was performed. Human neural stem cells were subjected to either ELL- or FHL-priming followed by a nine-day differentiation period in B27 media. Subsequently, the cells were double immunolabeled with antibodies against Hb9, an early marker for motor neurons and MAP2 (microtubule-associated protein 2), which marks mature differentiated neurons. We observed that ~35% of FHL-primed control cells expressed both Hb9 and MAP2 (Fig. 3D,F control). Upon inhibition of STAT3, it was increased to ~45% in FHL-primed 0.5 μM Stattic-treated cells (Fig. 3D,F) and 50% in FHL-primed cells treated with 0.25 μM Niclosamide (Fig. 3D, F). However, ELL-primed cells did not exhibit a significant increase in motor neuron specification upon STAT3 inhibition using either Stattic or Niclosamide (Fig. 3E, G). As graphically represented in Fig. 3G, ~20% of ELL-primed control cells co-localized for both Hb9 and MAP2. About 25% and 20% $HB9^{+}/MAP2^{+}$ cells were found in Stattic- and Niclosamide-treated groups, respectively. Our newly developed STAT3 inhibitor, HJC0149, with a much lower cellular toxicity and improved bioavailability [18,19], also exhibited similar increases in the Hb9 transcript level as well as the number of $Hb9^{+}/MAP2^{+}$ motor neurons in the presence of FHL (Fig. S3). Thus, we conclude that inhibition of STAT3 increased the transcript levels of Hb9 as well as the number of differentiated motor neurons only in FHL-primed cells but not in ELL-primed cells.

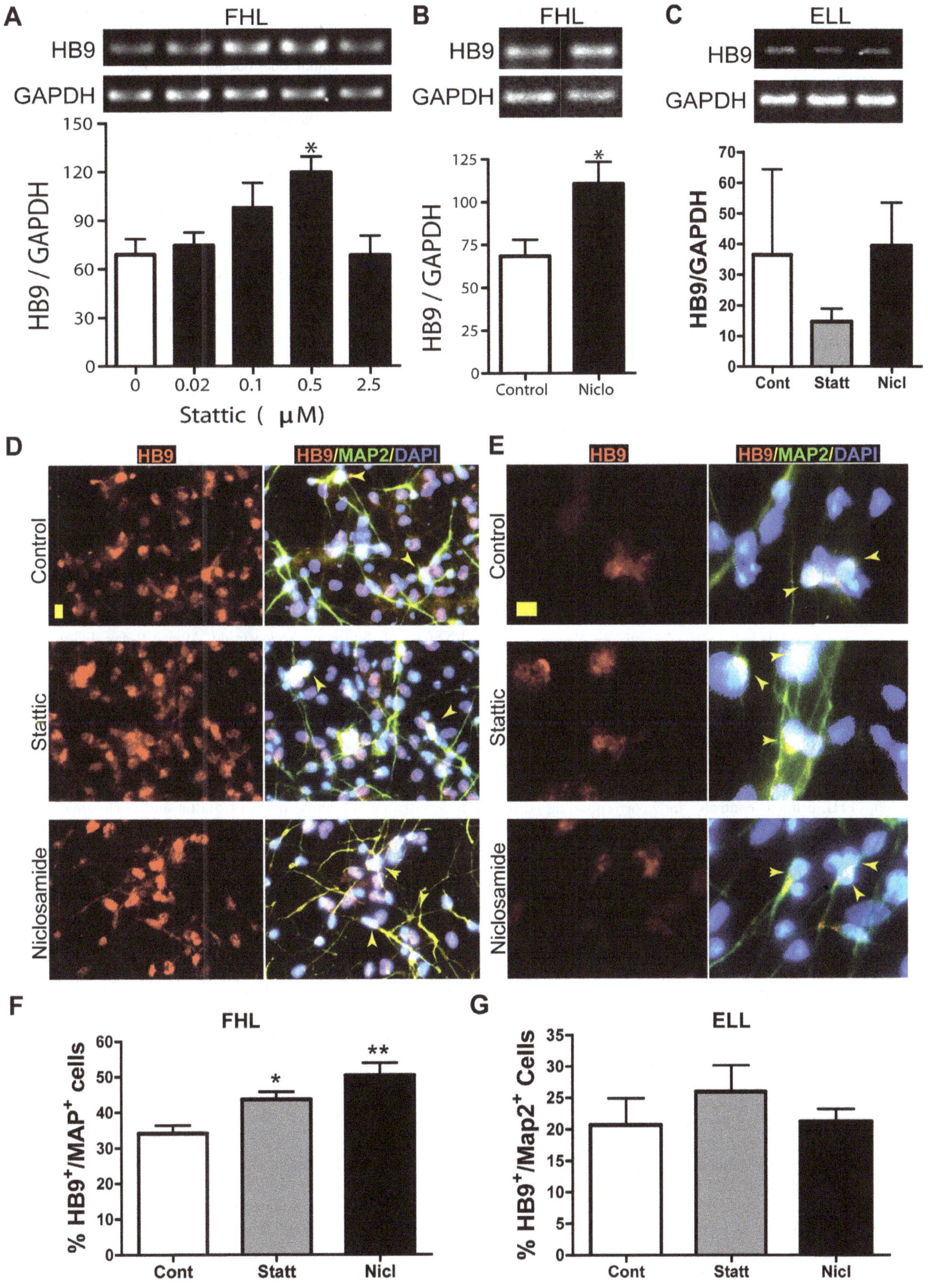
A
FHL
HB9
GAPDH
HB9 / GAPDH
150
120
90
60
30
0
*
0
0.02
0.1
0.5
2.5
Stattic (μM)
B
FHL
HB9
GAPDH
HB9 / GAPDH
125
100
75
50
25
0
*
Control
Niclo
C
ELL
HB9
GAPDH
HB9/GAPDH
70
60
50
40
30
20
10
0
Cont
Statt
Nicl
D
HB9
HB9/MAP2/DAPI
Control
Stattic
Niclosamide
E
HB9
HB9/MAP2/DAPI
Control
Stattic
Niclosamide
F
FHL
% HB9+/MAP+ cells
60
50
40
30
20
10
0
*
**
Cont
Statt
Nicl
G
ELL
% HB9+/Map2+ Cells
35
30
25
20
15
10
5
0
Cont
Statt
Nicl

Figure 3. Increased motor neuron differentiation in hNSCs by STAT3 inhibition. (**A–C**) Semi-quantitative RT-PCR analyses of the expression level of HB9 mRNA, a marker for spinal motor neurons, after a 4-day priming. GAPDH mRNA expression serves as internal control. In general, FHL-primed hNSCs (**A,B**) express more Hb9 mRNA than the corresponding ELL-primed cells (**C**). Hb9 mRNA levels are significantly increased in FHL-primed hNSCs treated with 0.5 μM Stattic (**A**) or 0.25 μM Niclosamide (**B**). In contrast, STAT3 inhibition does not alter HB9 mRNA expression in ELL-primed cells (**C**). Values are mean ± SEM (n = 3), *p<0.05, One-way ANOVA plus Tukey post- hoc tests (A and C) or Student's *t*-test (B). (**D–G**) Immunofluorescent staining of Hb9/MAP2-labeled motor neurons in hNSCs primed and inhibitor-treated for 4 days and differentiated in B27 for 9 days. Hb9 immunoreactivity is in general higher in FHL-primed than ELL-primed cells. Representative epifluorescent microscopic images show increased Hb9 and MAP2 immunoreactivity in FHL-primed hNSCs after treatment with Stattic (0.5 μM) and Niclosamide (0.25 μM) (**D**). Inhibition of STAT3, on the other hand, does not affect HB9/MAP2 labeling in ELL-treated cells (**E**). Arrowheads point to cells that are co-labeled with Hb9 and MAP2, and contain a DAPI-stained nucleus with cytoplasm extended into neurites. Scale bar: 10 μM (**F–G**) Quantitative analyses show that 0.5 μM Stattic significantly increase the percentage of $Hb9^+/MAP2^+$ cells in FHL-primed cells. **p*<0.05 by One-way ANOVA with Tukey post-hoc tests. hNSCs: human neural stem cells; ELL: EGF plus LIF and laminin; FHL: FGF2 plus heparin and laminin; Statt: Stattic; Nicl: Niclosamide.

Stattic and Niclosamide do not Affect Tyrosine Phosphorylation of STAT3 but Perturb its Nuclear Translocation

Tyrosine phosphorylation of STAT3 leads to its dimerization via phosphotyrosine interactions, which alters its conformation, allowing for target DNA binding and activation of downstream transcriptional targets. Thus, to identify the mechanism as to how Stattic and Niclosamide disrupt STAT3 pathway activity, we first hypothesized that these inhibitors may disrupt tyrosine phosphorylation of STAT3. To test that, we performed an immunoblot analysis of ELL- and FHL-primed hNSCs treated with various concentrations of Stattic and Niclosamide with an antibody specific to tyrosine 705-phosphorylated form of STAT3. As expected, we observed an overall increase in the levels of pSTAT3-Y705 in FHL-primed cells versus ELL-primed control cells (Fig. 4A,B. "0" panels). However, contrary to our expectations, there was no significant difference in the levels of pSTAT3-Y705 among various sub-lethal doses of Stattic or Niclosamide irrespective of whether they were primed with FHL or ELL (Fig. 4A,B). While a higher dose (2 μM) of Niclosamide resulted in decreased pSTAT3-Y705 levels, it was attributed to perturbed morphological changes (Fig. S2E,F) that indicate some unexplained underlying physiological changes and hence were not taken into consideration. The levels of pSTAT3-S727, total STAT3 and GAPDH (loading control) remained unchanged in ELL-primed, FHL-primed controls and corresponding drug treated cells (data not shown). Thus, Stattic and Niclosamide do not affect tyrosine phosphorylation of STAT3.

A recent study demonstrated that nuclear import of STAT3 occurs independent of tyrosine phosphorylation of STAT3 [21]. Therefore, we asked if nuclear translocation of tyrosine phosphorylated form of STAT3 was adversely affected in the presence of STAT3 inhibitors. If this was indeed the case, we expected to see decreased levels of nuclear tyrosine-phosphorylated STAT3 upon treatment with these STAT3 inhibitors. To test this, ELL- and FHL-primed hNSCs treated with 0.5 μM Stattic or 0.25 μM Niclosamide were immunostained with a phosphor-specific antibody against tyrosine-705 phosphorylated STAT3 and counter-stained for DAPI, a fluorescent dye that acts as a nuclear marker. We observed that in FHL-primed control cells, pTyr705-STAT3 was largely localized to the nucleus, although some of it was also observed in the cytoplasm (Fig. 4C). Interestingly, about 75% of Stattic-treated cells exhibited cytoplasmic localization of pSTAT3-Y705 and only about 25% had pSTAT3 in the nucleus (Fig. 4C,E). This block in nuclear transport was also observed in FHL-primed Niclosamide-treated cells (Fig. 4C). On the other hand, almost all of the ELL-primed control cells exhibited nuclear pSTAT3-Y705 (Fig. 4D) with the level of immunoreactivity much stronger than that in FHL-primed cell nuclei (Fig. 4C). Upon treatment with sub-lethal concentrations of Stattic or Niclosamide, ELL-primed cells exhibited no significant change in the amount of nuclear localized pSTAT3-Y705 when compared to ELL-primed control cells (Fig. 4D,F). Thus, Stattic and Niclosamide, block nuclear transport of pSTAT3-Y705, specifically in FHL-primed cells, but not in ELL-primed cells. This difference in subcellular localization correlates well with the increase in motor neuron specification only in STAT3 inhibitor-treated, FHL-primed cells. Taken together, it appears that through an unknown mechanism, increased levels of cytoplasmic tyrosine phosphorylated STAT3 may result in an increase in motor neurons.

STAT3 Inhibition in hNSCs Decreased $GFAP^+$ Astrocytes

Previous studies have shown that STAT3 binding to the glial fibrillary acidic protein (GFAP) promoter is essential for GFAP expression [22,23]. We hypothesized that reduced nuclear levels of STAT3 in FHL-primed Stattic or Niclosamide hNSCs should reduce GFAP expression and hence, the number of $GFAP^+$ astrocytes. To test that, we treated control, FHL- or ELL-primed hNSCs with Stattic or Nicloasmide. After a 9-day differentiation period, they were fixed and co-immunostained with antibodies against GFAP, an intermediate filament protein that marks mature astrocytes, and the nuclear marker, DAPI. It was observed that ~30% of FHL-primed control cells were positive for GFAP (Fig. 5A, D). FHL-primed hNSCs treated with 0.5 μM Stattic (Fig. 5B, D) or 0.25 uM Niclosamide (Fig. 5C, D) exhibited significantly reduced ratio of $GFAP^+$/DAPI (Fig. 5D). This clearly indicates that sub-lethal doses of Stattic and Niclosamide in the presence of FGF2, are sufficient to reduce GFAP expression and thereby, astroglial differentiation, most likely due to reduced nuclear pSTAT3-Y705.

Discussion

The main findings of our study are that 1) hNSCs primed with FGF2 had reduced levels of phosphorylated/activated STAT3; 2) Treatment of FGF2-primed, but not EGF-primed, hNSCs with specific pharmacological inhibitors of STAT3 enhanced motor neuron fate specification at the expense of astroglial differentiation; 3) The STAT3 inhibitors, Stattic and Niclosamide, do not inactivate STAT3 signaling by affecting STAT3 expression or its phosphorylation, but by blocking nuclear transport of activated STAT3.

FGF2 Reduced Levels of Phosphorylated STAT3

FGF2 is an essential neurogenic factor required for proliferation and differentiation of multipotent neural stem cells both during development and in the adult mouse brain [24,25]. Moreover, it is known that in the adult central nervous system (CNS), FGF2 is expressed in the neurogenic niches (the subventricular zone of the lateral ventricles–SVZ; and the subgranular zone of the hippocampal dentate gyrus–SGZ) and has been implicated in the control of adult neurogenesis based on changes in proliferation

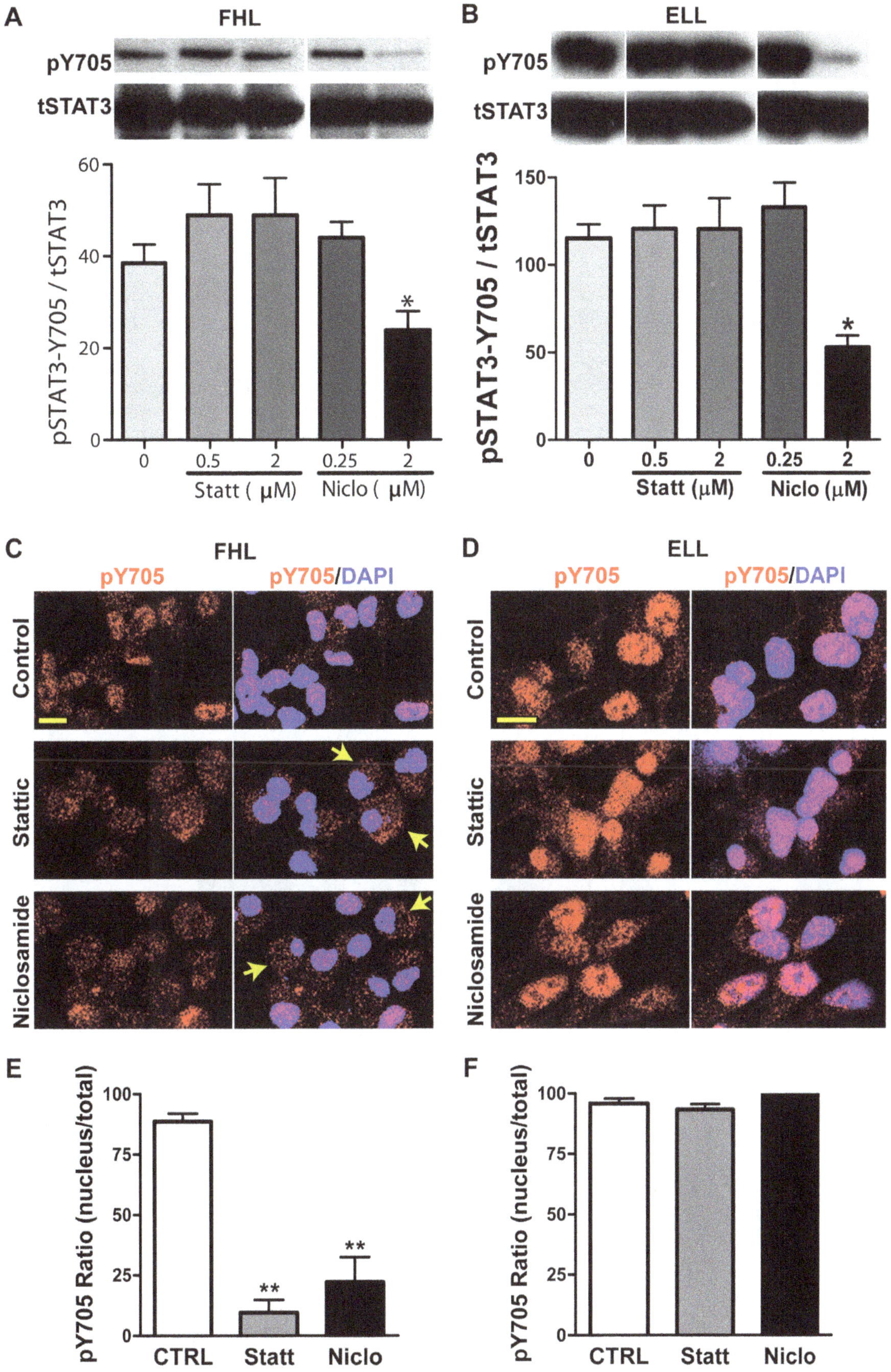
A
FHL
pY705
tSTAT3
pSTAT3-Y705 / tSTAT3
0
20
40
60
0
0.5
2
0.25
2
Statt (μM)
Niclo (μM)
B
ELL
pY705
tSTAT3
pSTAT3-Y705 / tSTAT3
0
50
100
150
0
0.5
2
0.25
2
Statt (μM)
Niclo (μM)
C
FHL
pY705
pY705/DAPI
Control
Stattic
Niclosamide
D
ELL
pY705
pY705/DAPI
Control
Stattic
Niclosamide
E
pY705 Ratio (nucleus/total)
0
25
50
75
100
CTRL
Statt
Niclo
F
pY705 Ratio (nucleus/total)
0
25
50
75
100
CTRL
Statt
Niclo

Figure 4. STAT3 phosphorylation in hNSCs treated with STAT3 inhibitors. (**A–B**): Western blot analyses of pSTAT3-Tyr705 (pY705) and total STAT3 (tSTAT3) in FHL- or ELL-primed hNSCs, with or without treatment of Stattic and Niclosamide for 24 hrs. GAPDH was used as loading control. Densitometric analysis was performed and normalized values of pSTAT3-Y705/tSTAT3 calculated from 3 independent experiments are graphically represented (Mean ± SEM). In general, FHL-primed hNSCs exhibit a much lower level of pY705 (**A**) than that in ELL-primed cells (**B**). STAT3 inhibitors, Stattic and Niclosamide at the doses showing no cytotoxicity, do not affect the phosphorylation of STAT3 at Y705 (pY705); whereas the cytotoxic dose of niclosamide resulted in a significant reduction of pY705 (n = 3, *$p<0.05$ by One-way ANOVA plus Tukey post-hoc tests). (**C–D**) Representative confocal images show the immunofluorescent staining of pY705 in hNSCs. Blue are nuclei counterstained with DAPI. pY705 (red) is localized mainly in nuclei of the FHL- or ELL-primed cells without STAT3 inhibitor treatment (Controls in **C** or **D**, respectively). Treatment with Stattic (0.5 μM) or Niclosamide (0.25 μM) decreases the nuclear translocation of activated STAT3 (pY705) in FHL- primed hNSCs (**C**), but not in ELL-primed cells (**D**). Scale bar, 10 μm. (**E–F**) Quantitative localization of pY705 STAT3 immunereactivity in the nucleus vs. in a whole cell. **$p<0.01$. One-way ANOVA with Dunnett post hoc tests. hNSCs: human neural stem cells; ELL: EGF plus LIF and laminin; FHL: FGF2 plus heparin and laminin; Statt: Stattic; Niclo: Niclosamide.

and differentiation of adult neural stem and progenitor cells [25,26]. The role of FGF2 in NSC propagation and proliferation both *in vivo* and *in vitro* is well established [26,27]. Previous studies from our lab demonstrated that FGF2 and EGF have differential effects on motor neuron fate specification in human fetal neural stem cells, achieved by fine modulation of phosphatidylinositol 3-kinase (PI3K)/Akt/glycogen synthase kinase 3β (GSK3β) signaling, independently of MAPK and PLC-γ pathway [15,20]. The current model to explain the differential effects of FGF2 and EGF on hNSCs is that FGF Receptor-induced Akt/GSK3β is lower than the corresponding EGF Receptor-induced Akt-GSK3β activation. This results in lowered phosphorylation of GSK3β at Ser9 and therefore, leads to increased transcription of Hb9, a crucial homeobox transcription factor crucial for the identity of postmitotic motor neurons, likely via Ngn2 phosphorylation/activation [20].

Interestingly, we found that priming hNSCs with FGF2 and heparin results in dramatic reduction in tyrosine phosphorylation of STAT3. It is known that STAT3 regulates the expression of GFAP, a key component of astrocytes. In early telencephalic neuroepithelial cells and postmitotic neurons, activation of GFAP expression is blocked by CpG methylation of its STAT3 binding sites, and demethylation of STAT3 binding sites leads to GFAP expression [22,23]. FGF2 regulates ciliary neurotrophic factor (CTNF)-mediated induction of GFAP expression via STAT3 binding but does not affect CNTF-induced STAT1/3 tyrosine-705 phosphorylation [28]. Thus, the reduction in tyrosine-705 phosphorylation of STAT3 that we observed upon FGF2-priming of hNSCs occurs via CNTF-independent mechanisms.

Blocking STAT3 Increases Motor Neuron Differentiation of FGF2-primed hNSCs

Our results demonstrate that optimal doses of pharmacological inhibitors of STAT3 in FGF2-primed hNSCs result in increased Hb9 mRNA expression and increased Hb9- and MAP2-positive mature neurons. At the same doses, Stattic and Niclosamide fail to

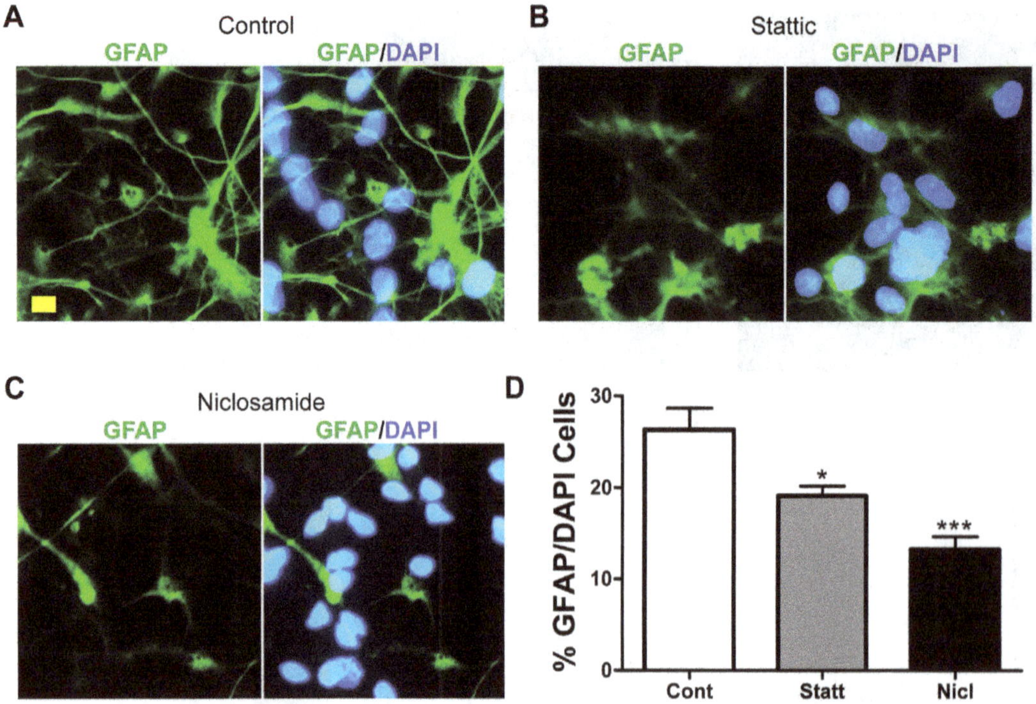

Figure 5. Astroglial differentiation in hNSCs treated with STAT3 inhibitors. Immunofluorescent staining is used to determine GFAP-labeled astrocytic differentiation in human neural stem cells (hNSCs) that were FHL-primed and inhibitor-treated for 4 days, and then differentiated in B27 for 9 days. (**A–C**) Representative epifluorescent microscopic images show GFAP immunoreactivity in FHL-primed hNSCs (**A**) or after treatment with Stattic (0.5 μM) (**B**) and Niclosamide (0.25 μM) (**C**). Scale bar, 10 μm. (**D**) Quantitative analyses show that 0.5 μM Stattic and 0.25 μM Niclosamide significantly decrease the percentage of GFAP^{+} cells. *$p<0.05$ and ***$p<0.001$ by One-way ANOVA with Tukey post-hoc tests.

promote motor neuron generation in EGF-primed hNSCs. This indicates that FGF2 together with STAT3 inhibition enhances motor neuron differentiation, whereas EGF blocks motor neuron differentiation, which further confirms our previous reports [15,20]. Alternatively, since we observed that ELL-primed hNSCs have very high levels of tyrosine phosphorylated/activated STAT3 to begin with, STAT3 inhibitors may be required at much higher concentrations to reduce pSTAT3 levels sufficiently to allow for motor neuron differentiation. However, such high concentrations result in pleiotropic effects including altered morphology, inhibited migration and even cytotoxicity. Thus, it appears that fine tuning of the STAT3 signaling pathway along with reduced toxicity, enhanced bioactivity and medical availability is necessary for modulating the gliogenic environment and enhancing endogenous neural repair. In an effort to explore new STAT3 inhibitors with higher specificity and bioavailability toward potential clinical usages, we have developed a new class of STAT3 inhibitors [18,19,27]. One of the compounds, HJC0149, increased HB9 mRNA expression and $HB9^+/Map2^+$ neuronal differentiation, and also decreased $GFAP^+$ astrogliogenesis of hNSCs with very little cytotoxicity (unpublished data).

Our data are consistent with previous reports in that STAT3 suppression or its conditional deletion in cultured neural stem cells promotes neurogenesis [11]. In those studies, Hb9 was not explored, and only the more generic MAP2 expression in differentiated neurons was assessed. Our study has thus demonstrated for the first time the role of the STAT3 pathway on Hb9 transcription and protein expression, which in vertebrates is specifically expressed in somatic motor neurons and is essential for distinguishing motor neuron/interneuron subtypes.

In previous studies, STAT3 was reduced either by inoculation of cultured rat embryonic brain neurospheres with adenovirus overexpressing a dominant negative form of STAT3 (Stat3F) [11] or by adenoviral infection of NSC prepared from STAT3-conditionally deleted mouse embryos with nuclear *Cre* recombinase [12]. In both cases, loss of STAT3 resulted in significant downregulation of Notch family members (Notch 1,2,3, hes5, Id3). In the developing CNS, Notch signaling preserves the progenitor pools and inhibits neurogenesis. Thus, it is plausible that increased Hb9 mRNA and protein expression that we observed upon STAT3 inhibition was a result of decreased Notch activity in human neural stem cells. However, the mechanism by which STAT3 activity could impact Notch signaling during neurogenesis remains to be determined.

In contrast to these studies, a recent finding suggests that STAT3 activation is needed for motor neuron differentiation during early development of the spinal cord [29]. This suggests that perhaps STAT3 performs different roles during neural stem cell maintenance and motor neuron differentiation. Alternatively, this provides further support for our hypothesis that maintaining precise spatial and temporal control *in vivo* and exact stoichiometric control of STAT3 under *in vitro* conditions is the key to obtaining maximum motor neuron differentiation. In addition, it is pertinent to note that the cellular environments during neurogenesis versus in injured/degenerating adult neurons are completely different and hence may not be directly comparable.

Stattic and Niclosamide Do Not Affect Phosphorylation of STAT3 but Perturb its Nuclear Translocation

We observed that treatment of hNSCs with pharmacological inhibitors, Stattic and Niclosamide, did not affect STAT3 phosphorylation status at either Tyr-705 or Ser-727. Typically, phosphorylation of STAT3 is considered the hallmark of the activated STAT3 signaling pathway. Although much effort has been made in developing STAT3 inhibitors that block its phosphorylation, there are known STAT3 inhibitors that block STAT3 pathway activity by disrupting other molecular steps. For instance, pyrimethamine affects STAT3 transcriptional activation without affecting its tyrosine phosphorylation [30].

Recent studies demonstrate that STAT3 is different from other members of the STAT family in that while tyrosine phosphorylation is critical for its DNA binding ability, nuclear import of STAT3 occurs independent of its phosphorylation status [21]. Consistent with this, we observed that upon treatment with Stattic and Niclosamide in FGF2-primed cells, nuclear localization of pSTAT3-Y705 was significantly reduced with a concomitant increase in its levels in the cytoplasm. Interestingly, ELL-primed cells exhibit a much higher baseline level of pSTAT3-Y705 nuclear localization, which was not changed by treatments with similar concentrations of Stattic or Niclosamide. Thus, we conclude that it is most likely that Stattic or Niclosamide inhibits STAT3 activity by blocking nuclear import and, presumably, by decreasing nuclear accumulation of pSTAT3-Y705, which somehow results in increased motor neuron specification.

STAT3 Inhibition Decreases $GFAP^+$ Astrocytes

Our results indicate that inhibition of STAT3 using optimal doses of STAT3 inhibitors, Stattic or Niclosamide, decreased $GFAP^+$ astrocyte populations in EGF- and FGF2-primed hNSCs. Activated STAT3 is an important cue for glial differentiation [12,31,32]. Various external cues like cytokines, CNTF, bone morphogenetic proteins, leukemia inhibitory factor, and Notch-Delta ligands activate the STAT3 pathway through JAK kinase [33,34] ERK [35], mTOR (Bone Morphogenetic Proteins) [36] or directly through Notch [37], which regulates GFAP expression by epigenetic chromatin remodeling. Moreover, it has been demonstrated that mouse cortical progenitors stimulated with FGF2 exhibit increased GFAP expression and astrocyte formation; this is due to hypermethylation of lysine4, and thereby increased STAT3 binding to the GFAP promoter [22,23,28]. Thus, it is plausible that in our paradigm of FGF2 priming followed by STAT3 inhibition, there is an insufficient nuclear pool of pSTAT3 to bind to GFAP promoter sites (owing to blocked nuclear import), which results in decreased GFAP expression and thereby, astroglial differentiation.

In summary, our study provides insights into how neural stem cells can be manipulated *in vitro* to obtain more motor neurons. We show that a combination of precise level of STAT3 activity, obtained by STAT3 inhibition along with increased FGF2 levels result in an enhanced generation of motor neurons. Presumably, this study will have broader implications to stem cell therapies designed to ameliorate the negative effects of spinal cord injury and ALS by increasing motor neuron production in a more favorable environment.

Supporting Information

Figure S1 Dose-dependent morphological effect of Stattic on ELL- and FHL-primed hNSCs. Representative phase contrast images of hNSCs following a 3-day priming in FHL (**A, C** and **E**) or ELL (**B, D** and **F**), with or without the treatment of a STAT3 inhibitor, Stattic. Low doses of Stattic (up to 2.5 μM) did not affect cell morphology. Scale bar, 20 μm.

Figure S2 Dose-dependent morphological effect of Niclosamide on ELL- and FHL-primed hNSCs. Representative phase contrast images of hNSCs after a 3-day priming in FHL (**A, C** and **E**) or ELL (**B, D** and **F**), with or without the treatment of a STAT3 inhibitor, Niclosamide. Low dose of Niclosamide (0.25 μM) did not affect cell morphology or cell viability. 2 μM Niclosamide not only blocked cell migration and inhibited process formation in both FHL and ELL conditions. Scale bar, 20 μm.

Figure S3 Increased motor neuron differentiation in hNSCs by a novel STAT3 inhibitor, HJC0149. (**A**) Chemical structure of HJC0149. (**B**) Semi-quantitative RT-PCR to determine the expression level of HB9 mRNA after 4-day priming. GAPDH used as an internal control. Hb9 mRNA levels are significantly increased in FHL-primed hNSCs treated with 0.5μM HJC0149 (HJC). Values are mean ± SEM (n = 3), *$p<0.05$, One-way ANOVA plus Bonferroni post-hoc tests. (**C**) Quantitative analyses show that 0.5μM HJC0149 significantly increase the %$Hb9^{+}/MAP2^{+}$ cells in FHL-primed cells by immunostaining. *$p<0.05$ compared to the control (CTRL), Student's *t* test. (**D–E**) Representative epifluorescent microscopic images to show HB9/MAP2-labeled motor neurons in hNSCs primed alone (**D**) and primed plus inhibitor-treated (**E**) for 4 days and differentiated in B27 for 9 days. Scale bar, 20 μm. DAPI, nuclear counterstain; HB9, transcription factor and motor neuron marker; MAP2, microtubule associated protein 2.

Acknowledgments

We thank Tiffany Dunn and William Green for technical support.

Author Contributions

Conceived and designed the experiments: RN VS RB JZ PW. Performed the experiments: RN VS RB JG H. Chan H. Chen. Analyzed the data: RN VS RB JG H. Chan PW. Contributed reagents/materials/analysis tools: H. Chen JZ. Wrote the paper: RN VS RB JG H. Chan YY JZ PW.

References

1. Howland DS, Liu J, She Y, Goad B, Maragakis NJ, et al. (2002) Focal loss of the glutamate transporter EAAT2 in a transgenic rat model of SOD1 mutant-mediated amyotrophic lateral sclerosis (ALS). Proc Natl Acad Sci USA 99: 1604–1609.
2. Bruijn LI, Miller TM, Cleveland DW (2004) Unraveling the mechanisms involved in motor neuron degeneration in ALS. Annu Rev Neurosci 27: 723–749.
3. Haidet-Phillips AM, Hester ME, Miranda CJ, Meyer K, Braun L, et al. (2011) Astrocytes from familial and sporadic ALS patients are toxic to motor neurons. Nat Biotechnol 29: 824–828. doi: 10.1038/nbt.1957.
4. Díaz-Amarilla P, Olivera-Bravo S, Trias E, Cragnolini A, Martínez-Palma L, et al. (2011) Phenotypically aberrant astrocytes that promote motoneuron damage in a model of inherited amyotrophic lateral sclerosis. Proc Natl Acad Sci USA 108: 18126–18131. doi: 10.1073/pnas.1110689108.
5. Yamauchi K, Osuka K, Takayasu M, Usuda N, Nakazawa A, et al. (2006) Activation of JAK/STAT signalling in neurons following spinal cord injury in mice. J Neurochem 96: 1060–1070.
6. Dominguez E, Rivat C, Pommier B, Mauborgne A, Pohl M (2008). JAK/STAT3 pathway is activated in spinal cord microglia after peripheral nerve injury and contributes to neuropathic pain development in rat. J Neurochem 107: 50–60. doi: 10.1111/j.1471-4159.2008.05566.x.
7. Okada S, Nakamura M, Katoh H, Miyao T, Shimazaki T, et al. (2006) Conditional ablation of Stat3 or Socs3 discloses a dual role for reactive astrocytes after spinal cord injury. Nat Med 12: 829–834.
8. Shibata N, Kakita A, Takahashi H, Ihara Y, Nobukuni K, et al. (2009) Activation of signal transducer and activator of transcription-3 in the spinal cord of sporadic amyotrophic lateral sclerosis patients. Neurodegener Dis 6: 118–126. doi: 10.1159/000213762.
9. Shibata N, Yamamoto T, Hiroi A, Omi Y, Kato Y, et al. (2010) Activation of STAT3 and inhibitory effects of pioglitazone on STAT3 activity in a mouse model of SOD1-mutated amyotrophic lateral sclerosis. Neuropathology 30: 353–360. doi: 10.1111/j.1440-1789.2009.01078.x.
10. Tsuda M, Kohro Y, Yano T, Tsujikawa T, Kitano J, et al. (2011) JAK-STAT3 pathway regulates spinal astrocyte proliferation and neuropathic pain maintenance in rats. Brain 134(Pt 4): 1127–1139. doi: 10.1093/brain/awr025.
11. Gu F, Hata R, Ma YJ, Tanaka J, Mitsuda N, et al. (2005) Suppression of Stat3 promotes neurogenesis in cultured neural stem cells. J Neurosci Res 81: 163–171.
12. Cao F, Hata R, Zhu P, Nakashiro K, Sakanaka M (2010) Conditional deletion of Stat3 promotes neurogenesis and inhibits astrogliogenesis in neural stem cells. Biochem Biophys Res Commun 394: 843–847. doi: 10.1016/j.bbrc.2010.03.092.
13. Qiu J, Cafferty WB, McMahon SB, Thompson SW (2005) Conditioning injury-induced spinal axon regeneration requires signal transducer and activator of transcription 3 activation. J Neurosci 25: 1645–1653.
14. Wu P, Tarasenko YI, Gu Y, Huang LY, Coggeshall RE, et al. (2002) Region-specific generation of cholinergic neurons from fetal human neural stem cells grafted in adult rat. Nat Neurosci 5: 1271–1278.
15. Jordan PM, Ojeda LD, Thonhoff JR, Gao J, Boehning D, et al. (2009) Generation of spinal motor neurons from human fetal brain-derived neural stem cells: role of basic fibroblast growth factor. J Neurosci Res 87: 318–332. doi: 10.1002/jnr.21856.
16. Schust J, Sperl B, Hollis A, Mayer TU, Berg T (2006) Stattic: a small-molecule inhibitor of STAT3 activation and dimerization. Chem Biol 13: 1235–1242.
17. Ren XM, Duan L, He QA, Zhang Z, Zhou Y, et al. (2010) Identification of Niclosamide as a New Small-Molecule Inhibitor of the STAT3 Signaling Pathway. ACS Med Chem Lett 1: 454–459. doi:10.1021/ml100146z.
18. Chen H, Yang Z, Ding C, Chu L, Zhang Y, et al. (2013) Fragment-based drug design and identification of HJC0123, a novel orally bioavailable STAT3 inhibitor for cancer therapy. Eur J Med Chem 62: 498–507. doi: 10.1016/j.ejmech.2013.01.023.
19. Chen H, Yang Z, Ding C, Chu L, Zhang Y, et al. (2013) Discovery of O-Alkylamino Tethered Niclosamide Derivatives as Potent and Orally Bioavailable Anticancer Agents. ACS Med. Chem Lett. 14; 4(2): 180–185.
20. Ojeda L, Gao J, Hooten KG, Wang E, Thonhoff JR, et al. (2011) Critical role of PI3K/Akt/GSK3β in motoneuron specification from human neural stem cells in response to FGF2 and EGF. PLoS One 6: e23414. doi: 10.1371/journal.pone.0023414.
21. Liu L, McBride KM, Reich NC (2005) STAT3 nuclear import is independent of tyrosine phosphorylation and mediated by importin-alpha3. Proc Natl Acad Sci USA 102: 8150–8155.
22. Takizawa T, Nakashima K, Namihira M, Ochiai W, Uemura A, et al. (2001) DNA methylation is a critical cell-intrinsic determinant of astrocyte differentiation in the fetal brain. Dev Cell 1: 749–758.
23. Cheng PY, Lin YP, Chen YL, Lee YC, Tai CC, et al. (2011) Interplay between SIN3A and STAT3 mediates chromatin conformational changes and GFAP expression during cellular differentiation. PLoS One 6: e22018. doi: 10.1371/journal.pone.0022018.
24. Tao Y, Black IB, DiCicco-Bloom E (1996) Neurogenesis in neonatal rat brain is regulated by peripheral injection of basic fibroblast growth factor (bFGF). J Comp Neurol 376: 653–663.
25. Werner S, Unsicker K, von Bohlen and Halbach O (2011) Fibroblast growth factor-2 deficiency causes defects in adult hippocampal neurogenesis, which are not rescued by exogenous fibroblast growth factor-2. J Neurosci Res 89: 1605–1617. doi: 10.1002/jnr.22680.
26. Rai KS, Hattiangady B, Shetty AK (2007) Enhanced production and dendritic growth of new dentate granule cells in the middle-aged hippocampus following intracerebroventricular FGF-2 infusions. Eur J Neurosci 26: 1765–1779.
27. Gritti A, Parati EA, Cova L, Frolichsthal P, Galli R, et al. (1996) Multipotential stem cells from the adult mouse brain proliferate and self-renew in response to basic fibroblast growth factor. J Neurosci 16: 1091–1100.
28. Song MR, Ghosh A (2004) FGF2-induced chromatin remodeling regulates CNTF-mediated gene expression and astrocyte differentiation. Nat Neurosci 7: 229–235.
29. Lee S, Shen R, Cho HH, Kwon RJ, Seo SY, et al. (2013) STAT3 promotes motor neuron differentiation by collaborating with motor neuron-specific LIM complex. Proc Natl Acad Sci USA 110: 11445–11450. doi: 10.1073/pnas.1302676110.
30. Walker SR, Frank DA (2012) Screening approaches to generating STAT inhibitors: Allowing the hits to identify the targets. JAKSTAT 1: 292–299.
31. Schubert KO, Naumann T, Schnell O, Zhi Q, Steup A, et al. (2005) Activation of STAT3 signaling in axotomized neurons and reactive astrocytes after fimbria-fornix transection. Exp Brain Res 165: 520–531.
32. Fukuda S, Abematsu M, Mori H, Yanagisawa M, Kagawa T, et al. (2007) Potentiation of astrogliogenesis by STAT3-mediated activation of bone morphogenetic protein-Smad signaling in neural stem cells. Mol Cell Biol 27: 4931–4937.
33. Kamakura S, Oishi K, Yoshimatsu T, Nakafuku M, Masuyama N, et al. (2004) Hes binding to STAT3 mediates crosstalk between Notch and JAK-STAT signalling. Nat Cell Biol 6: 547–554.

34. Bonni A, Sun Y, Nadal-Vicens M, Bhatt A, Frank DA, et al. (1997) Regulation of gliogenesis in the central nervous system by the JAK-STAT signaling pathway. Science 278: 477–483.
35. Rajan P, McKay RD (1998) Multiple routes to astrocytic differentiation in the CNS. J Neurosci 18: 3620–3629.
36. Rajan P, Panchision DM, Newell LF, McKay RD (2003) BMPs signal alternately through a SMAD or FRAP-STAT pathway to regulate fate choice in CNS stem cells. J Cell Biol 161: 911–921.
37. Gaiano N, Nye JS, Fishell G (2000) Radial glial identity is promoted by Notch1 signaling in the murine forebrain. Neuron 26: 395–404.

Permissions

All chapters in this book were first published in PLOS ONE, by The Public Library of Science; hereby published with permission under the Creative Commons Attribution License or equivalent. Every chapter published in this book has been scrutinized by our experts. Their significance has been extensively debated. The topics covered herein carry significant findings which will fuel the growth of the discipline. They may even be implemented as practical applications or may be referred to as a beginning point for another development.

The contributors of this book come from diverse backgrounds, making this book a truly international effort. This book will bring forth new frontiers with its revolutionizing research information and detailed analysis of the nascent developments around the world.

We would like to thank all the contributing authors for lending their expertise to make the book truly unique. They have played a crucial role in the development of this book. Without their invaluable contributions this book wouldn't have been possible. They have made vital efforts to compile up to date information on the varied aspects of this subject to make this book a valuable addition to the collection of many professionals and students.

This book was conceptualized with the vision of imparting up-to-date information and advanced data in this field. To ensure the same, a matchless editorial board was set up. Every individual on the board went through rigorous rounds of assessment to prove their worth. After which they invested a large part of their time researching and compiling the most relevant data for our readers.

The editorial board has been involved in producing this book since its inception. They have spent rigorous hours researching and exploring the diverse topics which have resulted in the successful publishing of this book. They have passed on their knowledge of decades through this book. To expedite this challenging task, the publisher supported the team at every step. A small team of assistant editors was also appointed to further simplify the editing procedure and attain best results for the readers.

Apart from the editorial board, the designing team has also invested a significant amount of their time in understanding the subject and creating the most relevant covers. They scrutinized every image to scout for the most suitable representation of the subject and create an appropriate cover for the book.

The publishing team has been an ardent support to the editorial, designing and production team. Their endless efforts to recruit the best for this project, has resulted in the accomplishment of this book. They are a veteran in the field of academics and their pool of knowledge is as vast as their experience in printing. Their expertise and guidance has proved useful at every step. Their uncompromising quality standards have made this book an exceptional effort. Their encouragement from time to time has been an inspiration for everyone.

The publisher and the editorial board hope that this book will prove to be a valuable piece of knowledge for researchers, students, practitioners and scholars across the globe.

List of Contributors

Karla Menezes, Aline Silva Cruz, João Ricardo Lacerda de Menezes, Maria Isabel Doria Rossi and Tatiana Coelho-Sampaio
Institute of Biomedical Sciences, Federal University of Rio de Janeiro, Rio de Janeiro, Rio de Janeiro, Brazil

Marcos Assis Nascimento and Juliana Pena Gon çalves
Institute of Biophysics Carlos Chagas Filho, Federal University of Rio de Janeiro, Rio de Janeiro, Rio de Janeiro, Brazil

Bianca Curzio and Martin Bonamino
National Institute of Cancer, Rio de Janeiro, Rio de Janeiro, Brazil

Radovan Borojevic
Excellion, Petrópolis, Rio de Janeiro, Brazil

Jaime L. Watson, Tamara J. Hala, Rajarshi Putatunda, Daniel Sannie and Angelo C. Lepore
Department of Neuroscience, Farber Institute for Neurosciences, Sidney Kimmel Medical College at Thomas Jefferson University, Philadelphia, Pennsylvania, United States of America

Haijun Chen and Jia Zhou
Department of Pharmacology and Toxicology, The University of Texas Medical Branch, Galveston, Texas, United States of America

Yongjia Yu
Department of Radiation Oncology, The University of Texas Medical Branch, Galveston, Texas, United States of America

Eloy Opisso and Josep Medina
Health Science Research Inst. of the "Germans Trias i Pujol" Found., Barcelona, Spain

Liuliu Pan, Hilary A. North, Vibhu Sahni, Su Ji Jeong, Tammy L. Mcguire and John A. Kessler
Department of Neurology, Northwestern University, Chicago, Illinois, United States of America

Eric J. Berns
Department of Biomedical Engineering, Northwestern University, Evanston, Illinois, United States of America

Samuel I. Stupp
Department of Materials Science and Engineering, Northwestern University, Evanston, Illinois, United States of America
Department of Chemistry, Northwestern University, Evanston, Illinois, United States of America. Department of Medicine and Institute for BioNanotechnology in Medicine, Northwestern University, Chicago, Illinois, United States of America

Roberta Barbizan, Mateus V. Castro and Alexandre L. R. Oliveira
Laboratory of Nerve Regeneration, Department of Structural and Functional Biology, University of Campinas - UNICAMP, Campinas, São Paulo, Brazil

Benedito Barraviera and Rui S. Ferreira Jr.
Center for the Study of Venoms and Venomous Animals (CEVAP), São Paulo State University (UNESP–Univ Estadual Paulista), Botucatu, São Paulo, Brazil

Anna Victoria Leonard and Emma Thornton
School of Medical Sciences, University of Adelaide, Adelaide, South Australia, Australia

Robert Vink
Division of Health Sciences, University of South Australia, Adelaide, South Australia, Australia

Mohor Biplab Sengupta and Debashis Mukhopadhyay
Biophysics and Structural Genomics Division, Saha Institute of Nuclear Physics, Kolkata, West Bengal, India

Mahashweta Basu and Pradeep K. Mohanty
Condensed Matter Physics Division, Saha Institute of Nuclear Physics, Kolkata, West Bengal, India

Sourav Iswarari
Department of Physical Medicine and Rehabilitation, Nil Ratan Sircar Medical College and Hospital, Kolkata, West Bengal, India

Kiran Kumar Mukhopadhyay, Krishna Pada Sardar and Biplab Acharyya
Department of Orthopaedic Surgery, Nil Ratan Sircar Medical College and Hospital, Kolkata, West Bengal, India

Marcus K. Giacci, Lachlan Wheeler, Sarah Lovett, Emma Dishington, Bernadette Majda, Carole A. Bartlett, Alan R. Harvey, Sarah A. Dunlop, Stuart Hodgetts and Melinda Fitzgerald
Experimental and Regenerative Neurosciences, The University of Western Australia, Crawley, Australia

Marcus K. Giacci, Carole A. Bartlett, Sarah A. Dunlop, Nathan S. Hart and Melinda Fitzgerald
School of Animal Biology, The University of Western Australia, Crawley, Australia

Marcus K. Giacci, Lachlan Wheeler, Sarah Lovett, Emma Dishington, Bernadette Majda and Stuart Hodgetts
School of Anatomy, Physiology and Human Biology, The University of Western Australia, Crawley, Australia

Emma Thornton, Elizabeth Harford-Wright, Anna Leonard4, Robert Vink and Corinna Van Den Heuvel
School of Medical Sciences, The University of Adelaide, Adelaide, Australia

Jan Provis and Riccardo Natoli
ANU Medical School and John Curtin School of Medical Research, The Australian National University, Canberra, Australia

Nathan S. Hart
Neuroecology Group, The Oceans Institute, The University of Western Australia, Crawley, Australia

Annemieke C. Scholten, Juanita A. Haagsma, Ed F. van Beeck and Suzanne Polinder
Department of Public Health, Erasmus University Medical Center, Rotterdam, The Netherlands

Martien J. M. Panneman
Research Department, Consumer and Safety Institute, Amsterdam, The Netherlands

SaÏd M'Dahoma, Sylvie Bourgoin, Valérie Kayser, Sandrine Barthélémy, Caroline Chevarin and Michel Hamon
Centre de Psychiatrie et Neurosciences, Institut National de la Santé et de la Recherche Médicale, INSERM U894, Université Paris Descartes, Paris, France
Neuropsychopharmacologie, Faculté de Médecine Pierre et Marie Curie, site Pitié-Salpétriére, Paris, France

Farah Chali and Didier Orsal
Laboratoire de Neurobiologie des Signaux Intercellulaires,
Centre National de la Recherche Scientifique, CNRS UMR 7101, Université- Pierre et Marie Curie, Paris, France

Sarah A. Figley, Yang Liu, Spyridon K. Karadimas, Kajana Satkunendrarajah, Peter Fettes and Michael G. Fehlings
Department of Genetics and Development, Toronto Western Research Institute, and Spinal Program, Krembil Neuroscience Centre, University Health Network, Toronto, Ontario, Canada

Sarah A. Figley, Spyridon K. Karadimas Martin Giedlin and Michael G. Fehlings
Institute of Medical Sciences, University of Toronto, Toronto, Ontario, Canada

S. Kaye Spratt, Gary Lee, Dale Ando and Richard Surosky
Department of Therapeutic Development, Sangamo BioSciences, Pt.Richmond, California, United States of America

Michael G. Fehlings
Department of Surgery, University of Toronto, Toronto, Ontario, Canada

Olivier Alluin, Hugo Delivet-Mongrain and Serge Rossignol
Multidisciplinary Team in Locomotor Rehabilitation of the Canadian Institutes of Health Research (CIHR) and Groupe de Recherche sur le Système Nerveux Central (GRSNC) of the Fonds de Recherche du Québec - Santé (FRQS), Department of Physiology, University of Montreal, Montreal, Quebec, Canada

Marie-Krystel Gauthier and Soheila Karimi-Abdolrezaee
The Department of Physiology and Pathophysiology and the Spinal Cord Research Center, University of Manitoba, Winnipeg, Manitoba, Canada

Michael G. Fehlings
Department of Surgery and Spinal Program, University of Toronto; Toronto Western Research Institute, University Health Network, Toronto, Ontario, Canada

Soheila Karimi-Abdolrezaee
Regenerative Medicine Program and Manitoba Institute of Child Health, Winnipeg, Manitoba, Canada

Nai-Feng Tian, Xu-Qi Hu, Xiao-Lei Zhang, Xiang-Yang Wang, Yong-Long Chi and Fang-Min Mao
Department of Orthopaedic Surgery, Second Affiliated Hospital of Wenzhou Medical University, Wenzhou, Zhejiang, China

Li-Jun Wu and Xin-Lei Wu
Institute of Digitized Medicine, Wenzhou Medical University, Wenzhou, Zhejiang, China,

Yao-Sen Wu
Department of Orthopaedics, Second Affiliated Hospital, School of Medicine, Zhejiang University, Hangzhou, Zhejiang, China

Xiao-Lei Zhang
Center for Stem Cells and Tissue Engineering, School of Medicine, Zhejiang University, Hangzhou, Zhejiang, China

Norman R. Saunders, Natassya M. Noor, Katarzyna M. Dziegielewska, Benjamin J. Wheaton, Shane A. Liddelow and Mark D. Habgood
Department of Pharmacology and Therapeutics, The University of Melbourne, Victoria, Australia

Shane A. Liddelow
Department of Neurobiology, Stanford University, Stanford, California, United States of America

David L. Steer
Department of Biochemistry and Molecular Biology, Monash University, Clayton, Victoria, Australia

C. Joakim Ek
Department of Neuroscience and Physiology, University of Gothenburg, Gothenburg, Sweden

Matthew J. Wakefield and Helen Lindsay
Walter and Eliza Hall Institute of Medical Research, Victoria, Australia

Matthew J. Wakefield
Department of Genetics, The University of Melbourne, Victoria, Australia

Helen Lindsay
Institute of Molecular Life Sciences, University of Zurich, Zurich, Switzerland

Jessie Truettner and W. Dalton Dietrich
The Miami Project to Cure Paralysis, University of Miami, Miller School of Medicine, Miami, Florida, United States of America

Robert D. Miller
Center for Evolutionary and Theoretical Immunology, Department of Biology, University of New Mexico, Albuquerque, New Mexico, United States of America

Shuo Tang, Zeyu Huang and Fuxing Pei
Department of Orthopaedics, West China Hospital, Sichuan University, Chengdu, China, 2 Department of Pain Medicine, Shenzhen Nanshan Hospital, Shenzhen, China

Xiang Liao
Department of Pain Medicine, Shenzhen Nanshan Hospital, Shenzhen, China

Bo Shi
Department of Orthopaedics, Mianyang Center Hospital, Mianyang, China

Yanzhen Qu and Xiaodong Guo
Department of Orthopaedics, Union Hospital, Tongji Medical College, Huazhong University of Science and Technology, Wuhan, China

Qiang Lin
Department of Orthopaedics, Guangdong hospital of traditional Chinese medicine, Guangzhou, China

Ursula Costa Eloy Opisso and Josep Medina
Guttmann Institute, Neurorehab. University inst. affil. with the UAB, Barcelona, Spain

Johana Tello Velasquez, Michelle E. Watts, Michael Todorovic, Lynnmaria Nazareth, Jenny A. K. Ekberg, Ronald J. Quinn and James A. St John
Eskitis Institute for Drug Discovery, Griffith University, Brisbane, Australia

Lynnmaria Nazareth and Jenny A. K. Ekberg
School of Biomedical Sciences, Queensland University of Technology, Brisbane, Australia

Erika Pastrana
Nature Communications, New York, New York, United States of America

Javier Diaz-Nido
Centro de Biologı´a Molecular Severo Ochoa, Madrid, Spain

Filip Lim
Universidad Autónoma de Madrid, Madrid, Spain

Josef Faller, Reinhold Scherer and Gernot R. Müller-Putz
Institute for Knowledge Discovery, Graz University of Technology, Graz, Austria

Rajalaxmi Natarajan, Vinamrata Singal, Richard Benes, Junling Gao, Hoi Chan and Ping Wu
Department of Neuroscience and Cell Biology, The University of Texas Medical Branch, Galveston, Texas, United States of America

Index

R

S

T

V

W

www.ingramcontent.com/pod-product-compliance
Lightning Source LLC
Chambersburg PA
CBHW080253230326
41458CB00097B/4412
9781632416841